AF882730

PHYSEO

We would like to extend a special thanks to the following individuals who have spent countless hours and support to make Physeo possible.

Adila Reddy

Alexandra Harding

Anne-Sophie van Wingerden
Medical Student
Columbia Vagelos College of Physicians and Surgeons

Anissa Liane Bayabos Amilhamja

Ayan Agarwal

Brianna Cocuzzo, MsC

Camelita Thrash

Christopher A. Price, MS

Irfan J. Ali, D.O.

Isabela Lorenzo, MS
Stritch School of Medicine
Loyola University Chicago

Dr. Jabran Wasti
House Officer, Dr. Ruth K.M. Pfau Civil Hospital
Karachi, Pakistan

Jae Cheol Bae
MD Candidate, Class of 2023
St. Matthew's University School of Medicine

Dr. James Nunn

Janet E. Lindsley, PhD
Professor, Biochemistry
Assistant Dean, Curriculum
Adjunct Professor, Nutrition and Integrative Physiology
University of Utah School of Medicine

Jennifer M. Locke, BA
MD Candidate

Julie A. Hansen
Class of 2022
St. George's University SOM

Marisol Cárdenas Calderón MD

Michelle M. Thomas

Lauren S. Faber, MD

Lauren Schwartz

Noon Isam Eldin Hassan Hagmusa, MBBS

Sarah Jaber, DO
Internal Medicine Physician

Sarah Manzoor
MD Candidate
Medical University of Lublin

Sibtain Hayee
MD Candidate
Medical University of Lublin

Sumit Raut
Mateo Betancourt Escobar
Universidad Autónoma de San Luis Potosí, Mexico

Syed Awais Ahmed, MD

Zachary Edwards, D.O.

TABLE OF CONTENTS

CARDIAC PATHOLOGY 140

PULMONARY & RESPIRATORY PATHOLOGY 188

ENDOCRINE PATHOLOGY 244

GENERAL PATHOLOGY

Section I - Growth Adaptations

I. Growth Adaptations
   A. Reversible cellular changes in attempt to adapt to stress
   B. Types of cellular changes associated with growth adaptations
      1. Size, number, phenotype, metabolic activity, functions
   C. Injury occurs if a cell is unable to adapt

II. Hypertrophy and Hyperplasia
   A. Increased organ size secondary to increase in stress
      1. Hypertrophy: increase in cell size
      2. Hyperplasia: increase in cell number
   B. Hypertrophy and hyperplasia generally occur together
   C. Permanent tissues (nervous, skeletal muscle, and cardiac muscle) only undergo hypertrophy and not hyperplasia

III. Hypertrophy and Hyperplasia: Mechanisms
   A. Hypertrophy: gene activation → formation of proteins → production of organelles and cell components
   B. Hyperplasia: growth factor stimulation → stem cell maturation

IV. Hypertrophy and Hyperplasia: Physiologic vs. Pathologic
   A. Physiologic hypertrophy: increases functional capacity of organs to meet the needs of body
   B. Pathologic hypertrophy: inappropriate actions of hormones/growth factors on target cells
   C. Pathologic hyperplasia can progress to dysplasia and ultimately, cancer

V. Atrophy
   A. Decreased organ size due to decrease in stress
   B. Mechanisms
      1. Decrease in the number of cells via apoptosis
      2. Decrease in the size of cells via ubiquitin proteasomal degradation pathway or autophagy

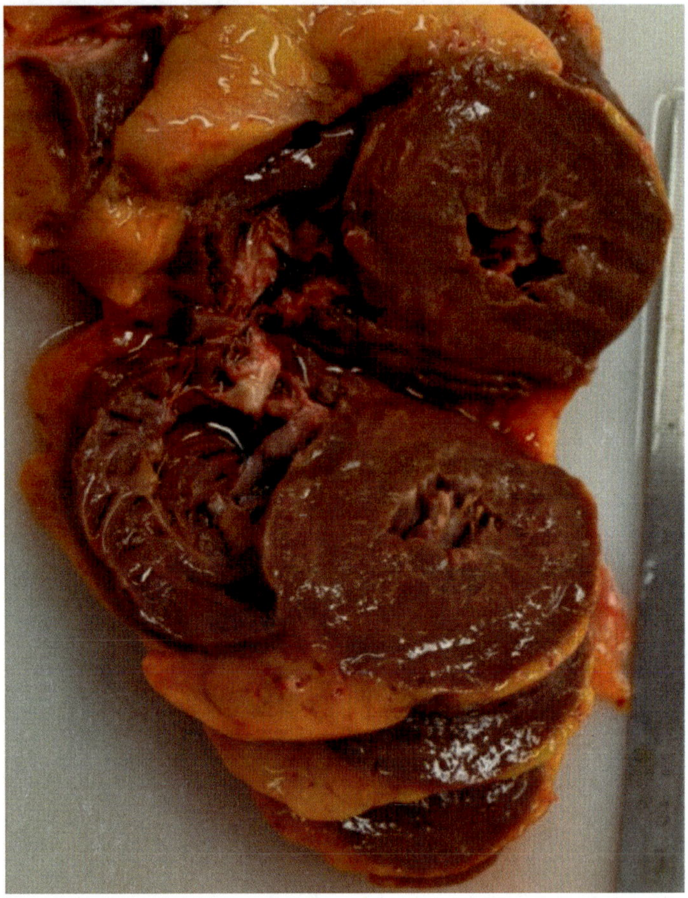

FIGURE 10.1.1 - Gross Specimen of Left Ventricular Hypertrophy

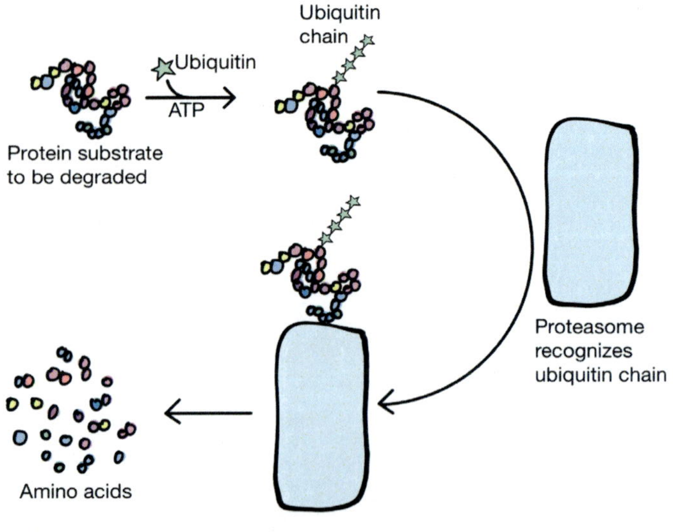

FIGURE 10.1.2 - Ubiquitin Proteasomal Degradation Pathway

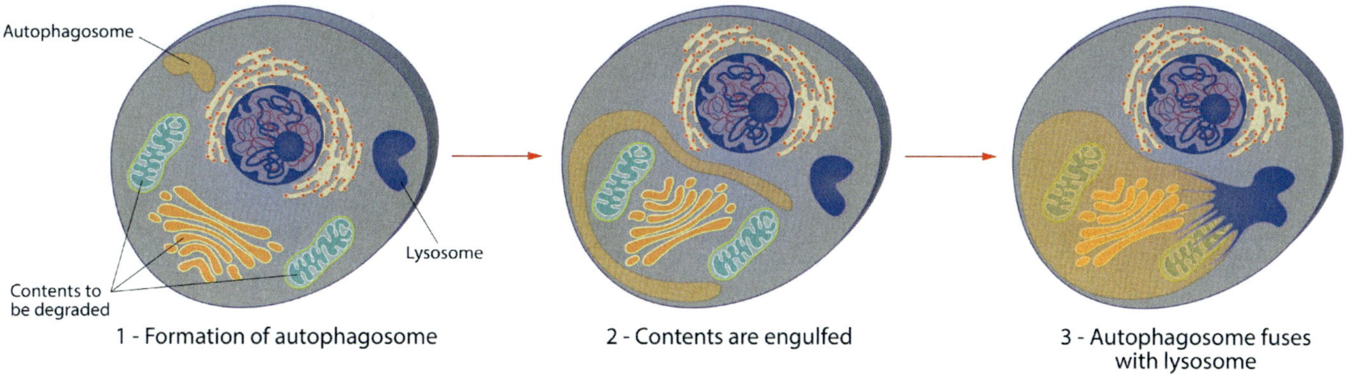

FIGURE 10.1.3 - Steps of Autophagy

VI. Atrophy: Physiologic vs. Pathologic
   A. Physiologic
      1. Seen in normal embryonic development
   B. Pathologic
      1. Decreased hormonal stimulation or nutrient/ blood supply
      2. Disuse atrophy
      3. Loss of innervation (denervation atrophy)
      4. Pressure atrophy

VII. Metaplasia
   A. Stress-induced reversible conversion from one cell type to another
   B. Stem cells reprogrammed to better handle stress
   C. Most commonly epithelial tissue
      1. Barrett's esophagus, vitamin A deficiency, myositis ossificans
   D. Usually progresses to dysplasia and cancer
      1. Exception: apocrine metaplasia of breast

VIII. Metaplasia: Barrett's Esophagus
   A. Non-keratinizing squamous epithelium damaged by acid reflux
   B. Chronic reflux → metaplasia to mucinous columnar epithelium
   C. Precancerous lesion with increased risk of esophageal adenocarcinoma

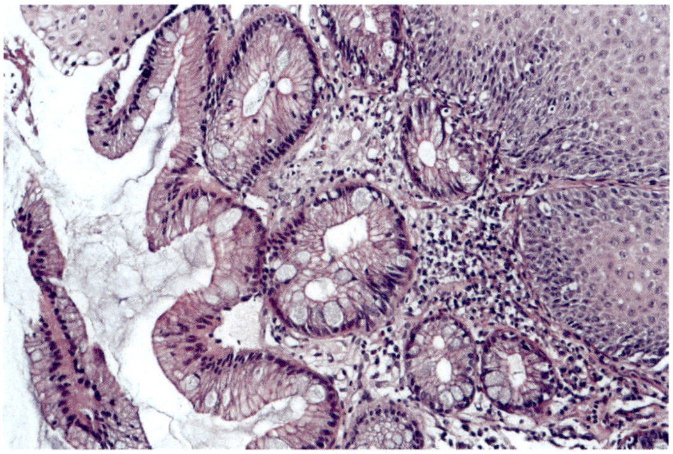

FIGURE 10.1.4 - Mucinous Columnar Epithelium

IX. Metaplasia: Vitamin A deficiency
   A. Vitamin A needed for differentiation of specialized epithelial surfaces
   B. Squamous lining of conjunctiva → stratified keratinizing squamous epithelium
   C. Keratomalacia

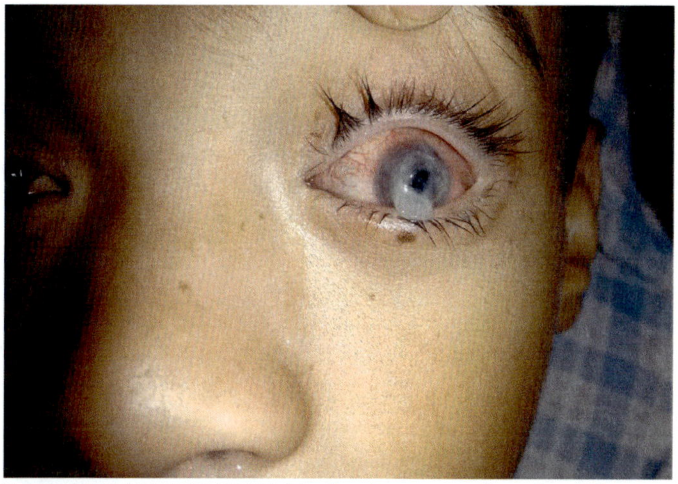

FIGURE 10.1.5 - Keratomalacia

X. Metaplasia: Myositis Ossificans
   A. Myositis ossificans
      1. Muscular tissue undergoes metaplasia to bone after injury due to erroneous healing process

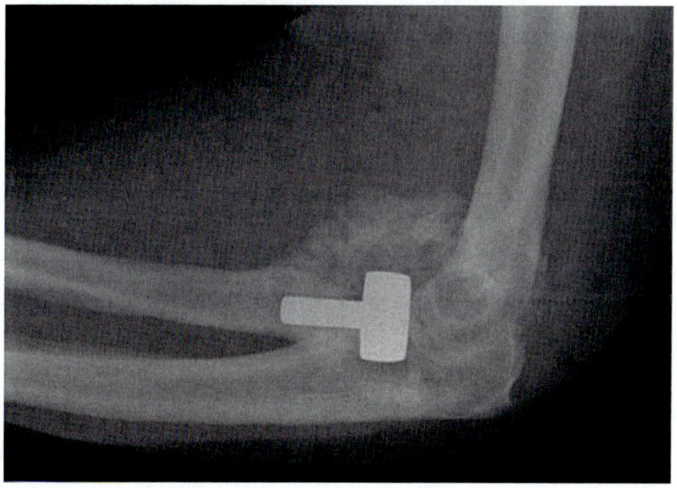

FIGURE 10.1.6 - Calcific Changes of Healing Muscle

XI. Dysplasia
   A. Disordered cell growth
   B. Not a true adaptive response
   C. Usually preceded by hyperplasia or metaplasia
   D. Non-neoplastic but can be pre-cancerous
   E. Reversible but unrelieved stress may yield carcinoma

XII. Dysplasia: Morphological changes
   A. Loss of tissue architecture
   B. Nuclear changes
      1. High nuclear-to-cytoplasmic ratio
      2. Clumped chromatin

REVIEW QUESTIONS

1. A 43-year-old male with a history of long-standing hypertension presents with shortness of breath, lightheadedness, and palpitations. Physical exam is significant for an S4 heart sound but otherwise unremarkable. Labs are all within normal limits. After thorough evaluation it is concluded that the patient's symptoms are due to pathologic changes involving thickening of the left ventricle. What type of growth adaptation is occurring in this patient's diseased organ?

   - The type of growth adaptation occurring is hypertrophy.
   - Based on the question stem, you may have been able to appreciate that the patient has left ventricular hypertrophy. If not, don't worry since we'll be covering the topic in great detail in our cardiology section.
   - For our purposes here, though, we're interested in the thickening of the left ventricle and the cellular mechanism by which it's happening. We want to know if cells in the left ventricle are simply getting larger, or if there are actually more cells.
   - Recalling that the three permanent tissues are neurons, skeletal muscle myocytes, and cardiac myocytes, you can confidently say that this is a case in which the cells are getting larger -- or hypertrophy, rather than hyperplasia. Hyperplasia doesn't happen in permanent tissues.

2. A 56-year-old male with a chronic cough, numerous respiratory infections, and a 40 pack-year smoking history presents with streaky blood in his sputum. Chest X-ray reveals hyperinflated lungs but no infiltrates or masses. Bronchoscopy is performed and samples of bronchial mucosa are biopsied. Microscopy reveals areas of stratified squamous epithelium. The pathogenesis of this patient's microscopic findings is most similar to which of the following conditions?

   A. Barrett esophagus
   B. Hypertrophic cardiomyopathy
   C. Streak ovary
   D. Cervical cancer

   - **The correct answer is A.**
   - This question states that we have a 56-year-old male with a chronic history of smoking. Also, microscopy reveals stratified squamous epithelium instead of normal ciliated columnar epithelium.
   - Since we would normally expect to see ciliated columnar epithelium in the respiratory tract, this is an example of metaplasia, making A the correct answer as it is the only example of metaplasia in the answer choices.
   - B is incorrect because hypertrophic cardiomyopathy, as we have discussed, is an example of hypertrophy.
   - C is incorrect because streak ovary is an example of hypoplasia.
   - D is incorrect because cervical cancer is not an example of a growth adaptation since it is an irreversible cancerous process.

Section II - Cell Injury

I. Cell Injury
   A. Changes in a cell that occur when a stress exceeds its ability to adapt

II. General Features
   A. Depends on: cell type affected, type of stress, severity
   B. Rapidly developing stress → injury
   C. Slowly developing stress → cellular adaptation (i.e. atrophy, hypertrophy, hyperplasia, metaplasia)
   D. Causes of stress are many (e.g. hypoxia, trauma, inflammation, genetic mutations, nutritional abnormalities)

III. Hypoxic Cellular Injury
   A. Insufficient oxygenation of tissues yielding decreased ATP production
   B. Impairs the last step of oxidative phosphorylation
   C. Major cause of hypoxia is ischemia

IV. Hypoxic Cellular Injury: Ischemia
   A. Inadequate blood flow to an organ results in an inadequate supply to meet oxygen demands.
   B. Mechanisms
      1. Decreased arterial perfusion (e.g. atherosclerosis)
      2. Decreased venous drainage (e.g. Budd-Chiari syndrome and testicular torsion)
      3. Generalized hypotension (e.g. shock)

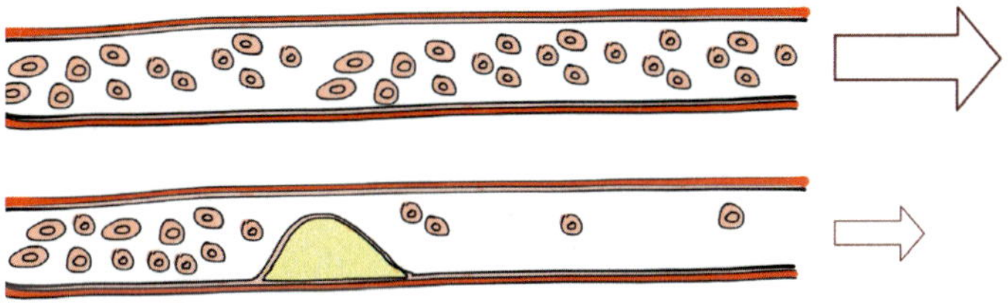

FIGURE 10.1.7 - Atherosclerosis

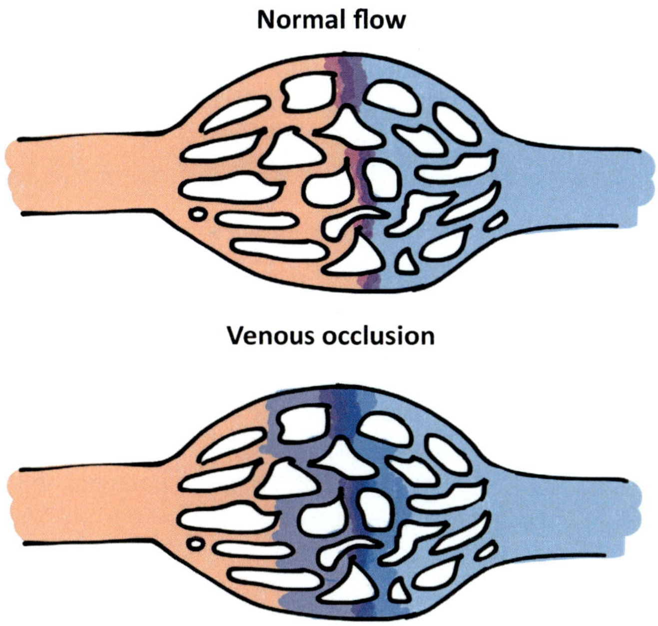

FIGURE 10.1.8 - Blood Flow in Venous Occlusion

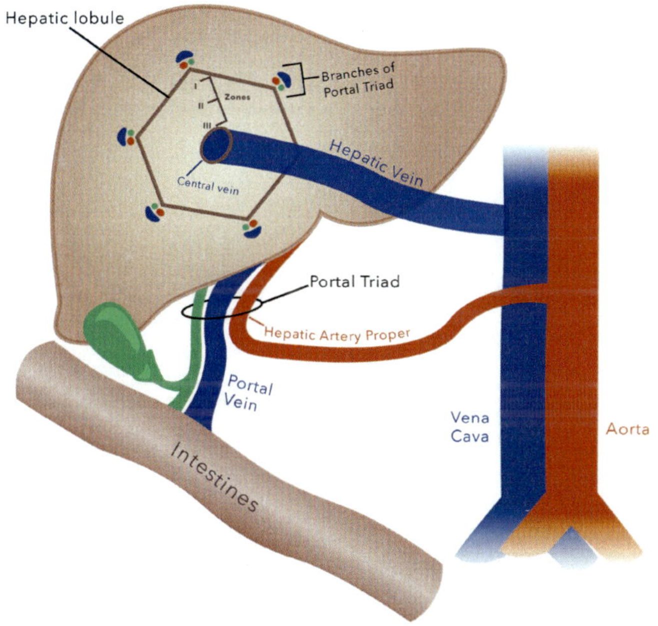

FIGURE 10.1.9 - Hepatic Blood Supply and Functional

V. Hypoxic Cellular Injury: Susceptible Organs
   A. Watershed areas: located between distal terminal branches of two different vascular territories
   B. Low-flow states: arterial insufficiency (e.g. diabetes, atherosclerosis) can cause non-occlusive ischemia
   C. Sustained hypoperfusion, especially in areas with high metabolic demand

Regions Susceptible to Ischemia (by Organ System)	
Brain	- Anterior, middle and posterior cerebral arteries - Specifically watershed areas (border zones)
Neurons	- Purkinje cells of cerebellum - Pyramidal cells (CA1) of hippocampus and neocortex (zones 3, 5, 6)
Heart	- Subendocardium of left ventricle
Liver	- Area around central vein (zone III)
Kidneys	- Straight segment of proximal tubule (medulla) - Thick ascending limb (medulla)
Colon	- Splenic flexure (Griffiths' point) - border zone of superior and inferior mesenteric arteries - Rectosigmoid junction (Sudeck's point) - Border zone of sigmoid arteries and superior rectal arteries

TABLE 10.1.1 - Ischemia Susceptible Regions

VI. Hypoxic Cellular Injury: Infarcts
   A. Result of the cellular response to ischemia
   B. Type of blood supply to organs relates to type of infarct
      1. End-arterial blood supply: kidney, spleen, heart → pale infarcts
      2. Dual blood supply: liver, lung, stomach → red infarcts
      3. Red infarcts also due to venous occlusion and reperfusion injuries

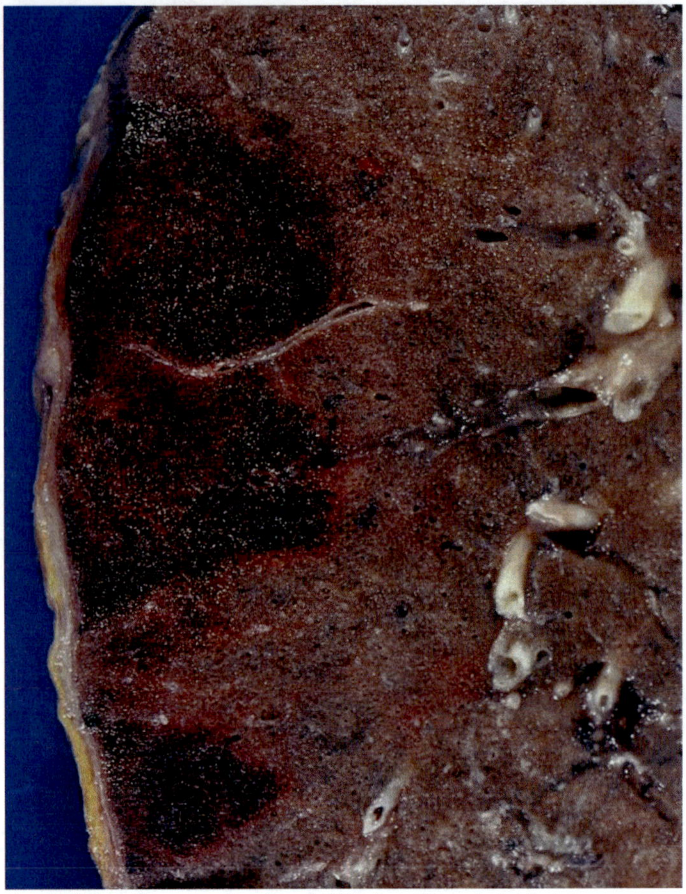

Photo Credit: https://commons.wikimedia.org/wiki/File:Recent_hemorrhagic_infarcts.jpg

FIGURE 10.1.10 - Red Infarcts of the Lung

VII. Reversible vs. Irreversible Injury
   A. Reversible
      1. Cell swelling
      2. Cellular integrity and function restored with oxygen restoration
   B. Irreversible
      1. Breakdown of plasma membrane
      2. Leads to cell death

VIII. Reversible Cell Injury: Swelling
   A. Impairment of the Na^+/K^+-ATPase → diffusion of sodium and water intracellularly
   B. Switch to anaerobic glycolysis → buildup of lactic acid→ decreased pH → denaturing of proteins
   C. Membrane blebbing
   D. Dissociation of ribosomes from rough ER → decreased protein synthesis

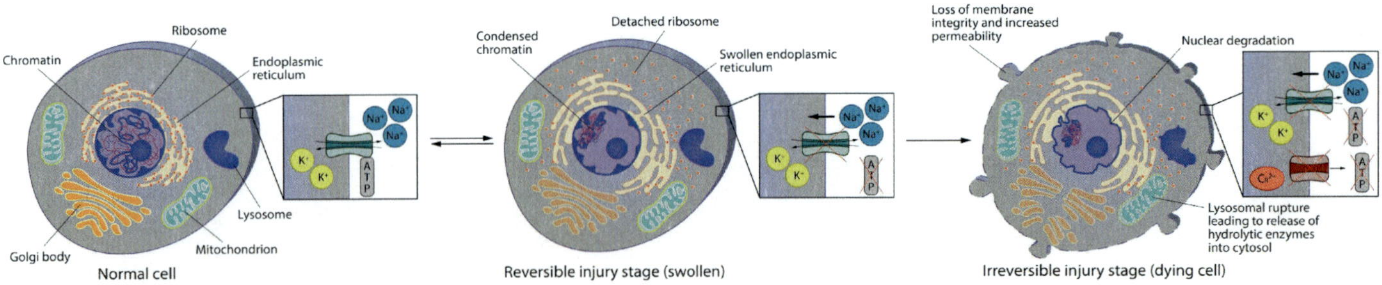

FIGURE 10.1.11 - Microscopic Changes of Cell Injury

IX. Irreversible Cellular Injury: Ca^{2+} Effects

A. Impairment of Ca^{2+} - ATPase pump → influx of Ca^{2+} into the cell
B. Activation of phospholipases → increases permeability of the cell
C. Activation of proteases → damages the cytoskeleton
D. Activates caspases directly → apoptosis

X. Irreversible Cellular Injury: Membrane Breakdown

A. Mitochondrial membrane damage → loss of electron transport chain and leakage of cytochrome c into cytosol → apoptosis
B. Rupture of lysosomes → hydrolytic enzymes leak into cytosol → autolysis
C. Nuclear degradation
D. End result → cell death

REVIEW QUESTIONS

1. What would be the gross appearance of an ischemic related infarct in the lungs?

- To imagine the ischemia from a gross pathology level, we have to think about the blood supply to that organ. Our question here asks about how the lungs would appear.
- For the lungs, the blood supply is not end-arterial and is actually dual. This will result in a red infarct.

2. A 48-year-old male with a history of "bothersome fast heart beats" presents with nausea, vomiting, flank pain, and blood in his urine that he saw this morning. His vital signs include a blood pressure of 168/74, a heart rate of 98 beats/min, and a low grade fever of 38.1ºC (100.6ºF). He denies any history of kidney issues or heart conditions. Gross pathology of a representation of the patient's kidney demonstrates a wedge-shaped pale infarct at the periphery. Which portion of his kidney was most vulnerable to the ischemia?

A. Thick ascending limb of loop of Henle
B. Distal convoluted tubule
C. Bowman's capsule
D. Renal cortex

- **The correct answer is A.**
- From the patient's complaints of nausea, vomiting and flank pain we should already be thinking of a pathology in the kidney. The high blood pressure as well as low grade fever should point us specifically to infarction in the kidney. As we learned and as confirmed by the gross pathology, the infarct was a pale infarct due to the kidney's end-arterial blood supply. The "bothersome heart beats" should make us think of possible atrial fibrillation that could be a cause of emboli that traveled to his kidney.
- Now we are at the arterial level and can recall what part of the kidney is most susceptible to ischemia, which points us to A. Due to their high perfusion rates and limited collateral circulation, the kidneys are particularly susceptible to embolic infarcts as we saw in our patient.
- The remaining answer choices provide portions of the kidney that are not as susceptible to ischemia as compared to the thick ascending limb of the loop of Henle.
- As a take-away, it's important to correlate pathology with physiology. Knowing the organs that have end-arterial blood supply can help you narrow down the pathology. In addition, knowing the watershed zones can help point you to the most susceptible regions.
- Finally, understanding the hallmarks of irreversible and reversible cellular injury can help you visualize what occurs at the cellular level due to injury like ischemia.

Section III - Apoptosis

I. Basic Principles
   A. Apoptosis is a type of cell death (includes apoptosis and necrosis)
      1. Cell nucleus is lost via nuclear condensation (pyknosis), fragmentation (karyorrhexis), and dissolution (karyolysis)
   B. Normal physiological process
   C. Energy dependent and genetically programmed
   D. Cell membrane remains intact
   E. Does not cause inflammation
   F. Examples of apoptosis
      1. Endometrial shedding during the menstrual cycle
      2. Tissue remodeling in embryogenesis (e.g. removal of cells to form spaces between fingers and toes)
      3. CD8+ T cell-mediated killing of virally infected cells

II. Morphology of Apoptosis
   A. Cell shrinks and becomes more eosinophilic
   B. Chromatin condenses (pyknosis)
   C. Cell membrane blebs and nucleus fragments (karyorrhexis)
   D. Apoptotic bodies containing the dissolved nucleus fragments break off from the cell and are removed by macrophages (karyolysis)

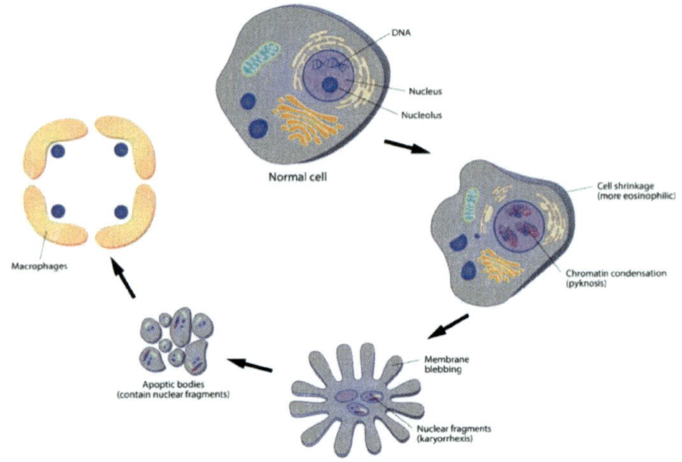

FIGURE 10.1.12 - Morphology of Apoptosis

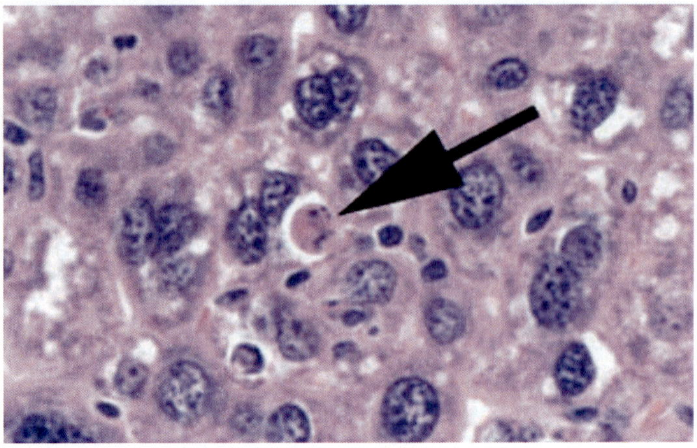

Photo Credit: Laboratory of Experimental Pathology, Division of Intramural Research, NIEHS (NIH) / Public domain

FIGURE 10.1.13 - Apoptotic Cell (Black Arrow)

III. Mechanisms
   A. Apoptosis is mediated by caspase enzymes
   B. These caspases activate proteases and endonucleases which degrade cell contents
   C. Caspases are activated by multiple pathways

IV. Intrinsic Mitochondrial Pathway
   A. Regulated by Bcl-2 family of proteins
   B. Bcl-2 is antiapoptotic
      1. Cellular injury, DNA damage, or decreased hormonal stimulation leads to inactivation of Bcl-2
      2. Bcl-2 inhibits BAX and BAK from complexing
   C. BAX and BAK are proapoptotic
      1. BAX and BAK complex forms pores in the inner mitochondrial membrane and release cytochrome C into the cytoplasm activation of → caspases

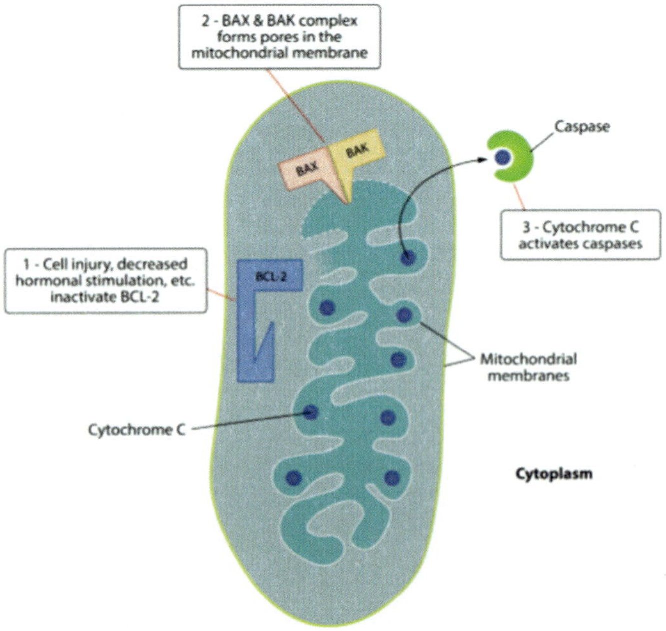

FIGURE 10.1.14 - Intrinsic Mitochondrial Pathway

V. Extrinsic ("Death Receptor") Pathway
   A. Ligand receptor interactions
      1. FasL binds to Fas death receptor (CD95) on the target cell → activation of caspases
      2. TNF-α binds to TNF receptor on the target cell → activation of caspases
   B. Example: thymic medullary negative selection

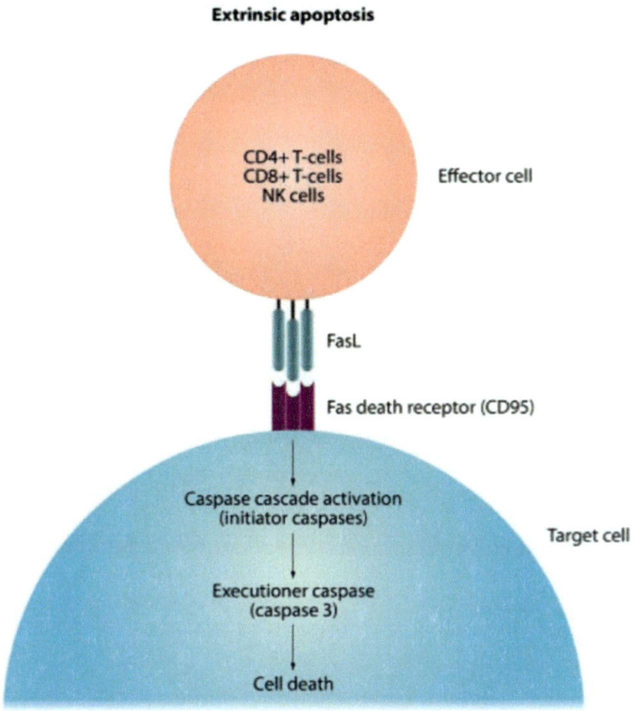

FIGURE 10.1.15 - Extrinsic Pathway of Apoptosis

VI. Cytotoxic CD8+ T-cell-Mediated Pathway
   A. Perforins secreted by CD8+ T-cell create pores in membrane of target cell
   B. Granzymes from CD8+ T-cell enter pores and activate caspases
   C. Example: CD8+ T-cell killing of virally infected cells is an example

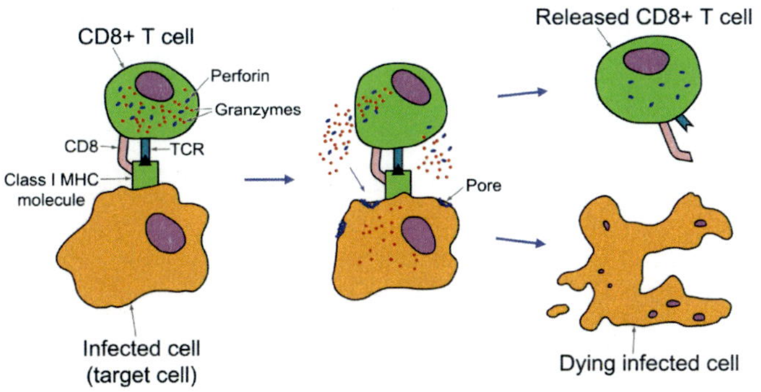

FIGURE 10.1.16 - CD8+ T-cell-Mediated Apoptosis

VII. Apoptosis Dysfunction
   A. Uncontrolled cell growth
   B. Example: Bcl-2 overexpression decreases caspase activation leading to tumor formation (e.g. follicular lymphoma t[14;18])

REVIEW QUESTIONS

1. A 16-year-old female with a history of Turner syndrome reports to your office with concern that she has never had a menstrual period. History reveals she is sexually active with one partner and does not use contraception. Laboratory analysis reveals elevated serum FSH. Urine beta-hCG is negative. Physical examination reveals normal pubic hair but no breast development. What underlying cellular mechanism is absent in this patient's endometrium leading to her amenorrhea?

   - **The correct answer is endometrial apoptosis.**
   - As stated previously, endometrial shedding during the menstrual period occurs due to apoptosis. In this patient with Turner syndrome and subsequent amenorrhea, apoptosis would not be occurring in the endometrium, i.e. would be absent.

2. A 49-year-old male presents with a 3-month history of painless cervical lymphadenopathy that he first noticed while showering. A lymph node biopsy is performed and histologic exam reveals an abundance of small, mononuclear cells forming follicle-like nodules. Immunohistochemical staining with anti-Bcl-2 antibody shows overexpression. Inhibition of which cellular pathway allows for uncontrolled proliferation and formation of these nodules?

   A. Release of cytochrome C from the mitochondria
   B. FasL binding Fas death receptor (CD95)
   C. Cytotoxic CD8+ T-cell-mediated apoptosis
   D. Ras-induced signal transmission

   - **The correct answer is A**
   - This patient's history of painless lymphadenopathy along with the overexpression of BCL-2 are indicative of a disease called follicular lymphoma. BCL-2 is an antiapoptotic that inhibits the formation of pores created by BAX and BAK in the inner mitochondrial membrane. It subsequently inhibits the release of cytochrome C from the inner mitochondrial membrane to the cytosol.
   - The intrinsic mitochondrial pathway (**FIGURE ###--Intrinsic Mitochondrial Pathway**), shows that stimuli such as cellular injury, decreased hormonal stimulation, etc. inactivate BCL-2. This allows BAX and BAK to form a proapoptotic complex, bind to the inner mitochondrial membrane, and create pores for cytochrome C. Cytochrome C in the cytosol is the cell's signal to self-destruct. This then activates the caspase enzymes.
   - B and C are incorrect because, although they are the other apoptotic pathways among the answer choices, they have nothing to do with BCL-2.
   - D is incorrect because, although Ras-induced signal transmission is a cellular signaling pathway, it is not involved in apoptosis and has nothing to do with BCL-2.

Section IV - Necrosis

I. Basic Principles
   A. Necrosis is a type of cell death (includes apoptosis and necrosis)
      1. Cell ceases to carry out functions
      2. Cell nucleus is lost via nuclear condensation (pyknosis), dissolution (karyolysis), or fragmentation (karyorrhexis)
   B. Occurs due to an underlying pathological process
   C. Death of a large number of cells

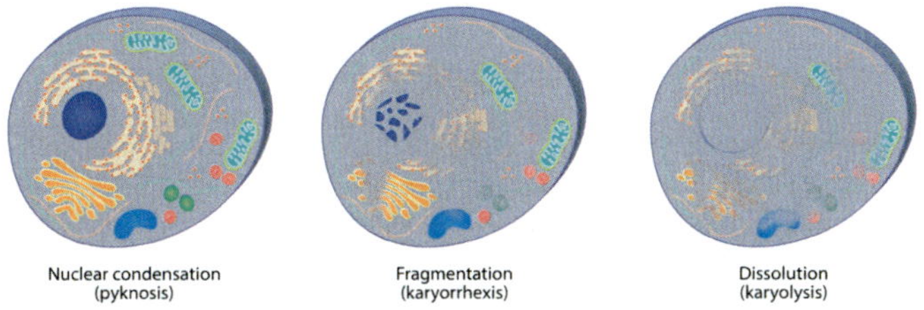

FIGURE 10.1.17 - Nuclear Changes in Necrosis

II. Mechanism of Necrosis
   A. Unregulated, unplanned form of cell death
   B. Cell membrane damaged → irreversible cell injury → cell death
   C. Escape of organelles through damaged membrane → inflammation
   D. Histologically, cells appear pink

III. Coagulative Necrosis
   A. A type of necrosis wherein the tissue architecture is temporarily preserved and remains firm due to coagulated proteins
   B. Gross appearance: wedge-shaped, pale area
   C. Microscopically: cell shape remains, nucleus disappears
   D. Cell death caused by a lack of blood flow or ischemia
   E. Any organ except the brain

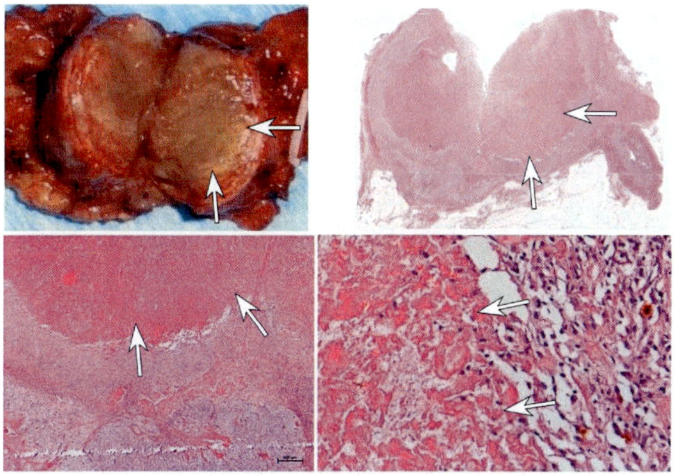

Photo Credit: Nobumasa Ohara, Yasuyuki Uemura, Naomi Mezaki, Keita Kimura, Masanori Kaneko, Hirohiko Kuwano, Katsuya Ebe, Toshio Fujita, Takeshi Komeyama, Hiroyuki Usuda, Yuto Yamazaki, Takashi Maekawa, Hironobu Sasano, Kenzo Kaneko & Kyuzi Kamoi / CC BY (https://creativecommons.org/licenses/by/4.0)

FIGURE 10.1.19 - Pheochromocytoma with Coagulative Necrosis

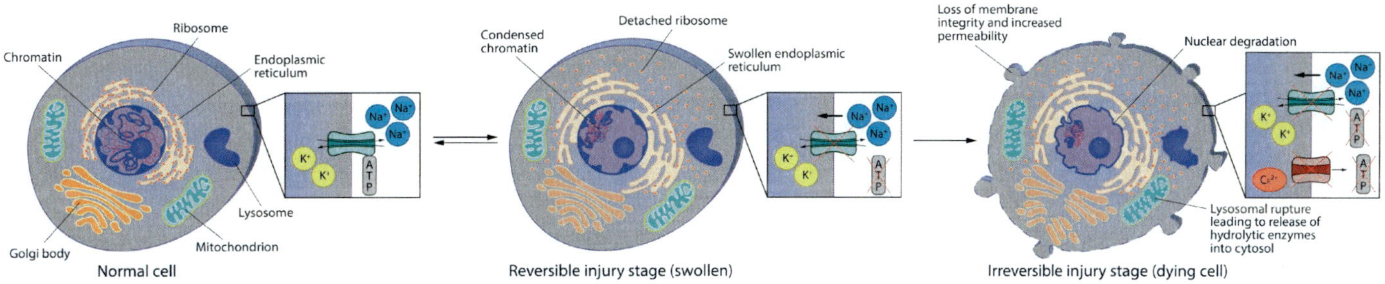

FIGURE 10.1.11 - Microscopic Changes of Cell Injury

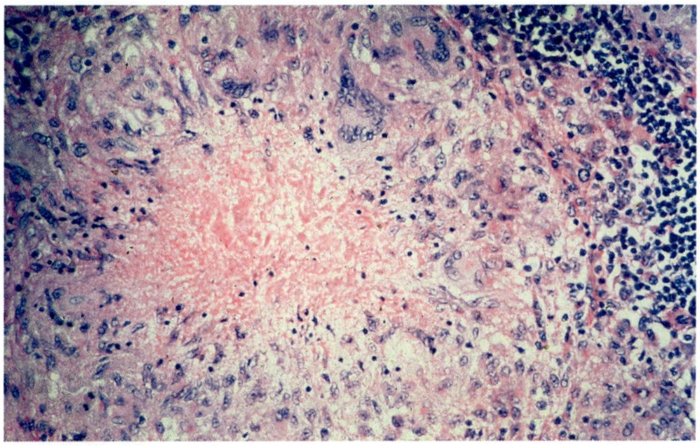

Photo Credit: Pulmonary tuberculosis - Necrotizing granuloma by Yale Rosen [CC BY-SA 2.0 (https://creativecommons.org/licenses/by-sa/2.0/)]

FIGURE 10.1.18 - Necrotizing Granuloma

IV. Liquefactive Necrosis
- A. Dead tissue becomes liquefied by enzymatic lysis of cells and proteins
- B. Brain infarctions as the brain contains proteolytic enzymes that digest tissues
- C. Also seen in pancreatitis and abscesses

V. Gangrenous Necrosis
- A. Multiple layers of tissue undergo coagulative necrosis, leading to a dry and shriveled appearance
- B. Loss of blood supply to distal limbs, particularly lower limbs and also the gastrointestinal tract
- C. Dry gangrene - similar to coagulative necrosis
- D. Wet gangrene - liquefactive necrosis superimposed on coagulative

VI. Caseous Necrosis
- A. Dead tissue has a soft, white appearance similar to cheese
- B. Combination of coagulative and liquefactive necrosis
- C. Seen in tuberculosis or fungal infections
- D. Granulomatous inflammation characterized by macrophages and lymphocytes

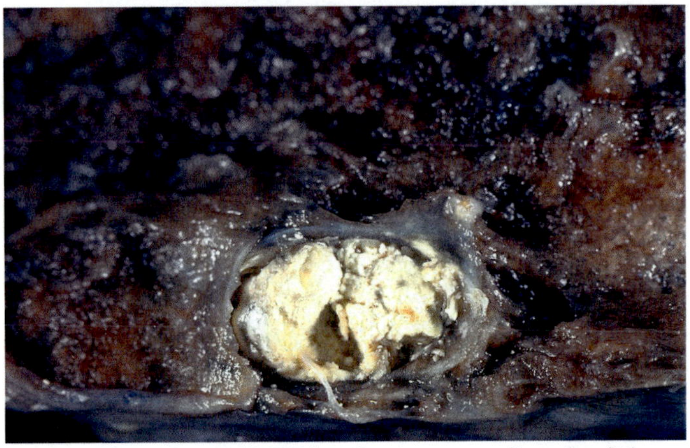

FIGURE 10.1.20 - Caseous Necrosis of the Lung

VII. Fat Necrosis
- A. Destruction of adipose tissue due to trauma or release of enzymes
- B. Non-enzymatic tissue (e.g. breast) or enzymatic tissue (e.g. pancreas)
- C. Fatty acids released combine with calcium via saponification
- D. Chalky-white appearance

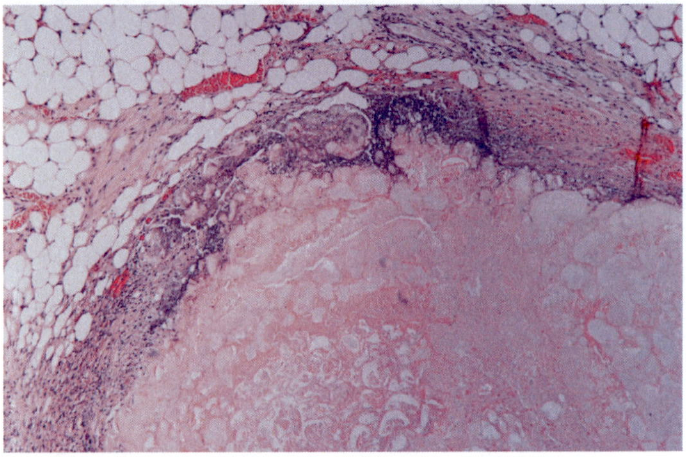

FIGURE 10.1.21 - Fat Necrosis in Pancreatitis

VIII. Fibrinoid Necrosis
- A. Antigen-antibody complexes and fibrin are deposited into blood vessel wall resulting in necrotic damage
- B. Bright pink blood vessel wall due to fibrin deposition
- C. Characteristic of vasculitis and malignant hypertension

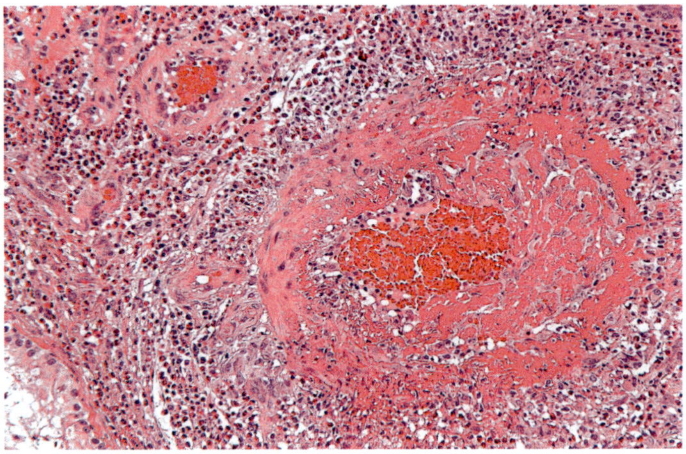

FIGURE 10.1.22- Fibrinoid Necrosis

REVIEW QUESTIONS

1. A 77-year-old man presents to the emergency department with right0sided weakness and difficulty speaking. Examination reveals right-sided hemiplegia and hemisensory loss. What type of necrosis would most likely be observed?

    - Hopefully from the question stem you've realized that the patient has had an ischemic stroke. This would explain the right-sided weakness, difficulty speaking, hemiplegia and hemisensory loss.
    - As the location of the infarct is the brain, we would expect to see liquefactive necrosis.

2. A 28-year-old woman is evaluated for nausea, abdominal pain and vomiting. Her heart rate is 120/min, blood pressure is 100/70 mmHg and temperature is 36.8ºC (98.2ºF). Lab results reveal that her ALT (alanine aminotransferase) levels are 3200 U/L (normal range: 7 - 56 U/L). A urine toxicology screen is positive for benzodiazepines. She tells the physician that she took 25 acetaminophen tablets each containing 325 mg of acetaminophen. Which of the following histopathological findings would most likely be found on biopsy of this patient's liver?

    A. Epithelioid cells with lymphocytes and Langerhans giant cells
    B. Eosinophilic cells with mononuclear cell infiltration
    C. Accumulation of fibrin-like material
    D. Small numbers of eosinophilic cells throughout the parenchyma

    - **The correct answer is B.**
    - From the question we can deduce that the patient has overdosed on acetaminophen. The maximum daily adult dose of acetaminophen is 4000 mg. So if the patient took 25 tablets of 325 mg each, she would have taken 8125 mg of acetaminophen, which is more than twice the maximum dose. It is important to remember that a major side effect of acetaminophen overdose is hepatotoxicity.
    - The patient presented with nausea, abdominal pain and vomiting, which can occur in acute liver injury, and her ALT levels are greatly elevated. The elevated ALT levels indicate damage to the hepatocytes, so in a liver biopsy we would expect to see option choice B. Eosinophilic cells with mononuclear cell infiltration.
    - Recall that in coagulative necrosis the cell retains its shape but loses its nucleus, making it appear very eosinophilic in a histological section. The main reason that B is the answer and not D is that the cells have undergone necrosis, not apoptosis. A hallmark of necrosis is the presence of inflammation, which is seen by the infiltration of monocytes. Additionally, apoptosis involves small numbers of cells.
    - C, which describes fibrinoid necrosis, is incorrect because for fibrin-like material to be found there would need to be damage to the blood vessels, not the hepatocytes.
    - A describes granulomatous inflammation and is incorrect because the patient does not have a tuberculous or fungal infection.

Section V - Free Radical Injury

I. Basic Principles
   A. Free radicals are highly reactive chemical species with an unpaired valence electron
   B. They are generated in physiological processes as well as pathological processes
   C. Free radicals cause cellular injury by adversely altering lipids, proteins, and DNA

II. Physiological Generation
   A. Occurs during oxidative phosphorylation in the electron transport chain
      1. Oxygen (O_2) serves as the final electron acceptor from cytochrome c oxidase (complex IV)
   B. Partial reduction of oxygen can form various reactive oxygen species
      1. Superoxide (O_2^-), hydrogen peroxide (H_2O_2), and hydroxyl radicals ($^{\bullet}OH$)

III. Pathological Generation
   A. Radiation exposure – converts water in tissues to hydroxyl radicals
   B. Drugs and toxins – hepatic P450 enzymes generate free radicals during drug metabolism (e.g. carbon tetrachloride → $CCl_3\bullet$)
   C. Cigarette smoke – partially responsible for harmful effects of smoking
   D. Inflammation – phagocytes generate superoxide (via NADPH oxidase) and hypochlorite ($OCl^{\bullet}$) during oxidative burst to kill microbes

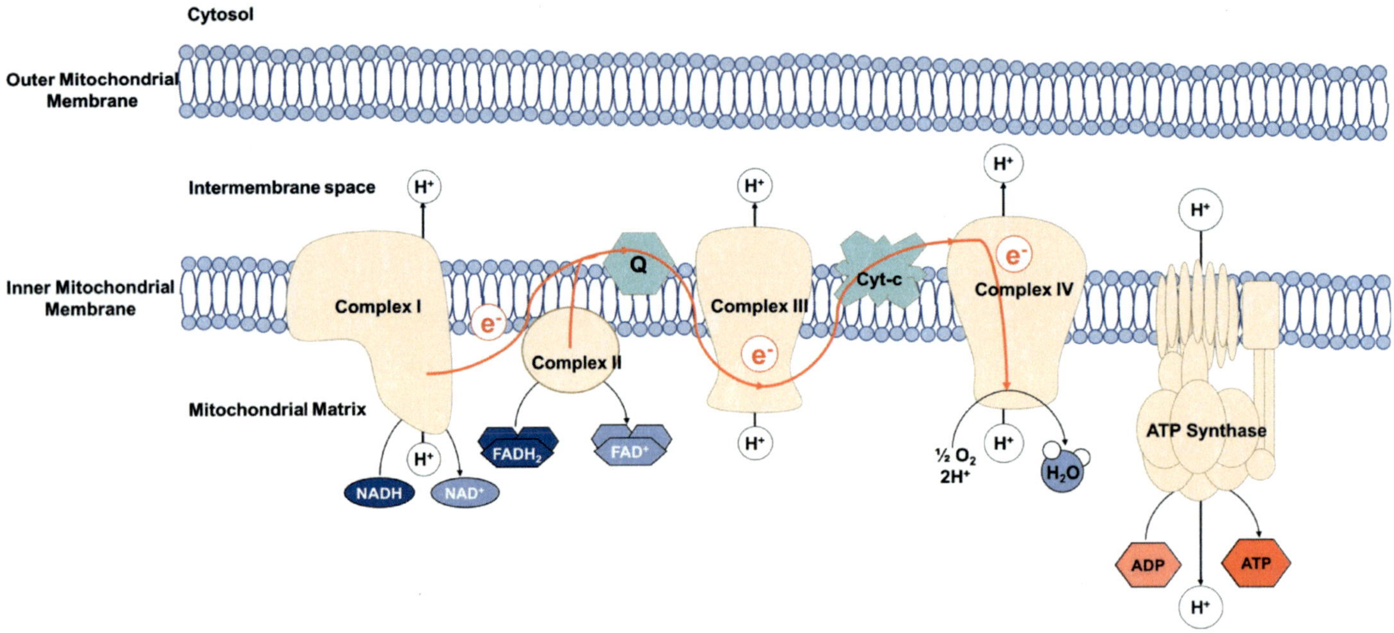

FIGURE 10.1.23 - Schematic of ElectronTransport Chain

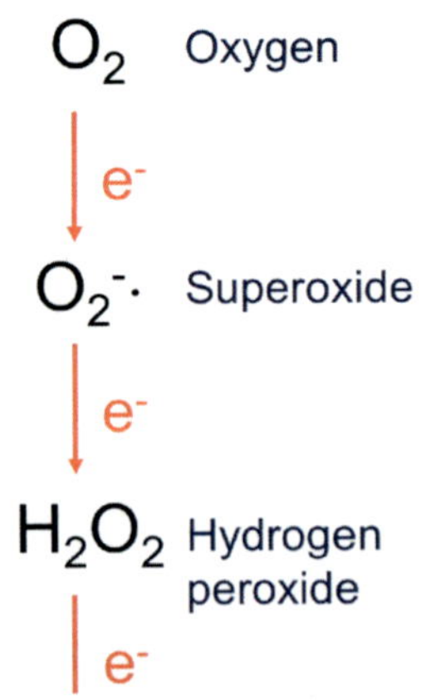

FIGURE 10.1.24 - Formation of Reactive Oxygen Species Through Partial Reduction of Oxygen

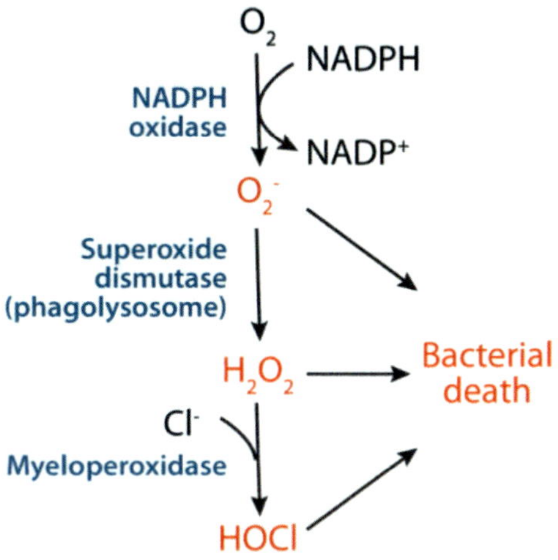

FIGURE 10.1.25 - Pathological Generation of Free Radicals From Oxidative Burst

IV. Pathological Generation of Free Radicals
  A. Metals – free iron, Fe^{2+}, generates hydroxyl radicals via Fenton reaction (copper also behaves similarly)
  B. $Fe^{2+} + H_2O_2 \rightarrow Fe^{3+} + OH^- + {}^{\bullet}OH$

V. Elimination of Free Radicals
  A. Spontaneous decay
  B. Metal binding proteins (e.g. ceruloplasmin, transferrin)
  C. Scavenging enzymes (e.g. glutathione peroxidase, catalase, superoxide dismutase)
  D. Antioxidants (e.g. vitamins, glutathione)

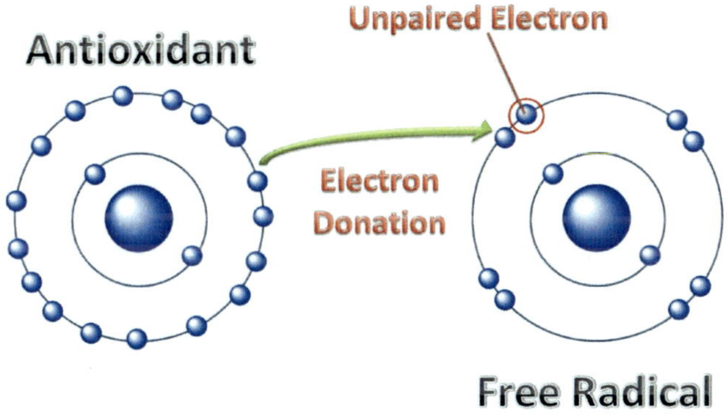

FIGURE 10.1.26 - Antioxidant Elimination of Free Radicals

VI. Examples of Free Radical Injury
  A. Acetaminophen overdose
    1. Acetaminophen is the most common cause of acute liver failure in the United States
    2. Hepatic P450 enzymes metabolize acetaminophen to NAPQI
    3. NAPQI overwhelms glutathione stores leading to formation of toxic free radicals
    4. Results in hepatotoxicity and may lead to massive hepatic necrosis

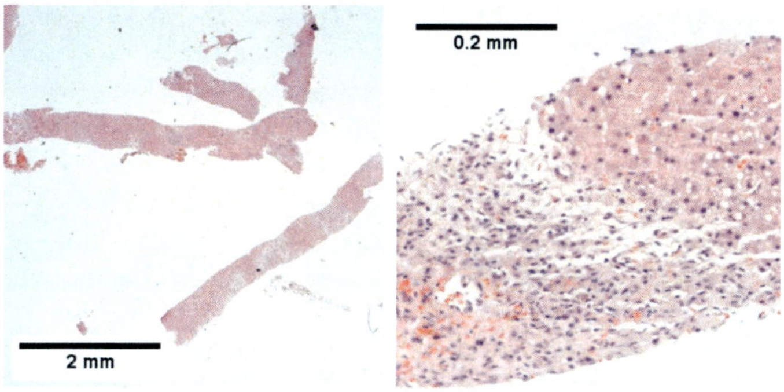

FIGURE 10.1.27 - Hepatic Necrosis from Acetaminophen Toxicity Taken in Low (Left) and High (Right) Magnification

  B. Oxygen toxicity via reperfusion injury
    1. Contributes to damage in myocardial and cerebral ischemia
    2. Cutting the blood supply to an organ results in ischemic damage (lack of oxygen)
    3. Return of blood to ischemic tissue results in production of O_2 - derived free radicals

REVIEW QUESTIONS

1. A 3-year-old boy in mild distress is brought to the clinic by his mother complaining that he has been coughing. He is tachypneic and has a fever of 38.3°C (101°F). Upon auscultation of the lung fields there are crackles and decreased breath sounds in the right middle lobe. His mother notes that he has been treated for pneumonia caused by *S. pneumoniae* three times in the past year with full resolution of symptoms each time. After neutrophil function testing, the patient is determined to have chronic granulomatous disease (a condition characterized by defective NADPH oxidase). This patient is at risk for recurrent infection due to dysfunction of what cellular process?

   - **The correct answer is oxidative burst.**
   - You are asked to determine the cause of the patient's recurrent infections given their diagnosis of chronic granulomatous disease, a condition characterized by defective NADPH oxidase. Neutrophils generate superoxide (via NADPH oxidase) and hypochlorite (OCl•) during oxidative burst to kill microbes, thus oxidative burst is defective.

2. A 49-year-old-man comes to the hospital complaining of lethargy for 2 months and a syncopal episode that occured yesterday. He notes that he is normally very active but now can barely seem to walk around the neighborhood. After further questioning it is discovered that the patient was recently diagnosed with diabetes. Physical examination reveals skin hyperpigmentation. An ECG shows sinus node dysfunction. Echocardiogram demonstrates dilation of the left ventricle. Vital signs are within normal limits. This patient's condition most likely resulted from which of the following processes?

   A. Tumor formation and metastasis
   B. Generation of hydroxyl free radicals
   C. CD8+ T-cell-mediated toxicity
   D. Ischemia-induced tissue damage

   - **The correct answer is B.**
   - The patient was recently diagnosed with diabetes and is compliant with his medication. The patient has an irregular heartbeat (likely indicating that he has an arrhythmia) and unusually pigmented skin. A patient in late adulthood with lethargy, weakness, diabetes, arrhythmia, and pigmented skin points towards hemochromatosis.
   - Iron overload can cause generation of hydroxyl free radicals via the Fenton reaction. The Fenton reaction characterizes how iron can lead to the generation of free radicals, which are harmful to fats, proteins, and DNA and cause cellular damage.
   - A is incorrect because hemochromatosis is not a type of cancer.
   - C and D are incorrect because CD8+ T-cellmediated toxicity and ischemia-induced tissue damage are not part of the pathological process here.

Section VI - Amyloidosis

I. Definition
   A. Deposition of misfolded protein in the extracellular space that causes damage to tissues

II. General Characteristics
   A. Misfolded protein in β-pleated structure
   B. Can be systemic or localized
   C. Positive Congo red histological stain
   D. Apple-green birefringence under polarized light

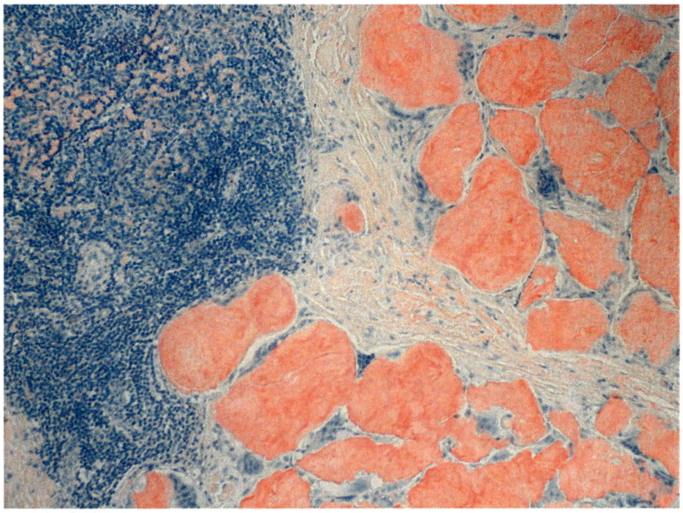

FIGURE 10.1.28 - Histological Slide Showing Amyloid Deposition Within a Lymph Node

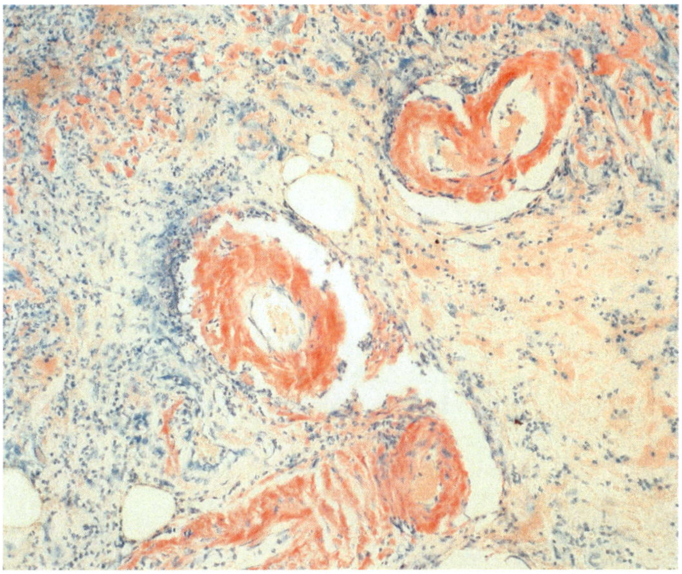

FIGURE 10.1.29 - Histological Slide Showing Amyloid Deposition Within Blood Vessels

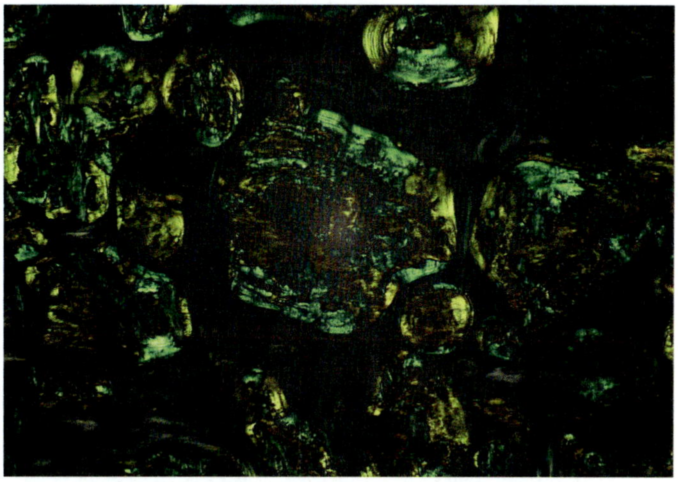

FIGURE 10.1.30 - Histological Image Of Lymph Node With Amyloid Deposits Under Polarized Light

III. Systemic Amyloidosis
   A. In multiple organs
   B. Primary or secondary
   C. Primary: deposition of AL (amyloid light chain) amyloid
      1. Deposition of AL amyloid, a protein derived from immunoglobulin light chain
      2. Caused by disorders of plasma cells (e.g. multiple myeloma)
      3. Increased production of light chain immunoglobulins → misfolded → deposition of AL amyloid
   D. Secondary: deposition of AA (amyloid-associated A protein) amyloid
      1. Derived from SAA (serum amyloid protein), an acute phase reactant
      2. Caused by chronic inflammation, infections, and malignancy
      3. Increased SAA mostly during inflammation→ defect in SAA degradation → increase in AA amyloid→ deposits in tissues
   E. Clinical Findings
      1. Variable (depends on organ involved)
      2. Kidney (most common organ involved in AA amyloid): asymptomatic proteinuria or clinically apparent nephrotic syndrome
      3. Heart: restrictive cardiomyopathy, arrhythmia or heart block
      4. Skin: waxy thickening, easy bruising, and purpura
      5. Other: hepatomegaly, neuropathy, large tongue, and malabsorption

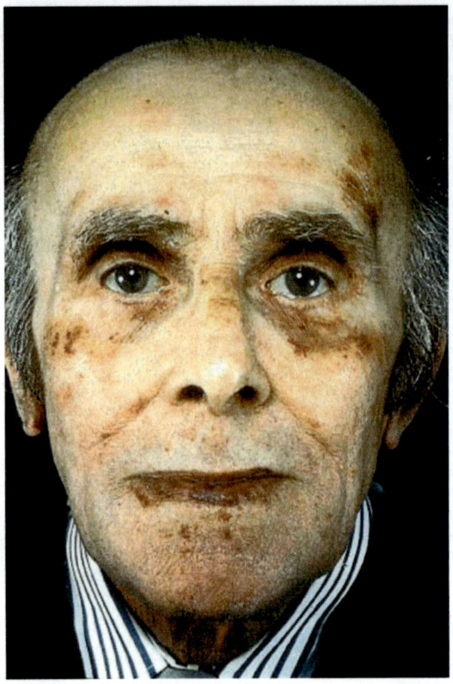

Photo Credit: Professor P N Hawkins / CC BY-SA (https://creativecommons.org/licenses/by-sa/3.0)

FIGURE 10.1.31 - Light Chain Amyloidosis With Purpura Around the Eyes

IV. Localized Amyloidosis
   A. Limited to a single organ
   B. Many subtypes
      1. Alzheimer disease
         a) Deposition of Aβ amyloid from β-APP (beta amyloid precursor protein)
         b) This gene is located on chromosome 21
      2. Age-related (senile) cardiac amyloidosis
         a) Deposition of normal transthyretin in myocardium
         b) Common autopsy finding, usually without clinical consequence

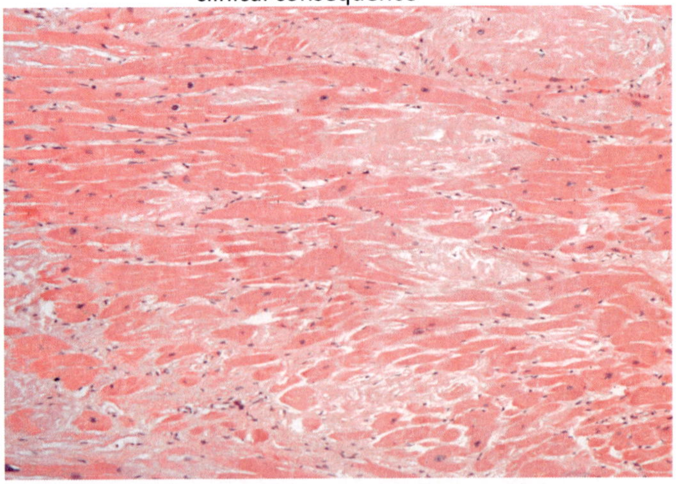

Photo Credit: Nephron / CC BY-SA (https://creativecommons.org/licenses/by-sa/3.0)

FIGURE 10.1.32 -Histological Slide of Senile Cardiac Amyloidosis

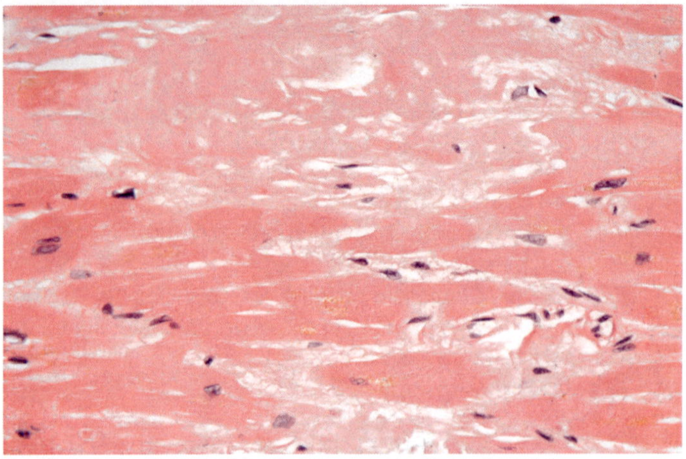

Photo Credit: Nephron / CC BY-SA (https://creativecommons.org/licenses/by-sa/3.0)

FIGURE 10.1.33 - Amyloid Deposits (Fluffy Pink Material) and Lipofuscin (Yellow Granular Material)

   C. Familial amyloid cardiomyopathy
      1. Deposition of mutated transthyretin protein (TTR)
      2. Different kinds of mutations → mutated TTR amyloid deposits in the heart → causes restrictive cardiomyopathy due to stiffening of the heart
      3. Familial disease (African Americans)
   D. Diabetes mellitus type II
      1. Amylin (derived from insulin) deposits into islets of the pancreas
      2. Peripheral tissue resistance to insulin → pancreas overproduces insulin → gets deposited in islets
   E. Dialysis-related amyloidosis
      1. Deposition of β2-microglobulin in joints
      2. Complication of long-term dialysis following end-stage renal failure
   F. Medullary carcinoma of the thyroid
      1. Tumor cells produce calcitonin that is deposited within the tumor
      2. Described as tumor cells dispersed in amyloid stroma
   G. Cerebral amyloid angiopathy
      1. Deposition of β-amyloid in the walls of the arteries in the brain
      2. Vessel weakening → increased risk for hemorrhagic stroke especially in elderly

V. Diagnosis
   A. Tissue biopsy
      1. AL and systemic amyloidosis: subcutaneous abdominal fat or rectal mucosa
      2. Localized amyloidosis: from the involved organs (e.g. kidney, thyroid)
   B. Congo red stain
   C. Polarized light with apple-green birefringence

VI. Treatment
   A. Once deposited, amyloid cannot be removed
   B. Transplantation of affected organ

REVIEW QUESTIONS

1. A 70-year-old patient with no history of recent trauma is brought to the emergency department due to sudden changes in vision and left-sided hemisensory loss that has lasted for about an hour. His symptoms have gradually worsened and he now presents with a new-onset headache. His CT shows multiple hemorrhages of varying size and age as well as an acute lobar bleed. He is not on blood thinners. What is the most likely cause of his multiple brain bleeds?

   - **The correct answer is cerebral amyloid angiopathy.**
   - This elderly patient experiences worsening acute neurological symptoms like vision changes and left-sided hemisensory loss. His CT shows multiple hemorrhages of varying size and age, which hints at an underlying condition that makes him susceptible to recurrent brain bleeds.

2. A 56-year-old man presents with 3 months of fatigue and back pain that is not associated with exercise or physical activity. On physical exam there is tenderness over the middle and lower back. Laboratory values show a hemoglobin level of 10.5 g/dL (13.5-17.5 g/dL) and serum calcium level of 12 mg/dL (8.4-10.2 mg/dL). Bone marrow aspirate shows abnormal plasma cells. This patient is at greatest risk of developing which of the following?

   A. Pericardial effusion
   B. Splenic rupture
   C. Immunoglobulin light chain deposition
   D. Alpha-helical deposits

   - **The correct answer is C.**
   - The patient has multiple myeloma that puts him at an increased risk of developing systemic amyloidosis. Primary amyloidosis occurs due to the systemic deposition of light chain amyloid and is mostly caused by plasma cell dyscrasias (abnormal or disordered plasma cells), such as multiple myeloma.
   - A is incorrect because, although some malignancies (such as lung and breast carcinomas) invade the pericardium, it is not typical of multiple myeloma.
   - B is incorrect because multiple myeloma doesn't cause severe splenic enlargement and subsequently put the patient at risk of splenic rupture.
   - D is incorrect because amyloidosis is characterized by beta-pleated sheet deposits, not alpha-helical deposits.

Section VII - Wound Healing

I. Basic Principles
  A. Accomplished by tissue regeneration and wound repair
    1. Degree of regeneration vs. repair often depends on tissue type
  B. Concurrent process with inflammation
    1. Shared mediators

II. Tissue Mediators
  A. Growth factors
    1. FGF: angiogenesis and skeletal development
    2. TGF-α: fibrosis
    3. TGF-β: fibrosis and angiogenesis
    4. VEGF: angiogenesis
    5. PDGF: fibroblast growth for collagen synthesis, vascular remodeling and smooth muscle cell migration
    6. EGF: cell growth via tyrosine kinases
  B. Matrix metalloproteinases: tissue remodeling

III. Regeneration
  A. Replaces a wound with native tissue

IV. Repair
  A. Occurs when regenerative cells are lost or regeneration cannot occur
  B. Replaces a wound with a scar
  C. Three phases

V. Regeneration vs. Repair
  A. Permanent tissues - cannot regenerate and are limited to repair: heart, skeletal muscle, and neurons
  B. Labile tissues - continuously regenerate: skin, bone marrow, large and small intestines
  C. Stable tissues - only regenerate when necessary: liver

VI. Normal Wound Healing
  A. New tissue deposition
  B. Primary intention
    1. Edges of wound are approximated
    2. Little to no scarring
  C. Secondary intention
    1. Edges of wound are not approximated
    2. Obvious scarring

Phase	Timing	Mediator(s)	Function
Inflammatory	-Up to 3 days after wound	-Platelets -Neutrophils -Macrophages	-Clot formation -Vessel permeability -Neutrophil migration -Clearing of debris (macrophages)
Proliferative	-Day 3 to weeks after wound	-Fibroblasts -Myofibroblasts -Endothelial cells -Keratinocytes -Macrophages	-Angiogenesis -Epithelial cell proliferation -Clot dissolution -Granulation tissue and type III collagen deposition (fibroblasts) -Wound contraction (myofibroblasts)
Remodeling	-1 week to months after wound	-Fibroblasts	-Replace pliable type III collagen with stronger type I collagen through collagenases (requires zinc)

TABLE 10.1.2 - Timeline of Wound Repair

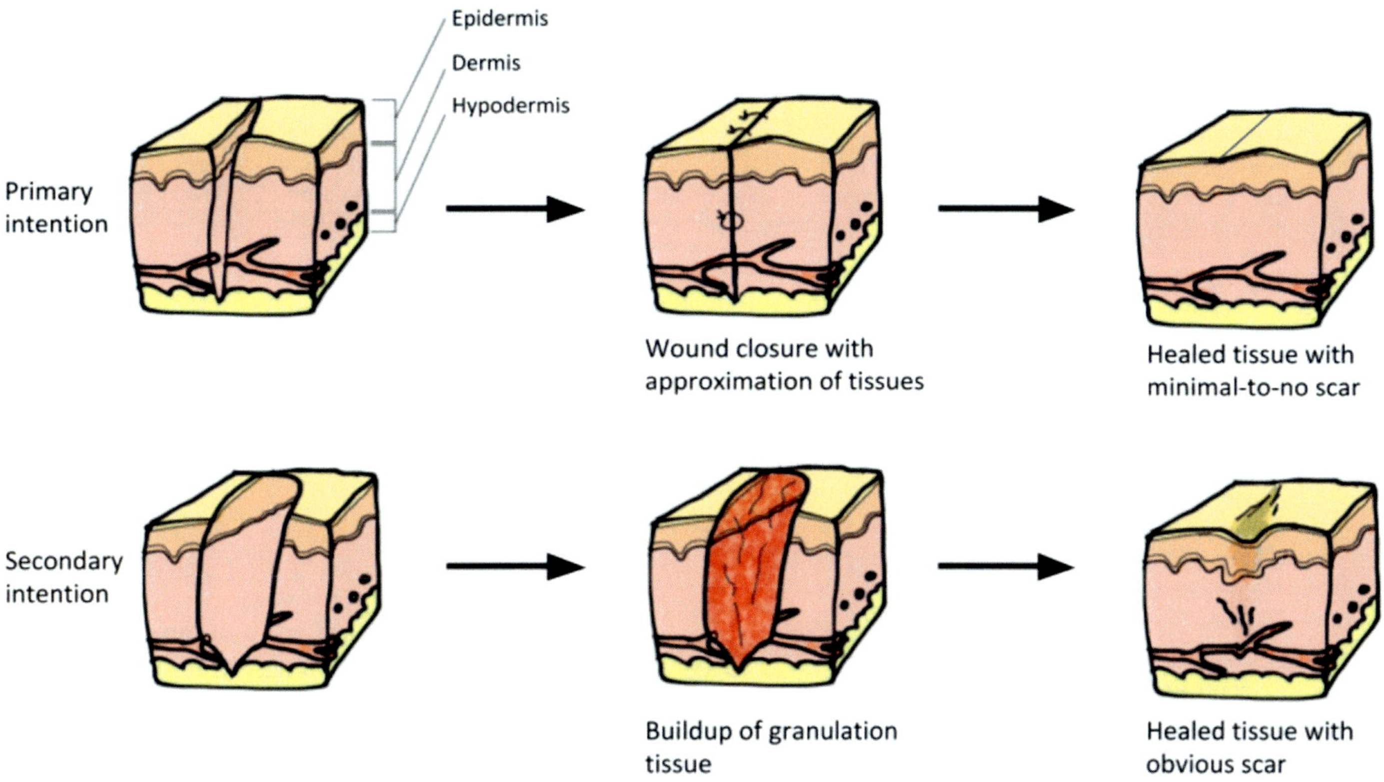

FIGURE 10.1.34 - Primary(Top) vs. Secondary (Bottom) Intention Wound Healing

VII. Abnormal Wound Healing
   A. Tertiary (delayed) wound healing
      1. Infection
      2. Vitamin C deficiency
      3. Copper deficiency
      4. Zinc deficiency
   B. Abnormal scarring
      1. Hypertrophic scarring: limited to wound borders
      2. Keloids: extend beyond wound borders
      3. TGF-β: hypertrophic scarring and keloids of lung, liver, and kidney

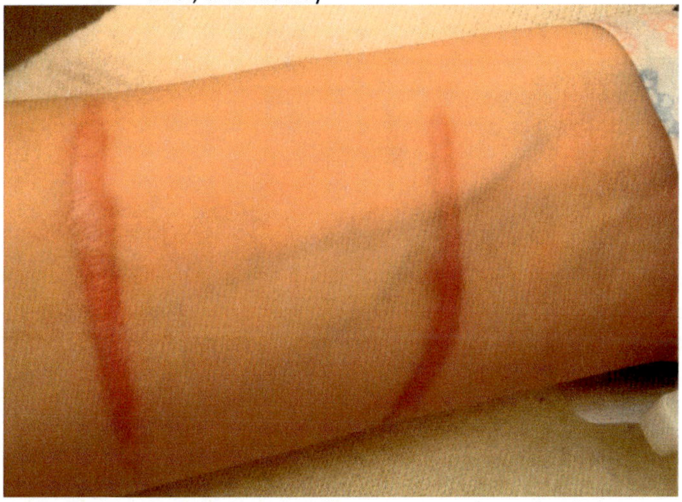

Photo Credit: User:Cgomez447 / CC BY-SA (https://creativecommons.org/licenses/by-sa/3.0)

FIGURE 10.1.35 - Hypertrophic Scar

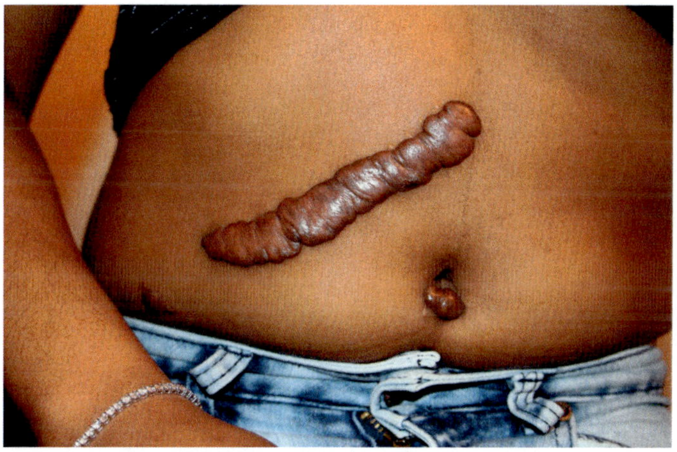

Photo Credit: Htirgan / CC BY-SA (https://creativecommons.org/licenses/by-sa/3.0)

FIGURE 10.1.36 - Keloid

   C. Examples
      1. Scurvy
      2. Ehlers-Danlos syndrome
      3. Osteogenesis imperfecta
      4. Diabetes

REVIEW QUESTIONS

1. A 22-year-old male cut the adductor pollicis muscle in his left hand while chopping vegetables. He initially went to the emergency department and was managed appropriately. Five days later he presents for follow up. Which phase of wound repair is likely occurring during this time?

- **The correct answer is repair is occurring.**
- There was damage to skeletal muscle, which is a permanent tissue. Therefore, the wound healing process that must occur in this situation is repair. It has been five days since the wound first occurred, meaning that it is in the proliferative phase of healing. This phase begins three days after a wounding incident and concludes several weeks later.
- Any of the following could occur during this time period: angiogenesis, epithelial cell proliferation, clot dissolution, granulation tissue deposition, type III collagen deposition, or wound contraction.

2. A 14-year-old African American girl presents with a large hyperpigmented rubbery lump on her left ear that appeared after getting her ears professionally pierced. She states that she cannot wear an earring on her left ear due to the lump. Vital signs are within normal limits and she appears to be in no distress. Which of the following is part of the pathophysiology of this clinical presentation?

   A. Zinc deficiency
   B. Vitamin C deficiency
   C. Excess collagen type III
   D. Deficient collagen type II
   E. Neutrophil migration

- **The correct answer is C.**
- The lesion is likely a keloid. The lesion is large enough to keep her from wearing an earring when a typical ear piercing is a tiny hole. This indicates that the scar has spread beyond the wound borders, a characteristic of a keloid. Keloids are formed during the remodeling phase of wound healing due to excess type III collagen formation.
- A and B are incorrect because they describe conditions that would cause tertiary wound healing.
- D is incorrect because type II collagen is found in hyaline cartilage and a deficiency of it is not part of a keloid's pathophysiology.
- E is incorrect because neutrophil migration is also not part of a keloid's pathophysiology.

Section VIII - Neoplasia

I. Basic Principles
  A. New tissue growth characterized by three properties
    1. Unregulated
    2. Irreversible
    3. Monoclonal (determined by studying G6PD isoenzymes)

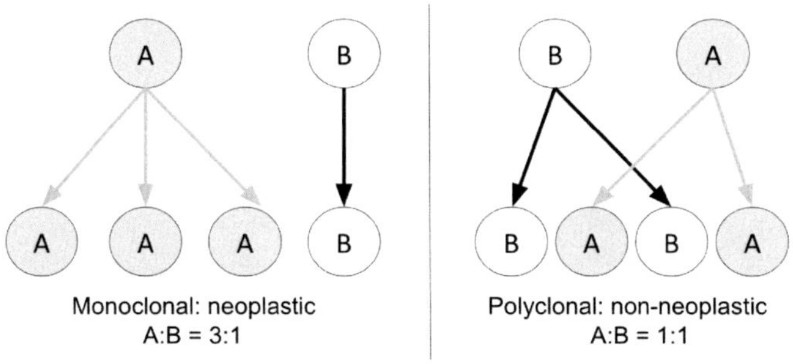

FIGURE 10.1.37 - Use of G6PD Isoenzymes to Determine Monoclonality

II. Nomenclature of Tumors
  A. Depends on
    1. Type of tissue from which tumor is derived
    2. Nature of tumor (benign or malignant)
  B. General Rules
    1. Benign tumors: "-oma" (e.g. fibroma, chondroma)
    2. Malignant tumors
      a) Mesenchymal: "-sarcoma" (e.g. fibrosarcoma, chondrosarcoma
      b) Blood-forming cells: "leukemia" or "lymphoma" (e.g. AML, Hodgkin's lymphoma)
      c) Epithelial origin: "-carcinoma" (e.g. squamous cell carcinoma, adenocarcinoma)

III. Screening
  A. Basics
    1. Diagnostic tests
      a) Screening (high sensitivity) vs. confirmatory (high specificity) tests
    2. Cancer shows clinical symptoms after approximately 30 cell divisions
    3. With each division → number of mutations increases
    4. Late-presenting cancer → more mutations
  B. Role of Screening
    1. Early detection of dysplasia (precancerous change) before it becomes carcinoma
    2. Early detection of cancers before clinical symptoms begin
    3. Efficacy is directly related to decrease in cancer-specific deaths

IV. Non-Neoplastic Growths
  A. Hamartoma
    1. Overgrowth of disorganized tissue indigenous to a particular site (e.g. birthmarks, pulmonary hamartomas)
  B. Choristoma
    1. Normal tissue in a foreign location (e.g. pancreatic tissue in stomach wall)

Screening Test	Cancer	Comments
Pap smear	- Cervical cancer	- Detects cervical dysplasia
Mammography	- Breast cancer	- Detects in situ breast cancer
Digital rectal exam	- Prostate carcinoma	- Detects benign prostatic hyperplasia
Hemoccult test and colonoscopy	- Colorectal carcinoma	- Detects colonic adenoma

TABLE 10.1.3 - Screening Tests for Early Detection of Cancer

REVIEW QUESTIONS

1. A 45-year-old woman with a 25-year history of chronic alcohol abuse presents with complaints of fatigue, weight loss, and abdominal pain with distension. Physical examination reveals hepatomegaly. Liver ultrasound shows a hyperechoic mass suggestive of a tumor. A sample is retrieved for biopsy, and the pathology report reveals that the tumor is a cancer of the hepatocytes. Using proper nomenclature, how would this cancer be named?

   - **The cancer should be named "hepatocellular carcinoma."**
   - Based on the path report, the tumor in this question is cancerous. Hepatocytes have an epithelial origin and are also known as the liver epithelial cells. Proper nomenclature for this cancer would thus require the suffix "-carcinoma."

2. A 30-year-old woman with no significant medical history presents to the office with complaints of weakness, significant weight loss and low-grade fever for 10 days. G6PD isoenzyme analysis is done and the number of cells with G6PD-A isoenzymes is found to be 400,000, while the number of cells with G6PD-B isoenzymes is found to be 100,000. Which of the following conditions is similar to the condition that the patient is suffering from?

   A. Prostatic carcinoma
   B. Benign prostatic hyperplasia
   C. Ventricular hypertrophy
   D. Barrett esophagus

   - **The correct answer is A**
   - The ratio of G6PD isoenzyme A and B is 4 to 1. Any ratio other than 1 to 1 suggests monoclonality, which is a feature of neoplastic cells. The patient must be suffering from a neoplastic condition. Prostatic cancer is the only one that signifies neoplastic growth.
   - B, C, and D are incorrect because benign prostatic hyperplasia, ventricular hypertrophy, and Barrett esophagus are examples of growth adaptations, and they show polyclonal growth.

Section IX - Carcinogenesis

I. Overview
  A. Basic principles
  B. Carcinogens
  C. Oncogenes and tumor suppressor genes
  D. Characteristics of carcinogenesis

II. Basic Principles
  A. Transformation of a normal cell into a cancer cell
  B. Occurs when cellular homeostasis is disrupted by hyperplasia and dysplasia
  C. Dysplasia is often caused by chronic hyperplasia and is responsible for the growth of preneoplastic cells
  D. Initiated by irreparable damage to DNA of stem cells by carcinogens

III. Oncogenes and Tumor Suppressor Genes
  A. Proto-oncogenes, tumor suppressor genes and apoptotic regulators are cell regulatory systems
  B. Mutation in proto-oncogenes → oncogene → uncontrolled growth
  C. Inactivated tumor suppressor gene → no regulation → tumor growth
  D. Mutation in one allele → oncogene
  E. Mutation of both alleles → inactivated tumor suppressor gene

Carcinogenic Category	Example	Associated Cancer
Natural carcinogens	- Aflatoxin B1	- Hepatocellular carcinoma
Anti-cancer drugs	- Alkylating agents	- Leukemia/lymphoma
Metals	- Arsenic - Nickel	- Liver angiosarcoma, lung carcinoma, and squamous cell carcinoma of skin - Lung carcinoma
Silicate minerals	- Asbestos - Silica	- Bronchogenic carcinoma and mesothelioma - Lung carcinoma
Acetaldehyde	- Alcohol	- Carcinoma of esophagus, stomach, and liver
Chlorinated hydrocarbons	- Vinyl chloride	- Liver angiosarcoma
Cigarette smoke	- Polycyclic aromatic hydrocarbons (e.g. benzopyrene) - Aromatic amines (e.g. naphthylamine) - Nitrosamines	- Lung carcinoma and gastrointestinal carcinoma - Transitional cell carcinoma of bladder - Carcinoma of nasal cavity, esophagus, stomach, and pancreas
Oncogenic microbes	- EBV - HBV and HCV - HPV (high-risk subtypes 16, 18) - HHV-8 - HTLV-1 - *H. pylori*	- Burkitt lymphoma, Hodgkin lymphoma, nasopharyngeal carcinoma, and CNS lymphoma in immunocompromised patients (e.g., AIDS) - Hepatocellular carcinoma - Squamous cell carcinoma of vulva, vagina, cervix, and anus; penile carcinoma - Kaposi sarcoma - Adult T-cell leukemia/lymphoma - Stomach adenocarcinoma and MALT lymphoma
Ionizing radiation	- X-rays, nuclear reactions, and radiotherapy	- Papillary thyroid carcinoma, CML, and AML
Non-ionizing radiation	- UV rays	- Basal cell carcinoma, squamous cell carcinoma, and melanoma

TABLE 10.1.4 - Carcinogens

Proto-oncogene	Action	Mechanism	Associated Cancer
PDGFB	- Encodes platelet-derived growth factor - Physiological role in blood vessel growth	- Autocrine loop → overexpression	- Astrocytoma
ERBB1/EGFR	- Tyrosine kinase - Encodes epidermal growth factor receptor	- Amplification	- Glioblastoma, adenocarcinoma of lung, and head and neck carcinomas
ERBB2/HER2/neu	- Tyrosine kinase	- Amplification	- Breast carcinoma and ovarian carcinoma
RET	- Encodes neural growth factor receptor	- Point mutation	- Multiple endocrine neoplasia (MEN) 2A, 2B, medullary thyroid cancer, and pheochromocytoma
BCL-2	- Anti-apoptotic molecule	- T(14;18)	- Follicular B-cell lymphoma
KIT	- Encodes stem cell growth factor receptor	- Point mutation	- Gastrointestinal stromal tumor
RAS genes	- GTP-binding protein	- Point mutation	- Carcinoma of lung, colon, and pancreas -Melanoma, and lymphoma
ABL	- Tyrosine kinase	- T(9;22) → BCR-ABL gene	- CML and some types of ALL
BRAF	- Serine/threonine kinase	- Point mutation	- Melanoma
ALK	- Tyrosine kinase	- Chromosome 2 translocation - Chromosome 2 inversion → fusion gene EML4-ALK	- Large cell lymphoma and non-small cell lung cancer
c-MYC	- Transcription factor	- T(8;14)	- Burkitt lymphoma
N-MYC	- Transcription factor	- Amplification	- Neuroblastoma
L-MYC	- Transcription factor	- Amplification	- Small cell lung cancer
CCND1 (cyclin D1)	- Cyclin	- T(11;14)	- Mantle cell lymphoma
CDK4	- Cyclin-dependent kinase	- Amplification	- Melanoma

TABLE 10.1.5 - Proto-Oncogenes

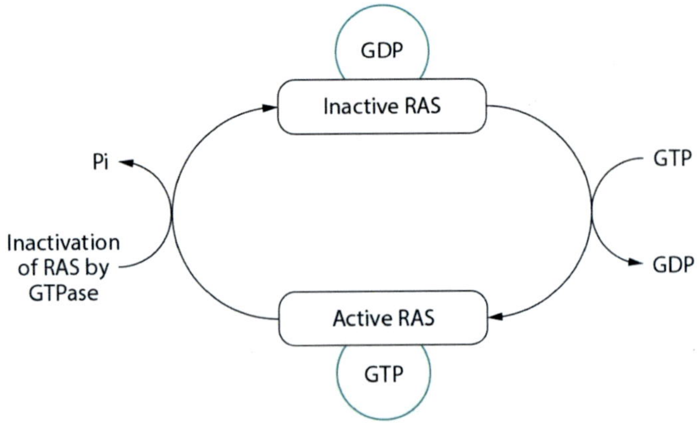

FIGURE 10.1.38 - RAS Inactivation

Tumor suppressor gene	Action	Associated cancer
APC	- Negatively regulates β-catenin by signaling for its breakdown	- Familial adenomatous polyposis, colorectal carcinoma, and melanoma
BRCA1, BRCA2	- Encodes proteins involved in DNA repair	- Breast carcinoma and ovarian carcinoma
NF1	- Encodes tumor-suppressor protein neurofibromin	- Neurofibromatosis type 1 which can lead to development of neuroblastomas and sarcomas
MEN1	- Encodes tumor-suppressor protein menin	- MEN 1, parathyroid, pituitary, and pancreatic adenomas
RB	- Encodes tumor-suppressor protein retinoblastoma (Rb)	- Retinoblastoma and osteosarcoma
VHL	- Inhibits hypoxia inducible factor 1a (HIF1a)	- Von Hippel-Lindau (VHL) disease - Renal cell cancer (can be caused by VHL disease)
WT1	- Encodes Wilms tumor protein which regulates gene activity	- Wilms tumor
TP53	- Encodes tumor protein 53 (p53)	- Most human carcinomas - Li-Fraumeni syndrome (development of carcinomas and sarcomas at a young age)

TABLE 10.1.6 - Tumor Suppressor Genes

IV. Characteristics of Carcinogenesis
   A. All cancer cells have certain characteristics that distinguish them from normal cells
   B. Replicative immortality, sustained angiogenesis, resistance to apoptosis, evasion of immune surveillance
   C. Cancer cells have high telomerase activity → preservation of telomeres → cell immortality
   D. Stimulate neo-angiogenesis by producing FGF and VEGF
   E. Neo-angiogenesis ensures growth of tumor by providing oxygen and nutrients as well as growth factors for new tumor cells
   F. Evade host immune system by decreasing expression of MHC class I → cancer cell is undetected by cytotoxic CD8+ cells

REVIEW QUESTIONS

1. A 54-year-old construction worker comes into the office after being told by his employer that a project they worked on 15 years ago tested positive for asbestos. He is concerned about his risk of developing cancer. Which cancer is he at greatest risk of developing?
    - **He is at greatest risk for developing Bronchogenic carcinoma (most common malignancy associated with asbestos exposure).**
    - Mesothelioma is also possible, but less likely.

2. A 45-year-old male has a lymph node biopsy performed for persistent lymphadenopathy. Histologic examination reveals small lymphocytes in a follicular pattern, which show over expression of the *BCL2* gene. What does this gene normally inhibit?
    - ***BCL2* gene normally inhibits apoptosis and the cell death cascade.**

3. A 29-year-old woman is evaluated for a breast lump. Her heart rate is 100/min., blood pressure is 100/70 mmHg and temperature is 36.8ºC (98.2ºF). The patient's mother died of a brain tumor at age 45 and her 16-year-old brother was recently diagnosed with osteosarcoma of his right knee. Breast examination reveals a 3 cm, firm spherical mass that moves with pectoral contraction. Which of the following gene mutations is the most likely cause of this patient's condition?

    A. APC
    B. TP53
    C. BRCA2
    D. PDGFB

    - **The correct answer is B.**
    - This is a young patient (29 yo) with a breast lump.
    - Her mother died from a brain tumor at a relatively young age (45).
    - Her 16-year-old brother was diagnosed with an osteosarcoma.
    - The patient's family history of sarcoma and brain tumors is suggestive of Li-Fraumeni syndrome, meaning that the patient has a high risk of developing cancer at a young age.
    - "Patients with Li-Fraumeni syndrome have a high risk of cancer diagnosed before age 45, as well as having a first-degree relative (such as a parent or sibling) diagnosed with any cancer before age 45.
    - Li-Fraumeni syndrome occurs due to mutations in the *BTP53* gene, which encodes for tumor-suppressor protein TP53.

Section X - Tumor Progression

I. Basic Principles
   A. The accumulation of DNA mutations in cells results in tumor formation
   B. Over time these tumors will grow, invade, and spread

II. Mechanisms
   A. Adjacent epithelial cells are attached to one another by a variety of adhesion molecules (e.g. E-cadherin)
   B. Downregulation of E-cadherin in tumor cells
   C. Disruption of cell-to-cell adhesion → tumor spread
   D. Basement membrane destruction via collagenase
   E. Attachment to fibronectin in the extracellular matrix → spread to local structures
   F. Invasion of vascular/lymphatic spaces → metastasis

III. Routes of Metastasis
   A. Lymphatic spread
   B. Hematogenous spread
   C. Seeding of body cavities

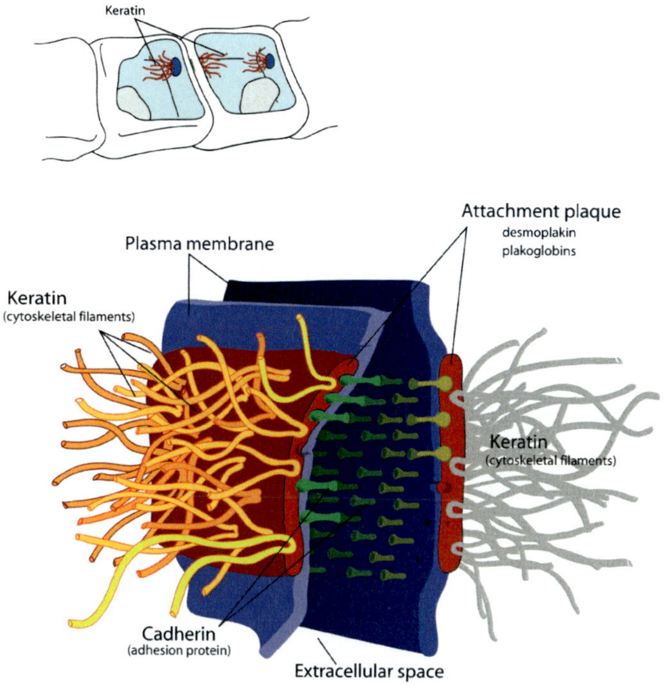

Photo Credit: LadyofHats / Public domain

FIGURE 10.1.40 - Junction Between Epithelial Cells at a Macroscopic (Top) and Microscopic (Bottom) Level

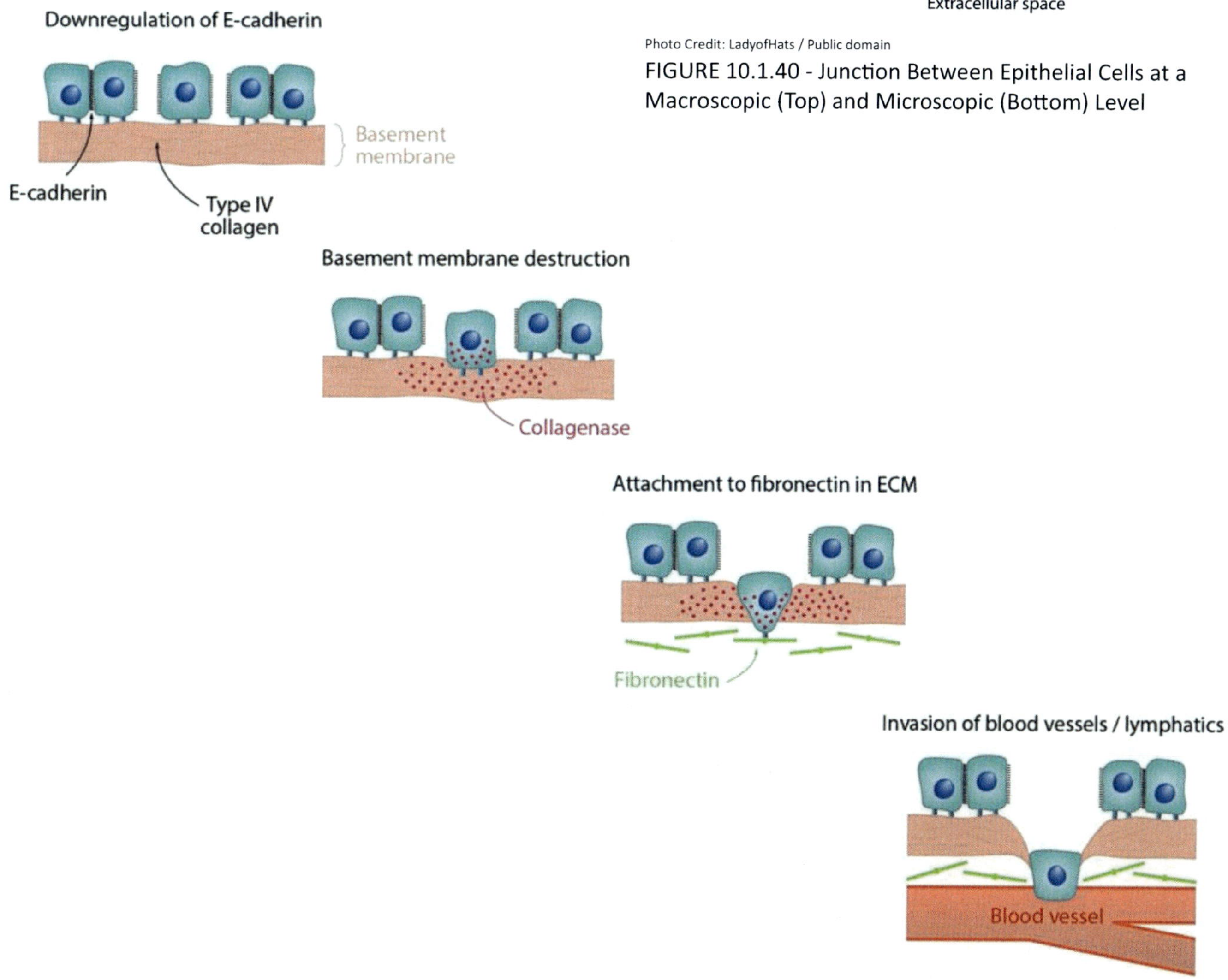

FIGURE 10.1.39 - Mechanism of Tumor Proliferation

IV. Lymphatic Spread
   A. Characteristic of carcinomas (malignant tumors of epithelial origin)
   B. Initially spreads to draining lymph nodes
   C. Later uses lymphatics to metastasize throughout the body

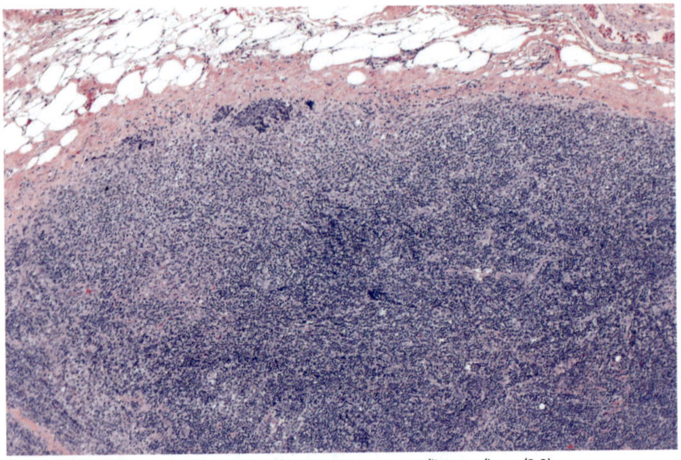

FIGURE 10.1.41 - Carcinoma Spreading to a Lymph Node

V. Hematogenous Spread
   A. Characteristic of most sarcomas
   B. Four carcinomas spread hematogenously (not via lymphatics)
      1. Renal cell carcinoma
      2. Hepatocellular carcinoma
      3. Follicular carcinoma of the thyroid
      4. Choriocarcinoma

VI. Seeding of Body Cavities
   A. Characteristic of ovarian carcinoma
   B. Involvement of the peritoneum (omentum) is referred to as 'omental caking'
   C. Ovaries have direct access to peritoneum and spread via peritoneal fluid

REVIEW QUESTIONS

1. A 68-year-old woman with a past medical history of hypertension and type II diabetes mellitus presents to the clinic complaining of left breast fullness and swelling in her left arm. The patient is a retired teacher. On exam, she has a palpable mass in the upper outer quadrant of her left breast and non-pitting edema in the left upper extremity. Subsequent mammography shows a mass and a biopsy is performed confirming invasive ductal carcinoma. Sentinel lymph node biopsy indicates spread to axillary lymph nodes. Downregulation of which of the following proteins by the cancer cells is necessary for this invasion of the lymphatics?

   A. Integrin
   B. Fibronectin
   C. E-cadherin
   D. Actin

- **The correct answer is C.**
- The patient complained of left breast fullness and swelling in her left arm and given the diagnosis of invasive ductal carcinoma, the cancer has metastasized to the lymphatics. Tumor cells downregulate production of E-cadherin. E-cadherin attaches adjacent cells and is characteristically downregulated by tumor cells, which leads to dissociation of adjacent cells and predisposes the cancer cells to the processes of invasion and metastasis.
- Choices A, B and D are incorrect because while they are all proteins that are involved in cellular adhesion, they serve to adhere cells to the basement membrane, not to each other. Furthermore, they are generally upregulated in many cancers.

Section XI - Clinical Features of Neoplasia

		Benign	Malignant
General characteristics	Growth rate	- Slow	- Rapid
	Border	- Regular with distinct margins (well circumscribed)	- Irregular (poorly circumscribed)
	Mobility	- Mobile	- Fixed
Macroscopic Features	Shape	- Spherical/ovoid	- Usually amorphous
	Secondary changes	- Uncommon	- Ulceration, necrosis, or bleeding
Microscopic Features	Cellular growth	- Organized (maintained polarity)	- Disorganized
	Nuclei	- Normal, uniform nuclei	- Dysmorphic nuclei with high nuclear-to-cytoplasmic ratio
	Mitotic activity	- Minimal	- High
	Resemblance to native tissue	- Yes	- No
	Invasive	- No	- Yes (through the basement membrane)
	Metastatic potential	- None	- High

TABLE 10.1.7 - Differences Between Benign and Malignant Tumors

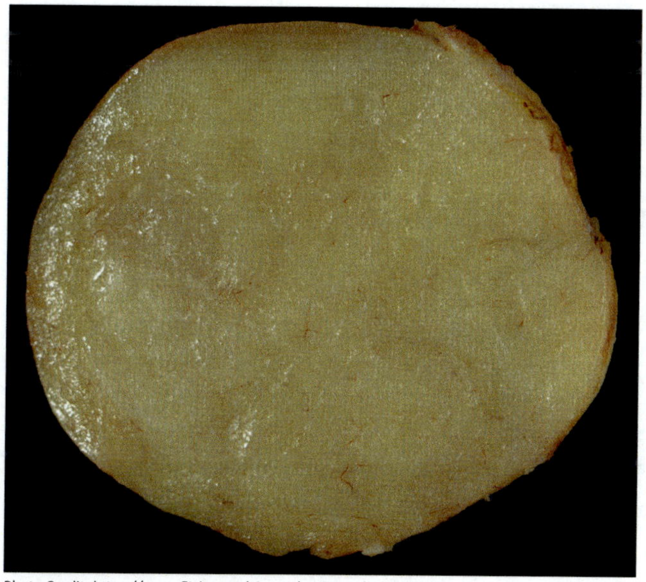

Photo Credit: https://www.flickr.com/photos/euthman/4544443708

FIGURE 10.1.42 - Subcutaneous Lipoma

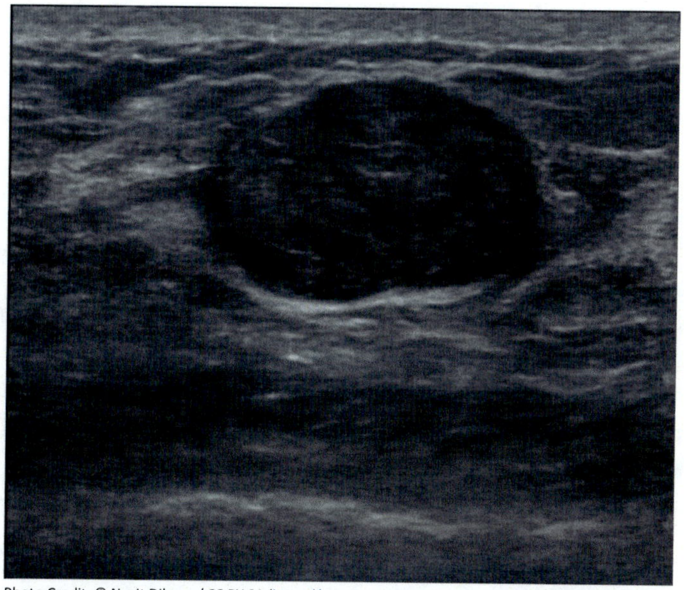

Photo Credit: © Nevit Dilmen / CC BY-SA (https://creativecommons.org/licenses/by-sa/3.0)

FIGURE 10.1.43 - Ultrasound of Fibroadenoma of the Breast

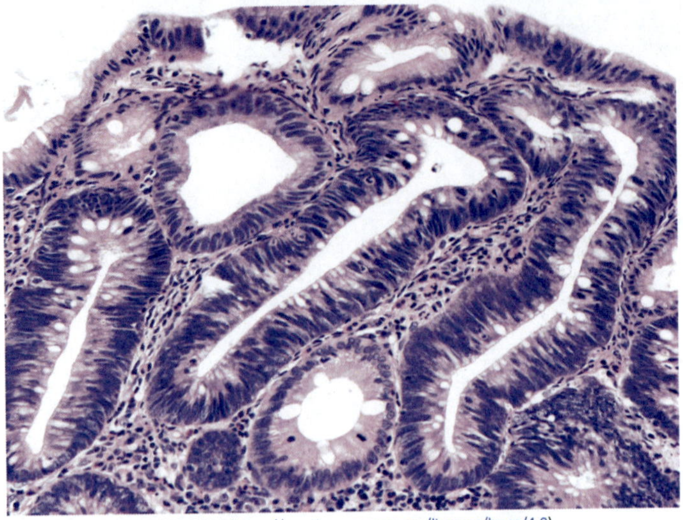

FIGURE 10.1.44- Adenomatous Polyp of the Colon

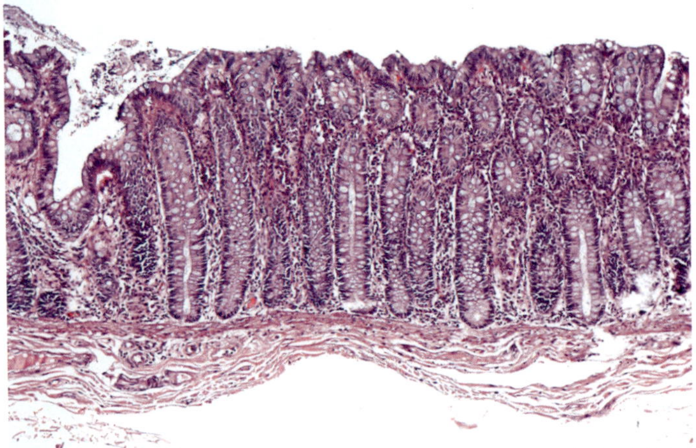

FIGURE 10.1.45 - Normal Histology of the Colon

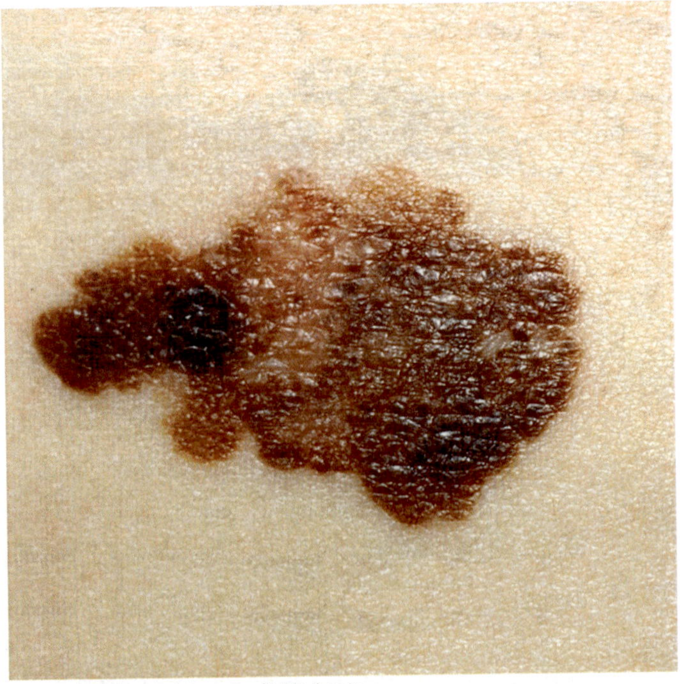

Photo Credit: Unknown photographer / Public domain

FIGURE 10.1.46 - Malignant Melanoma

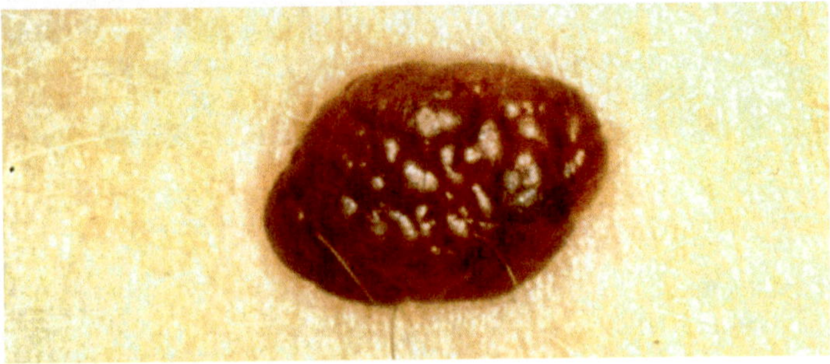

Photo Credit: Unknown photographer / Public domain

FIGURE 10.1.47 - Benign Mole

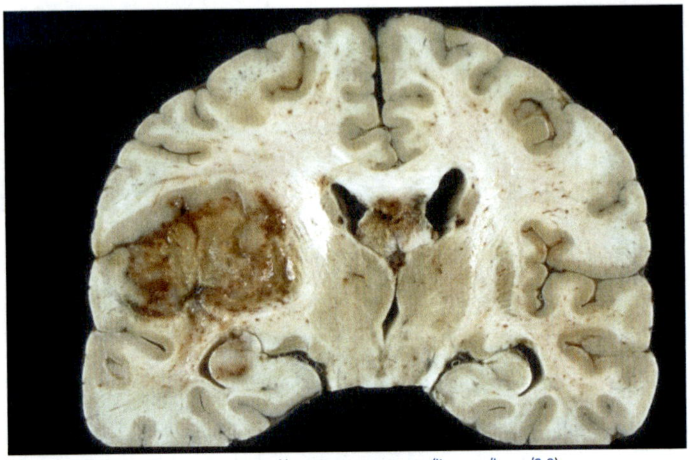

FIGURE 10.1.48 - Glioblastoma Multiforme

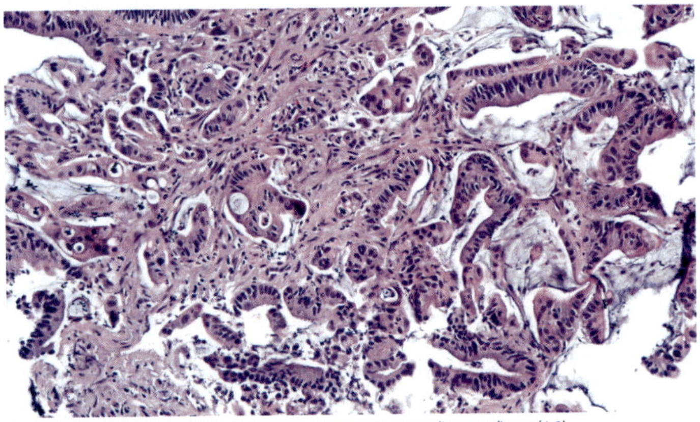

FIGURE 10.1.49 - Adenocarcinoma of the Colon

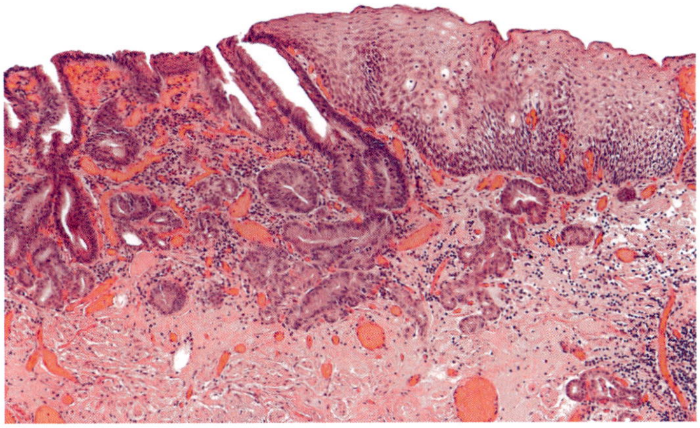

FIGURE 10.1.50 - Adenocarcinoma (Left) and Normal Epithelium (Right) of the Esophagus

I. Immunohistochemical Stains
   A. Immunohistochemistry stain helps classify tumors
   B. Intermediate filaments such as keratin (epithelium), vimentin (mesenchyme), desmin (muscle), GFAP (neuroglia), and neurofilament (neurons)
   C. Others such as chromogranin A and neural cell adhesion molecule (neuroendocrine) and S-100 (melanoma, schwannoma)

II. Serum Tumor Markers
   A. Substances found at higher levels in the blood, urine, or body tissue of some people with cancer
   B. Not for diagnosis
      1. Useful for screening, predicting response to therapy, and monitoring recurrence
   C. Examples include PSA (prostate carcinoma), AFP (hepatocellular or yolk sac tumors)

III. Grading
   A. Description of a tumor based on how differentiated it is under the microscope
   B. Resembles normal tissue → well differentiated (low grade) → good prognosis
   C. Little resemblance to normal tissue → poorly differentiated (high grade) → poor prognosis
   D. Grade 1-4

IV. Staging
   A. Size and extent of the tumor
   B. Tumor location, number, and regional lymph node involvement
   C. Important for prognosis
   D. TNM staging:
      1. T→ tumor size
      2. N→ lymph node involvement
      3. M→ distant metastasis

REVIEW QUESTIONS

1. A patient comes to the hospital due to an enlarging neck mass. The patient says that she has had it for a while, but that it has recently grown in size. On physical examination, the mass is mobile and well-circumscribed. Palpation of the mass does not elicit pain and there is no redness, ulceration, or change in the overlying skin. Is this mass most likely benign or malignant?

   - **This mass is most likely benign.**
   - This patient has a mass that has been stable for a while but has now grown in size. Upon examination, it is found to be mobile and well-circumscribed, both of which are benign features. It's painless on palpation, so it's less likely to be caused by an infection or inflammation. The fact that there's no visible redness, ulceration or change in the overlying skin is reassuring.
   - From the description of the mass, we can say that it is most likely benign. However, any suspicious mass must undergo thorough examination to confirm whether it is benign or malignant.
   - A biopsy and or other definitive diagnostic measures are needed as clinical features alone will almost never be definitive when it comes to cancer.

2. A 65-year-old man with a 50 pack-year smoking history presents with right-sided flank pain, hematuria and weight loss. A CT scan of the abdomen shows a right-sided renal mass. A biopsy reveals cells with clear cytoplasm. Which of the following is necessary to determine the tumor grade in this patient?

   A. Involvement of regional lymph nodes
   B. Degree of differentiation
   C. Response to chemotherapy
   D. Invasion of surrounding tissues

   - **The correct answer is B.**
   - This question basically asks what determines the grading of the tumor. Recall that grading of a tumor depends on how differentiated it looks under the microscope. That means how different it is from the normal tissue.
   - If it has high resemblance to the normal tissue, it's well differentiated and vice versa.
   - A is incorrect because it refers to the staging and not the grading of a tumor.
   - C and D are incorrect because neither the response to chemo nor the invasion of surrounding tissue play a factor in the grading of a tumor.

RENAL/NEPHROLOGICAL PATHOLOGY

Section I - Acute Renal Failure

Type	Etiology	Clinical Findings
Prerenal azotemia	- Decreased blood flow to kidneys (heart failure, hypotension) - NSAIDs in patients with intravascular volume depletion	- Urine osmolality >500 mOsm/kg - FENa <1% - Serum BUN/creatinine ratio >15
Postrenal azotemia	- Obstruction of urinary tract downstream of kidney	- Urine osmolality <350 mOsm/kg - FENa: varies - Early: <1% - Late: >2% - Serum BUN/creatinine ratio: varies - Early: >15 - Late: <15
Intrinsic azotemia	- Acute tubular necrosis - Acute interstitial nephritis	- Urine osmolality <350 mOsm/kg - FENa >2% - Serum BUN/creatinine ratio <15

TABLE 10.2.1 - Types of Acute Renal Failure

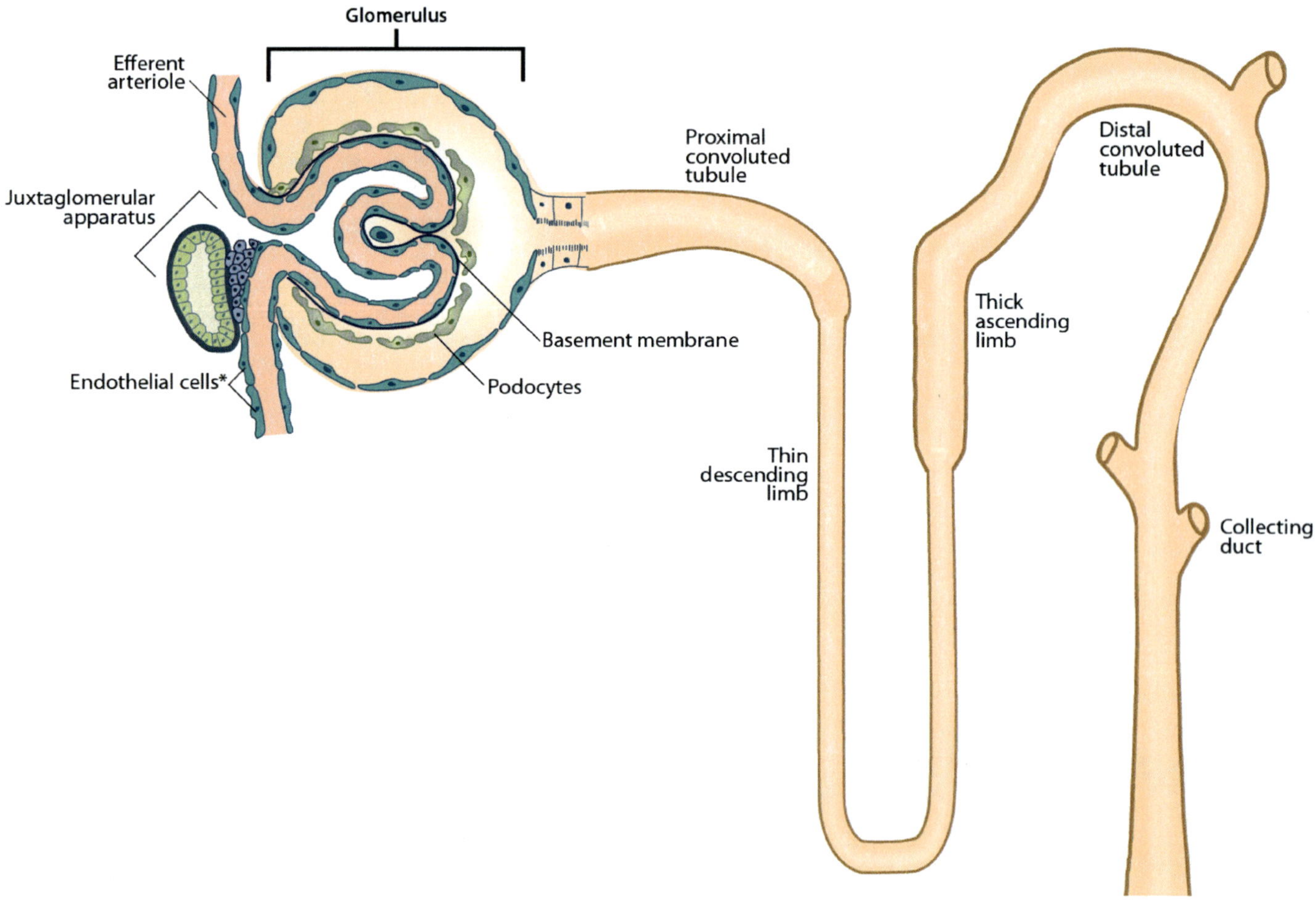

FIGURE 10.2.1 - Anatomy of the Nephron

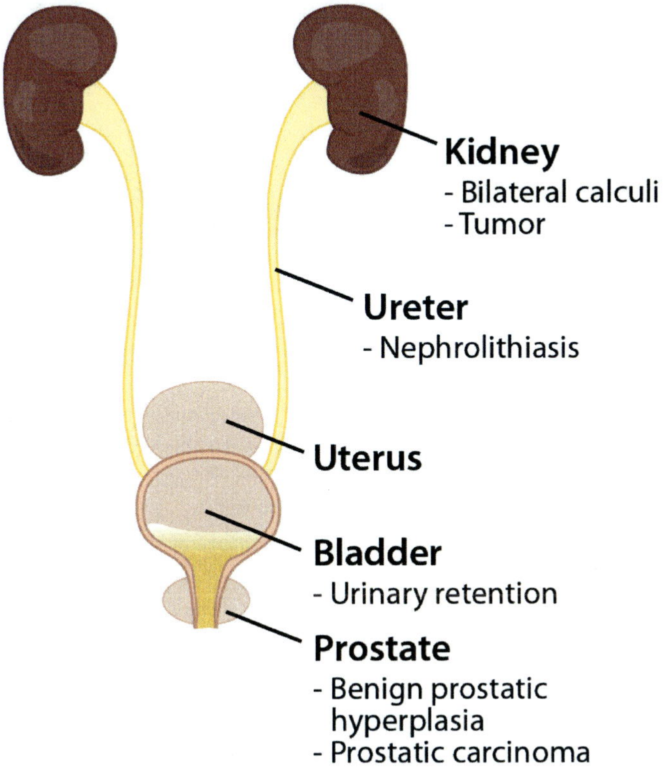

FIGURE 10.2.2 - Causes of Postrenal Azotemia

I. Acute Tubular Necrosis: Pathophysiology
   A. Ischemic
      1. Decreased blood supply → necrosis of tubules → death of tubular cells that slough into tubular lumen
      2. Proximal tubule and medullary segment of thick ascending limb are particularly susceptible to ischemic damage
   B. Nephrotoxic
      1. Toxic agents → necrosis of tubules (aminoglycosides, myoglobinuria, heavy metals, ethylene glycol, radiocontrast dye, urate)
      2. Proximal tubule is particularly susceptible

II. Acute Tubular Necrosis: Clinical findings
   A. Decreased GFR
   B. Oliguria
   C. Brown, granular casts

III. Acute Tubular Necrosis: Stages
   A. Inciting event (24-36 hours)
   B. Maintenance phase (1-3 weeks)
      1. Oliguric: risk of hyperkalemia, metabolic acidosis, uremia
   C. Recovery phase: GFR improves
      1. Polyuria
      2. Hypokalemia
      3. Re-epithelialization of tubules

IV. Acute Interstitial Nephritis: Pathophysiology
   A. Drug-induced hypersensitivity involving interstitium and tubules
      1. NSAIDs, penicillin, diuretics, proton pump inhibitors, rifampin, quinolones, sulfonamides
   B. May be secondary to systemic infections (*Mycoplasma*) or autoimmune diseases (Sjögren syndrome, SLE, sarcoidosis)

V. Acute Interstitial Nephritis: Clinical Findings
   A. Oliguria
   B. Fever
   C. Rash days to weeks after starting a drug
   D. Eosinophiluria
   E. White blood cell casts
   F. Progression to renal papillary necrosis

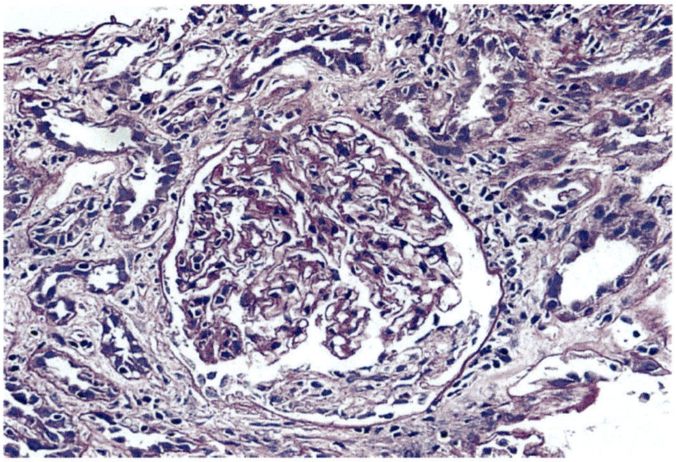

Photo Credit: Libertas Academica (citing Figure 2 of An Unusual Presentation of Classic Idiopathic Polyarteritis Nodosa as Acute Interstitial Nephritis, in Clinical Medicine Insights: Case Reports, first author Ravi Sunderkrishnan) / CC BY (https://creativecommons.org/licenses/by/2.0)

FIGURE 10.2.3 - Acute Interstitial Nephritis

VI. Renal Papillary Necrosis
   A. Necrosis of renal papillae
   B. Presents with gross hematuria and flank pain
   C. Causes
      1. Diabetes mellitus
      2. Chronic analgesic abuse
      3. Sickle cell trait or disease
      4. Severe acute pyelonephritis

REVIEW QUESTIONS

1. A 62-year-old man presents with a 2-day history of shortness of breath. His blood pressure is 73/53 mmHg. Physical examination reveals bilateral jugular vein distension and pitting edema. Laboratory studies include the following:
    - BUN of 60 mg/dL (normal: 7-20 mg/dL)
    - Creatinine of 3 mg/dL (normal: 0.6-1.2 mg/dL)
    - Glucose of 100 mg/dL (normal: <100 mg/dL)
    - Sodium of 137 mEq/L (normal: 135-145 mEq/L)

What is the pathophysiology of this patient's laboratory values?

- **These are signs of congestive heart failure.**
- The laboratory studies show a BUN of 60 and a creatinine of 3. This gives a BUN/creatinine ratio of 20, which is greater than 15. This patient could have either prerenal azotemia or early postrenal azotemia.
- Given the patient's CHF symptoms and elevated BUN/creatinine ratio it is most likely that the patient has prerenal azotemia. The pathophysiology of prerenal azotemia is decreased blood flow to the kidneys, leading to a decreased GFR, oliguria, and azotemia.

2. A 70-year-old woman with a history of hypertension, diabetes, and osteoarthritis presents to the emergency department with periorbital edema, a maculopapular rash on her chest, and fever. Urinalysis shows mild proteinuria and eosinophils. What is the most likely cause of this patient's symptoms?

- **These symptoms and physical findings are consistent with acute interstitial nephritisdiagnosis.**
- We are told that the patient has a history of HTN, diabetes, and osteoarthritis. With this history, she is likely taking many medications.
- Of the patient's past medical history, drugs treating HTN and osteoarthritis are most likely to cause acute interstitial nephritis. Her symptoms are likely due to either diuretic use in treatment of hypertension or NSAID use in treatment of osteoarthritis.

3. A 48-year-old woman presents with chest pain. Physical examination reveals low blood pressure, cool extremities, and elevated jugular venous pressure. Her urine output is decreased. Urine microscopy reveals brown, granular casts. Which of the following lab findings supports a diagnosis of acute tubular necrosis?

    A. Fractional Na^+ excretion = 0.5%
    B. Serum BUN/creatinine ratio = 16
    C. Urine osmolality = 250 mOsmol/kg H_2O
    D. Eosinophils in urine

- **The correct answer is C.**
- A and B are incorrect because a FENa<1% and serum BUN/creatinine ratio >15 are findings for prerenal azotemia. Given the brown granular casts, the patient most likely has intrinsic azotemia.
- D is incorrect because eosinophils are found in the urine in acute interstitial nephritis, another cause of intrinsic azotemia. Acute interstitial nephritis would present with a fever, rash, and white blood cell casts. This patient's brown, granular casts makes her more likely to have acute tubular necrosis.

Section II - Chronic Renal Failure

I. Basic Principles
   A. Gradual, irreversible decline in kidney function
   B. Decline in renal filtration leads to excess retained nitrogenous waste products and electrolyte disturbances

II. Causes
   A. Glomerular diseases
      1. Focal segmental glomerulosclerosis
      2. Membranous nephropathy
   B. Diabetes mellitus
      1. Hyperglycemia → hyaline arteriolosclerosis → hyperfiltration
   C. Hypertension
      1. Vessel narrowing → hypofiltration

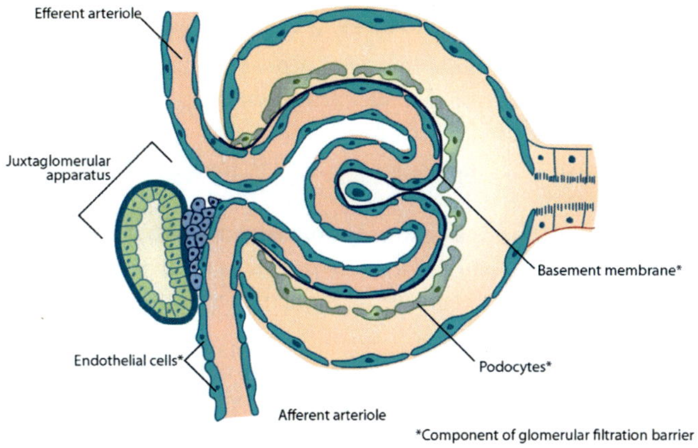

FIGURE 10.2.4 - Cross-Section of Glomerulus

III. Features
   A. Uremia: nausea, anorexia, pericarditis, platelet dysfunction, encephalopathy with asterixis, deposition of urea crystals in skin (uremic frost).Na^+/H_2O retention (HF, pulmonary edema, hypertension)
   B. Hyperkalemia
   C. Metabolic acidosis (↓ NH_4^+ excretion and ↓ HCO_3^- formation)
   D. Anemia

IV. Renal Osteodystrophy
   A. Hyperphosphatemia, hypocalcemia, and failure of vitamin D hydroxylation → 2° hyperparathyroidism
   B. Presents with bone pain
   C. If untreated can progress to 3° hyperparathyroidism (parathyroid glands no longer respond to serum calcium) → elevated PTH → hypercalcemia → subperiosteal thinning of bones

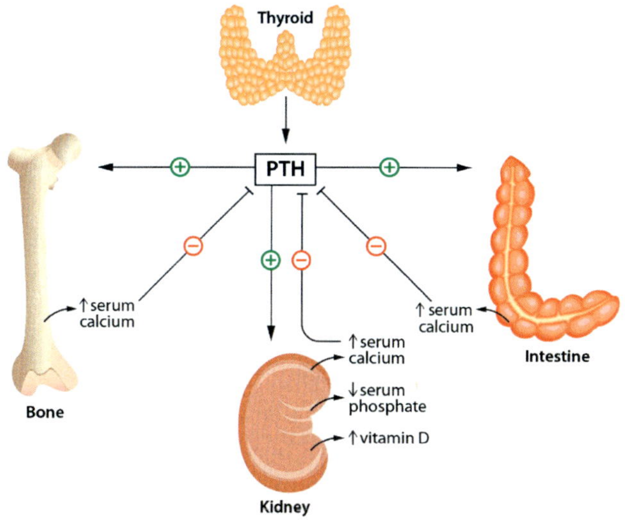

FIGURE 10.2.5 - Thyroid Physiology

V. Treatment
   A. Dialysis
      1. Can cause cysts with shrunken kidneys → increased risk of renal cell carcinoma
   B. Renal transplant

REVIEW QUESTIONS

1. A 57-year-old male with a history of hypertension presents to the emergency room with nausea, vomiting, chest pain, dyspnea on exertion, and dizziness. His chest pain has been present for 2-3 days and is described as burning and worse on inspiration. On physical examination, his skin is pale with numerous areas of bruising. Lung auscultation reveals bilateral rales. Chest X-ray shows moderate cardiomegaly with increased pulmonary vascular markings. Assuming the parathyroid glands are still able to respond appropriately to serum calcium, what are the most likely serum findings in this patient?

   A. ↓ PTH, ↓ Ca^{2+}, ↓ phosphate, ↓ vitamin D
   B. ↑ blood pH
   C. ↑ PTH, ↓ Ca^{2+}, ↑ phosphate, ↓ vitamin D
   D. ↑ erythropoietin concentration

- **The correct answer is C.**
- This man presents with dyspnea on exertion, chest pain that's burning and worse on inspiration, bilateral rales, and cardiomegaly with increased pulmonary vascular markings.
- This tells us that he has pulmonary edema.
- He also presents with nausea, anemia (skin is pale), and platelet dysfunction (numerous areas of bruising).
- This indicates uremia.
- The serum findings that are most consistent with his chronic renal failure are high PTH, low calcium, high phosphate, and low vitamin D
- If you were thinking about tertiary hyperparathyroidism, you might have been expecting the calcium level to be elevated.
- However, we aren't suspecting tertiary hyperparathyroidism in this patient because we are specifically told that the parathyroid glands are still able to respond appropriately to serum calcium.
- Remember, in chronic renal failure, the kidneys are damaged and they can't perform their normal functions, including reabsorbing calcium, converting vitamin D to its active form, and excreting phosphate.
- Without these functions, the patient's serum will be low in calcium and vitamin D and have high phosphate.
- This signals to the thyroid to release PTH, leading to hyperparathyroidism secondary to kidney damage.
- This increase in PTH is not able to properly stimulate the kidneys in chronic renal failure.
- So this excess PTH will primarily act on the bone, pulling calcium from the bone.
- So again, we'd expect high PTH, low calcium, high phosphate, and low vitamin D.
- A is incorrect because renal osteodystrophy presents with hypocalcemia, hyperphosphatemia, and low vitamin D that leads to hyperparathyroidism.
- B is incorrect because chronic renal failure is complicated by metabolic acidosis, which would present with a low blood pH.
- D is incorrect because chronic renal failure is complicated by anemia due to a low erythropoietin concentration.

Section III - Nephrotic Syndrome

I. Definition
   A. Glomerular disorders identified by proteinuria (>3.5 g/day)
      1. "Frothy" urine
      2. Represented as 2+ or 3+ protein in urine

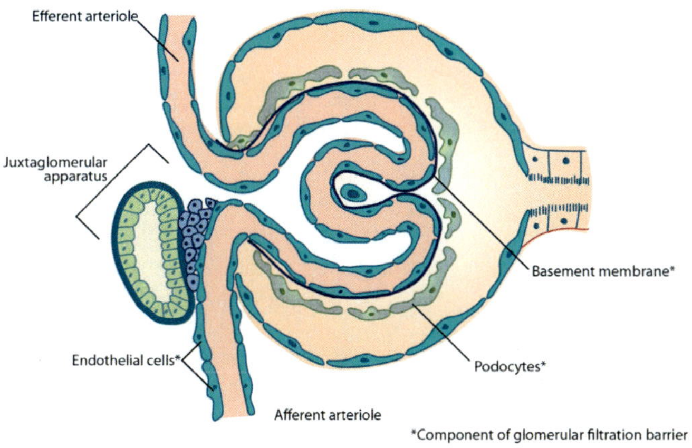

FIGURE 10.2.4 - Cross-Section of Glomerulus

II. Pathophysiology
   A. Glomerular injury→ podocyte disruption
      1. Impairment of charge barrier → inappropriate filtration

III. Clinical Findings
   A. Hypoalbuminemia → pitting edema
   B. Hypogammaglobulinemia → increased risk of infection
   C. Loss of antithrombin III → hypercoagulability → renal vein thrombosis
   D. Hyperlipidemia and hypercholesterolemia → fatty casts in the urine

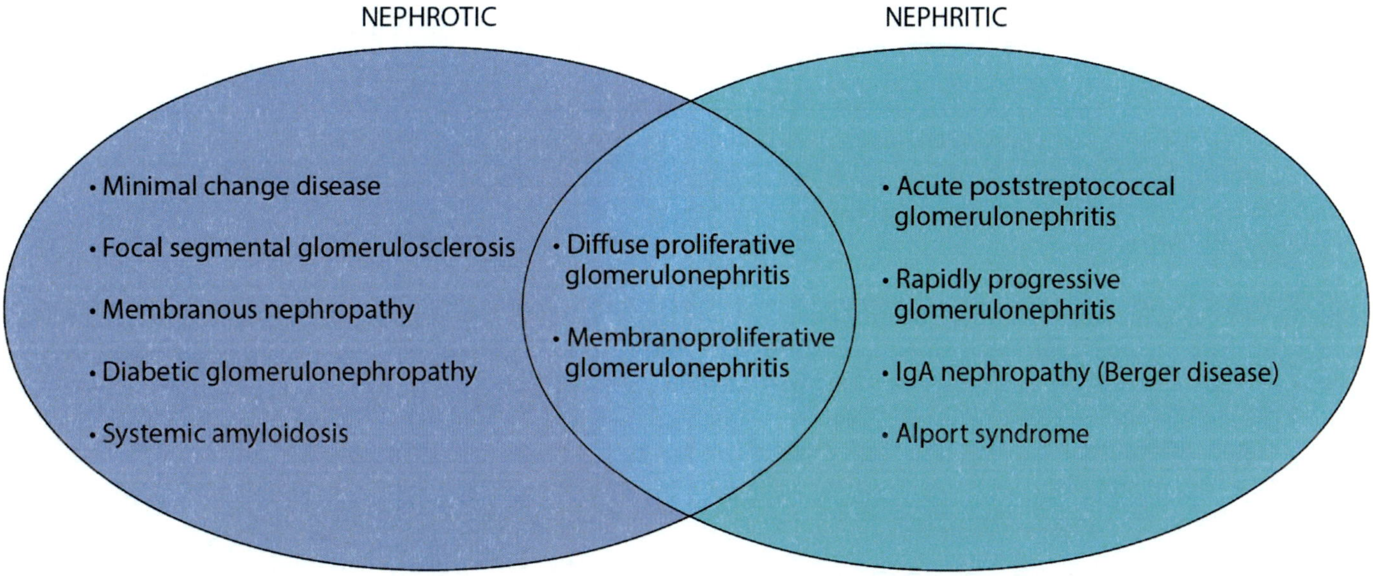

FIGURE 10.2.6 - Nephrotic vs. Nephritic Syndrome

Condition	Pathophysiology	Associated Conditions	Biopsy Findings
Minimal change disease	- Most common cause of nephrotic syndrome in children - Usually idiopathic - Triggered by recent infection, NSAIDs, immunization, or immune stimulus	- Hodgkin lymphoma	- H&E: normal - Electron microscopy: effacement of foot processes - Immunofluorescence: negative
Focal segmental glomerulosclerosis	- Most common cause of nephrotic syndrome in Hispanics and African Americans - Idiopathic	- HIV - Heroin use - Sickle cell disease	- H&E: focal and segmental sclerosis - Electron microscopy: effacement of foot processes - Immunofluorescence: may be positive for nonspecific focal deposits of IgM, C3, and C1
Membranous nephropathy	- Usually idiopathic - Antibodies to phospholipase A2 receptor	- Hepatitis B or C - Syphilis - Solid tumors - SLE - Drugs (NSAIDs, gold, and penicillamine)	- H&E: thick glomerular basement membrane - Electron microscopy: subepithelial deposits with "spike and dome" appearance - Immunofluorescence: granular due to IgG and C3 deposits
Diabetic glomerulonephropathy	- Hyperglycemia → hyaline arteriolosclerosis → high GFR → microalbuminuria	- Diabetes mellitus	- Sclerosis of the mesangium - Formation of Kimmelstiel-Wilson nodules
Systemic amyloidosis	- Amyloid deposits in the mesangium		- Apple-green birefringence under polarized light with Congo red stain - Amyloid deposits in mesangium

TABLE 10.2.2 - Types of Nephrotic Syndrome

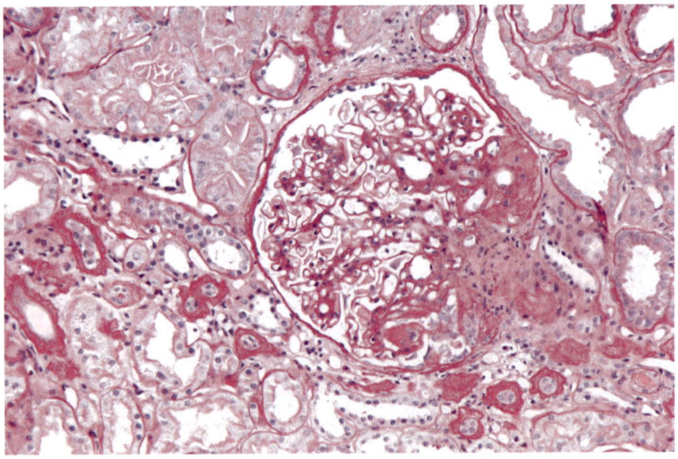

FIGURE 10.2.7 - Focal Segmental Glomerulosclerosis

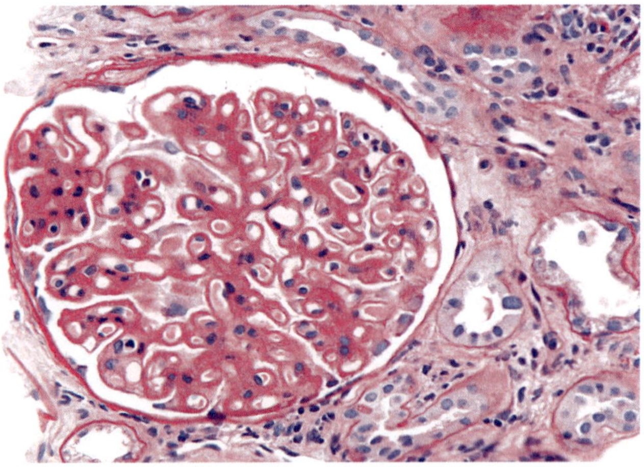

FIGURE 10.2.8 - Membranous Nephropathy

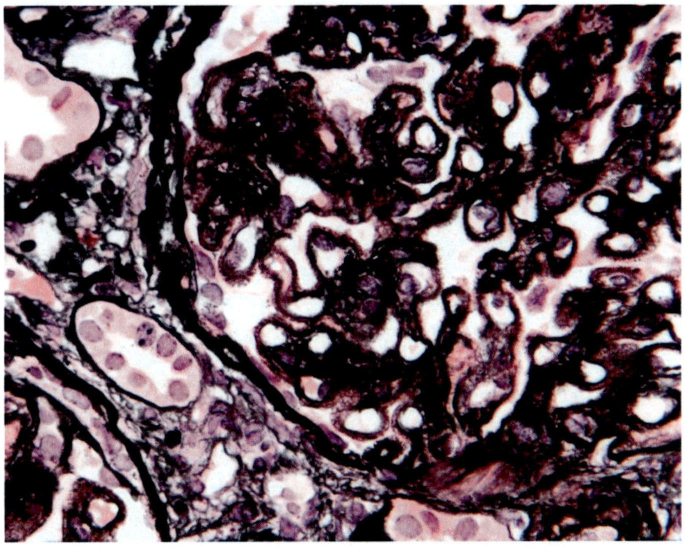

FIGURE 10.2.9 - Membranous Nephropathy Under Silver Stain

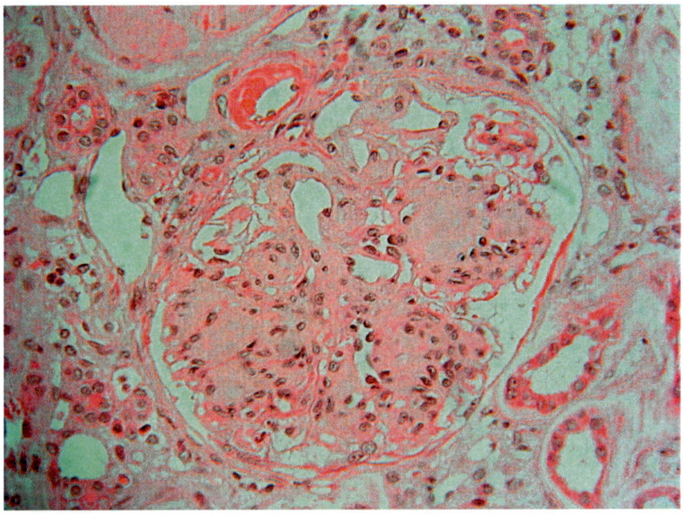

FIGURE 10.2.10 - Kimmelstiel-Wilson Nodules

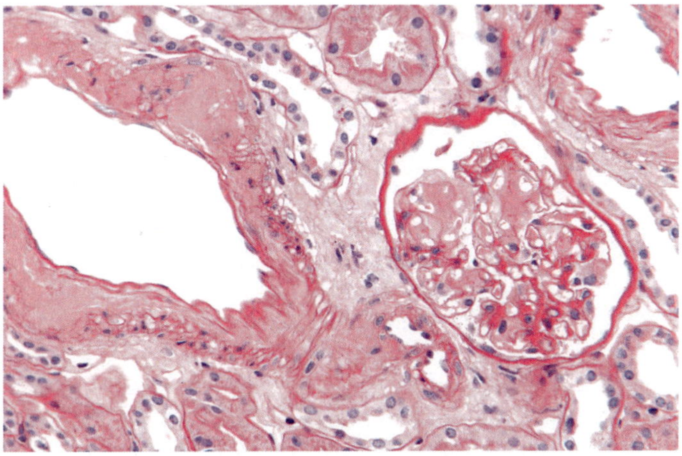

FIGURE 10.2.11 - Amyloid Deposits in Mesangium

REVIEW QUESTIONS

1. An 8-year-old boy is brought to the office due to swelling of the hands and feet. Two weeks ago, the patient was treated for anaphylaxis following a bee sting. He mentions that his pants feel tighter than usual. The patient's urine has also become frothy. Physical examination reveals lungs that are clear to auscultation. What other condition is most likely associated with the patient's disorder?
   - **The most likely diagnosis is minimal change disease.**
   - Minimal change disease is the most common cause of nephrotic disease in children and often presents following an immune stimulus - like anaphylaxis in this case.
   - The patient presents with edema, This shows as swelling of the hands, feet, and legs [pants feel tighter] (following a bee sting). He also has proteinuria (frothy urine). The other condition associated with minimal change disease is Hodgkin lymphoma.

2. A 42-year-old man with a history of Wilson's disease comes to the office for evaluation of progressive generalized edema and weight gain for the past several weeks. Mild ascites is present. There is bilateral lower extremity pitting edema to the knees. Urinary protein excretion is 6.0 g over 24 hours. A kidney biopsy is ordered. What is the most likely finding on electron microscopy?
   - **Membranous nephropathy presents with subepithelial deposits with "spike and dome" appearance on electron microscopy.**
   - A 42-year-old man presents with progressive generalized edema, weight gain and proteinuria (urinary protein excretion = 6.0g/24hr). With these signs, we can determine that he has nephrotic syndrome. Now we have to figure out the cause of his nephrotic syndrome.
   - We are told that he has a history of Wilson's disease. Recall that Wilson's disease is treated with penicillamine. Penicillamine is a secondary cause of membranous nephropathy.

3. A 67-year-old woman comes to the physician with a 5-month history of fatigue, recurrent urinary tract infections, and dysuria. Physical examination shows 2+ pitting edema of the lower legs and ankles. Kidney biopsy shows Kimmelstiel-Wilson nodules. What is the initial cause of this patient's renal findings?
   - Diabetic glomerulonephropathy is due to non-enzymatic glycosylation of the vascular basement membrane following hyperglycemia.
   - So here we have a woman with fatigue, recurrent UTIs, dysuria, and pitting edema. Kidney biopsy shows Kimmelstiel-Wilson nodules. Taken together, this points to nephrotic syndrome due to diabetes mellitus.

4. A previously healthy 35-year-old man complains of recent fatigue and swelling of his feet and ankles. He also notes puffy eyes. Physical exam reveals an afebrile man with lower extremity edema extending to the knee, periorbital edema, and a small amount of ascites. Urinalysis reveals 4+ protein and oval fat bodies. 24-hour urine protein is 6.0 g. A day later he develops right flank pain. What is the most likely cause of the patient's most recent symptom?

   A. Antithrombin III deficiency
   B. Low oncotic pressure
   C. Capillary injury
   D. Bacterial infection

   - **The correct answer is A.**
   - A 35-year-old man presents with fatigue, swelling of his feet and ankles, and puffy eyes. Urinalysis reveals 4+ protein and oval fat bodies. From these signs, we can determine that he has nephrotic syndrome.
   - Also, a day after the initial symptoms, he presents with right flank pain. In the context of nephrotic syndrome, this is highly suspicious for renal vein thrombosis. Renal vein thrombosis is a complication of nephrotic syndrome, due to loss of antithrombin III in the urine. The question asked for the cause of his most recent symptom, which is the right flank pain.
   - B is incorrect because low oncotic pressure causes edema and hyperlipidemia, which do not directly cause flank pain.
   - C is incorrect because the capillaries are not damaged in nephrotic syndrome.
   - D is incorrect because bacterial infections do not cause nephrotic syndrome.

Section IV - Nephritic Syndrome

I. Pathophysiology
   A. Glomerular disorders identified by glomerular inflammation and bleeding
   B. Glomerular inflammation → capillary swelling → leakage of RBCs, proteins, and electrolytes → decrease in GFR → retention of nitrogenous waste, creatinine, salt, and water

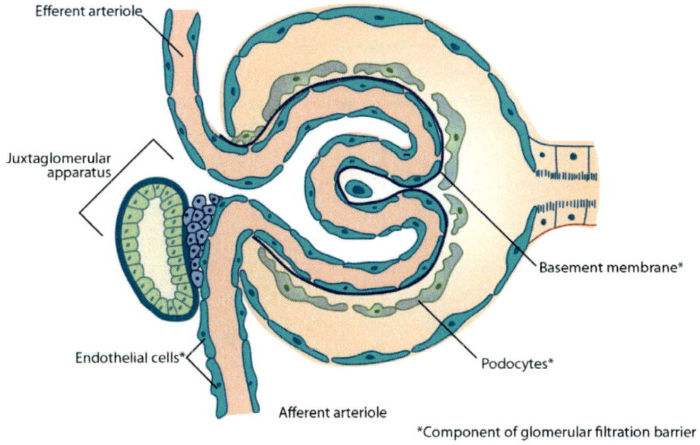

FIGURE 10.2.4 - Cross-Section of Glomerulus

II. Clinical Findings
   A. Limited proteinuria (<3.5 g/day)
   B. Salt retention
      1. Periorbital edema and hypertension
   C. RBC casts with dysmorphic RBCs in urine (hematuria)
   D. May lead to acute kidney injury (oliguria, ↓ GFR, ↑ serum BUN or Cr)

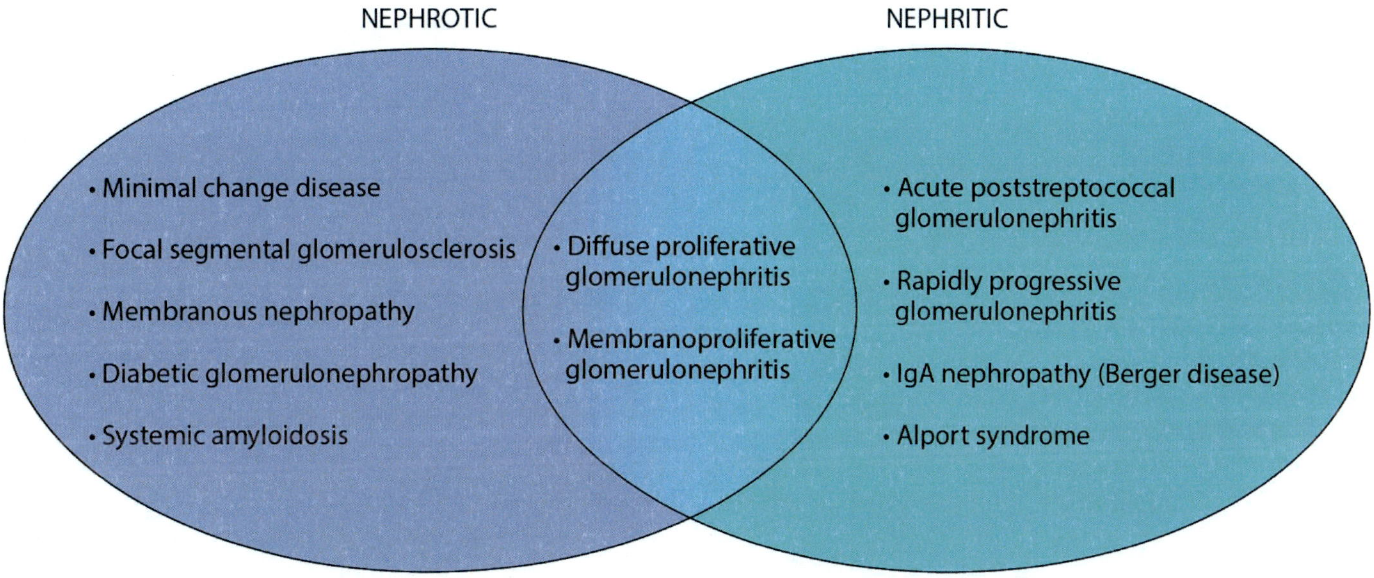

FIGURE 10.2.6 - Nephrotic vs. Nephritic Syndrome

Glomerular Disorder	Pathophysiology	Clinical Findings	Biopsy Findings
Poststreptococcal Glomerulonephritis (PSGN)	- Arises after group A streptococcal infection of skin or pharynx - IgM, IgG and C3 deposit along glomerular basement membrane	- Hematuria 2-3 weeks after infection - Decreased C3 and total complement levels - May progress to rapidly progressive glomerulonephritis in adults	- EM: subepithelial "humps" - IF: granular - H&E: hypercellular, inflamed glomeruli
IgA Nephropathy (Berger Disease)	- Most common nephropathy worldwide - IgA immune complex deposition in mesangium	- Presents in childhood as episodic gross or microscopic hematuria with RBC casts - Usually seen days after mucosal infection	- IF: IgA immune complex deposition in mesangium
Alport Syndrome	- X-linked defect in type IV collagen	- Isolated hematuria - Sensory hearing loss - Ocular disturbances	- H&E: thinning and splitting of glomerular basement membrane - EM: "basket weave"
Rapidly Progressive Glomerulonephritis	- Goodpasture syndrome - Granulomatosis with polyangiitis, microscopic polyangiitis, and Churg-Strauss syndrome - Diffuse proliferative glomerulonephritis	- Nephritic syndrome that progresses to renal failure in weeks to months	- H&E: crescent moon shape - IF: varies

TABLE 10.2.3 - Types of Nephritic Syndrome

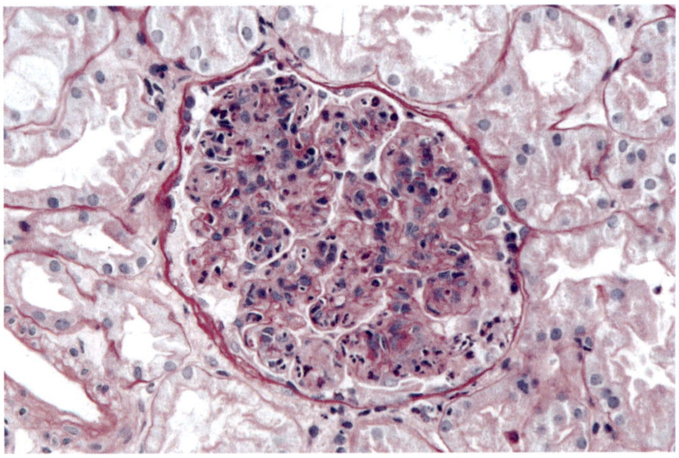

FIGURE 10.2.12 - Post-Streptococcal Glomerulonephritis

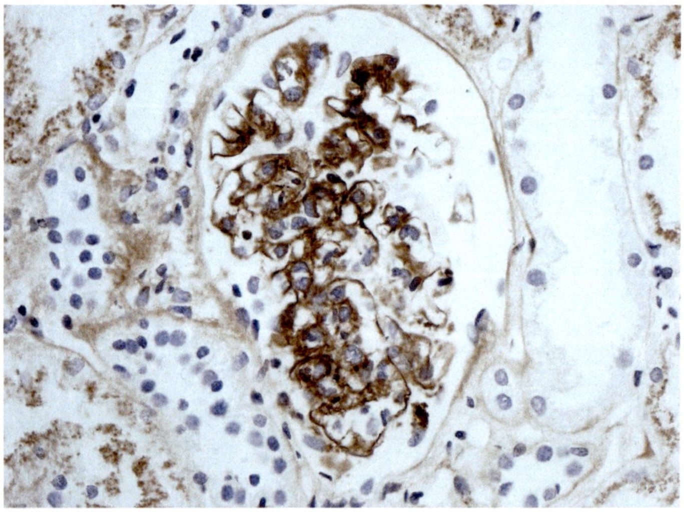

FIGURE 10.2.13 - Immunostain of IgA Nephropathy

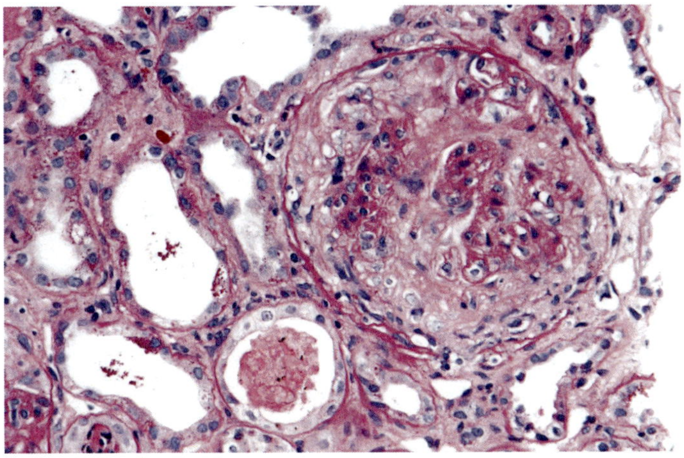

FIGURE 10.2.14 - Rapidly Progressive Glomerulonephritis

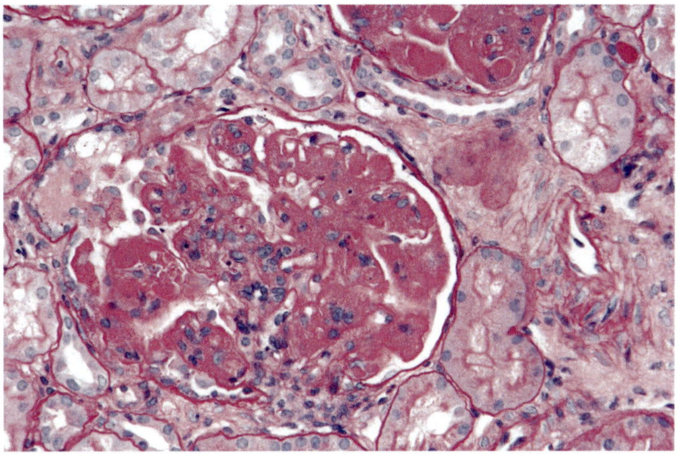

FIGURE 10.2.15 - Diffuse Proliferative Glomerulonephritis

III. Goodpasture Syndrome
   A. Antibodies against alpha-3 chain of type IV collagen in glomerular and alveolar basement membranes
   B. Presents with hematuria and hemoptysis
   C. Linear immunofluorescence staining pattern
   D. Treatment: plasmapheresis

IV. Vasculitides
   A. Negative immunofluorescence
   B. Granulomatosis with polyangiitis: c-ANCA
   C. Microscopic polyangiitis: p-ANCA
   D. Churg-Strauss syndrome: p-ANCA

V. Diffuse Proliferative Glomerulonephritis
   A. Most common type of renal disease in SLE
   B. May progress to rapidly progressive glomerulonephritis
   C. H&E: "wire-looping" of capillaries
   D. EM: subendothelial deposits
   E. IF: granular IgG and C3 deposition

VI. Membranoproliferative Glomerulonephritis
   A. H&E: thick glomerular basement membrane, "tram-track" appearance
   B. IF: granular, due to immune complex deposition
   C. Type I: subendothelial
      1. Associated with HBV and HCV
   D. Type II: dense deposit disease
      1. Intramembranous deposits
      2. C3 nephritic factor

REVIEW QUESTIONS

1. A 21-year-old woman with a history of type I diabetes mellitus develops gross hematuria. Her only medication is daily insulin injections. Four days ago, she experienced diarrhea, cramps, nausea, vomiting, and a one-day fever. What is the most likely diagnosis?

   - **The most likely diagnosis given this information is IgA nephropathy.**
   - The gross hematuria strongly points to nephritic syndrome, but not a specific type of nephritic syndrome. You're not able to make a diagnosis based only on the presence of hematuria.
   - However, there are other clues. Four days ago, she had gastroenteritis, as evidenced by her diarrhea, cramps, nausea, vomiting, and fever, and gastroenteritis is a mucosal infection.
   - Remember that IgA nephropathy presents with episodic gross or microscopic hematuria with RBC casts, usually days after mucosal infection.

2. A 26-year-old previously healthy man comes to the office with a 3-week history of dyspnea, cough, and hemoptysis preceded by an upper respiratory tract infection. Urinalysis shows proteinuria and hematuria with dysmorphic red blood cells. Bilateral pulmonary infiltrates are seen on chest X-ray. Antibodies directed against what structure is most likely to be associated with this patient's condition?

   - **This patient likely has antibodies directed against the alpha-3 chain of type IV collagen.**
   - A 26-year old previously healthy man presents with a history of dyspnea, cough and hemoptysis. He also has proteinuria and hematuria with dysmorphic red blood cells.
   - These are symptoms of Goodpasture syndrome, which is associated with antibodies against alpha-3 chain of type IV collagen.

3. A 27-year-old woman comes to the office with a 2-year history of skin problems worsened by exposure to sunlight. She also has fatigue and recurrent episodes of pain in her wrists and ankles over the past year. Physical examination reveals red patches with scaling on both cheeks. Urinalysis is positive for 4g of protein and red blood cell casts. A renal biopsy specimen is most likely to show which of the following?

   A. Thickened capillary loops
   B. Tram-track appearance of basement membrane
   C. IgA antibodies in the mesangium
   D. Crescent formation

   - **The correct answer is D.**
   - This young woman's history of skin problems that are worsened by exposure to sunlight, fatigue, pain in wrists and ankles, and red patches with scaling on both cheeks. This strongly points to a diagnosis of SLE.
   - Remember that SLE can cause both nephrotic syndrome (membranous nephropathy) and nephritic-nephrotic syndrome (diffuse proliferative glomerulonephritis). We are told that she has proteinuria that is >3.5 grams (4 grams) and red blood cell casts. This indicates a nephritic-nephrotic syndrome.
   - So, this woman most likely has diffuse proliferative glomerulonephritis, which can progress to rapidly progressive glomerulonephritis. On biopsy, you would expect to see crescents, as this is characteristic of diffuse proliferative glomerulonephritis.
   - A is incorrect because thickened capillary loops are found in membranous nephropathy, a nephrotic syndrome where RBC casts are not seen.
   - B is incorrect because tram-track appearance of the basement membrane is seen in membranoproliferative glomerulonephritis. This is a nephritic-nephrotic syndrome, like diffuse proliferative glomerulonephritis, but it is not associated with lupus.
   - C is incorrect because IgA antibodies depositing in the mesangium characterizes IgA nephropathy, a nephritic syndrome that is most common in children and is not associated with lupus.

Section V - Urinary Tract Infections (UTIs)

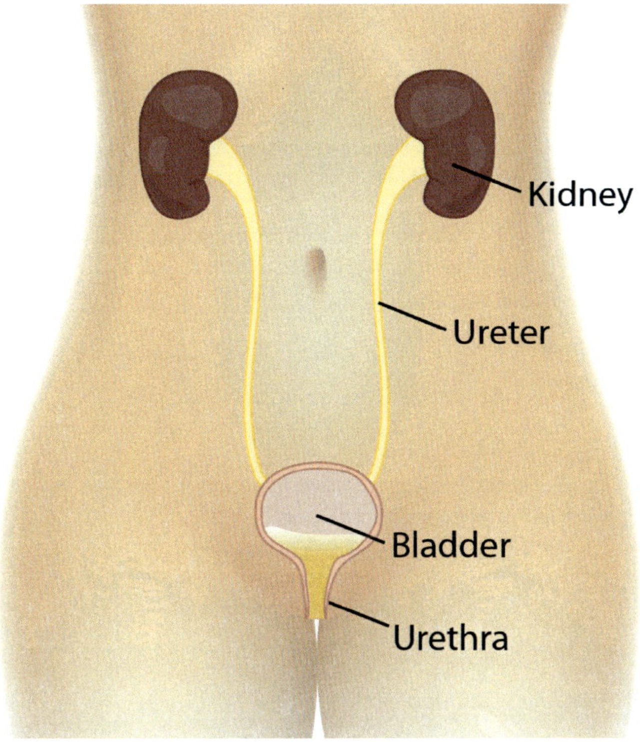

FIGURE 10.2.16 - Anatomy of the Urinary Tract

I. Risk Factors
   A. Females > males
   B. Postmenopause
   C. Sexual intercourse
   D. Catheter use
   E. Congenital abnormalities: vesicoureteral reflux
   F. Urinary stasis: neurogenic bladder, pelvic organ prolapse, benign prostatic hyperplasia, prostate cancer

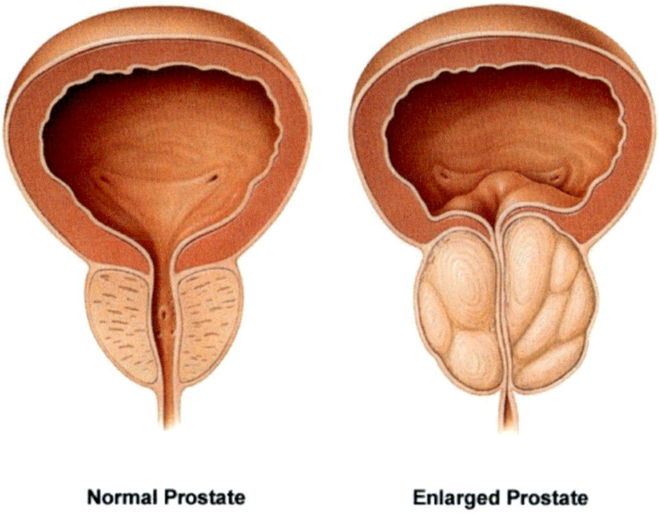

FIGURE 10.2.18 - Gross Pathology of Enlarged Prostate

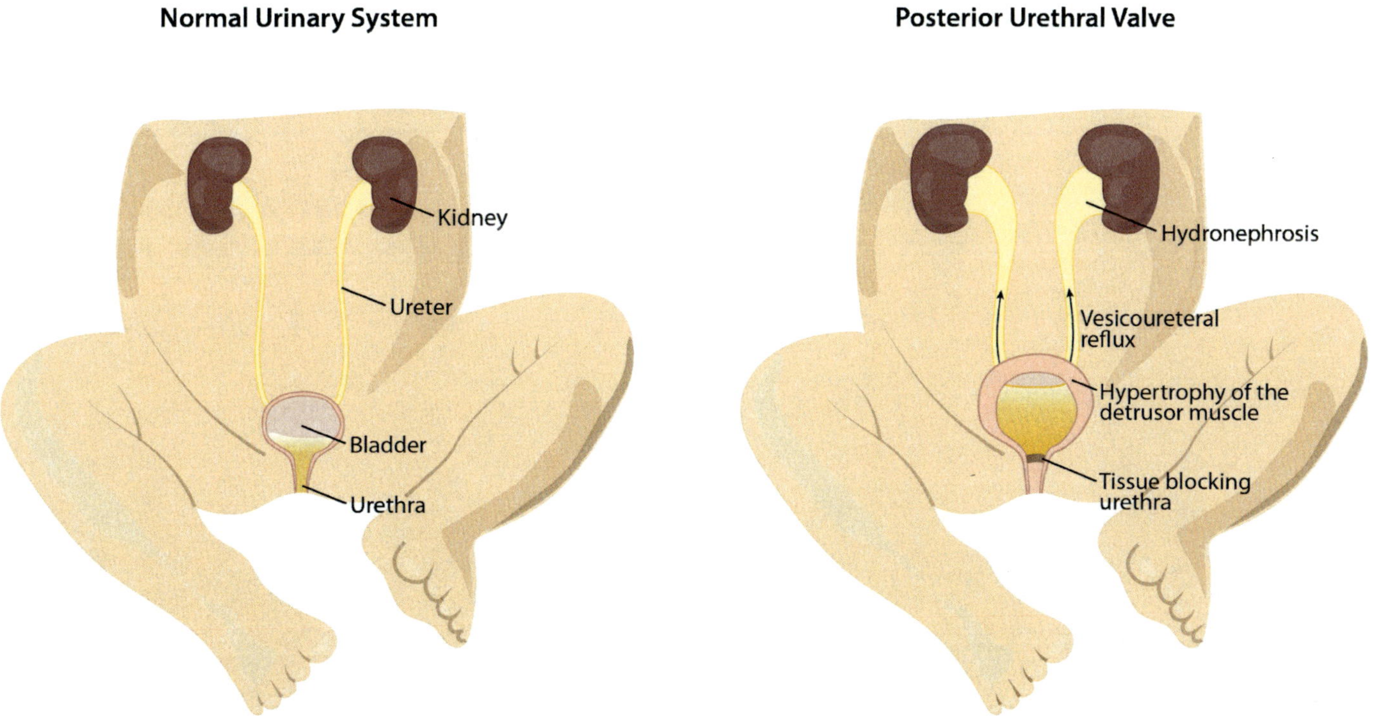

FIGURE 10.2.17 - Pathology of Posterior Urethral Valve

II. Vesicoureteral Reflux
   A. Congenital abnormality
   B. Causes urine to reflux from bladder to kidneys
   C. Risk of infection and kidney damage

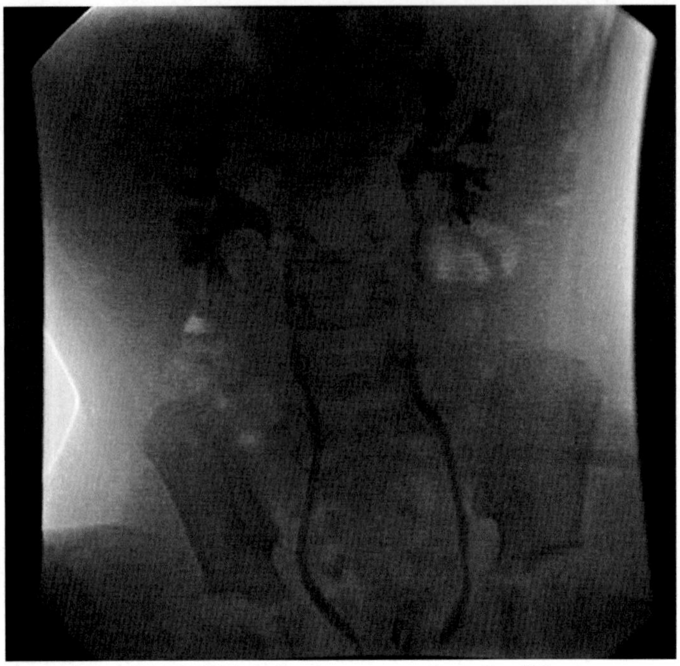

FIGURE 10.2.18 - Voiding Cystourethrogram in Bilateral Urethral Reflux

III. Labs
   A. Urinalysis (UA)
      1. Nitrites (gram neg. bacteria)
      2. Pyuria (leukocyte esterase, WBCs)
      3. +/- blood
   B. Culture
      1. >100,000 colony-forming units
      2. If asymptomatic, do not treat

IV. Urethritis
   A. Symptoms: dysuria, urinary frequency, urethral discharge
      1. May be asymptomatic
   B. Labs: sterile pyuria
      1. UA shows leukocyte esterase / WBCs
      2. Culture does not grow bacteria
   C. Causes: gonorrhea, chlamydia

V. Cystitis
   A. Symptoms: dysuria, urinary frequency, urinary urgency, no fever/chills
   B. Labs: nitrites, pyuria, +/- blood, positive culture
   C. Cause: bacteria
      1. E. coli
      2. Staphylococcus saprophyticus

VI. Acute Pyelonephritis
   A. Symptoms: cystitis plus fever, chills, nausea, vomiting, back/flank pain
   B. Physical exam: CVA tenderness
   C. Labs: cystitis plus WBC casts, leukocytosis on CBC
   D. CT: perinephric stranding
   E. Cause: *E. coli*

VII. Chronic Pyelonephritis
   A. Develops after multiple episodes of acute pyelonephritis
   B. Inflammation, scarring, atrophy → irreversible damage to kidney → possible end-stage renal disease
   C. Risk factors: vesicoureteral reflux, chronic obstruction

REVIEW QUESTIONS

1. A 23-year-old woman comes to the emergency room with complaints of dysuria and urinary frequency for the past three days. Overnight she began having chills. Past medical history is unremarkable. She is not sexually active. Blood pressure is 110/70, heart rate is 90, and temperature is 101.3°F (38.5°C). Physical exam is positive for right sided CVA tenderness. CBC reveals mild leukocytosis. What finding on UA is most concerning for pyelonephritis as opposed to cystitis?

- **The correct answer is WBC casts.**
- This is a young woman with symptoms of dysuria and frequency. She also has chills, which are a systemic symptom. Her vital signs are stable, but she is febrile. She also has right CVA tenderness and leukocytosis. This should make you concerned for acute pyelonephritis.
- The question wants to know what finding on UA is most concerning for pyelonephritis. UA will likely show things that you also see in cystitis, such as nitrites or pyuria. However, WBC casts are more specific to pyelonephritis.

2. A 4-year-old girl comes to the pediatrician because of two episodes of "bladder infections" with fevers. She is currently asymptomatic. A CBC and metabolic panel are within normal limits. She has a radiographic study done that shows substantial retrograde flow of contrast from the bladder to the right ureter and kidney. She is started on prophylactic antibiotics. Which of the following might be seen on kidney biopsy if this patient does not get treated?

   A. Severe hydronephrosis
   B. Hypertrophy of the right kidney
   C. Carcinoma in situ
   D. Tubular atrophy
   E. No scarring of the parenchyma

- **The correct answer is D.**
- This is a child with two episodes of pyelonephritis who is currently asymptomatic. She has normal kidney function as evidenced by her metabolic panel. She has a study that shows "substantial retrograde flow of contrast from the bladder to the right ureter and kidney." This should help you figure out that she has vesicoureteral reflux.
- As we know, vesicoureteral reflux puts her at risk for chronic pyelonephritis if the reflux causes her to get repeated infections. The question is asking what you might see on kidney biopsy if the patient developed chronic pyelonephritis. We know that chronic pyelonephritis can cause irreversible kidney damage, including scarring, inflammation, and atrophy.
- A is incorrect because hydronephrosis is not a microscopic diagnosis. Remember that we were specifically asked what would be seen on the kidney biopsy.
- B is incorrect because the damaged kidney would not be hypertrophic; it would be scarred and atrophic.
- C is incorrect because the presentation of recurring infections leads us to chronic pyelonephritis. We aren't given any evidence that should make us suspicious of kidney cancer.
- E is incorrect because there would be scarring.

Section VI - Nephrolithiasis

I. Overview
   A. Definition
   B. Risk factors
   C. Presentation
   D. Types of stones

II. Definition
   A. "Kidney stones"
   B. Deposition of urinary solute, forming a calculus

III. Risk Factors
   A. High solute concentration
   B. Low urinary volume

IV. Presentation
   A. Nonspecific symptoms: nausea, vomiting
   B. Hematuria
      1. Free RBCs of normal morphology
   C. Unilateral, waxing and waning (colicky) pain
      1. Obstruction at ureteropelvic junction → flank or upper abdominal pain
      2. Obstruction at ureterovesical junction → lower abdominal pain

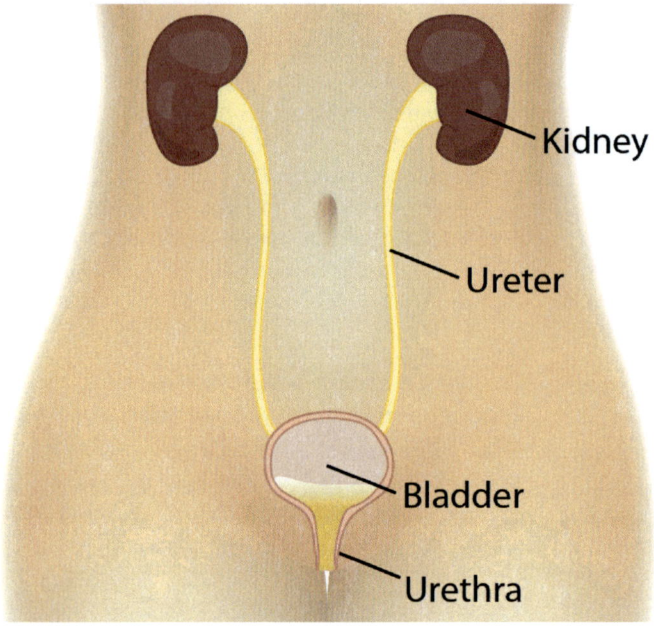

FIGURE 10.2.16 - Anatomy of the Urinary Tract

Stone type	Associations	Causes	Treatment
Calcium oxalate or calcium phosphate	- Most common - Adults - Oxalate: radiopaque envelopes - Phosphate: radiopaque prisms	- Hypercalciuria - Hypercalcemia (hyperparathyroidism) - Hypocitraturia (distal RTA) - Idiopathic	- Hydrochlorothiazide (increased calcium reabsorption)
Ammonium magnesium phosphate (struvite)	- Recurrent UTIs - Staghorn calculi - Radiopaque coffins	- Infection with urease-expressing bacteria (*Proteus*, *Klebsiella*)	- Surgical removal of staghorn calculi - Treatment of infection to prevent recurrence
Uric acid	- Gout - Radiolucent rhomboids - Uric acid crystals on microscopy	- Increased uric acid excretion (gout, myeloproliferative disorders, leukemia) - Increased urine uric acid concentration (hot, arid climates; dehydration) - Low urine pH (chronic diarrhea)	- Hydration - Alkalinization of urine (potassium bicarbonate or potassium citrate) - Allopurinol (for gout)
Cystine	- Rare - Children - Staghorn calculi - Radiopaque hexagons	- Cystinuria	- Hydration - Alkalinization of urine (potassium bicarbonate or potassium citrate)

TABLE 10.2.4 - Types of Nephrolithiasis

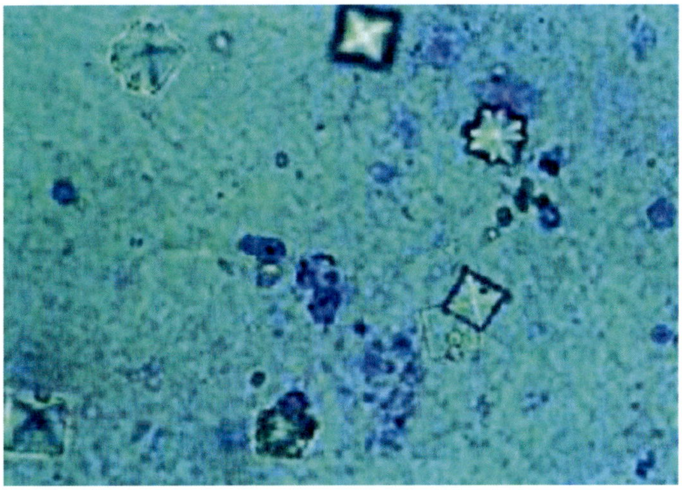

Photo Credit: NASA/JSC / Public domain

FIGURE 10.2.19 - Calcium-Oxalate Crystals on Urine Microscopy

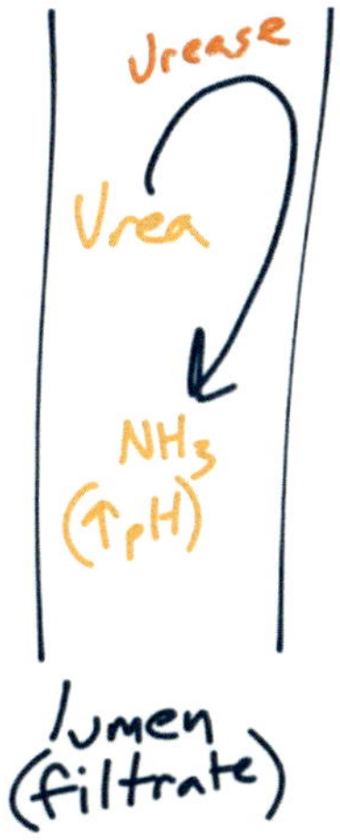

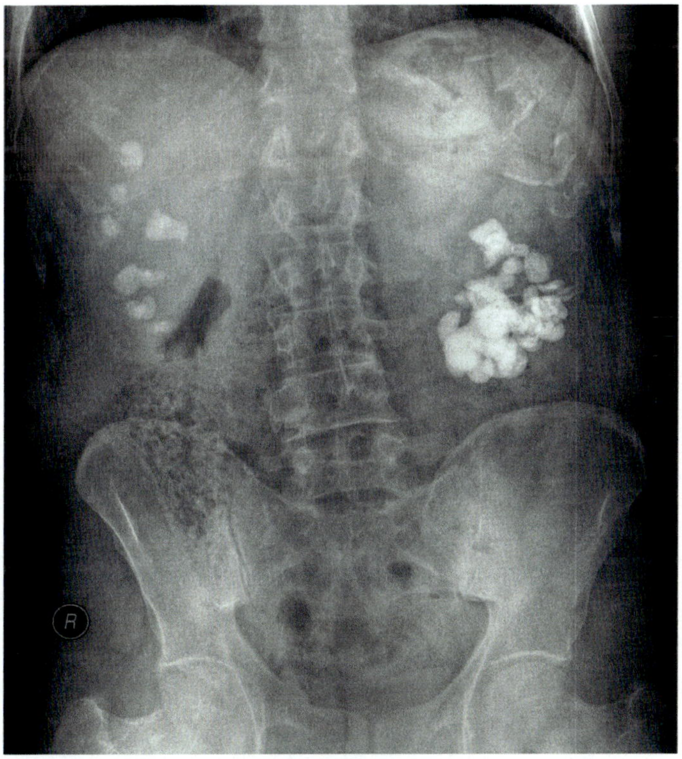

Photo Credit: © Nevit Dilmen / CC BY-SA (https://creativecommons.org/licenses/by-sa/3.0)

FIGURE 10.2.20 - Staghorn Calculi From Struvite Crystals

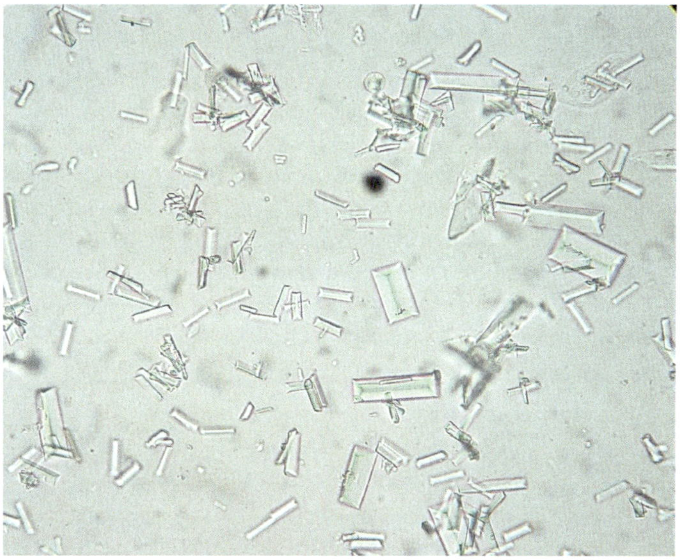

Photo Credit: Joel Mills / CC BY-SA (http://creativecommons.org/licenses/by-sa/3.0/)

FIGURE 10.2.21 - Struvite Crystals on Urine Microscopy

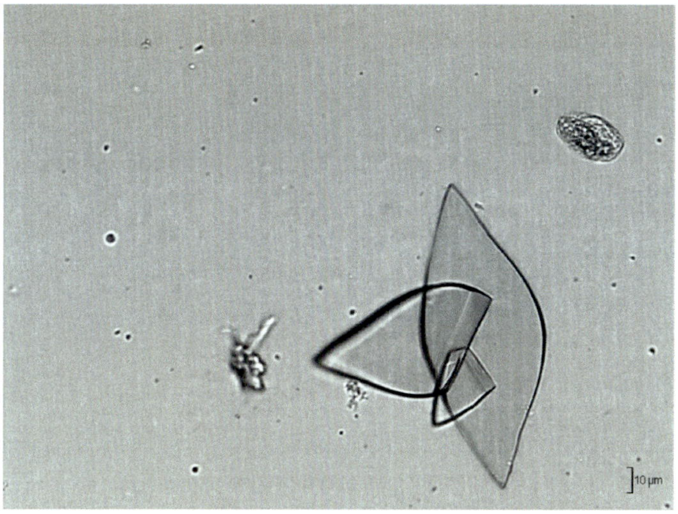

Photo Credit: Doruk Salancı / CC BY-SA (https://creativecommons.org/licenses/by-sa/3.0)

FIGURE 10.2.22 - Uric Acid Crystals (Rhomboid) on Urine Microscopy

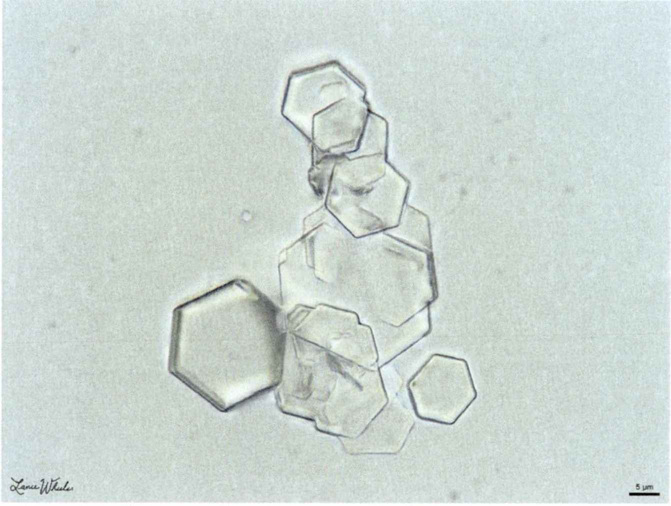

Photo Credit: Lance Wheeler / CC BY-SA (https://creativecommons.org/licenses/by-sa/4.0)

FIGURE 10.2.23 - Cystine Crystals on Urine Microscopy

REVIEW QUESTIONS

1. A 55-year-old woman presents with right flank pain on and off for the past 4 days. She has a history of recurrent urinary tract infections. Her temperature is 39.3° C (102.8° F), blood pressure is 90/55 mmHg, heart rate is 106 beats/min, and respiratory rate is 24 breaths/min. Physical exam confirms mild right flank tenderness. A radiograph reveals the presence of a radiopaque substance within the renal calyces and pelvis. What type of infectious organism is the likely cause of her current symptoms?
    - **This patient likely has ammonium magnesium phosphate (struvite) stones caused by urease-positive organisms such as *Proteus* and *Klebsiella*.**
    - She presents with waxing and waning right flank pain and a radiopaque obstruction, both of which point to nephrolithiasis.
    - The patient's history of recurrent UTIs, fever, and low blood pressure mean that the cause of her nephrolithiasis is most likely infectious.

2. A 27-year-old man presents to the emergency room with severe dehydration. He recently had a surgical resection due to ulcerative colitis and has been having complications with excess output from his ileostomy. Physical exam shows mild left flank pain. X-ray shows no evidence of nephrolithiasis. Ultrasound examination shows a 4 mm stone lodged in the left ureter. Which of the following explains the mechanism of nephrolithiasis in this patient?

    A. Increased urine calcium due to undiagnosed hyperparathyroidism
    B. Low urine pH due to bicarbonate loss
    C. *Proteus mirabilis* infection
    D. Increased uric acid excretion due to gout

    - **The correct answer is B.**
    - This patient has excess ileostomy output (i.e. diarrhea), which means that he is losing bicarbonate. This will result in a low urine pH
    - The combination of a negative radiograph and a positive ultrasound indicates that there is a radiolucent stone.
    - These findings are most consistent with a uric acid stone.
    - A is incorrect because increased urine calcium describes calcium stones. While these are the most common type of stone that causes nephrolithiasis, this patient's symptoms are more consistent with uric acid stones.
    - C is incorrect because *Proteus* infections are associated with ammonium magnesium phosphate stones. Patients with these types of stones will also have a history of recurrent UTIs, which is not present in this patient. Plus, ammonium magnesium stones would likely have been visualized on radiograph, as they are radiopaque.
    - D is incorrect because the symptoms are not consistent with gout.

Section VII - Renal Neoplasia

I. Angiomyolipoma
  A. Benign
  B. Comprised of vessels (angio), smooth muscle (myo), and fat (lipoma)
  C. Incidental finding on CT scan
    1. Majority are isolated
    2. Minority associated with tuberous sclerosis (bilateral, multiple)
  D. Treatment: typically not needed

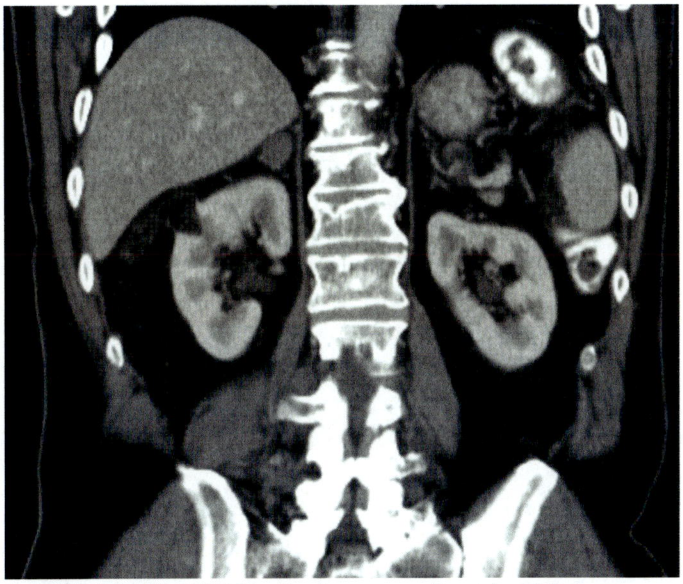

FIGURE 10.2.24 - Sagittal Abdominal CT of Isolated Angiomyolipoma

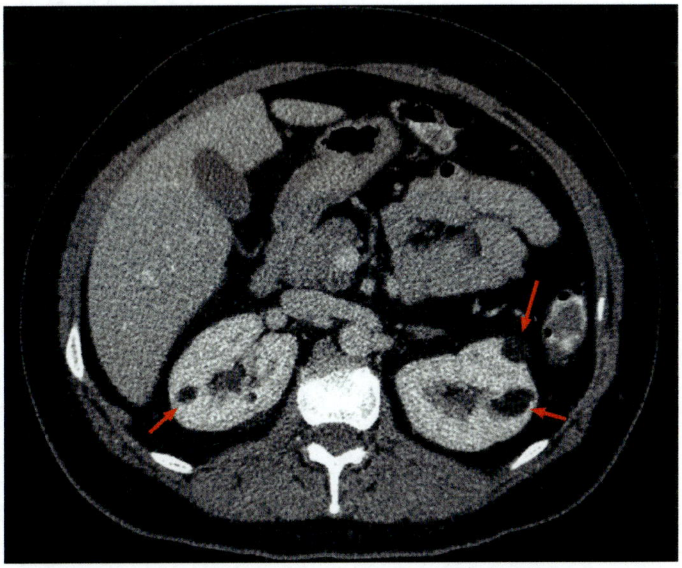

FIGURE 10.2.25 - Axial Abdominal CT of Angiomyolipoma

II. Wilms Tumor
  A. Malignant tumor in toddlers
  B. Inactivation of WT1 or WT2 genes on chromosome 11
  C. Triad: large flank mass, hypertension, and hematuria
  D. Treatment: nephrectomy
  E. Sporadic (majority)
  F. Part of syndrome (minority)
    1. WAGR: Wilms tumor, aniridia, genitourinary abnormalities, mental retardation
    2. Beckwith-Wiedemann: hemihypertrophy, macroglossia, organomegaly, omphalocele

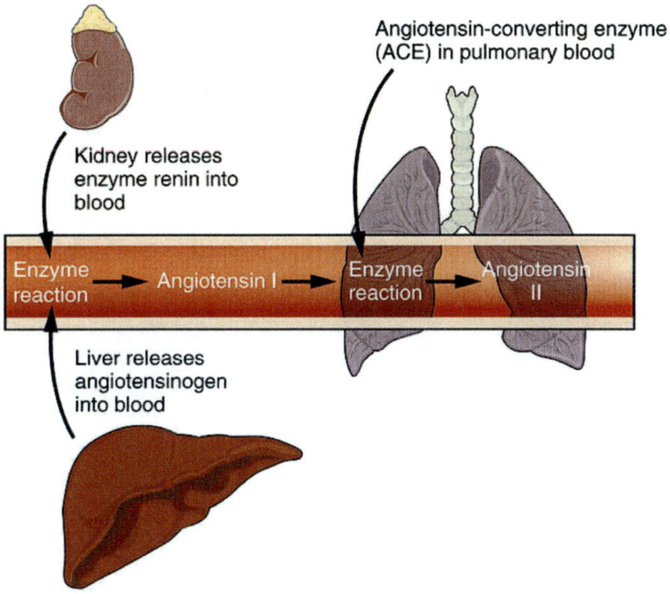

FIGURE 10.2.26 - Renin-Angiotensin-Aldosterone

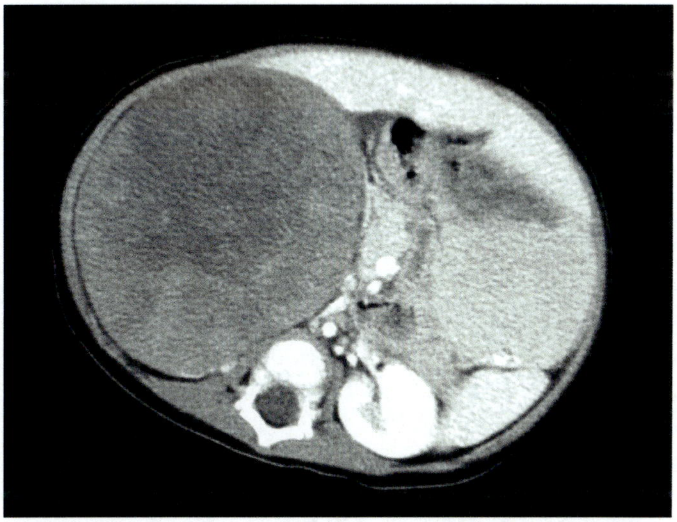

FIGURE 10.2.27 - Axial Abdominal CT of Wilms Tumor

III. Renal Cell Carcinoma
   A. Malignant growth in one or both kidneys
   B. 60 years and older
   C. Risk factors: cigarette smoking, hypertension, obesity, von Hippel-Lindau
   D. Most common: clear cell carcinoma
   E. Incidental finding

IV. Renal Cell Carcinoma: Clinical Presentation
   A. Triad (9% of patients): hematuria, mass, and flank pain
   B. Scrotal varicocele (11% of patients):
   C. Paraneoplastic syndromes possible

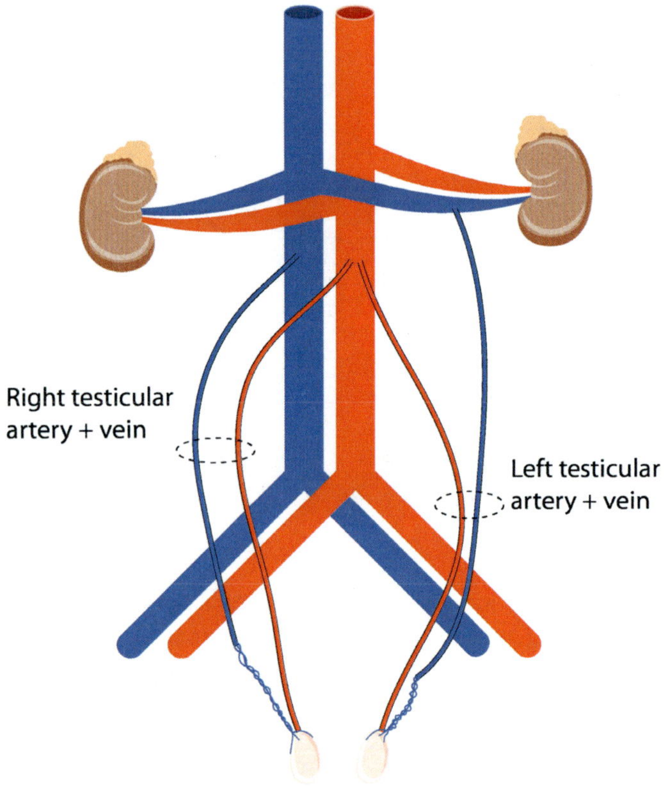

FIGURE 10.2.28 - Vascular Supply of Testicles and Scrotum

V. Paraneoplastic Syndrome
   A. Can vary significantly depending on the hormone produced
   B. Examples:
      1. ↑ ACTH → Cushing syndrome (similar to small cell lung cancer)
      2. ↑ EPO → polycythemia
      3. ↑ renin → hypertension
      4. ↑ PTHrP → hypercalcemia
      5. Many more are possible
   C. Renal Cell C'arcinoma: morphology
      1. Gross: gold or yellow due to high lipid composition
      2. Histology: clear cells with abundant cytoplasm due to high lipid content

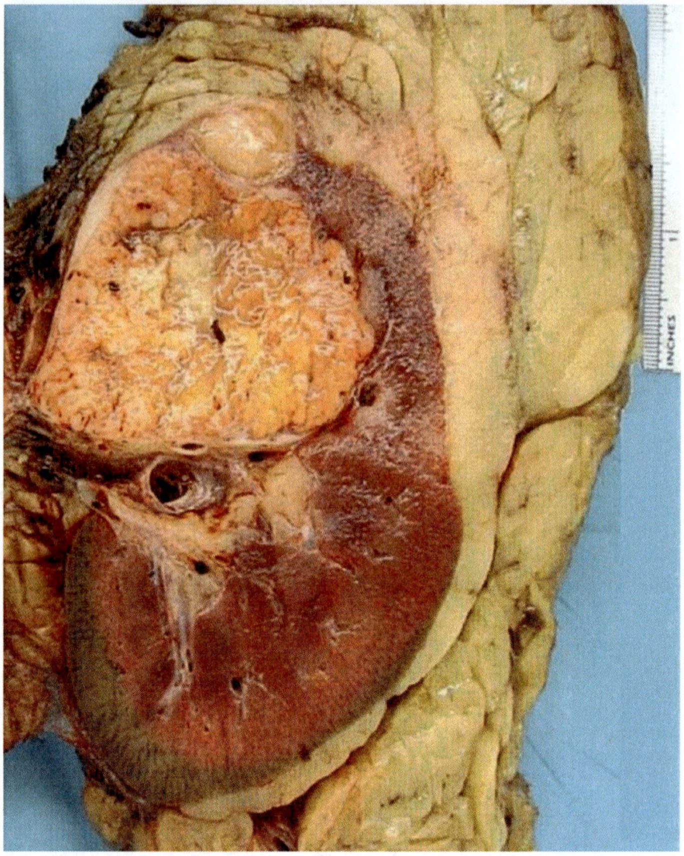

FIGURE 10.2.29 - Gross Pathology of Renal Cell Carcinoma

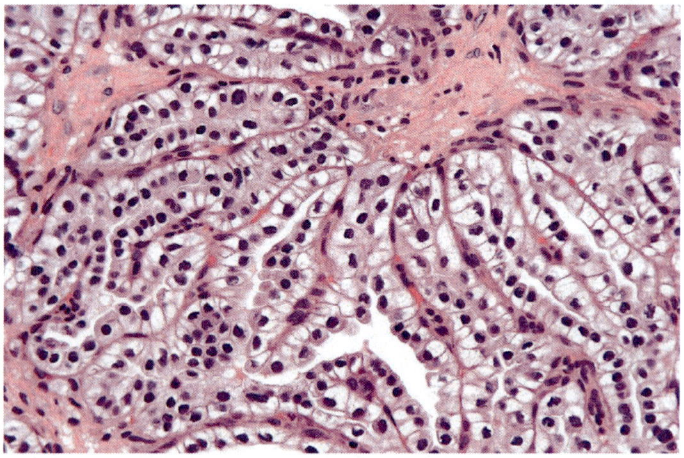

FIGURE 10.2.30 - Clear Cell Renal Cell Carcinoma

VI. Renal Cell Carcinoma: Staging and Treatment
   A. TNM staging:
      1. T = tumor → size and extent of primary tumor
      2. N = lymph node involvement
      3. M = metastasis
   B. Treatment: partial or total nephrectomy
   C. Typically resistant to radiation or chemotherapy

REVIEW QUESTIONS

?

1. A 58-year-old male presents to the clinic after a mass on his right kidney was identified following a CT scan for abdominal pain. He is otherwise healthy. He does not smoke. Vital signs are stable. His BMI is 24. He denies fever, chills, weight loss, or bone pain. A biopsy of the kidney mass reveals blood vessels, smooth muscle, and fat. What is the most likely diagnosis?

    A. Clear cell renal cell carcinoma
    B. Wilms tumor
    C. Angiomyolipoma
    D. Abscess

- **The correct answer is C.**
- This is a 58-year-old male with an incidental finding of a mass on his right kidney. Biopsy shows blood vessels, smooth muscle, and fat. This should make you think of an angiomyolipoma.
- A is incorrect because clear cell carcinoma would show clear cells, not vessels, muscle, or fat. Additionally, smoking and obesity are risk factors for renal cell cancer, so this information doesn't raise the suspicion of angiomyolipoma.
- B is incorrect as this is an adult male with an incidental finding.
- D is incorrect because this patient shows no signs of infection. Remember, he denies fever and chills.

Section VIII - Lower Urinary Tract Carcinoma

I. Urothelial (Transitional Cell) Carcinoma
  A. Malignant proliferation of urothelial lining (normal lining)
  B. Most common lower urinary tract cancer
  C. Risk factors
    1. Cigarette smoking (naphthylamine)
    2. Long term use of phenacetin or cyclophosphamide
    3. Occupational exposure (azo dyes, rubber, plastic, leather)

II. Urothelial Carcinoma: Clinical Features
  A. Older adults
  B. Painless hematuria
  C. Multifocal and recurring tumors
    1. Entire urothelium mutated via field defect

III. Urothelial Carcinoma: Tumor Pathways
  A. Flat tumors
    1. High grade tumor → invasion
    2. p53 mutations
  B. Papillary tumors
    1. Low grade tumor → high grade tumor → invasion
    2. Not associated with p53 mutations

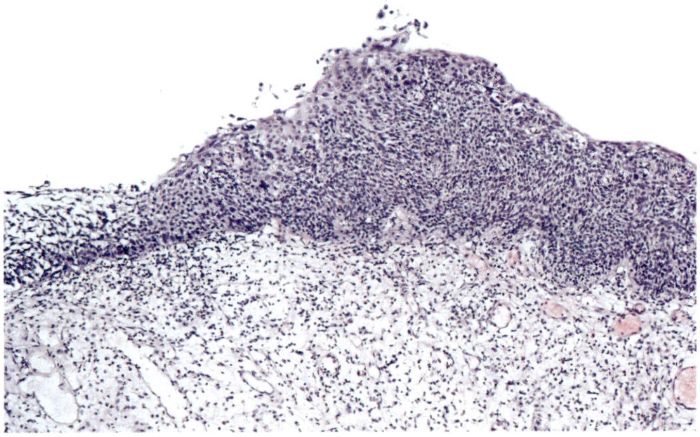

Photo Credit: CoRus13 / CC0

FIGURE 10.2.31 - Flat Tumor of Urothelial Carcinoma

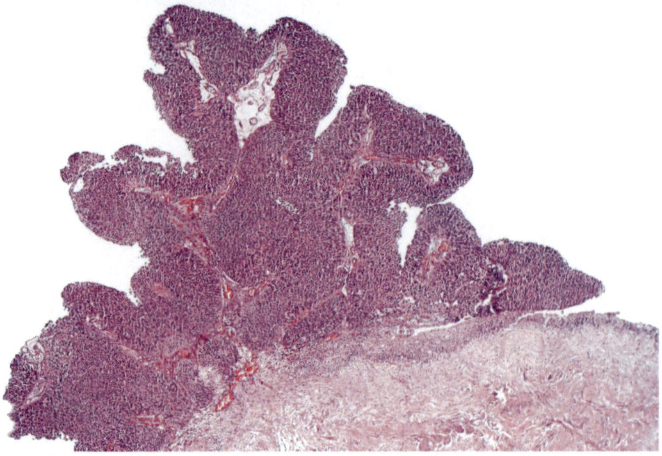

Photo Credit: CoRus13 / CC0

FIGURE 10.2.32 - Papillary Tumor of Urothelial Carcinoma

IV. Squamous Cell Carcinoma of the Bladder
  A. Malignant proliferation of squamous cells
    1. Follows squamous metaplasia
  B. Painless hematuria
  C. Risk factors:
    1. Chronic cystitis (older females)
    2. *Schistosoma haematobium* infection (Middle Eastern males)
    3. Chronic nephrolithiasis

V. Adenocarcinoma of the Bladder
  A. Malignant proliferation of glands
  B. May arise from various tissues
    1. Urachal remnant: tumor at dome of bladder
    2. Cystitis glandularis: chronic inflammation → glandular metaplasia
    3. Exstrophy: caudal portion of anterior abdominal wall not formed

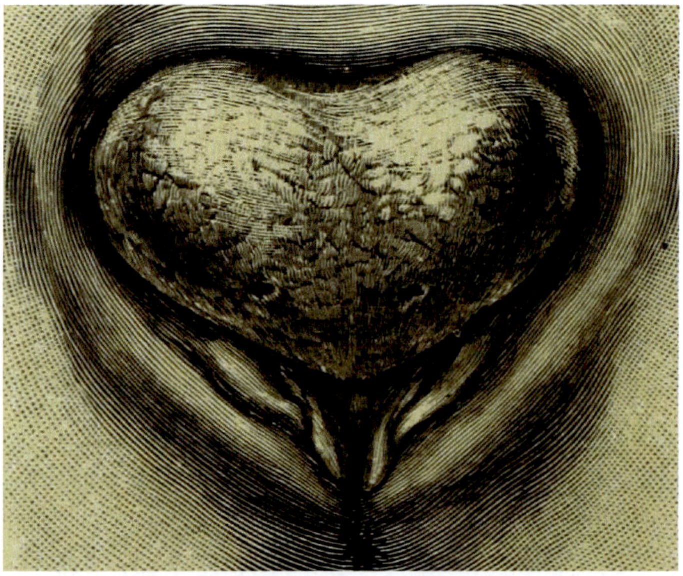

Photo Credit: Bland-Sutton. https://www.flickr.com/photos/internetarchivebookimages/14591734167/

FIGURE 10.2.33 - Bladder Exstrophy

REVIEW QUESTIONS

1. A 58-year-old woman presents to the emergency department complaining about blood in her urine. She denies any pain while urinating. She has been working at a hair salon for the past 30 years. After a thorough workup, she is diagnosed with urothelial carcinoma. What was the most likely risk factor contributing to the development of urothelial carcinoma in this patient?

    - **The correct answer is exposure to azo dyes.**
    - We're told that the patient has developed urothelial carcinoma. Her hematuria is consistent with this, especially since her hematuria is painless.
    - We know that she has worked at a salon for the past 30 years, so it is likely that she came in contact with products containing azo dyes
    - Recall that certain occupational hazards, such as exposure to azo dyes, rubber, plastic, and leather, are common risk factors for developing urothelial carcinoma

2. A 63-year-old Egyptian male complains of painless blood in his urine over the past 2 weeks. He has a history of a parasitic infection after swimming in the Nile River, for which he was prescribed praziquantel, but has been noncompliant. A cystoscopy is performed and a biopsy is taken of the bladder tissue. What type of epithelium will likely be observed in the biopsy specimen?

    A. Columnar epithelium
    B. Squamous epithelium
    C. Glandular epithelium
    D. Cuboidal epithelium

    - **The correct answer is B.**
    - From the question we know that the patient has painless hematuria. In an older patient, painless hematuria should raise suspicion for cancer. The patient has a medical history of a parasitic infection. He acquired this while in the Middle East and was prescribed praziquantel for it. This should make you think of an infection with *Schistosoma haematobium*. A *Schistosoma haematobium* infection is a risk factor for squamous cell carcinoma.
    - The question is essentially what epithelial abnormality is associated with squamous cell carcinoma. Recall that the bladder normally has a urothelial lining. However, an insult such as a *Schistosoma* infection can lead to squamous metaplasia. When this occurs, we can see a growth of squamous epithelium replacing the normal urothelial epithelium. Prolonged metaplasia in the bladder can eventually lead to squamous cell carcinoma.
    - A is incorrect because you wouldn't expect columnar metaplasia in this patient, who most likely has squamous cell carcinoma.
    - C is incorrect because glandular epithelium is seen in adenocarcinoma of the bladder, something we would not expect in our patient with a *Schistosoma* infection.
    - D is incorrect because cuboidal epithelium is not associated with carcinoma of the bladder.

REPRODUCTIVE PATHOLOGY

Section I - Penis

I. Peyronie's Disease
   A. Definition: curvature in the penis (varying degrees)
   B. Cause: tunica albuginea plaque
   C. Symptoms: curvature with erection, erectile dysfunction, pain, and anxiety
   D. Treatment: traction, collagenase injections, and surgery

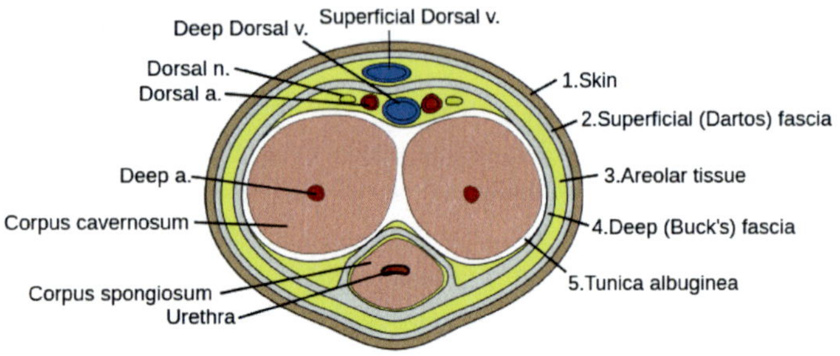

FIGURE 10.3.1 - Cross-Section of a Penis

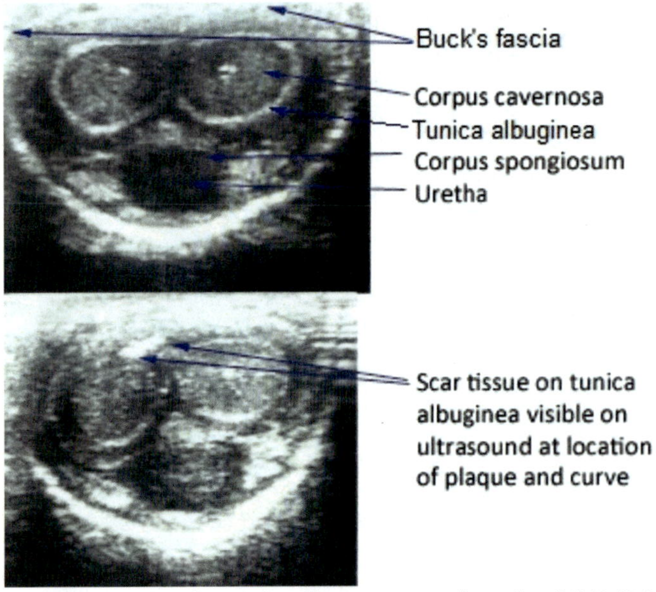

FIGURE 10.3.2 - Coronal Ultrasound Showing Normal Anatomy (Top) and a Plaque in the Tunica Albuginea (Bottom)

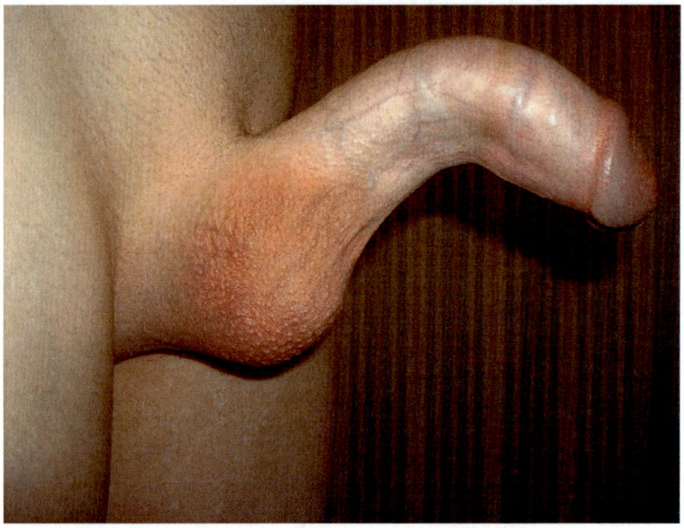

FIGURE 10.3.3 - Peyronie's Disease

II. Ischemic Priapism
   A. Priapism: persistent erection lasting over 4 hours
   B. Ischemic priapism: erection caused by low blood flow
   C. Cause: sickle cell disease and medications (e.g. sildenafil, trazodone)
   D. Symptoms: severe pain with an erect, rigid penis
   E. Treatment: corporal aspiration, intracorporeal injection (phenylephrine), and surgery

III. Cancer
   A. Squamous cell carcinoma is most common
   B. May be preceded by precancerous lesion
   C. Risk factors: uncircumcised and high risk HPV infection (strains 16 and 18)
   D. Treatment: surgery (penectomy)

REVIEW QUESTIONS

1. A 17-year-old male presents to the emergency room complaining of an erection that has lasted 4 hours and is associated with severe pain. He has a known history of sickle cell disease. Physical exam reveals a rigid phallus that is exquisitely tender to touch without deformity. Which of the following is the most appropriate next step?

    A. Emergency surgery
    B. Intracorporeal injection of phenylephrine
    C. Intracorporeal injection of epinephrine
    D. Intracorporeal injection of saline
    E. Observation

- **The correct answer is B.**
- This is a 17-year-old male presenting with a painful, sustained erection lasting more than four hours who has a known history of sickle cell disease. This should raise concern for ischemic priapism. His physical exam is consistent with priapism and there are no signs of trauma or penile fracture. The most appropriate next step is intracorporeal injection of a sympathomimetic drug. Phenylephrine is the drug of choice for ischemic priapism because it is relatively specific for alpha receptors, which minimizes side effect risk.
- A is incorrect because surgery is the treatment of choice only after failure of aspiration and intracorporeal injection.
- C is incorrect because epinephrine would not be the drug of choice.
- D is incorrect because saline would not be therapeutic.
- E is incorrect because priapism, without treatment, causes irreversible penile damage.

Section II - Testicle

I. Cryptorchidism
   A. Testicle does not fully descend into scrotum
   B. Very common

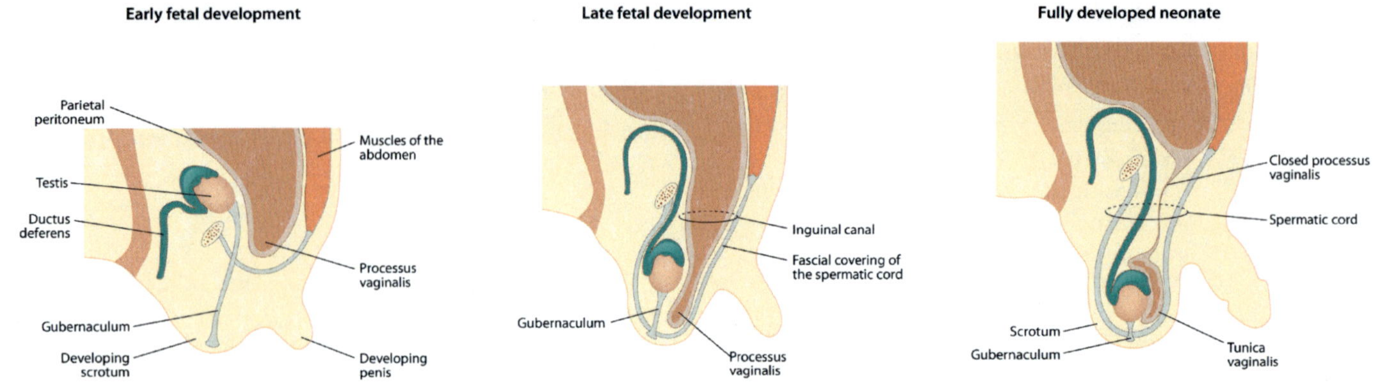

FIGURE 10.3.4 - Normal Descent of the Testicles

   C. High core body heat → cellular damage
      1. Increased risk of atrophy, infertility, and testicular cancer
   D. Some resolve spontaneously
      1. If not resolved by 6 months → surgery
      2. Surgery reduces risk of atrophy, infertility, and cancer

II. Hydrocele
   A. Fluid accumulation between visceral and parietal layers of tunica vaginalis
   B. Causes
      1. Congenital: processus vaginalis fails to close
      2. Adults: idiopathic or reactive

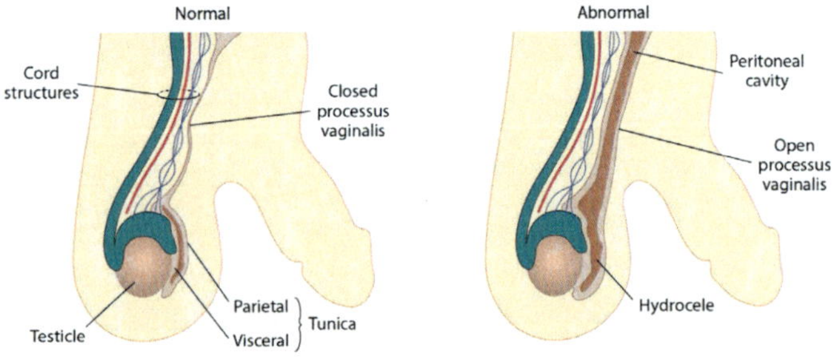

FIGURE 10.3.5 - Normal Anatomy (Left) and Congenital Hydrocele (Right)

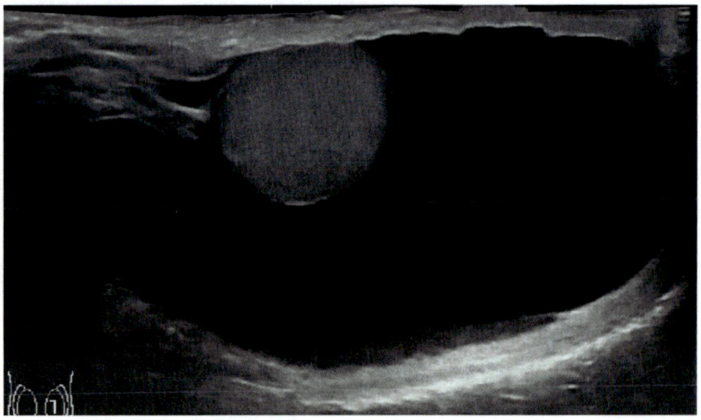

Photo Credit: Mikael Häggström, M.D. - Author info - Reusing imagesWritten informed consent was obtained from the individual, including online publication. / CC0

FIGURE 10.3.6 - Ultrasound of Hydrocele

   C. Physical exam
      1. Scrotal swelling
      2. ransilluminates with light
   D. Treatment
      1. Congenital: no intervention; spontaneous resolution
      2. Adults: if reactive treat underlying cause, if idiopathic and painful consider surgery

III. Varicocele
   A. Dilation of veins in the pampiniform plexus
   B. Due to poor drainage or faulty/absent valves
   C. Physical exam: "bag of worms" appearance
   D. Risks: atrophy and infertility
   E. Treatment: electrive surgery

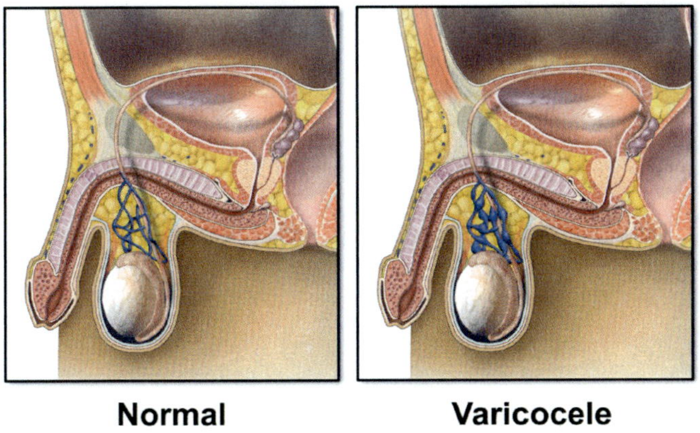

FIGURE 10.3.7 - Varicocele

IV. Orchitis
   A. Inflammation of the testicle
   B. Teenagers: viral
      1. Mumps virus
   C. Young adults: sexually transmitted
      1. *Chlamydia trachomatis* (D-K)
      2. *Neisseria gonorrhoeae*
   D. Older adults: spread from UTI
      1. *E. coli* and
      2. *Pseudomonas*
   E. Teenagers and young adults: risk of atrophy or infertility
   F. Treatment
      1. Bacterial: antibiotic
      2. Viral: supportive care (anti-inflammatory medications)

V. Torsion
   A. Twisting of the testicle and spermatic cord
   B. Veins collapse → congestion of the testicle → hemorrhagic death of testicle
   C. Physical exam: severe testicular pain, horizontal testicle, and absent cremasteric reflex
   D. Ultrasound: lack of blood flow to testicle
   E. Treatment: emergency surgery

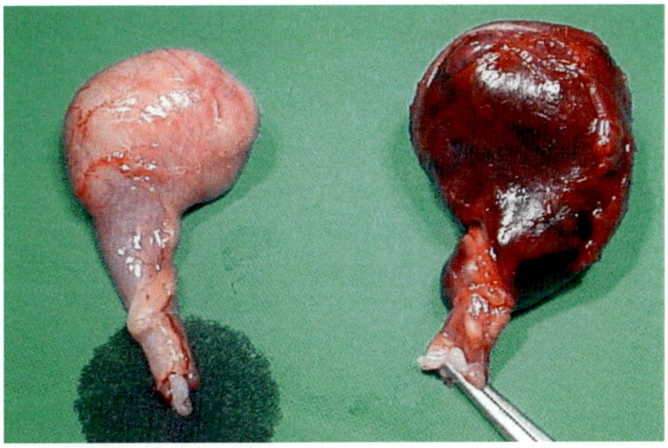

FIGURE 10.3.8 - Normal Testicle (Right) and Hemorrhagic Testicle (Left)

REVIEW QUESTIONS

1. A 15-year-old male presents to the emergency department with 3 hours of severe pain in his scrotum. On physical exam his scrotum is exquisitely tender to palpation and his left testicle appears horizontal. His scrotal ultrasound with Doppler is shown below, which shows no blood flow in the testicle. What is the next best step in treatment?

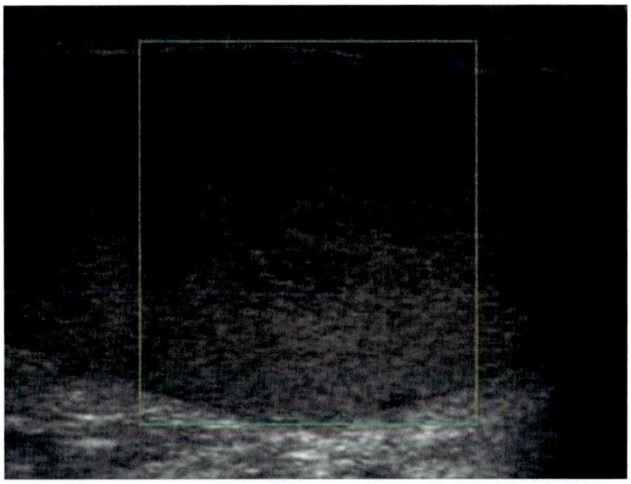

FIGURE 10.3.9 - Scrotal Ultrasound with Doppler

   A. CT scan of the pelvis
   B. Emergent corrective surgery
   C. Exploratory laparotomy
   D. Antibiotics
   E. STD testing

- **The correct answer is B.**
- This is a 15-year-old male who has severe pain in his scrotum. His physical exam is significant for tenderness to palpation and a left testicle lying horizontally. A scrotal ultrasound is ordered and shows no blood flow in the testicle, creating concern for testicular torsion. The correct treatment for testicular torsion is an emergency surgery to correct the torsion and fix the testicle in the scrotum.
- A is incorrect because torsion is a clinical diagnosis and requires emergency surgery.
- C is incorrect because the testicle is in the scrotum and an exploratory abdominal surgery would be inappropriate in this case.
- D is incorrect because torsion is not a bacterial disease requiring antibiotics.
- E is incorrect because torsion is not a sexually transmitted infection.

Section III - Testicular Tumors

I. Overview
   A. Epidemiology
   B. Clinical presentation
   C. Risk factors
   D. Diagnosis and treatment
   E. Subtypes
      1. Germ cell tumors
      2. Sex-cord stromal tumors
   F. Lymphoma

II. Epidemiology
   A. Most common tumors in males 15-35 years
   B. 10% of all cancer deaths worldwide

III. Clinical Presentation
   A. Unilateral, painless testicular mass
   B. Discomfort, heaviness, and dull aching lower abdominal pain
   C. Scrotal examination
      1. Firm, solid testicular mass
      2. Cannot be transilluminated

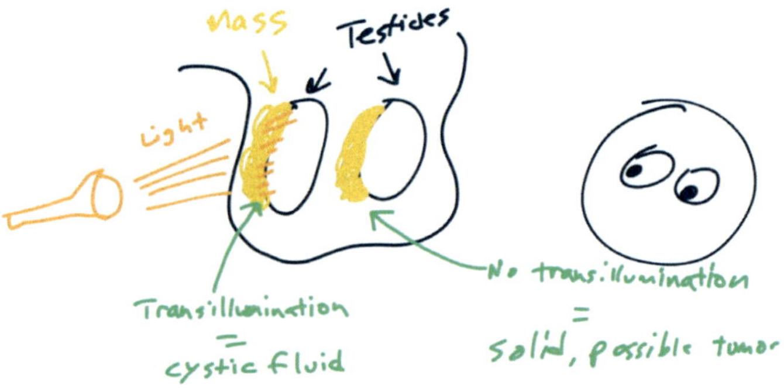

FIGURE 10.3.10 - Transillumination vs. Absent Transillumination

IV. Risk Factors
   A. Cryptorchidism: undescended testis
   B. Klinefelter syndrome (47, XXY)
   C. Family history

V. Diagnosis and Treatment
   A. Diagnosis: bilateral scrotal ultrasound
      1. Biopsy contraindicated (high risk of seeding to inguinal lymph nodes and scrotal skin)
   B. Treatment: radical inguinal orchiectomy
      1. Chemotherapy or radiotherapy

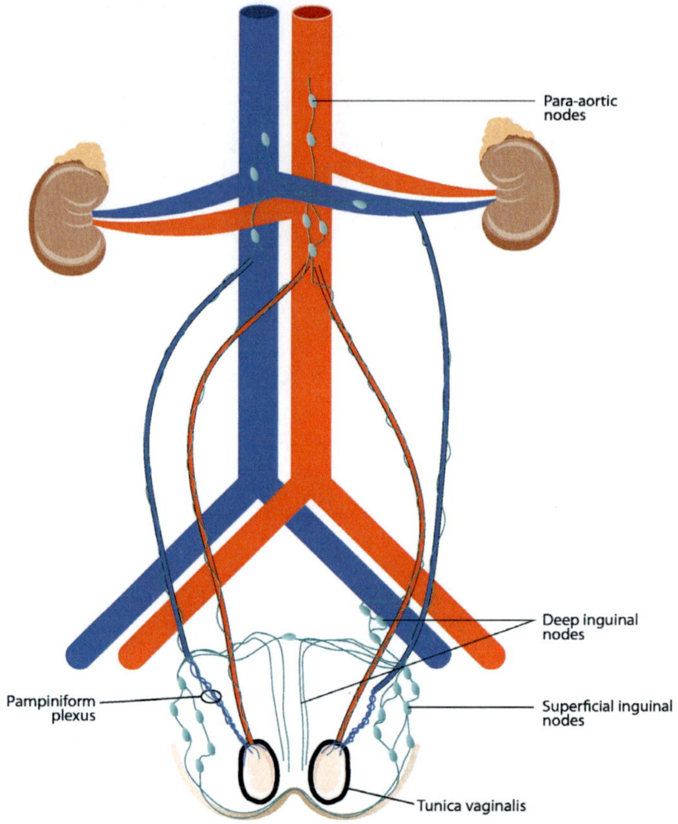

FIGURE 10.3.11 - Anatomy of Male Urogenital Tract

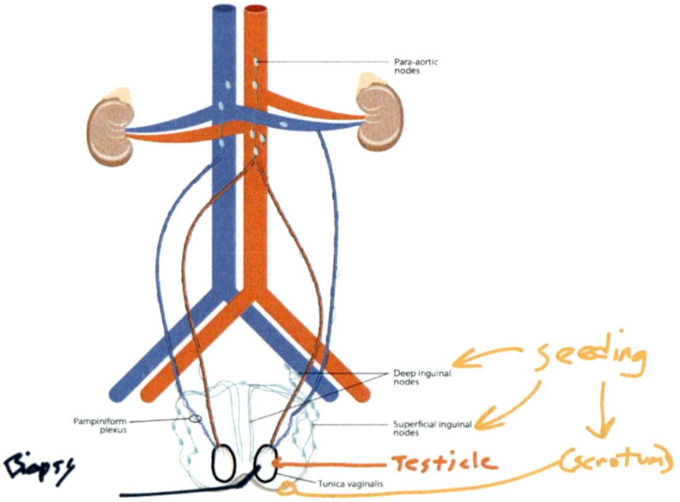

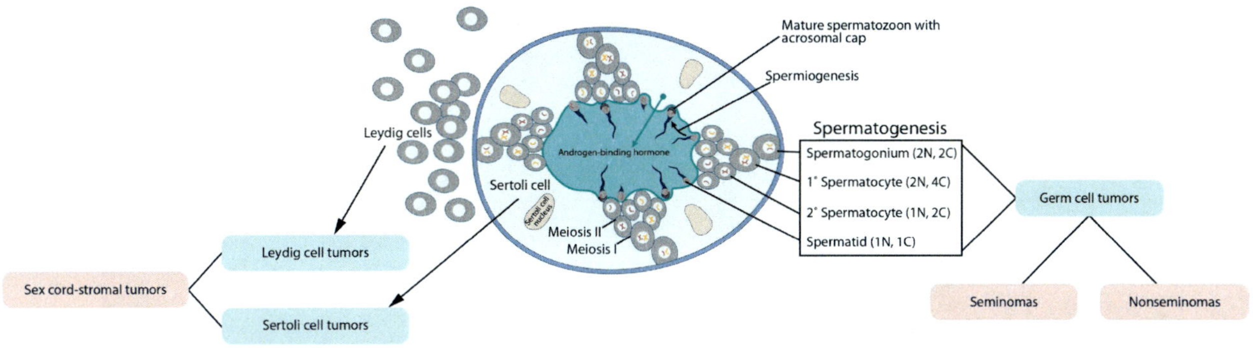

FIGURE 10.3.12 - Cross-Section of Seminiferous Tubules

Tumor	Description	Morphology	Features	Markers
Seminomas				
Seminoma	- 50% of all testicular tumors - Counterpart to the female dysgerminoma - Cells resembling primordial germ cells	- Sheets of uniform cells poorly demarcated into lobules by fibrous septa - No hemorrhage or necrosis	- Bulky masses - Radiosensitive - Metastasize late (via lymphatics) - Better prognosis than nonseminomas	- ↑ β-hCG (sometimes)
Nonseminomas				
Nonseminomas	- Less prevalent - Differentiated or undifferentiated germ cells		- Not radiosensitive - Metastasize early (hematogenous) - Poor prognosis	
Yolk sac tumor (endodermal sinus)	- Resembles yolk sac elements	- Schiller-Duval bodies (resemble primitive glomeruli)	- Most common in infants and children up to age 3 - Good prognosis	- ↑ AFP
Choriocarcinoma	- Contains trophoblastic tissue (syncytiotrophoblast and cytotrophoblast)	- No testicular enlargement - Hemorrhage/necrosis	- Hyperthyroidism - Gynecomastia	- ↑ β-hCG
Teratoma (malignant in males)	- Derivatives of 2 or 3 germ layers	- Neural tissue - Cartilage - Muscle	- Any age - Mature and immature - Benign in children - Malignant in adults	- ↑ AFP - ↑ β-hCG (sometimes)
Embryonal carcinoma	- Growth of cells in alveolar or tubular patterns (glands)	- Smaller than seminomas - Hemorrhage/necrosis	- Ages 20-30	- ↑ AFP (when mixed) - ↑ β-hCG (sometimes)
Sex Cord-Stromal Tumors				
Leydig cell tumors	- Usually benign	- Large, round cells with prominent nuclei and abundant pink cytoplasm - Reinke crystals (⅓ of cases)	- Ages 20-60 - May secrete androgens and estrogens - Gynecomastia in adults - Precocious puberty in children	
Sertoli cell tumors	- Benign	- Cells form cordlike structures and tubules	- Do not secrete any hormone	

TABLE 10.3.1 - Seminomas and Nonseminomas

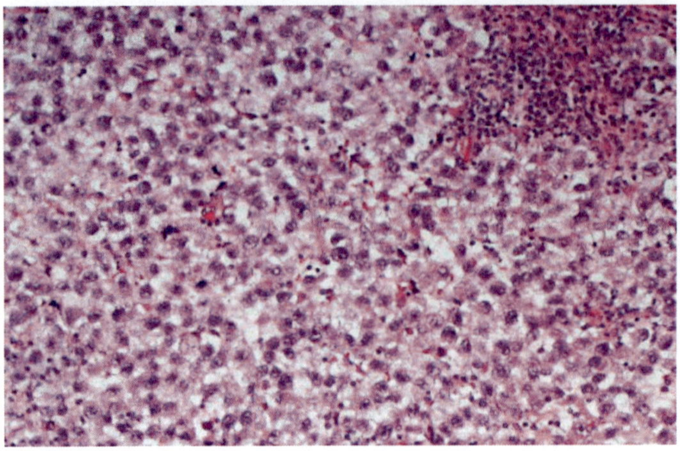

FIGURE 10.3.13 - Seminoma (Histology)

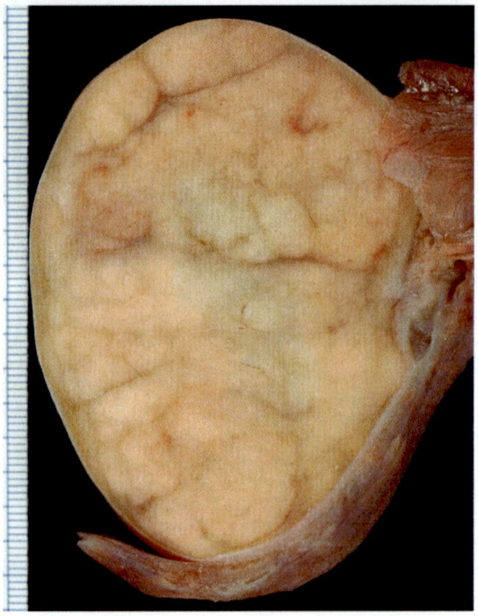

FIGURE 10.3.16 - Seminoma (Gross)

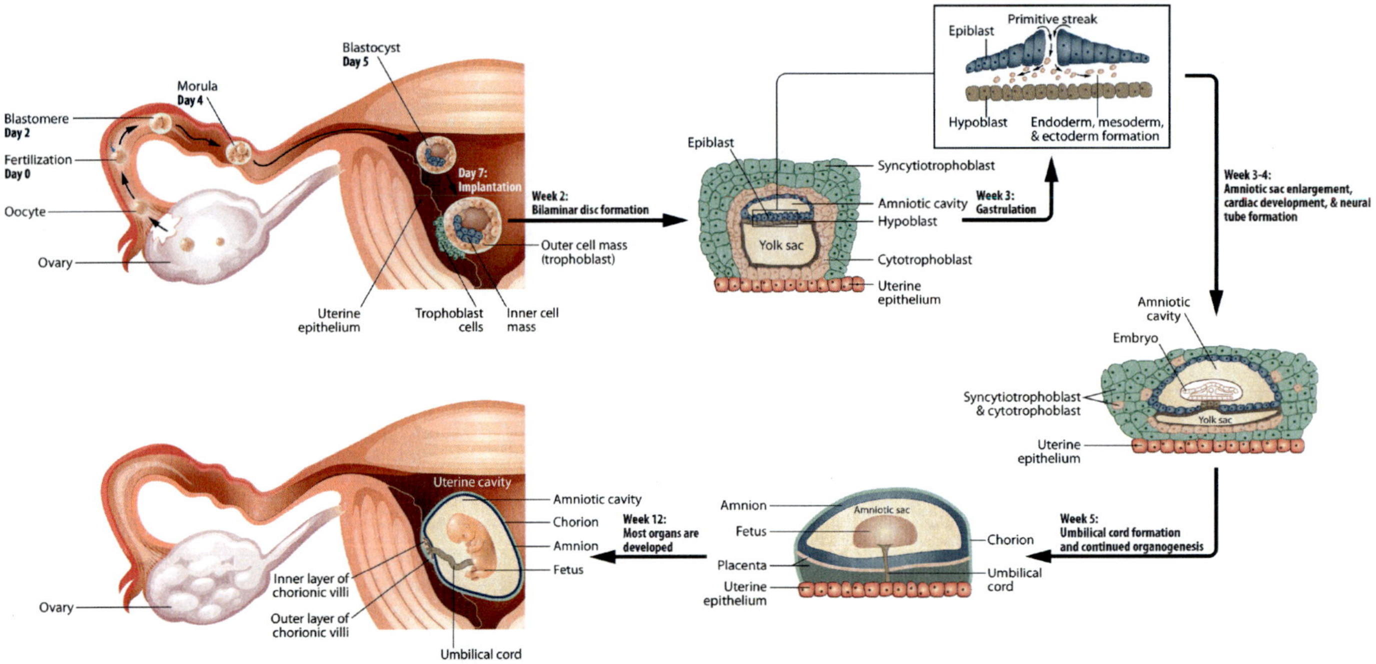

FIGURE 10.3.14 - Nonseminoma Tumor Marker Overview

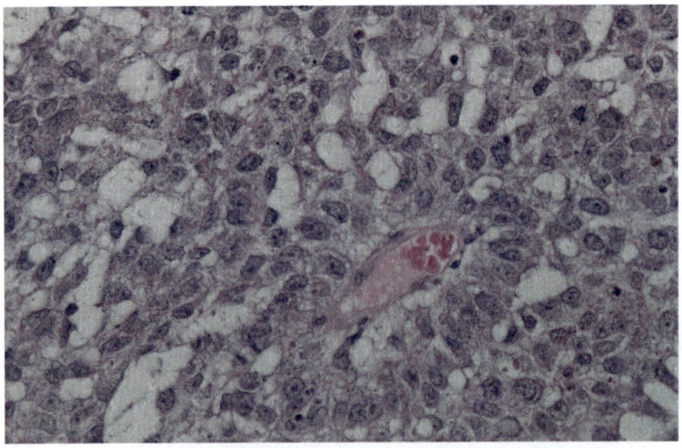

FIGURE 10.3.15 - Yolk Sac Tumor (Histology)

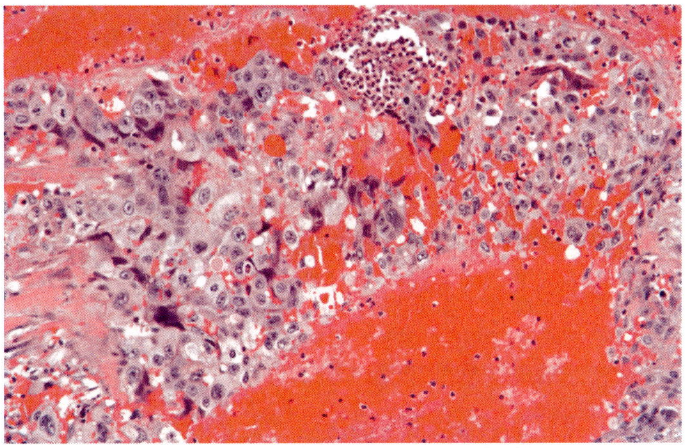

FIGURE 10.3.17 - Choriocarcinoma Testicular Tumor (Histology)

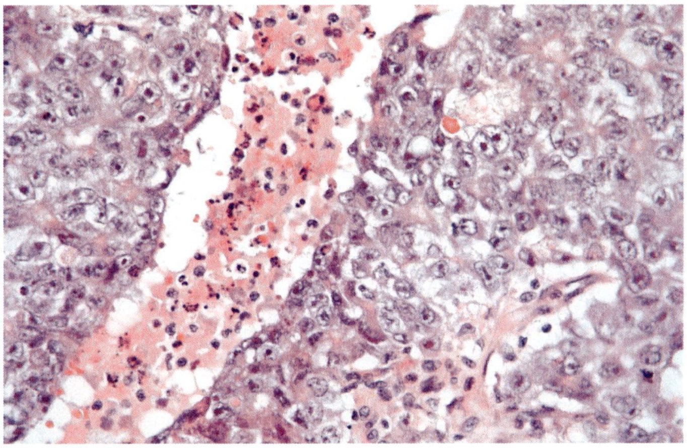

FIGURE 10.3.18 - Embryonal Carcinoma (Histology)

VI. Mixed Tumors
  A. 60% of testicular tumors consist of more than one pattern
  B. Prognosis depends on the more aggressive component

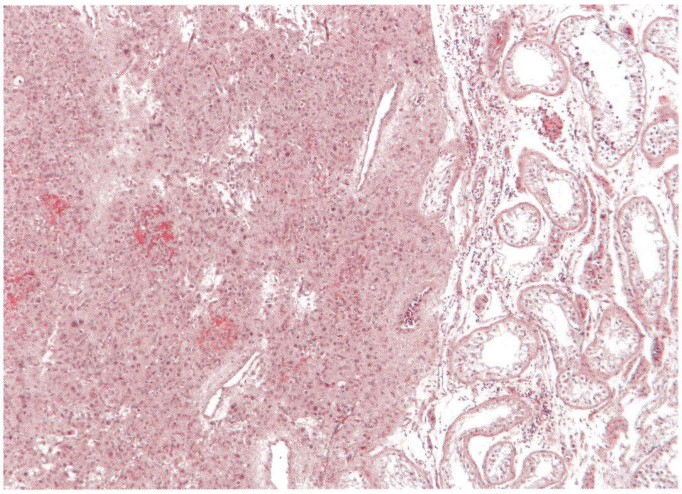

FIGURE 10.3.19 - Leydig Cell Tumor (Histology)

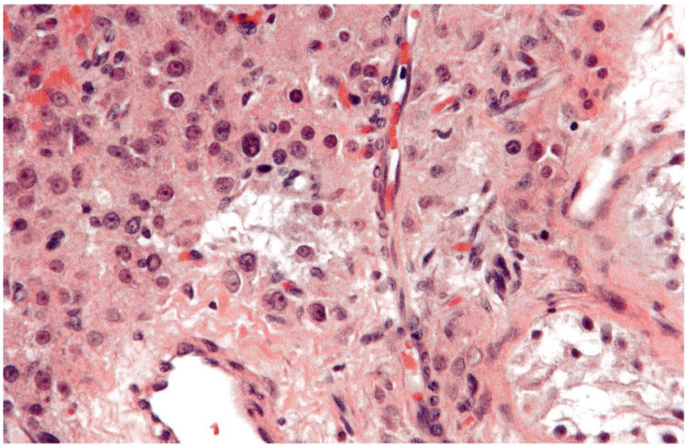

FIGURE 10.3.20 - Embryonal Carcinoma at High Magnification

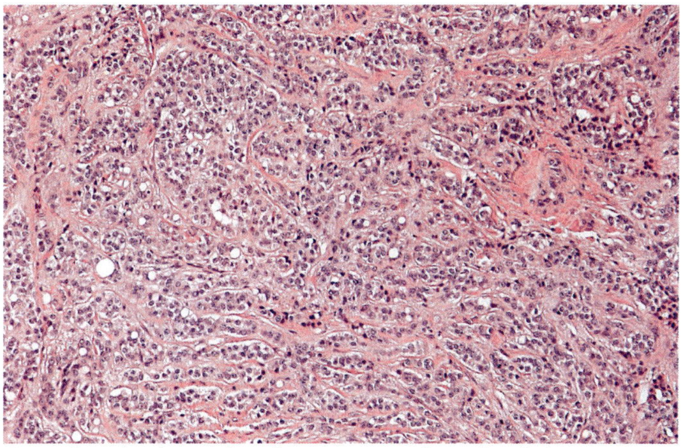

FIGURE 10.3.21 - Sertoli Cell Tumor

VII. Lymphoma
  A. Usually a secondary tumor
  B. Usually bilateral
  C. Diffuse large B-cell lymphoma
  D. Most common testicular neoplasm in men > 60 years

REVIEW QUESTIONS

1. A 25-year-old male presents with complaints of a painless right testicular mass. There is no history of recent trauma. Vitals are within normal limits. Other than the testicular mass, he is asymptomatic. On physical examination, a nontender, solid right testicular mass is palpated. The mass does not transilluminate. Inguinal lymph nodes are not palpable. On ultrasound, a hypoechoic mass is observed within the right testicle. What is the most likely diagnosis?

   - **The answer here is testicular cancer.**
   - The fact that the mass does not transilluminate indicates that it is solid (not fluid-filled).
   - Testicular tumors are most common in males ages 15 to 30 and the patient in the question stem is 25 years old.
   - Testicular tumors are painless, such as the mass that this patient presents with.

2. A 25-year-old male presents to the office with complaints of nervousness, sweating, heat intolerance, and unintentional weight loss. He has also noticed left testicular enlargement. He does not complain of any dragging sensation or pain in his lower abdomen. Physical examination reveals diffuse enlargement of the thyroid gland and a nontender left testicular mass that does not transilluminate. Laboratory examination reveals decreased TSH level. Which of the following is the most likely diagnosis?

   A. Leydig cell tumor
   B. Sertoli cell tumor
   C. Yolk sac tumor
   D. Choriocarcinoma

   - **The correct answer is D.**
   - The fact that the mass does not transilluminate supports the diagnosis of a testicular neoplasm.
   - The decreased serum TSH level indicates a paraneoplastic cause of hyperthyroidism.
   - A is incorrect because Leydig cell tumors do not cause hyperthyroidism. Instead, they can secrete androgens or estrogens, causing precocious puberty in children or gynecomastia in adults.
   - B is incorrect because Sertoli cell tumors are mostly hormonally silent and don't cause hyperthyroidism.
   - C is incorrect because yolk sac tumors occur in infants and young children up to the age of 3 years and do not cause hyperthyroidism.

Section IV - Prostate

I. Anatomy

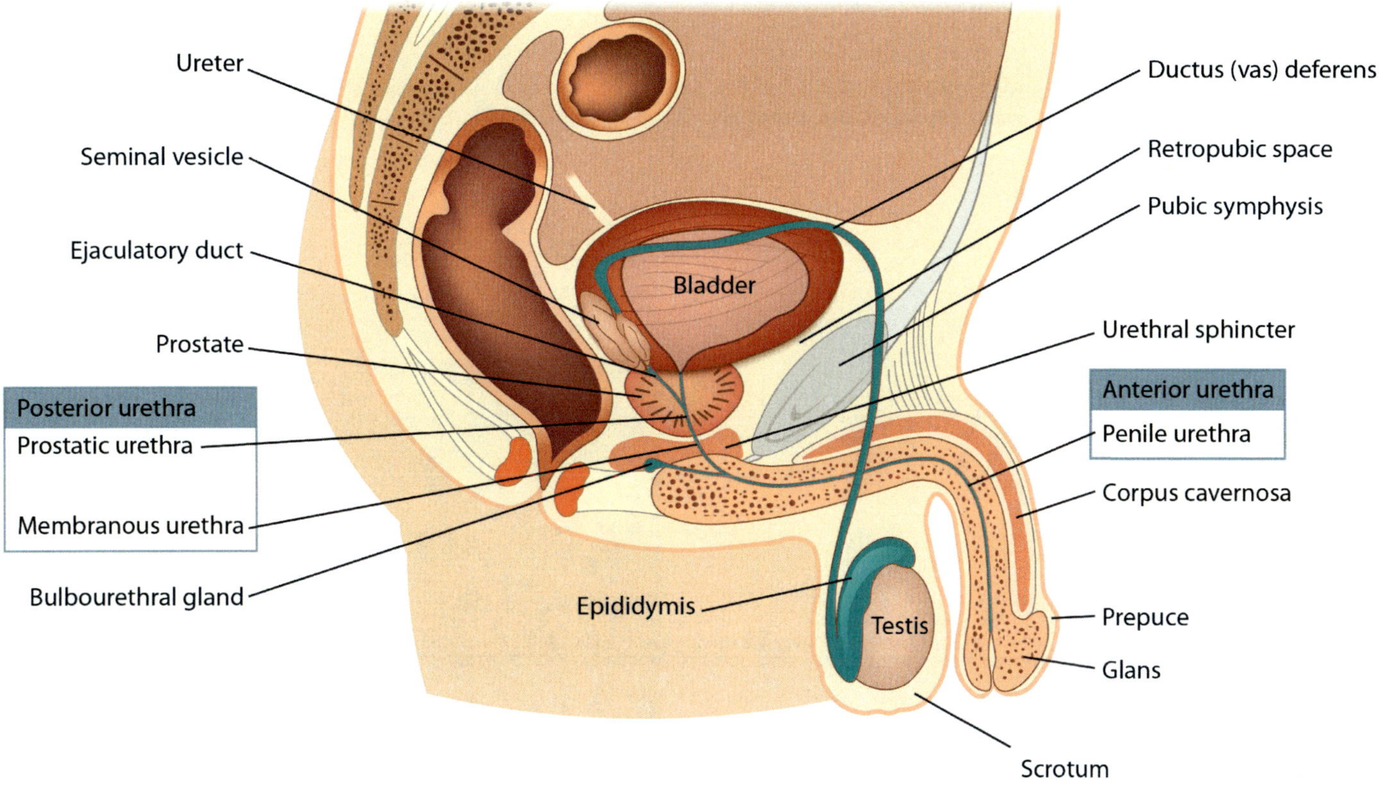

FIGURE 10.3.22 - Male Reproductive Anatomy

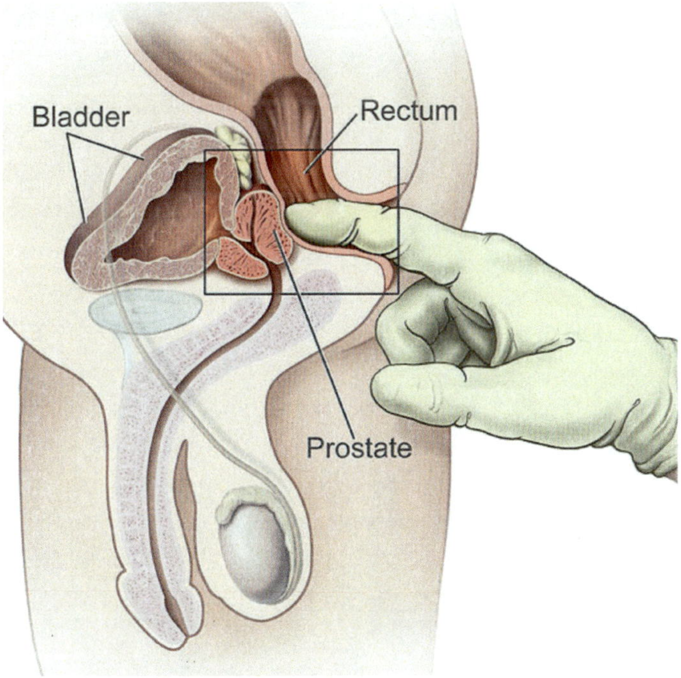

Photo Credit: Unknown author / Public domain

FIGURE 10.3.23 - Digital Rectal Exam

II. Acute Prostatitis
   A. Acute inflammation of the prostate
   B. Often bacterial
      1. Young men: *Chlamydia trachomatis* and *Neisseria gonorrhoeae*
      2. Older men: *E. coli*
   C. Presentation: dysuria, fever, chills, "boggy" and tender prostate
   D. Labs: leukocytosis, pyuria, bacteriuria, and elevated PSA
   E. Treatment: antibiotics

III. Chronic Prostatitis
   A. Chronic inflammation of the prostate
   B. Causes
      1. Bacterial
      2. Noninfectious: trauma, chemical irritation, and radiation
   C. Symptoms: dysuria, pelvic pain, and pain on ejaculation
   D. Labs: pyuria, elevated PSA, and negative urine culture

IV. Benign Prostatic Hyperplasia

A. Basics

1. Benign excessive growth of prostate tissue

B. Hormone-mediated overgrowth

1. Common in older men
2. Symptoms: urinary frequency, nocturia, weak stream, straining, and urinary retention
3. Digital rectal exam shows smooth, large prostate without nodules
4. Labs: elevated PSA, +/- microscopic hematuria

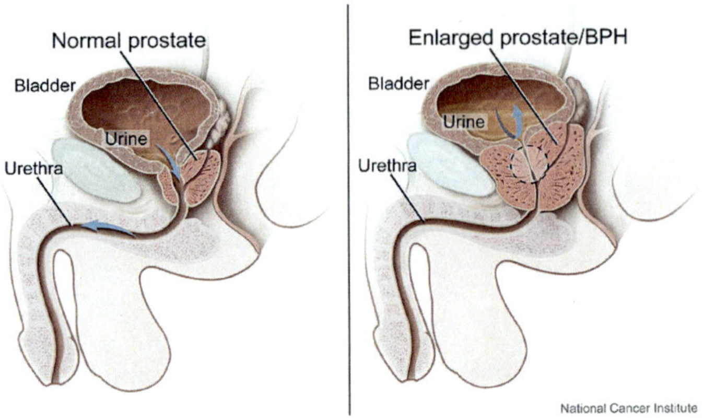

Photo Credit: Alan Hoofring (Illustrator) / Public domain

FIGURE 10.3.24 - Normal Anatomy (Left) and Benign Prostatic Hyperplasia (Right)

C. Complications

1. Due to urinary retention
   a) Damage to bladder muscle
   b) Urinary tract infections
   c) Hydronephrosis → irreversible kidney damage

D. Treatment

1. Medical
   a) Alpha-1 adrenergic receptor blockers (tamsulosin): relax smooth muscle of bladder and prostate → improve urine flow
   b) 5-alpha-reductase inhibitors (finasteride): decrease production of dihydrotestosterone → decrease prostate growth
2. Surgical: transurethral resection of prostate

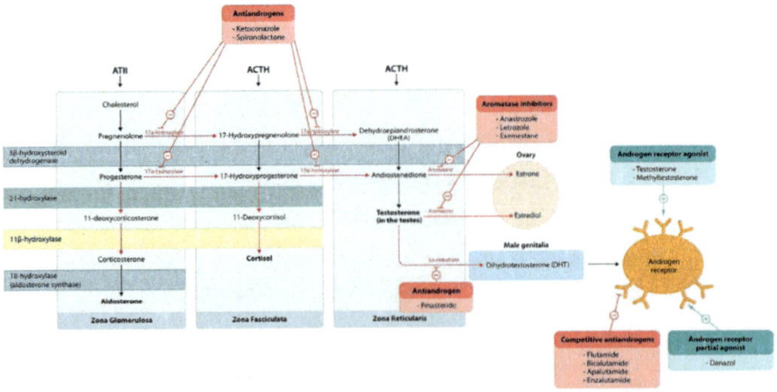

FIGURE 10.3.25 - Steroid Synthesis Pathway

V. Prostate Cancer

A. Basics

1. Most common cancer in men
2. Often asymptomatic
3. Identified by screening with PSA and digital rectal exam
   a) Guidelines debated
   b) American Urologic Association: screen men ages 55 to 69
4. Diagnosed by biopsy

B. Metastasis

1. May spread to bones (e.g. spine, pelvis)
   a) Osteoblastic lesions → bone pain
   b) Elevated alkaline phosphatase

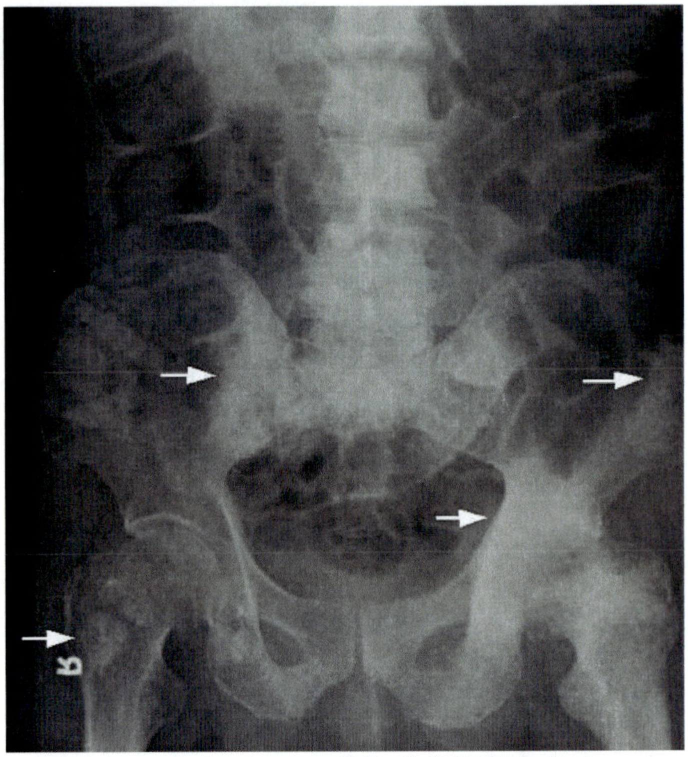

Photo Credit: Wan-Hsiu Liao, Sheng-Hsiang Lin and Tsu-Tuan Wu / CC BY-SA (https://creativecommons.org/licenses/by-sa/2.0)

FIGURE 10.3.26 - X-ray of Male Pelvis Showing Osteoblastic Lesions (White Arrows)

C. Treatment

1. Treatment algorithm is complicated
   a) Hormone therapy
   b) Radiation
   c) Surgical resection

REVIEW QUESTIONS

1. A 60-year-old male comes to the clinic complaining of progressive difficulty urinating. He says that for the past year he has noticed increased urinary frequency, but feels like he has to strain to urinate and that his stream is weak. He gets up to urinate 5 times at night. He is not sexually active. He denies fever, dysuria, or gross hematuria. Rectal exam reveals an enlarged, smooth prostate without nodules. Urinalysis is within normal limits. Serum PSA is normal. He is started on a medication that relaxes smooth muscle in the bladder. What receptor is targeted by this medication?

    A. Alpha-1 adrenergic
    B. Alpha-2 adrenergic
    C. Alpha-3 adrenergic
    D. Beta-1 adrenergic
    E. Beta-2 adrenergic

- **The correct answer is A.**
- This is a 60-year-old male who presents with difficulty urinating, increased urinary frequency, straining, and a weak stream. He also has significant nocturia at 5 times per night. He denies fever and dysuria, which lowers the concern for acute urinary tract infection. He also denies gross hematuria, which lowers the concern for a bladder cancer mass causing obstruction. His DRE shows an enlarged, smooth prostate without nodules and his serum PSA is normal. This is consistent with BPH. The medicine he was started on belongs to the class of alpha blockers that target alpha-1 adrenergic receptors, such as tamsulosin.
- B is incorrect because alpha-2 receptors are not found on the bladder or prostate smooth muscle.
- C is incorrect as alpha-3 receptors are not a type of adrenergic receptor
- D is incorrect because beta-1 receptors are primarily found on the heart and do not regulate bladder relaxation.
- E is incorrect because beta-2 receptors, while found on some smooth muscle, are not a target for BPH therapy.

Section V - Inflammatory Conditions of the Breast

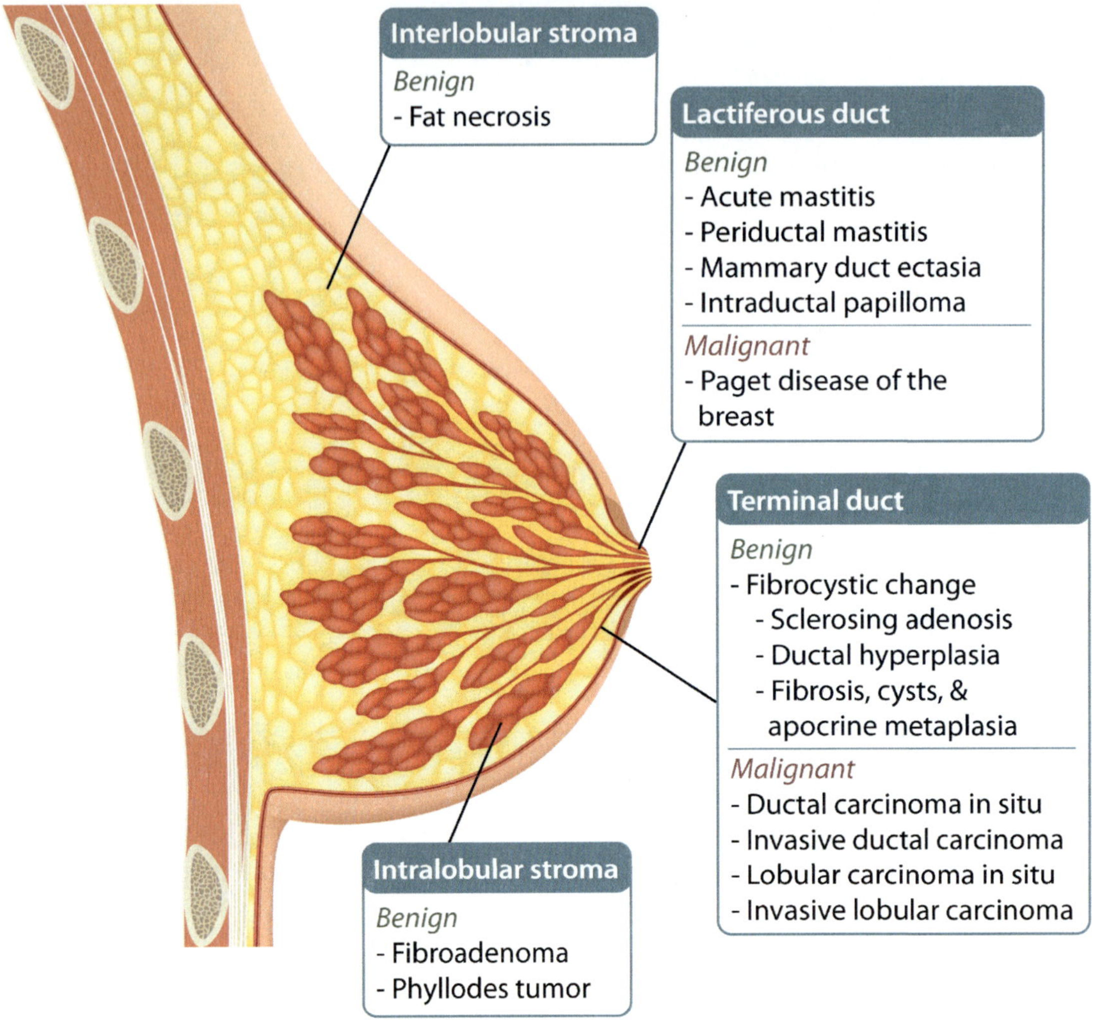

FIGURE 10.3.27 - Tumors Associated with Structural Components of the Breast

Location	Type	Definition	Associations	Clinical findings
Lactiferous ducts	- Acute mastitis	- Bacterial infection of the breast (*S. aureus*)	- Breastfeeding	- Erythematous breast - Purulent nipple discharge
	- Periductal mastitis	- Inflammation of the subareolar ducts	- Smokers	- Subareolar mass - Nipple retraction
	- Mammary duct ectasia	- Inflammation with dilation (ectasia) of the subareolar ducts	- Multiparous postmenopausal women	- Periareolar mass - Green-brown nipple discharge - Chronic inflammation with plasma cells on biopsy
Interlobular stroma	- Fat necrosis	- Necrosis of breast fat	- Trauma	- Mass on physical exam - Abnormal calcification on mammography - Necrotic fat with calcifications and giant cells on biopsy

TABLE 10.3.2 - Inflammatory Conditions of the Breast

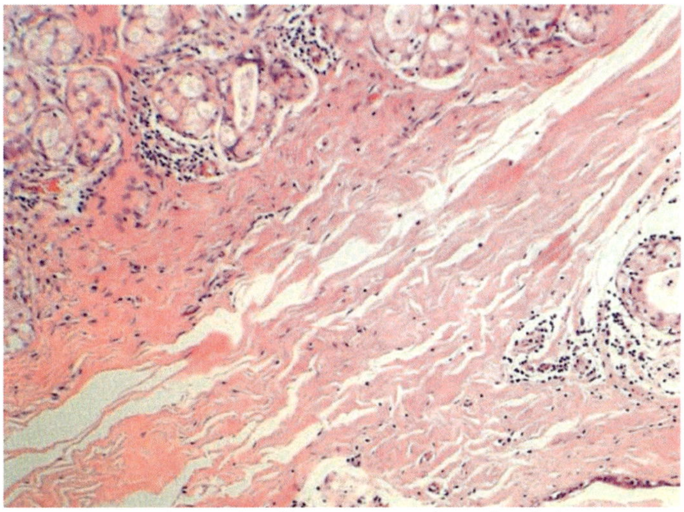

Photo Credit: Sarahkayb / CC BY-SA (https://creativecommons.org/licenses/by-sa/4.0)

FIGURE 10.3.28 - Mammary Duct Ectasia

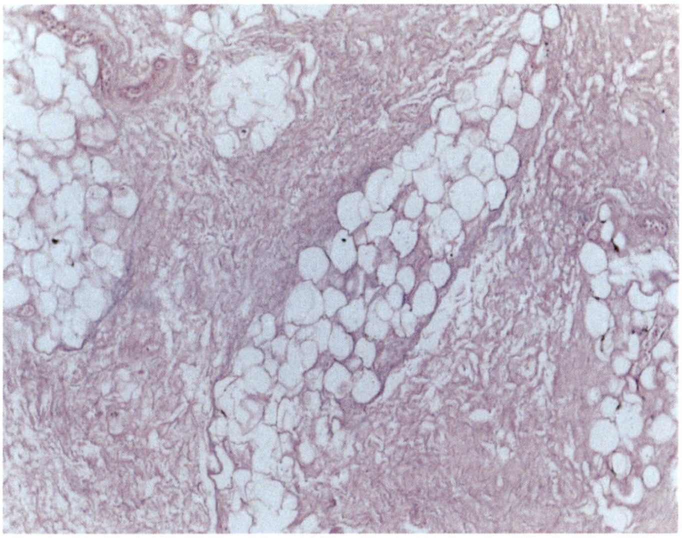

Photo Credit: Calicut Medical College / CC BY-SA (https://creativecommons.org/licenses/by-sa/4.0)

FIGURE 10.3.29 - Fat Necrosis

REVIEW QUESTIONS

1. A 25-year-old woman presents with a 2.0 cm mass in the upper right quadrant of her right breast that she discovered while showering. She denies a history of trauma. A biopsy reveals necrotic fat with calcification. What is the most likely diagnosis?

    A. Acute mastitis
    B. Fat necrosis
    C. Mammary duct ectasia
    D. Periductal mastitis

- **The correct answer is B.**
- A 25-year-old woman presents with a 2.0 cm mass in the upper right quadrant of her right breast
- She denies a history of trauma, but biopsy reveals necrotic fat with calcification.
- Remember that trauma is not always evident in cases of fat necrosis, but that doesn't mean that it did not occur.
- A is incorrect because acute mastitis does not present with a mass or necrotic fat with calcification.
- C is incorrect because mammary duct ectasia presents with a periareolar mass. Since that is the case, we'd expect pathology to be around the nipple, not in the upper right quadrant, as we see in this patient.
- D is incorrect because periductal mastitis presents with a mass just below the nipple.

Section VI - Benign Tumors and Fibrocystic Changes

I. Definition
   A. Growth of fibrosis and cysts in the breast
   B. Most common in premenopausal women 20-50 years old

II. Clinical Findings
   A. Vague irregularity of breast tissue
   B. Usually in the upper outer quadrant
   C. Premenstrual breast pain or lumps

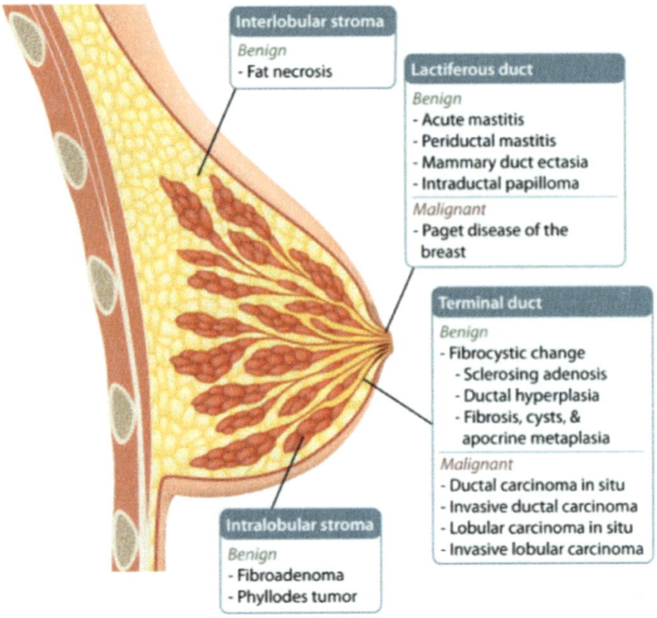

FIGURE 10.3.27 - Tumors Associated with Structural Components of the Breast

III. Subtypes
   A. Fibrosis, cysts, and apocrine metaplasia
      1. No increased risk for carcinoma
   B. Ductal hyperplasia and sclerosing adenosis
      1. Two times increased risk for carcinoma
   C. Atypical hyperplasia
      1. Five times increased risk for carcinoma

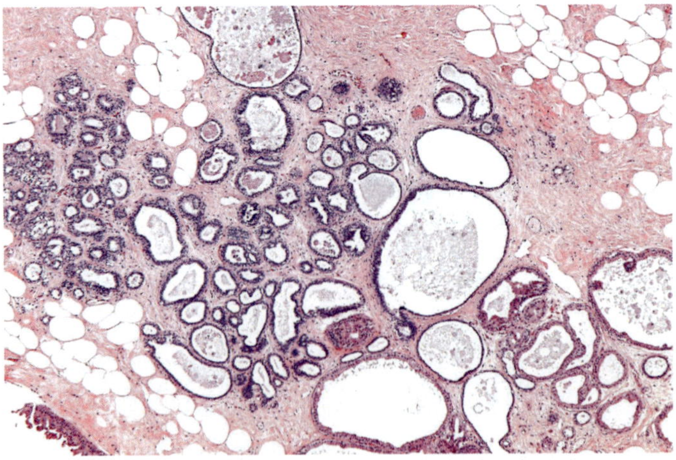

FIGURE 10.3.30 - Fibrocystic Breast Changes with Apocrine Metaplasia (H&E Stain, Low Magnification)

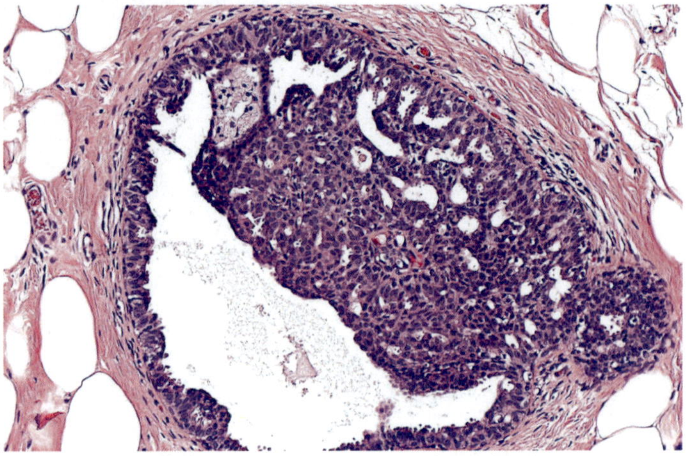

FIGURE 10.3.31 - Proliferative Fibrocystic Changes, Usual Ductal Hyperplasia and Florid Epithelial Hyperplasia (H&E Stain)

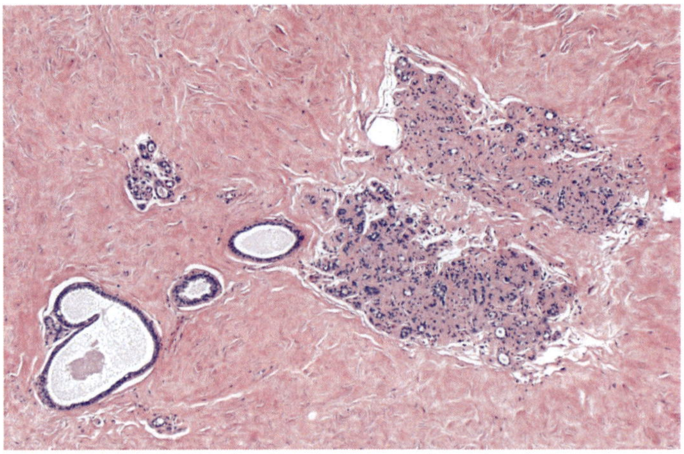

FIGURE 10.3.32 - Sclerosing Adenosis of the Breast (H&E Stain)

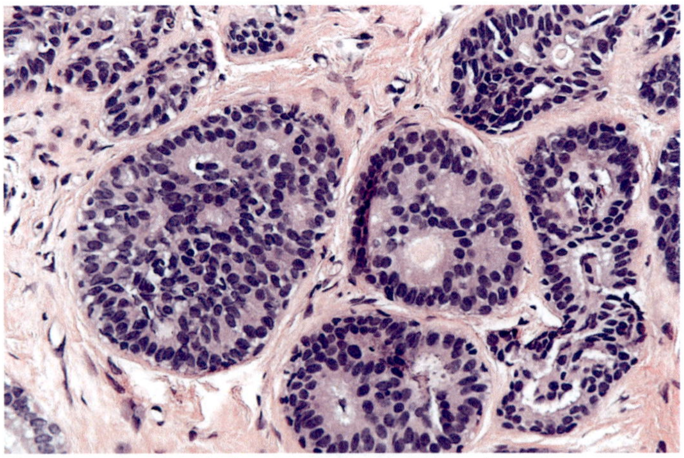

FIGURE 10.3.33 - Atypical Ductal Hyperplasia on Breast Core Biopsy (H&E Stain, Very High Magnification)

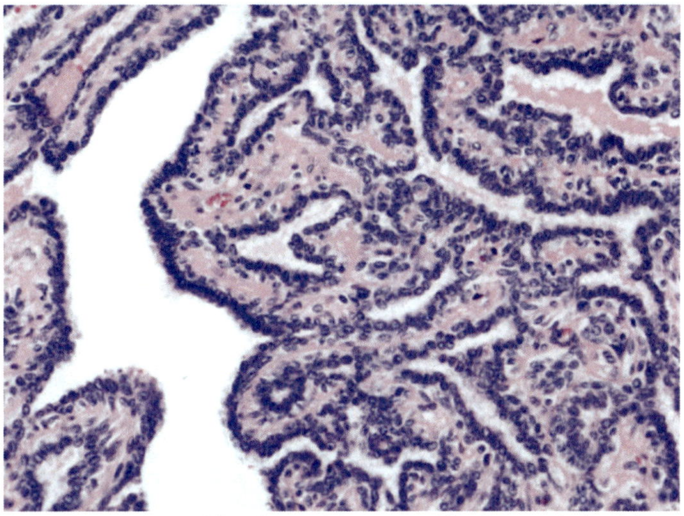

FIGURE 10.3.34 - Intraductal Papilloma of the Breast on Excisional Biopsy (H&E Stain)

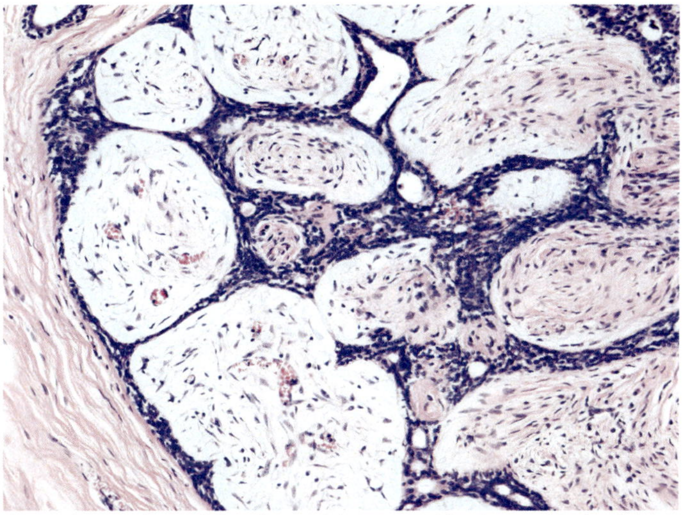

FIGURE 10.3.35 - Breast Fibroadenoma on Core Needle Biopsy (H&E Stain)

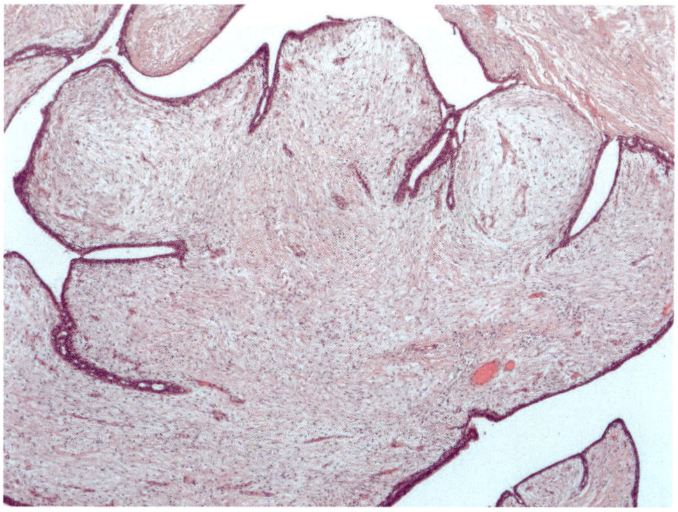

FIGURE 10.3.36 - Benign Phyllodes Tumor of the Breast (H&E Stain, Low Magnification)

Type	Definition	Clinical Findings
Intraductal papilloma	- Small fibroepithelial tumor within lactiferous ducts - Located beneath areola	- Bloody nipple discharge - Premenopausal women - Histology: fibrovascular projections lined by epithelial (luminal) and myoepithelial cells
Fibroadenoma	- Tumor of fibrous tissue and glands - Most common benign breast tumor in premenopausal women	- Well-circumscribed, mobile, marble-like mass - Grows during pregnancy - May be painful during menstrual cycle - Histology: benign-appearing cellular or myxoid stroma that encircles epithelial-lined granular and cystic spaces
Phyllodes tumor	- Fibroadenoma-like tumor with overgrowth of fibrous component	- Postmenopausal women - Histology: leaf-like projections

TABLE 10.3.3 - Benign Tumors of the Breast

REVIEW QUESTIONS

1. A 45-year-old woman presents with a lump in her right breast. She has not noticed nipple discharge, skin changes, or alteration in the lump's size. She is perimenopausal. Physical examination reveals a nontender, slightly moveable, 2.0-cm mass in her right breast. She notes the mass is only painful during her menstrual cycle. Where is the mass mostly likely located?

   A. Lactiferous duct
   B. Terminal duct
   C. Intralobular stroma
   D. Interlobular stroma

- **The correct answer is C.**
- A 45-year-old perimenopausal woman presents with a nontender, slightly moveable, 2.0-cm mass in her right breast that is only painful during her menstrual cycle. Given these findings, this woman most likely has a fibroadenoma.
- Fibroadenoma is a benign condition that is found in and affects the intralobular stroma. It presents with a well-circumscribed, mobile, marble-like mass that may be painful during the menstrual cycle.
- A is incorrect because intraductal papillomas occur in the lactiferous duct and would present with a bloody nipple discharge. We are told that she hasn't noticed any nipple discharge.
- B is incorrect because fibrocystic change occurs in the terminal duct. Fibrocystic change does not present as a moveable mass.
- D is incorrect because fat necrosis occurs in the interlobular stroma. Fat necrosis is not painful during menstruation.

Section VII - Breast Cancer

I. Basic Principles
   A. Second most common cause of cancer mortality in women
   B. Risk factors
      1. Nonmodifiable factors
         a) Female, first-degree relative with breast cancer, early menarche or late menopause, age
      2. Modifiable factors
         a) Obesity (due to ↑ estrogen)

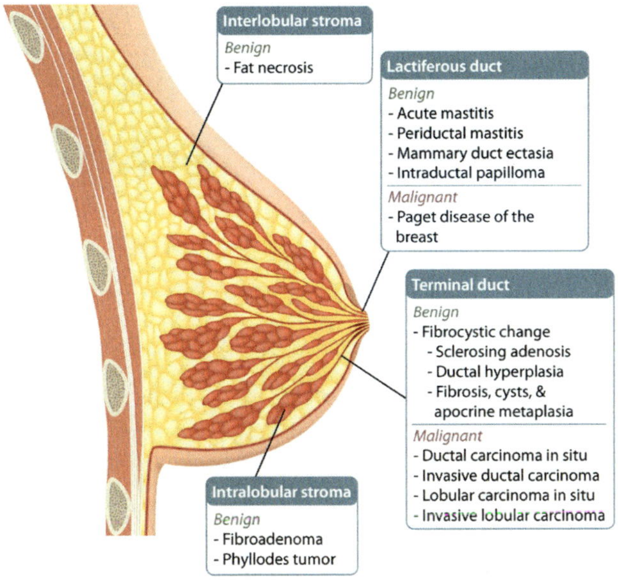

FFIGURE 10.3.27 - Tumors Associated with Structural Components of the Breast

Type	Pathophysiology	Clinical Findings	Subtypes
Ductal carcinoma in situ (DCIS)	- Malignant proliferation of cells in ducts - No basement membrane invasion	- Mammography: calcification - Biopsy: neoplastic cells fill ductal lumen	- Cribriform - Comedo - Paget disease of breast
Invasive ductal carcinoma	- Basement membrane invasion	- Firm, fibrous, "rock-hard" mass with sharp margins - Dimpling of skin or retraction of nipple (advanced) - Biopsy: duct-like structures in desmoplastic stroma	- Tubular carcinoma - Mucinous carcinoma - Medullary carcinoma - Inflammatory carcinoma
Lobular carcinoma in situ (LCIS)	- Malignant proliferation of cells in lobules - No basement membrane invasion	- Discohesive cells lacking E-cadherin - Multifocal, bilateral	
Invasive lobular carcinoma	- Invasive carcinoma lacking desmoplastic response	- Grows in a single-file pattern - Signet-ring morphology - ↓ in E-cadherin expression - Bilateral with multiple lesions	
Hereditary breast cancer	- Autosomal dominant BRCA1 and BRCA2 mutations	- Multiple first-degree relatives with breast cancer - Young age - Multiple tumors	
Male breast cancer	- Associated with BRCA2 mutation, Klinefelter syndrome	- Subareolar mass in older males - Nipple discharge	- Histology: invasive ductal carcinoma

TABLE 10.3.4 - Malignant Breast Cancers

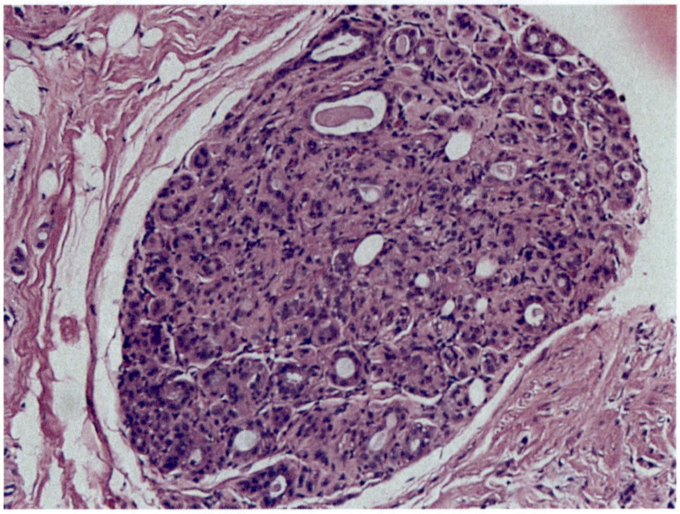

FIGURE 10.3.37 - Cribriform-Type Ductal Carcinoma in Situ of Breast

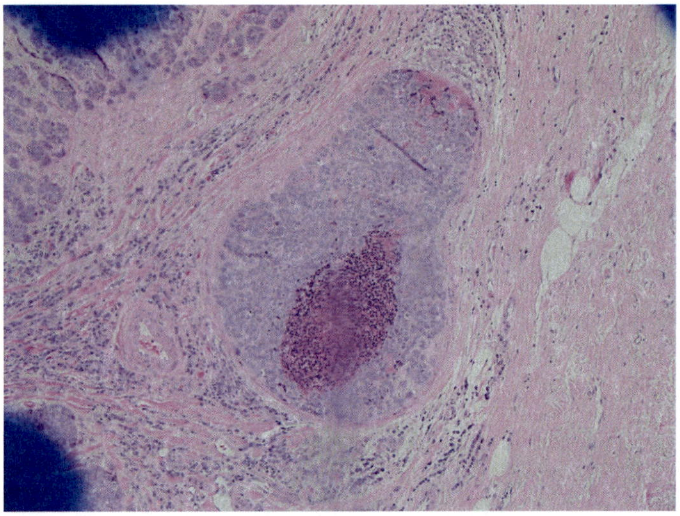

FIGURE 10.3.38 - High-Grade Ductal Carcinoma in Situ with Central Comedo-Type Necrosis

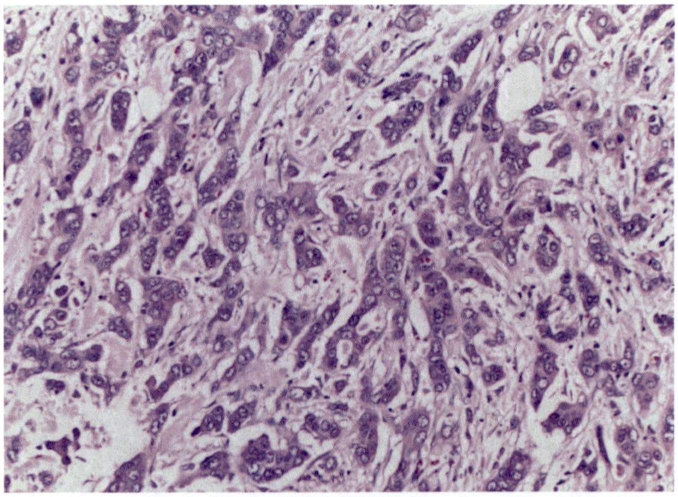

FIGURE 10.3.39 - Malignant Epithelium with Tubules and Solid Sheets Infiltrating into Desmoplastic Stroma

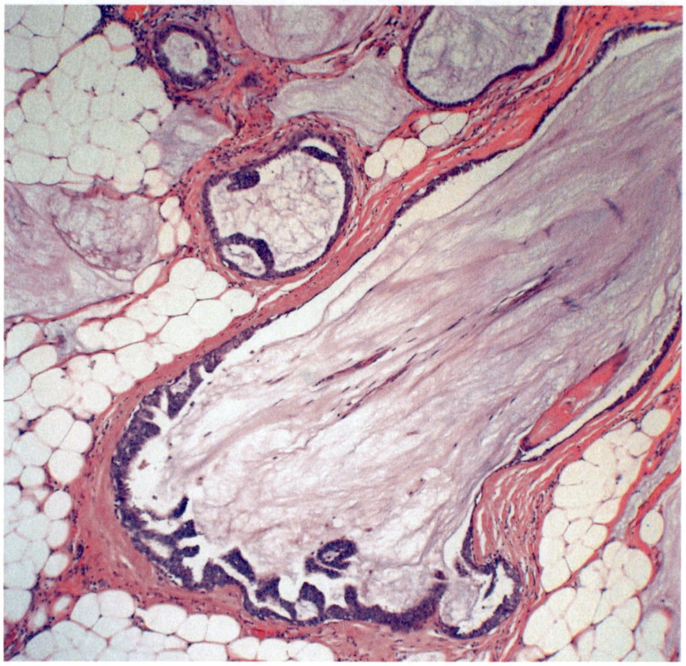

FIGURE 10.3.40 - Mucinous-Type Ductal Carcinoma in Situ of the Breast Showing Mucin Extravasation

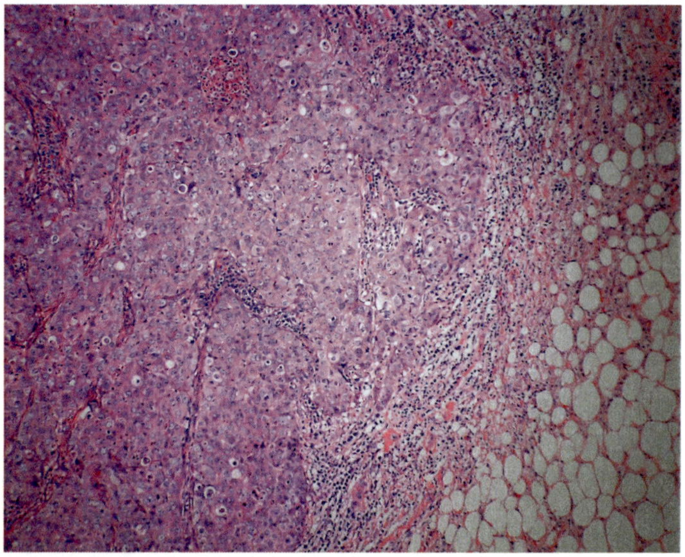

FIGURE 10.3.41 - Medullary Carcinoma of the Breast

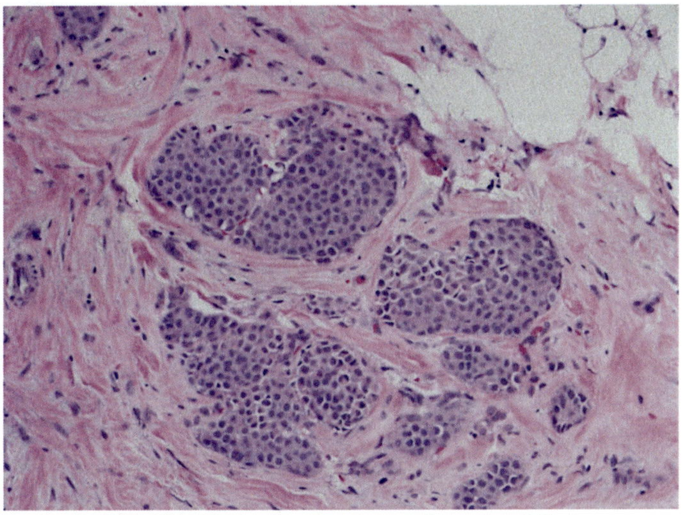

Photo Credit: Difu Wu. / CC BY-SA (https://creativecommons.org/licenses/by-sa/3.0)

FIGURE 10.3.45 - Lobular Carcinoma in Situ

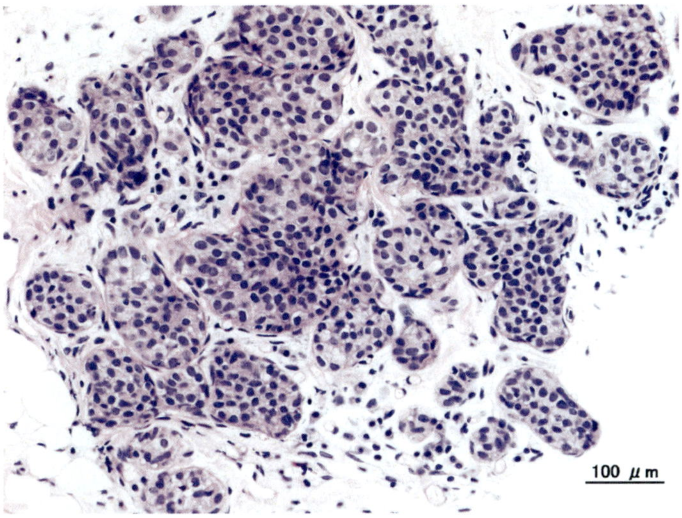

Photo Credit: KGH / CC BY-SA (http://creativecommons.org/licenses/by-sa/3.0/)

FIGURE 10.3.43 - Focal Lobular Growth Pattern in Infiltrating Ductal Carcinoma in Situ

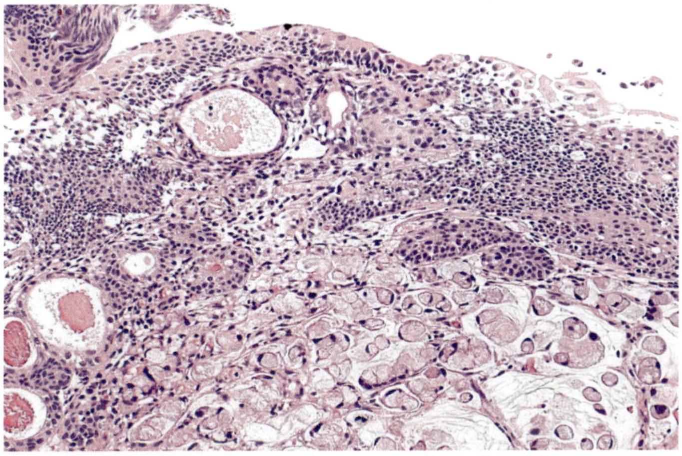

Photo Credit: Nephron / CC BY-SA (https://creativecommons.org/licenses/by-sa/3.0)

FIGURE 10.3.44 - Signet Ring Cell Carcinoma of the Urinary Bladder

II. Paget Disease of the Breast
  A. DCIS that extends up lactiferous ducts to involve nipple skin
  B. Presentation: nipple ulceration, erythema
  C. Almost always associated with underlying carcinoma of breast

III. Tubular Carcinoma
  A. Well-differentiated tubules that lack myoepithelial cells

IV. Mucinous Carcinoma
  A. Abundant extracellular mucin
  B. Older women

V. Medullary Carcinoma
  A. Large, high-grade cells growing in sheets
    1. Lymphocytes, plasma cells
  B. Presentation: well-circumscribed mass
    1. Can mimic fibroadenoma on mammography
  C. Increased incidence in *BRCA1* carriers

VI. Inflammatory Carcinoma
  A. Dermal lymphatics
  B. Presentation
    1. Inflamed, swollen breast with no discrete mass
    2. Peau d'orange appearance

VII. Prognostic Factors
  A. Prognosis based on TNM staging
  B. Metastasis is most important prognostic factor
  C. Spread to axillary lymph nodes is most useful prognostic factor

VIII. Predictive Factors for Treatment
  A. Estrogen and progesterone receptor → anti-estrogenic agents
    1. Tamoxifen, raloxifene
  B. HER2/neu gene amplification → trastuzumab
  C. Triple negative tumors: negative for estrogen receptor, progesterone receptor, and *HER2*/neu gene amplification
    1. Poor prognosis
    2. African American females

REVIEW QUESTIONS

1. A 63-year-old woman presents with persistent swelling and tenderness in her left breast. She was treated with antibiotics for four weeks, but there was no change in her condition. Physical exam reveals a swollen, tender, red, and warm area on the left breast adjacent to the areola. Nipple retraction is also present. What is the most likely etiology of the patient's symptoms?
    - **The answer is dermal lymphatic channel invasion by cancer cells.**
    - The patient is a 63-year-old postmenopasual woman. She has swelling and tenderness in her left breast that could not be relieved with antibiotics along with nipple retraction. This makes infection less likely and inflammation more likely.
    - The most likely diagnosis is inflammatory carcinoma, which is due to dermal lymphatic channel invasion by cancer cells.

2. A 54-year-old woman presents with a lump in her left breast. Physical exam reveals a firm, "rock hard" mass in the upper outer quadrant. Biopsy reveals infiltrating glandular structures lined by poorly differentiated cells and surrounded by desmoplastic stroma. Which subtype of the most likely diagnosis is associated with a BRCA1 mutation?
    - **The correct answer is medullary carcinoma.**
    - A 54-year old woman presents with a firm lump in the upper outer quadrant of her left breast that is described as "rock hard." Biopsy reveals infiltrating glandular structures lined by poorly differentiated cells and surrounded by desmoplastic stroma. This description is highly suspicious of invasive ductal carcinoma.
    - The subtypes of invasive ductal carcinoma are tubular carcinoma, mucinous carcinoma, medullary carcinoma, and inflammatory carcinoma. Of these subtypes, only medullary carcinoma is associated with a BRCA1 mutation.

3. A 45-year-old woman undergoes radical mastectomy for breast carcinoma. Examination reveals metastatic involvement of 4 out of 12 axillary lymph nodes. Immunohistochemistry is positive for estrogen receptors. The estrogen receptor status of breast carcinoma is most likely associated with which of the following clinicopathologic factors?

    A. Diagnostic subtype of carcinoma
    B. Prognosis and treatment
    C. Staging of carcinoma
    D. Likelihood of spread to distant organs

    - **The correct answer is B.**
    - A woman undergoes a mastectomy for breast carcinoma. The carcinoma has metastasized to 4 out of 12 of the axillary lymph nodes, and immunohistochemistry is positive for estrogen receptors.
    - Estrogen receptors, progesterone receptors, and HER/neu gene are used as predictive factors for a patient's response to treatment.
    - A is incorrect because the diagnostic subtype of the carcinoma is not associated with immunohistochemistry (IHC) finding. Subtypes are determined by biopsy findings.
    - C and D are incorrect because the staging of a carcinoma, as well as the likelihood of spread to distant organs, is determined by TNM staging.

Section VIII - Vulva

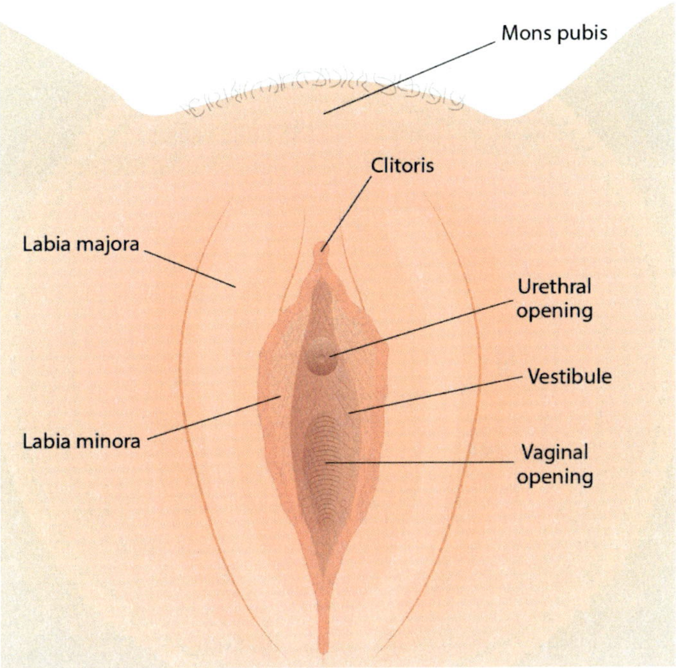

FIGURE 10.3.45 - Vulva

I. Bartholin Cyst
   A. Fluid-filled cyst of Bartholin gland
      1. Due to obstruction of Bartholin duct
      2. Inflammation due to infection or STD
   B. Occurs in women of reproductive age
   C. Unilateral, painful lesion within the lower vestibule

II. Condyloma
   A. Painless genital warts
      1. Sexually transmitted
   B. Condyloma acuminatum (most common): cauliflower buds
      1. HPV serotypes 6 or 11
      2. Koilocytes
   C. Condyloma latum: flat papules due to secondary syphilis
   D. Rarely progress to carcinoma

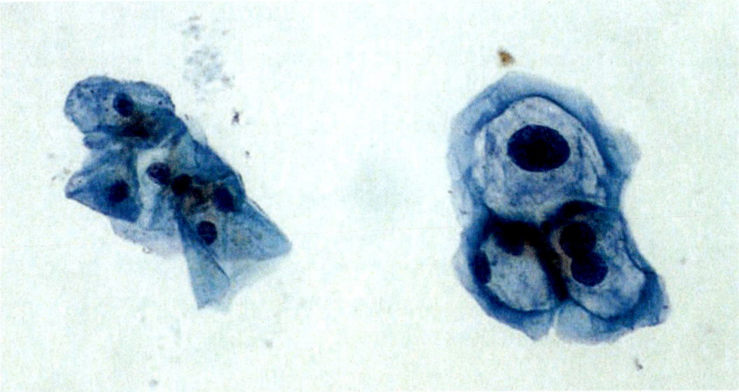

Photo Credit: Photomicrograph by Ed Uthman, MD. 20 July 2006 Euthman 20:24, 29 November 2006 (UTC) / Public domain

FIGURE 10.3.46 - Normal Cervical Cells (Left) and Koilocytes (Right)

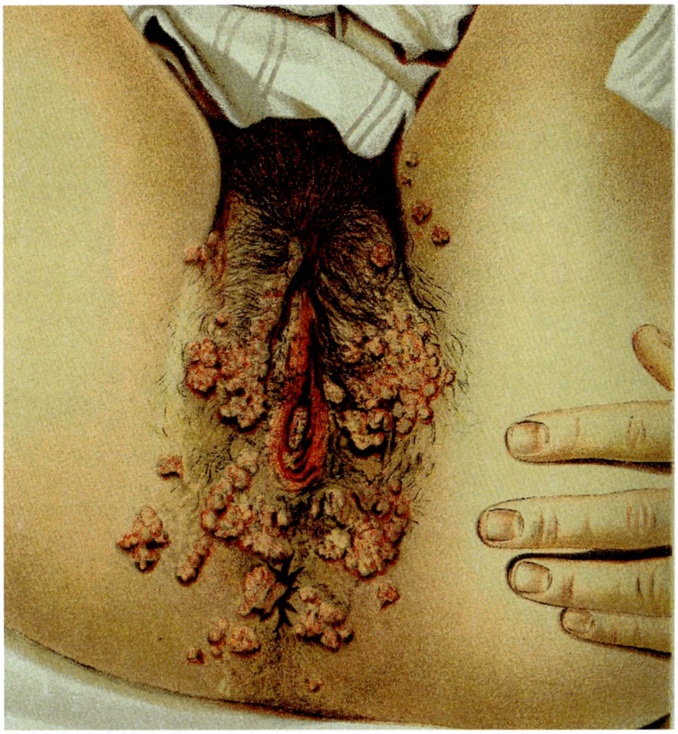

Photo Credit: Samuel Goodwin. https://www.flickr.com/photos/internetarchivebookimages/14597932160

FIGURE 10.3.47 - Condyloma Acuminatum

III. Lichen Sclerosis
   A. Thinning of vulvar epidermis with fibrosis of dermis
      1. "Parchment-like" epidermis
      2. Vulvar leukoplakia
   B. May be associated with autoimmunity
   C. Most commonly present in postmenopausal women
   D. Benign
      1. Minor risk of squamous cell carcinoma

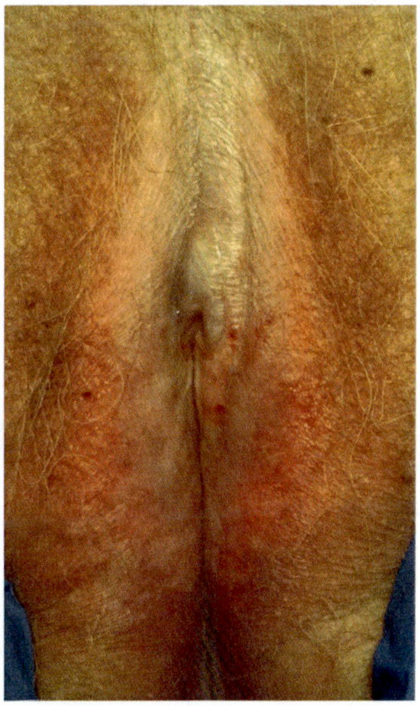

Photo Credit: Mikael Häggström / CC0

FIGURE 10.3.48 - Lichen Sclerosus

IV. Lichen Simplex Chronicus
   A. Hyperplasia of vulvar epithelium
      1. Thick, leathery skin with leukoplakia
   B. Due to excessive scratching from chronic irritation
      1. Insect bites, scars, and atopic dermatitis
   C. Benign
      1. No increased risk of squamous cell carcinoma

V. Vulvar Carcinoma
   A. Squamous cell carcinoma
   B. HPV serotypes 16 or 18
      1. Dysplasia: vulvar intraepithelial neoplasia (VIN)
   C. Chronic lichen sclerosus
      1. Women > 70 years of age
   D. Presents with leukoplakia
   E. Biopsy required to confirm neoplastic growth

VI. Extramammary Paget Disease
   A. Malignant epithelial cells within vulvar epidermis
      1. Carcinoma *in situ*
   B. Presentation: erythema, pruritus, vulvar ulcers
   C. No underlying malignancy

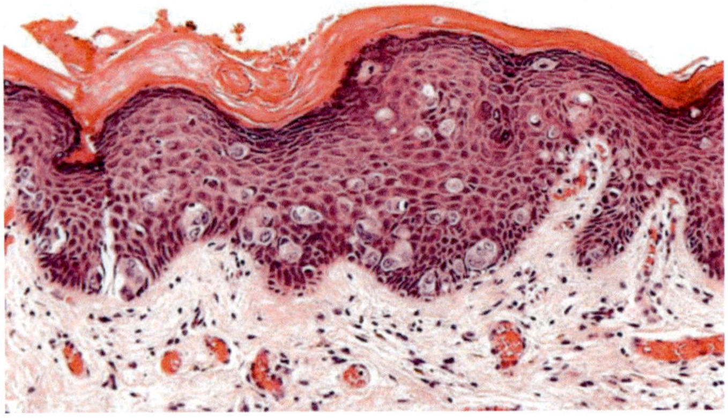

FIGURE 10.3.49 - Extramammary Paget Disease

Stain	Extramammary Paget Disease	Melanoma
S100	-	+
Keratin	+	-
PAS	+	-

TABLE 10.3.6 - Immunohistochemical Stains to Differentiate Between Extramammary Paget Disease and Melanoma

REVIEW QUESTIONS

1. A 27-year-old woman with a history of repeated gonococcal infections presents to the office complaining of pain during sexual intercourse. A physical examination reveals a unilateral tender mass. Which vulvar region was most likely affected?

- **The correct answer is the labia majora.**
- The patient has had past gonorrhea infections and now is having pain during intercourse. This, coupled with the finding of a painful mass on one side, is suggestive of a Bartholin cyst. Bartholin cysts can arise due to an infection and their presence hinders the proper lubrication of the vagina, meaning that patients often present with complaints of painful intercourse. Bartholin cysts are found in the lower one third of the labia majora.

2. A 32-year-old sexually active woman presents to her gynecologist's office for a routine examination. Pelvic examination reveals white patches around her vulvar region. She notifies the doctor that she always feels itchy, and this is relieved when she rubs or scratches her skin. A biopsy reveals regular growth of squamous cells. Which of the following findings would most likely be seen in this patient?

   A. Thin epidermis
   B. Thick epidermis
   C. Vulvar intraepithelial neoplasia
   D. Fibrosis of the dermis

- **The correct answer here is B.**
- We know that the patient has vulvar leukoplakia, or white patches, which is seen in lichen sclerosus, lichen simplex chronicus, and vulvar carcinoma. The biopsy shows no irregular growth, which eliminates vulvar carcinoma. The patient also reveals that she scratches and rubs her vulvar region a lot. This is also consistent with lichen simplex chronicus. Lichen simplex chronicus is caused by hyperplasia of the vulvar epithelium, which causes thickening of the skin. Physical presentation of lichen simplex chronicus involves a thick epidermis and is due to hyperplasia of the epithelium, which results from excessive scratching from chronic irritation.
- A is incorrect because a thin epidermis is a characteristic of lichen sclerosis.
- C is incorrect because vulvar intraepithelial neoplasia is a characteristic of vulvar carcinoma.
- D is incorrect because fibrosis of the dermis is seen in lichen sclerosis.

Section IX - Vagina

I. Embryonal Rhabdomyosarcoma
   A. Also known as sarcoma botryoides
   B. Malignant proliferation of rhabdomyoblasts (undifferentiated skeletal muscle)
      1. Stains positive for desmin
   C. Most common in toddlers < 6
   D. Presentation: grape-like vaginal mass
      1. Vaginal bleeding

II. Clear Cell Adenocarcinoma
   A. Malignant
      1. Adeno → glands
      2. Carcinoma → malignant
      3. Clear cell → abundant clear cytoplasm
   B. Risk factor: DES exposure *in utero*
      1. DES: synthetic estrogen previously prescribed to prevent miscarriage or premature birth

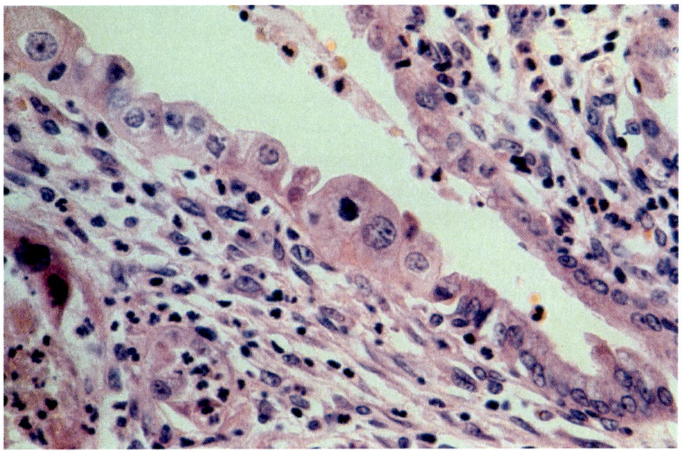

Photo Credit: Unknown photographer / Public domain

FIGURE 10.3.50 - Clear Cell Adenocarcinoma of the Vagina

III. Squamous Cell Cancer
   A. Most commonly secondary to cervical squamous cell cancer
   B. Risk factor: high-risk HPV infection (subtypes 16, 18)
   C. Prevention: HPV vaccine

REVIEW QUESTIONS ?

1. A 2-year-old female presents to the pediatrician with her father. Her father is concerned because he saw blood in her diaper. He also noticed a new "bulge" coming from the patient's vagina. Her vital signs are stable. Physical exam is remarkable for a grape-like mass protruding from the vagina. Biopsy of this mass would most likely show which of the following characteristics?

   A. Positive S100 stain
   B. Positive gram stain
   C. Glandular cells with abundant clear cytoplasm
   D. Positive desmin stain
   E. Positive Tzanck smear

- **The correct answer is D.**
- This is a 2-year-old female presenting with vaginal bleeding and a bulge from her vagina. Physical exam shows a grape-like mass protruding from the vagina, which should make you think of embryonal rhabdomyosarcoma. Rhabdomyosarcomas are a malignant proliferation of immature skeletal muscle cells and stain positive for desmin, an intermediate filament in muscle cells.
- A is incorrect because S100 is a protein found in cells that derive from the neural crest.
- B is incorrect because this is not a bacterial infection.
- C is incorrect because glandular cells with abundant clar cytoplasm is associated with clear cell adenocarcinoma of the vagina.
- E is incorrect because positive Tzank smear would be associated with herpes viruses.

Section X - Cervix

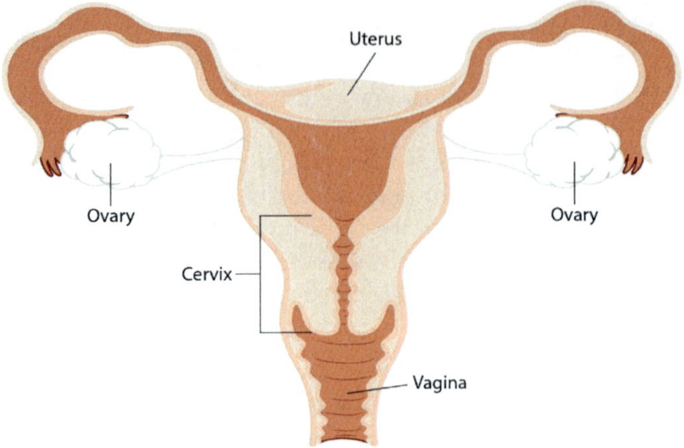

FIGURE 10.3.51 - Normal Female Reproductive Anatomy

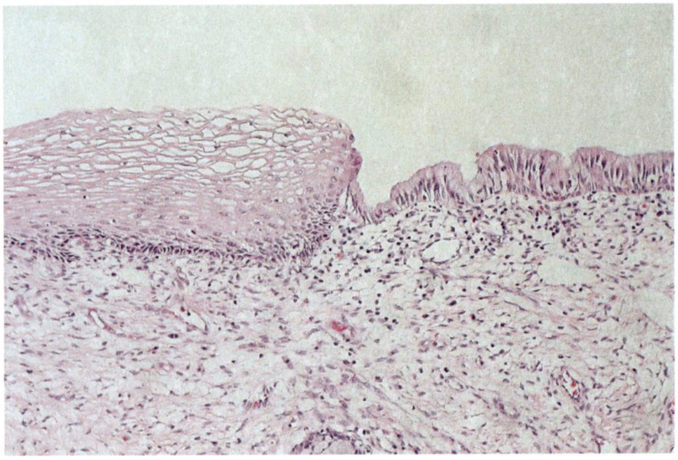

Photo Credit: Ed Uthman. https://www.flickr.com/photos/euthman/4796821432

FIGURE 10.3.52 - Transformation Zone of the Cervix

I. Cervical Intraepithelial Neoplasia
   A. Dysplasia of cervical epithelium that arises due to high-risk serotype HPV infection (produces proteins E6 and E7)
   B. Begins at basal layer of transformation zone and extends outward
   C. Characterized by
      1. Loss of normal cell maturation
      2. High nuclear-to-cytoplasm ratio
      3. Koilocytic change

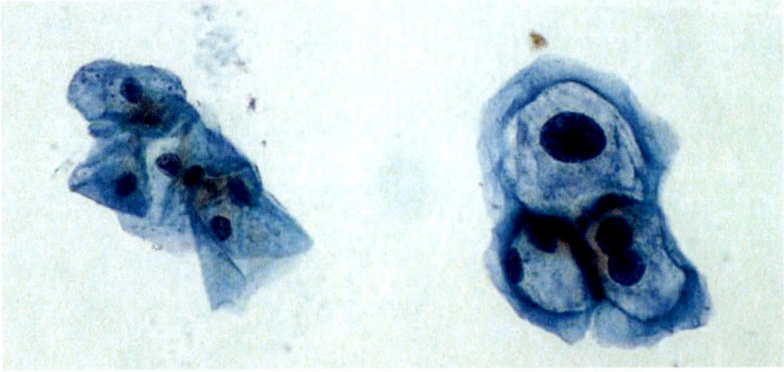

Photo Credit: Photomicrograph by Ed Uthman, MD. 20 July 2006 Euthman 20:24, 29 November 2006 (UTC) / Public domain

FIGURE 10.3.46 - Normal Cervical Cells (Left) and Koilocytes (Right)

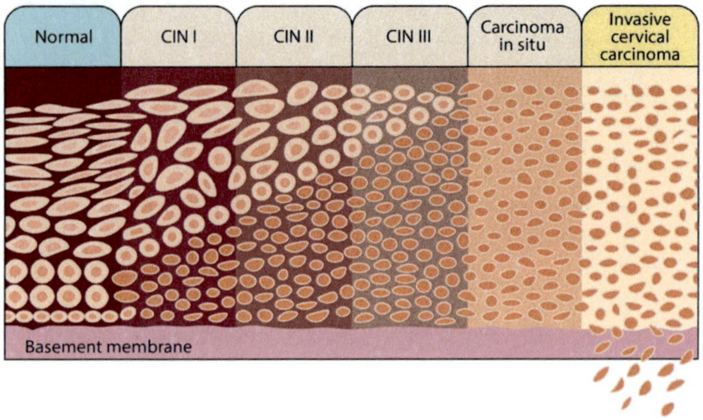

FIGURE 10.3.53 - Degrees of Cervical Intraepithelial Neoplasia

II. Cervical Carcinoma
   A. Basics
      1. Carcinoma in situ: earliest stage of cervical carcinoma
      2. Invasive cervical carcinoma: tumor invasion of basement membrane
      3. Middle-aged women (ages 40-50)
      4. Usually asymptomatic or some vaginal bleeding (postcoital)
      5. Types:
         a) Squamous cell carcinoma (80%)
         b) Adenocarcinoma (15%)
   B. Risk Factors
      1. Multiple sexual partners (HPV infection)
      2. History of sexually transmitted disease
      3. Immunodeficiency (e.g. HIV/AIDS, transplant)
      4. Tobacco use
      5. Early onset of sexual activity
   C. Complications
      1. Invasion into bladder → hydronephrosis with postrenal failure
         a) Most common cause of death

III. Prevention and Screening
   A. Basics
      1. Gardasil vaccine to prevent HPV
      2. Regular use of condoms
      3. Routine screening helps identify dysplasia before it progresses into carcinoma
         a) Screening via Pap smear
         b) Performed every 3 years starting at age 21
         c) Development of carcinoma from CIN takes 10-20 years

B. Pap Smear
1. Cells scraped from transformation zone and viewed under microscope
   a) CIN I → mild dysplasia (low grade)
   b) CIN II → moderate/severe dysplasia (high grade)
   c) CIN III → severe dysplasia (high grade)
2. Routine Pap smears responsible for marked reduction in morbidity and mortality due to cervical carcinoma

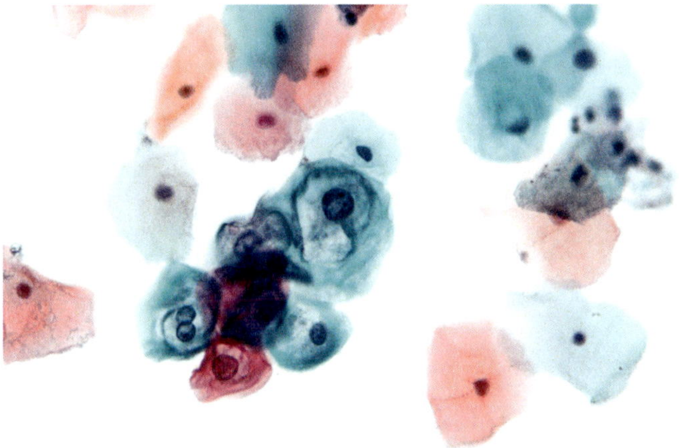

FIGURE 10.3.54 - Abnormal Cervical Cells

3. False negatives may result from inadequate sampling of the transformation zone
4. Limited efficacy for cervical adenocarcinoma screening
   a) Despite Pap smear screening, incidence of cervical adenocarcinoma has not decreased significantly

REVIEW QUESTIONS

1. A 26-year-old woman comes to the clinic for her first gynecological examination. She has a history of HIV and has been noncompliant with her medication. She has had one sexual partner in her lifetime and uses condoms consistently. Her mother had cervical cancer and died at age 46. She does not drink alcohol or smoke tobacco. A Pap smear reveals high grade cervical dysplasia. What is the strongest risk factor for the development of cervical dysplasia in this patient?
   A. Family history of cervical cancer
   B. Age at first intercourse
   C. Immunosuppression
   D. Nulliparity

- **The correct answer is C.**
- The patient's Pap smear revealed high grade cervical dysplasia. We can conclude that she has either CIN II or CIN III. The patient also has HIV and has been noncompliant with her treatment, which makes immunosuppression the correct answer. Immunodeficiency is a risk factor for the development of cervical carcinoma. HIV coinfection with HPV allows HPV to persist because these patients are not able to mount a strong enough immune response against HPV. This leads to the development of cervical carcinoma.
- Choice A is incorrect because family history of cervical cancer is not one of the risk factors associated with the development of cervical dysplasia. There is no genetic component to cervical dysplasia or cancer since it is mainly caused by a persistent HPV infection, which is normally sexually transmitted.
- Choice B is incorrect because she has only had one sexual partner throughout her life. This makes her unlikely to have had her first intercourse before the age of 18. Although it could be a possibility that the patient had had sexual intercourse before the age of 18, answer choice C is still a better answer to this question since it references HIV instead of her age of first intercourse.
- Choice D is incorrect because the number of times a woman has given birth is not a risk factor for the development of cervical dysplasia or carcinoma.

Section XI - Endometrium

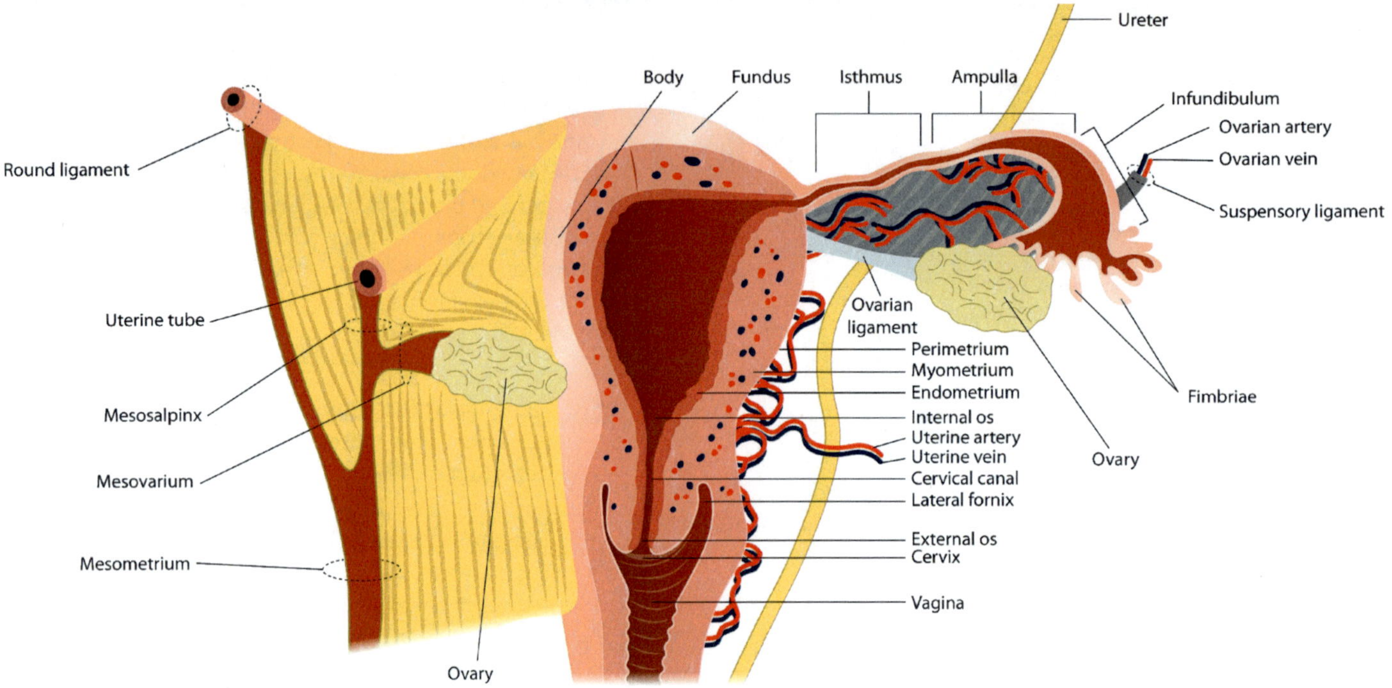

FIGURE 10.3.55 - Uterus

I. Asherman Syndrome
   A. Scar tissue (adhesions) and/or fibrosis of endometrium
      1. Overaggressive dilation and curettage of intrauterine cavity
   B. Clinical findings
      1. Amenorrhea
      2. Pelvic pain
      3. Decreased fertility or recurrent pregnancy loss

II. Anovulatory Cycle
   A. Lack of ovulation
   B. High estrogen without balance of progesterone
   C. Amenorrhea or oligomenorrhea

III. Acute Endometritis
   A. Endometrial inflammation due to bacterial infection
      1. Products of conception not properly removed
   B. Clinical findings
      1. Fever
      2. Abnormal uterine bleeding
      3. Pelvic pain

IV. Chronic Endometritis: Clinical findings
   A. Chronic endometrial inflammation
   B. Presentation
      1. Abnormal uterine bleeding
      2. Pain
      3. Infertility
   C. Biopsy: lymphocytes and plasma cells

V. Chronic Endometritis: Causes
   A. Retained products of conception
   B. Chronic pelvic inflammatory disease
   C. IUDs
   D. Tuberculosis

VI. Endometriosis: Pathophysiology
   A. Non-neoplastic endometrial-like glands and stroma outside of the endometrium
   B. The underlying cause is uncertain, but several theories exist
      1. Retrograde menstruation
      2. Metaplastic transformation
      3. Lymphatic transport

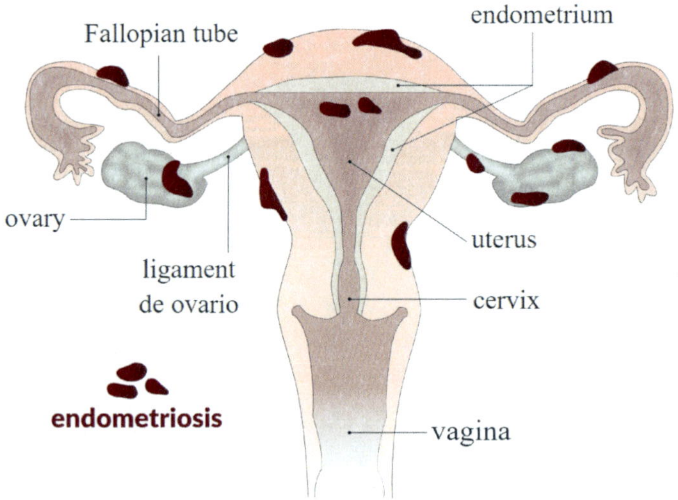

FIGURE 10.3.56 - Endometriosis

VII. Endometriosis: Clinical Findings
   A. Implants classically appear as yellow-brown "gunpowder" nodules
   B. Manifests as pain
      1. Ovary (chocolate cysts) → dysmenorrhea
      2. Uterine ligaments → pelvic pain
      3. Fallopian tube mucosa → ectopic pregnancy
      4. Pouch of Douglas → pain with defecation
      5. Bladder wall → pain with urination

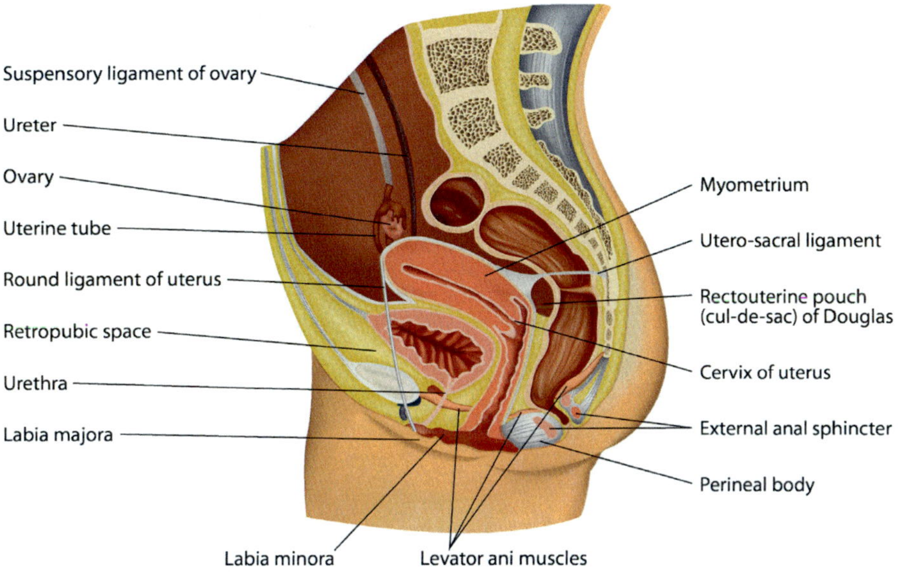

FIGURE 10.3.57 - Pelvic Female Anatomy

VIII. Endometriosis: Complications
   A. Infertility
   B. Increased risk of carcinoma at site of implantation, especially ovary

IX. Endometrial Polyp
   A. Well-circumscribed hyperplastic collection of endometrial tissue
      1. Extends into the endometrial cavity
   B. Painless abnormal uterine bleeding
   C. Side effect of tamoxifen

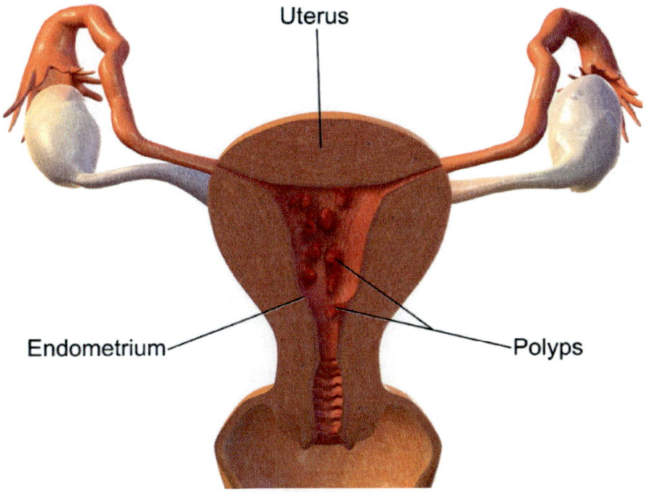

FIGURE 10.3.58 - Endometrial Polyp

X. Endometrial Hyperplasia: Pathophysiology
   A. Abnormal endometrial gland proliferation due to unopposed estrogen
   B. Causes
      1. Obesity
      2. Polycystic ovary syndrome
      3. Estrogen replacement therapy
      4. Granulosa cell tumor
      5. Anovulatory cycle

XI. Endometrial Hyperplasia: Clinical Findings
   A. Postmenopausal vaginal bleeding
   B. Histology
      1. Simple or complex hyperplasia
      2. With or without atypia
      3. Simple hyperplasia with atypia progresses to cancer in 30% of cases
         a) Normal gland-to-stroma ratio and irregular glands
      4. Complex hyperplasia without atypia progresses to cancer in < 5% of cases
      5. Increased gland-to-stroma ratio due to increased glandular crowding

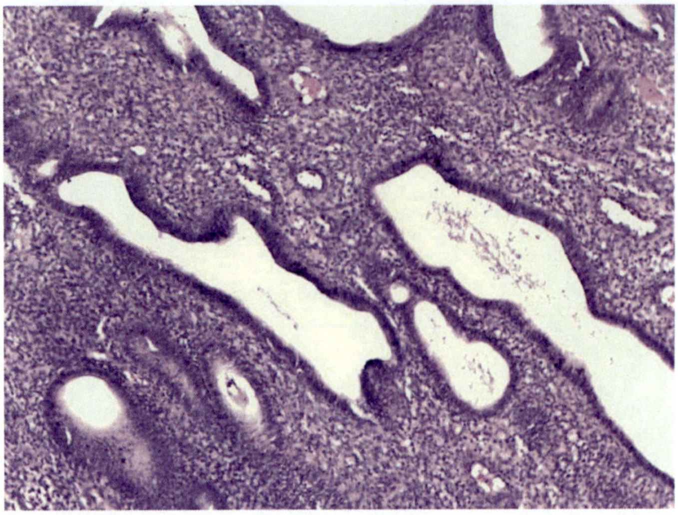

Photo Credit: Calicut Medical College / CC BY-SA (https://creativecommons.org/licenses/by-sa/4.0)

FIGURE 10.3.59 - Simple Endometrial Hyperplasia

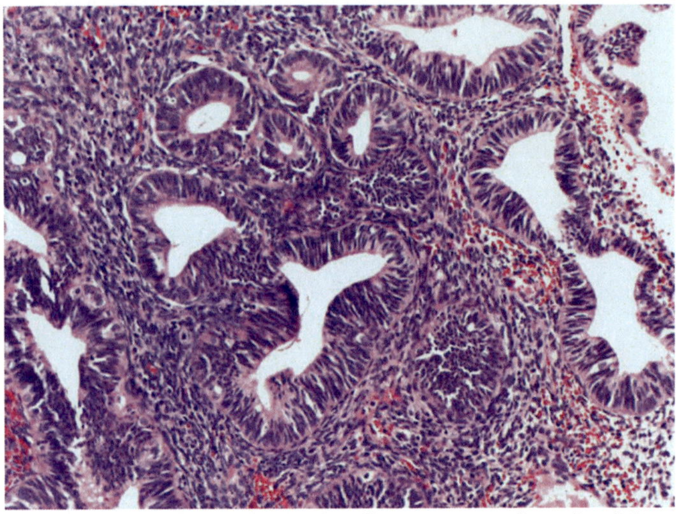

Photo Credit: Calicut Medical College / CC BY-SA (https://creativecommons.org/licenses/by-sa/4.0)

FIGURE 10.3.60 - Complex Endometrial Hyperplasia

XII. Endometrial Carcinoma
   A. Malignant proliferation of endometrial glands
   B. Causes
      1. Endometrial hyperplasia
      2. Sporadic

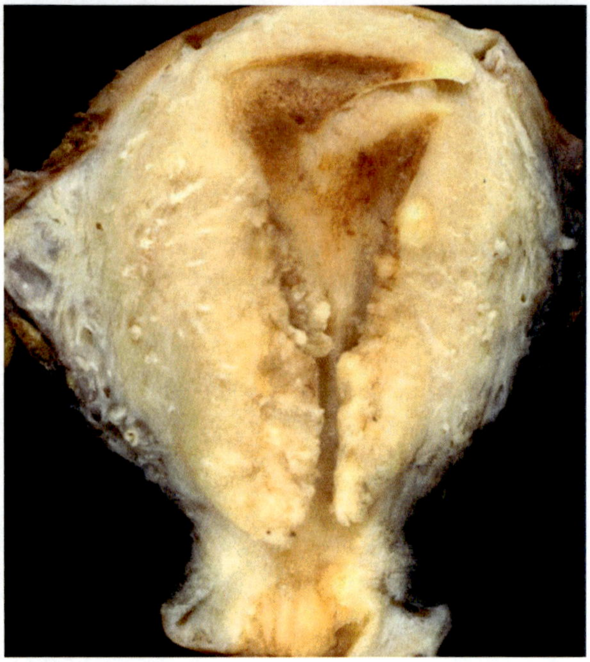

Photo Credit: Ed Uthman via Flickr (CC BY SA 2.0)

FIGURE 10.3.61 - Endometrial Carcinoma

XIII. Endometrial Carcinoma: Hyperplasia
   A. Loss of PTEN or mismatch repair proteins → cell growth
   B. Risk factors
      1. Early menarche/late menopause
      2. Nulliparity
      3. Infertility with anovulatory cycles
      4. Obesity
   C. Histology: endometrioid

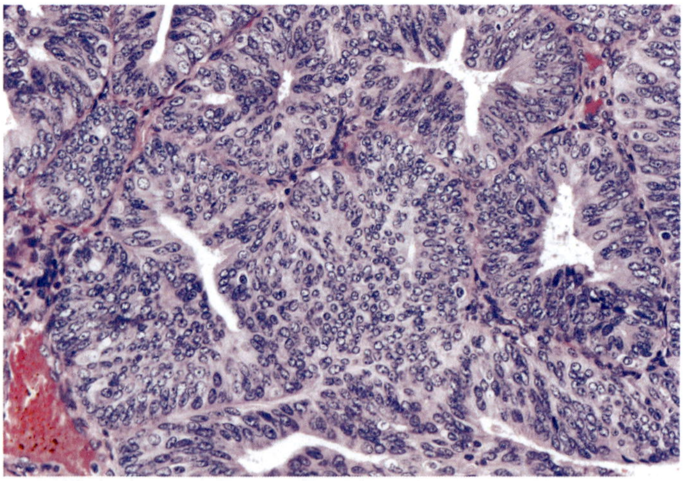

Photo Credit: No machine-readable author provided. KGH assumed (based on copyright claims). / CC BY-SA (http://creativecommons.org/licenses/by-sa/3.0/)

FIGURE 10.3.62 - Endometrial Carcinoma (Hyperplasia)

XIV. Endometrial Carcinoma: Sporadic
   A. Arises in atrophic endometrium with no precursor lesion
   B. P53 mutation is common
   C. Aggressive
   D. Histology: serous with papillary structures and psammoma bodies

REVIEW QUESTIONS

1. A 45-year-old multigravid woman presents with pelvic pain that is worse immediately before and during her menstrual period. A pelvic ultrasound shows ovarian cysts. Biopsy of the cysts reveals endometrial-like glands and stroma. What is the most likely underlying cause of these findings?

    - **The answer is endometriosis due to retrograde menstruation.**
    - A woman presents with dysmenorrhea and ovarian cysts.
    - Biopsy of the ovaries reveals endometrial-like glands and stroma.
    - Given these findings, the patient's diagnosis is most likey endometriosis. The most likely underlying cause of her endometriosis is retrograde menstruation.
    - We can make that conclusion based on the finding of endometrial glands and stroma in the ovaries and dysmenorrhea, which is a common clinical finding for endometriosis.

2. A 32-year-old woman with a history of hyperlipidemia and hypertension presents with fertility concerns. Menarche was at age 10. Her normal menstrual cycle occurs only 6 months out of the year. BMI is 37 kg/m^2. Physical exam reveals acne and thick hair growth on the upper lip and chin. This patient is at greatest risk for a condition that involves which of the following?

    A. Ectopic endometrial tissue
    B. Plasma cells in the endometrium
    C. Increased endometrial gland-to-stroma ratio
    D. Adhesions and fibrosis of the endometrium

    - **The correct answer is C.**
    - An obese (BMI is 37) woman presents with fertility concerns.
    - We learn she had early menarche (age 10), oligomenorrhea (menstrual cycle occurs only 6 months out of the year), acne, and hirsutism (thick hair growth on the upper lip and chin).
    - From these findings, we can determine that the patient has polycystic ovarian syndrome.
    - Next, we need to identify what each of these options refer to.
    - Ectopic endometrial tissue describes endometriosis.
    - Plasma cells in the endometrium describes chronic endometritis.
    - Increased endometrial gland to stroma ratio describes hyperplasia.
    - Adhesions and fibrosis of the endometrium describes Asherman syndrome.
    - PCOS can lead to endometrial hyperplasia due to unopposed estrogen levels.
    - Most women with PCOS are obese because adipose tissue contains aromatase. Aromatase converts androgens to estrogen. In obesity where there's an increase in adipose tissue, there will be an increase in aromatase and estrogen.
    - This leads to abnormal endometrial gland proliferation.
    - And how can you identify this abnormal growth? As mentioned earlier, hyperplasia can be normal gland-to-stroma ratio with irregular glands, or even increased gland to stroma ratio.
    - A is incorrect because this describes endometriosis and PCOS is not a risk factor for endometriosis.
    - B is incorrect because this describes chronic endometritis.
    - D is incorrect because this describes Asherman syndrome.

Section XII - Myometrium

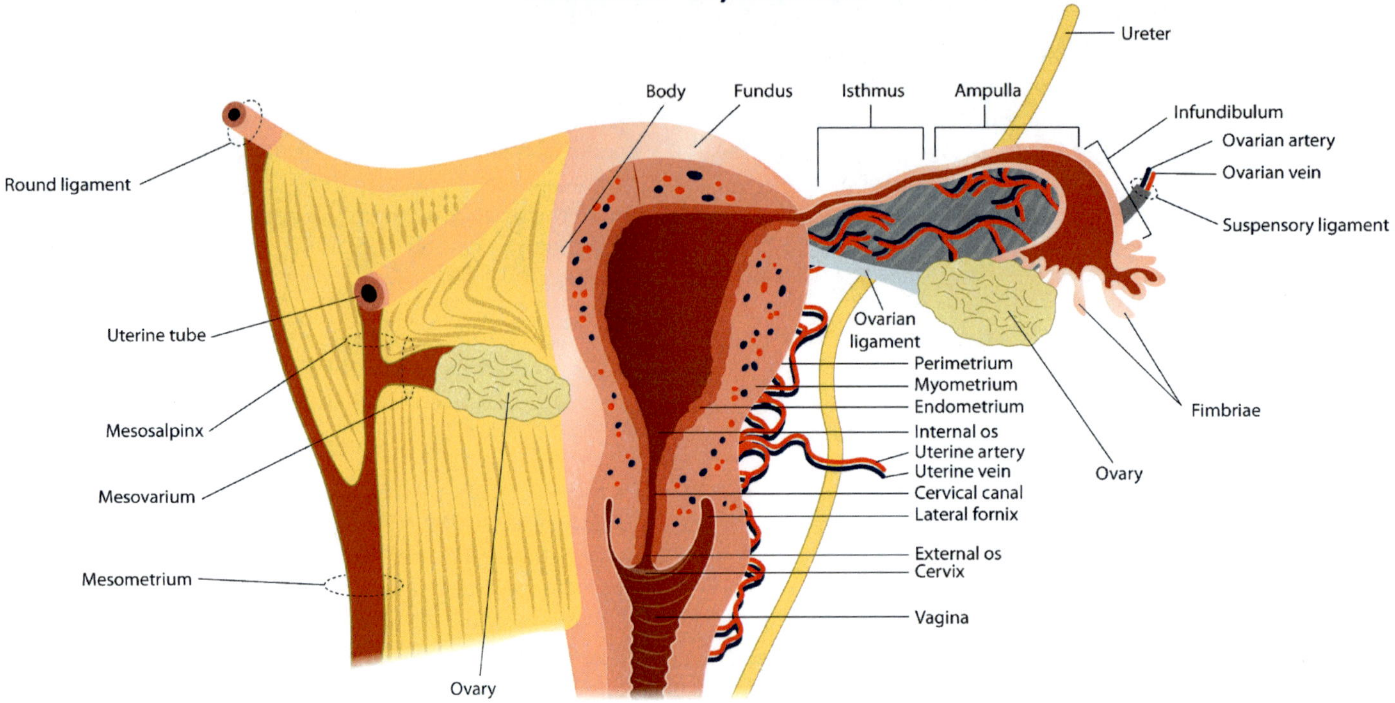

FIGURE 10.3.55 - Uterus

I. Adenomyosis
   A. Endometriosis of myometrium
      1. Extension of endometrial tissue into myometrium
   B. Dysmenorrhea and thickened myometrium

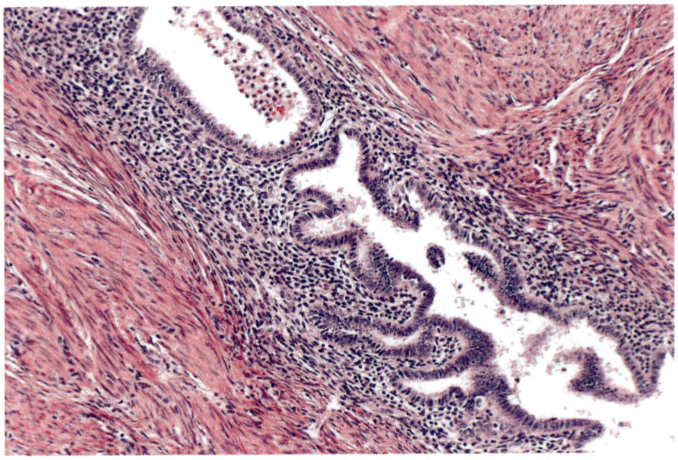

FIGURE 10.3.63 - Adenomyosis

II. Leiomyoma (Fibroids)
   A. Benign neoplastic proliferation of myometrium smooth muscle
      1. Most common tumor in females
      2. Estrogen-sensitive
   B. Usually asymptomatic
      1. Possible abnormal uterine bleeding, infertility, and a pelvic mass
      2. Severe bleeding → iron deficiency anemia
   C. Multiple, well-demarcated, "whorled masses"

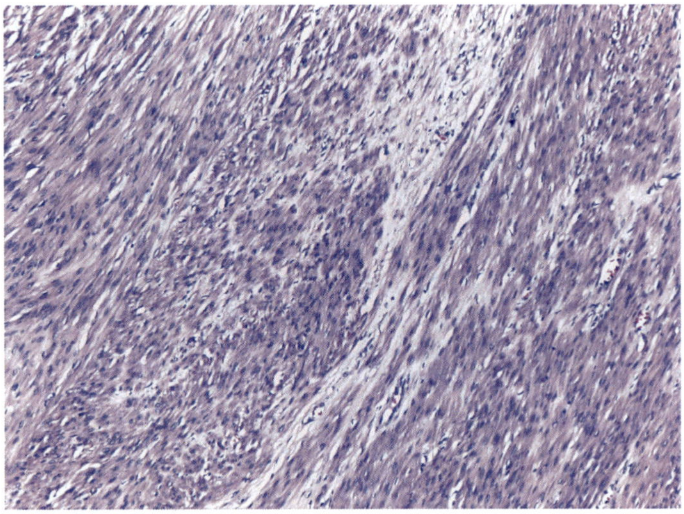

FIGURE 10.3.64 - Leiomyoma (Fibroid Uterus)

III. Leiomyosarcoma
   A. Malignant proliferation of smooth muscle of the myometrium
      1. Arises *de novo*
      2. Postmenopausal women
   B. Gross: single lesion with areas of necrotic tissue and hemorrhage
   C. Histology: necrosis, cellular atypia, and mitotic activity

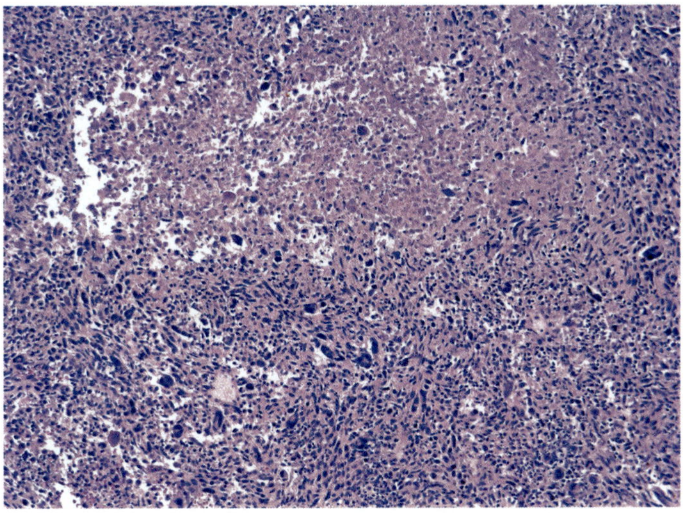

FIGURE 10.3.65 - Leiomyosarcoma

REVIEW QUESTIONS ?

1. A 36-year-old woman with a history of 5 previous spontaneous abortions and chronic pelvic pain presents with fertility concerns. Ultrasound of the uterus reveals a smoothly marginated, submucosal, 5-cm mass on the fundus, as well as multiple small, well-circumscribed subserosal and submucosal masses in the myometrium. Which of the following findings is most likely on microscopic examination of the uterine masses?

   A. Heterogeneous cells with components of endoderm and ectoderm
   B. Whorling pattern of well-differentiated cells
   C. Poorly differentiated cells with abundant atypical mitoses
   D. Moderately differentiated cells with a striated pattern

- **The correct answer is B.**
- We have a premenopausal woman with fertility concerns and chronic pelvic pain.
- Ultrasound reveals multiple masses in the myometrium.
- From this information the patient most likely has fibroids or leiomyomas.
- Leiomyomas are benign neoplastic proliferations of the myometrial smooth muscle. They usually appears as a whorled mass on histologic examination.
- A is incorrect because this describes a teratoma, not a leiomyoma.
- C is incorrect because this describes a leiomyosarcoma, which present with a single lesion and are typically seen in postmenopausal women.
- D is incorrect because this refers to skeletal muscle with a striated pattern, which is more consistent with a rhabdomyosarcoma. And Leiomyomas involve smooth muscle, not skeletal muscle.

Section XIII - Polycystic Ovary Syndrome

I. Definition
   A. Many ovarian follicular cysts due to hormone imbalance
   B. Associated with
      1. Acanthosis nigricans
      2. Obesity

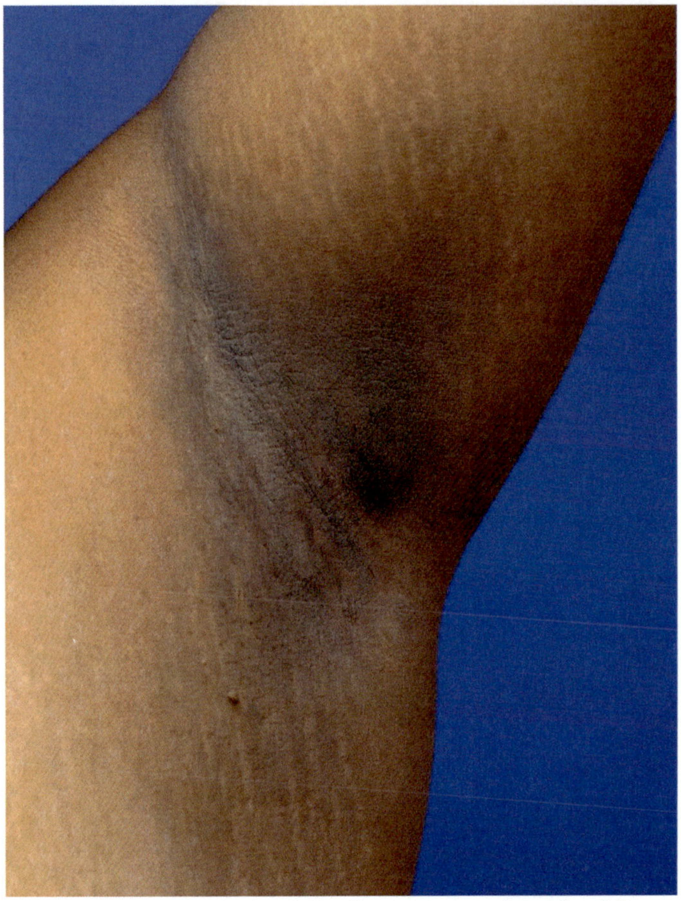

Photo Credit: Mark F. Brady; Prashanth Rawla (https://creativecommons.org/licenses/by-sa/4.0)

FIGURE 10.3.66 - Acanthosis Nigricans

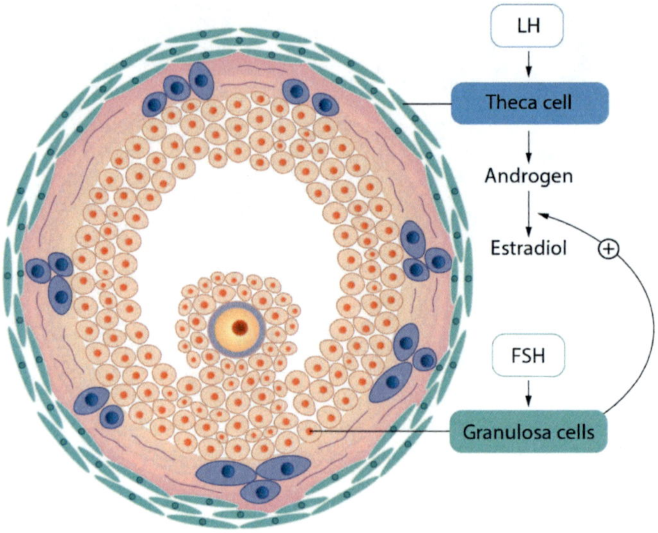

FIGURE 10.3.67 - Theca and Granulosa Cells

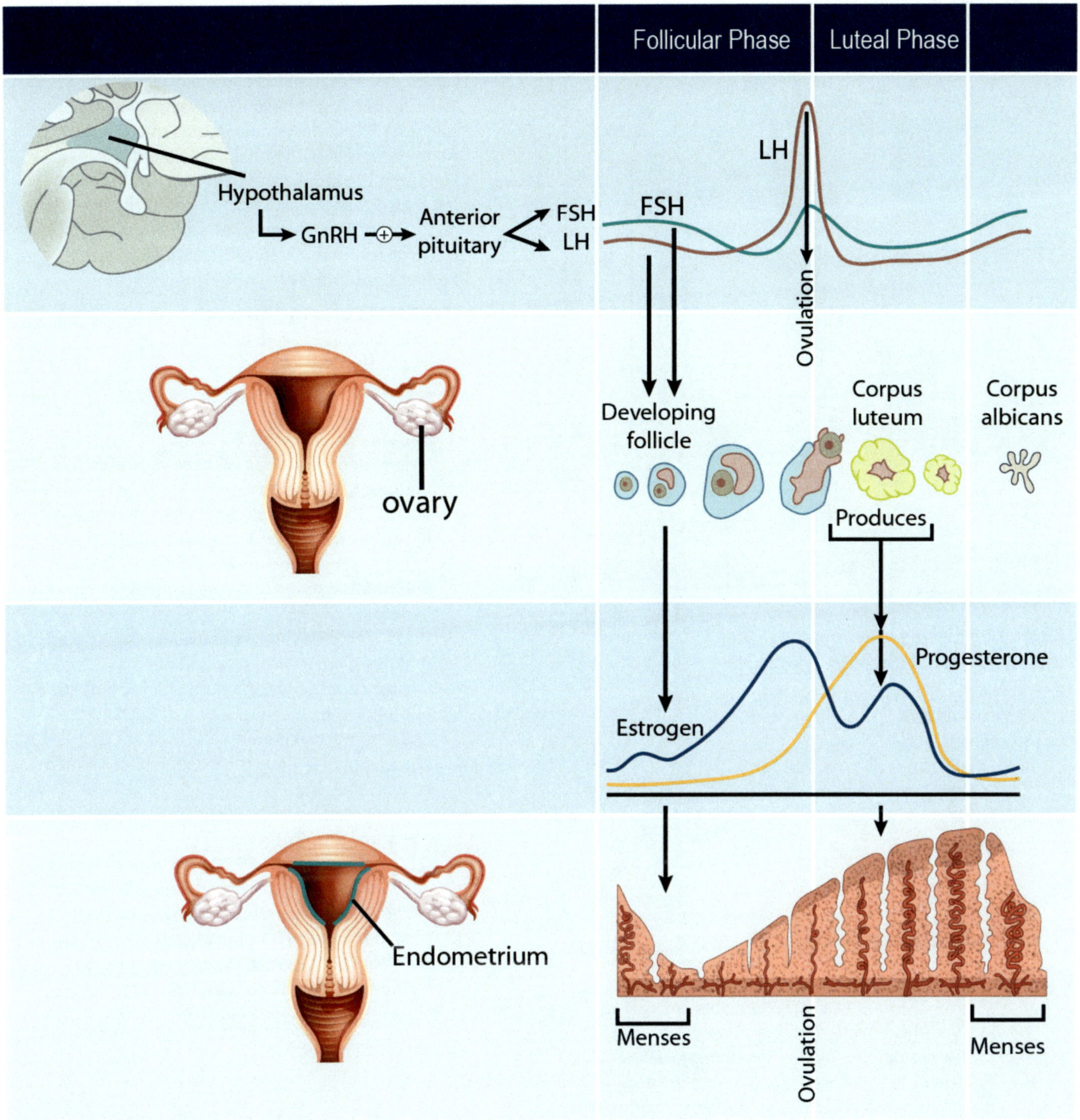

FIGURE 10.3.68 - Ovulation Overview

II. Pathophysiology
   A. Elevated insulin → GnRH gene overexpression → elevated LH levels → elevated LH to FSH ratio → elevated androgens (↑ theca cell stimulation)

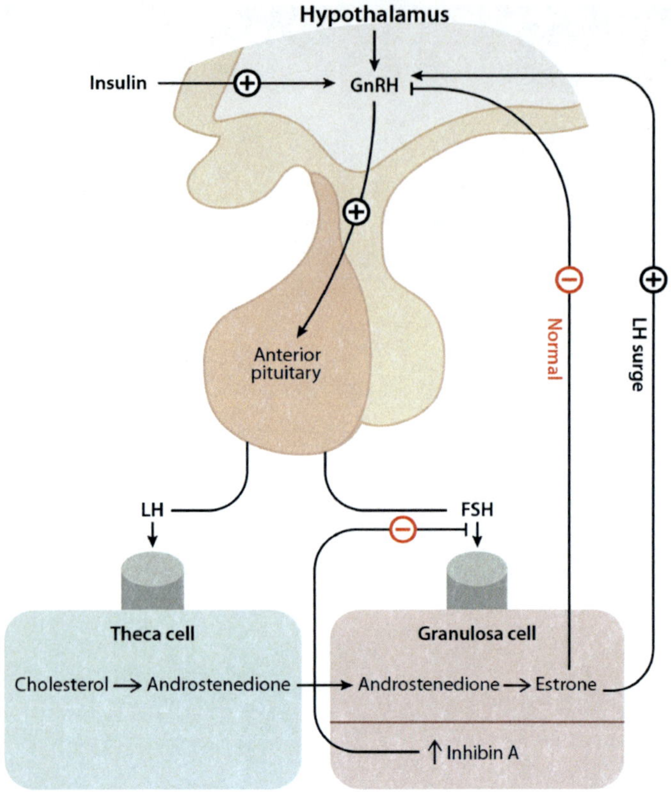

FIGURE 10.3.69 - Hypothalamic Interactions with Anterior Pituitary, Theca Cells, and Granulosa Cells

III. Clinical Findings
    A. Elevated LH/FSH ratio
    B. Amenorrhea/oligomenorrhea
    C. Enlarged, bilateral cystic ovaries
    D. Acne
    E. Hirsutism

IV. Complications
    A. Infertility
    B. Endometrial carcinoma

V. Treatment
    A. Treatment for infertility (i.e. anovulatory cycles)
        1. Weight reduction
        2. Letrozole (first-line) or clomiphene (second-line)
    B. Treatment for androgenicity (e.g. hirsutism)
        1. Oral contraceptives (also prevents endometrial hyperplasia)
        2. May consider spironolactone or finasteride

REVIEW QUESTIONS

1. A 25-year-old sexually active woman with a history of type II diabetes mellitus and hypertension presents to her gynecologist because of vaginal spotting for one year. Physical exam reveals an obese abdomen. An endometrial biopsy yields abundant tissue. Following the biopsy, the patient is lost to follow-up for eight years. She is now brought to the emergency department after fainting at home. Her hemoglobin is 5 g/dL (normal: 12-15 g/dL). What additional finding is most likely?

    A. Elevated FSH/LH ratio
    B. Increased scalp hair growth
    C. Infertility
    D. Diabetic ketoacidosis

- **The correct answer is C.**
- **This patient likely has PCOS complicated by endometrial carcinoma.**
- PCOS is the most likely underlying pathology based on her age (25), the fact that she is sexually active, and a biopsy yielding abundant endometrial tissue (indicating endometrial hyperplasia).
- PCOS is further supported by other associated findings (type II DM, HTN, and obesity).
- Vaginal spotting is not a normal finding of PCOS, but it could be a complication of PCOS (i.e. endometrial carcinoma).
- The patient's anemia is likely due to continued vaginal bleeding.
- A is incorrect because PCOS presents with an elevated LH to FSH ratio.
- B is incorrect because PCOS can cause hirsutism, which presents with male hair distribution, particularly male pattern baldness. Increased scalp hair growth is not expected.
- D is incorrect because this patient has type II diabetes. Diabetic ketoacidosis is typically associated with type I diabetes.

Section XIV - Surface Epithelial Tumors of the Ovary

I. Basic Principles
   A. 3% of all female cancers
   B. US: 5th most common cause of cancer deaths in females

II. Clinical Presentation
   A. Late presentation
   B. Weight loss and loss of appetite
   C. Most common adnexal (pelvic) mass in females > 55 years
   D. Abdominal pain and distention
   E. Bowel changes: constipation and obstruction
   F. Bladder changes: urinary frequency
   G. Ascites
   H. Pleural effusion

III. Risk Factors
   A. ↑ ovulation (age and nulliparity)
   B. Endometriosis
   C. PCOS
   D. Genetic factors: *BRCA1* or *BRCA2* mutations, Lynch syndrome (HNPCC), and family history

IV. Protective Factors
   A. ↓ ovulation
      1. OCPs
      2. Pregnancy
      3. Breastfeeding
      4. Tubal ligation

V. Treatment
   A. Surgical excision
   B. Chemotherapy
   C. Sometimes radiotherapy

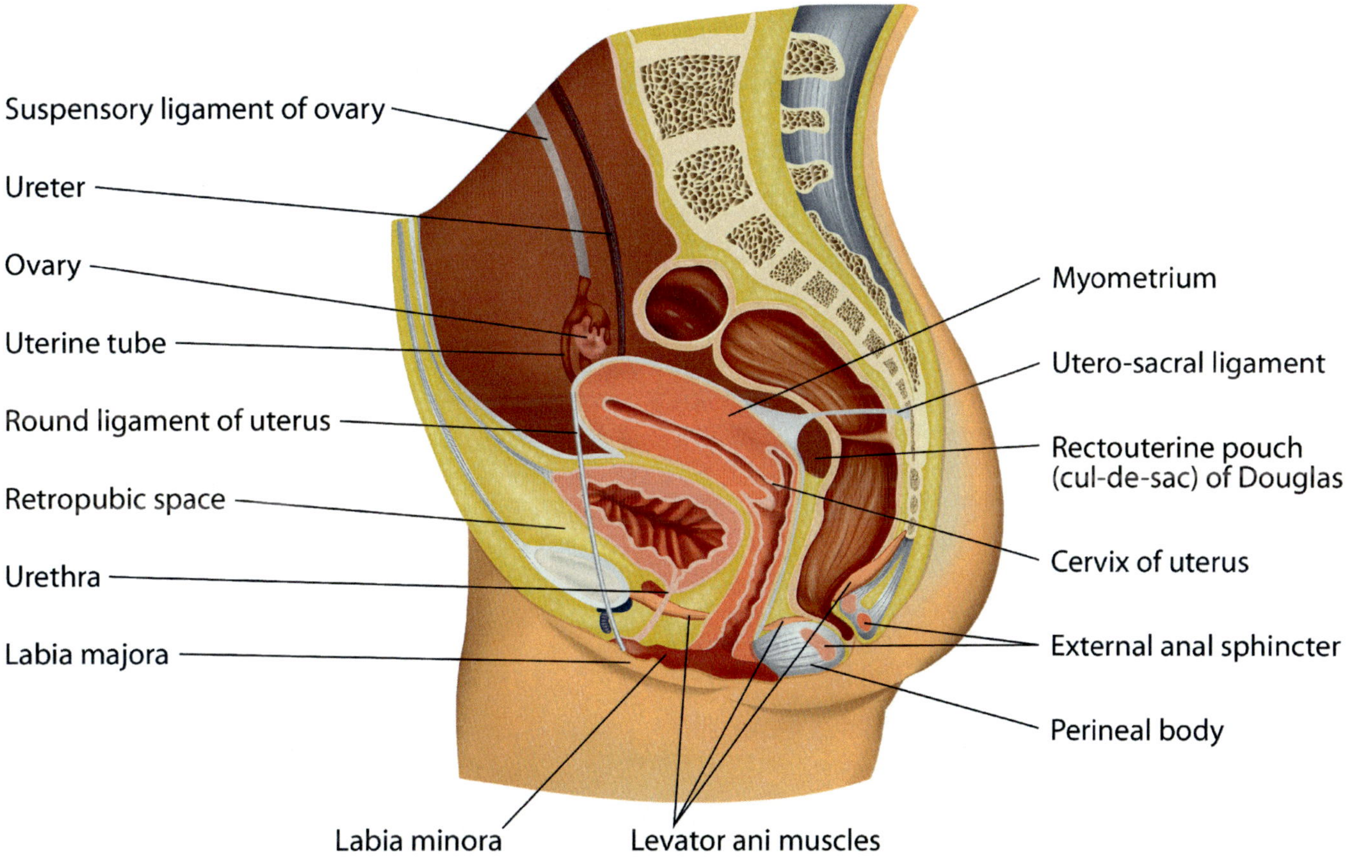

FIGURE 10.3.57 - Pelvic Female Anatomy

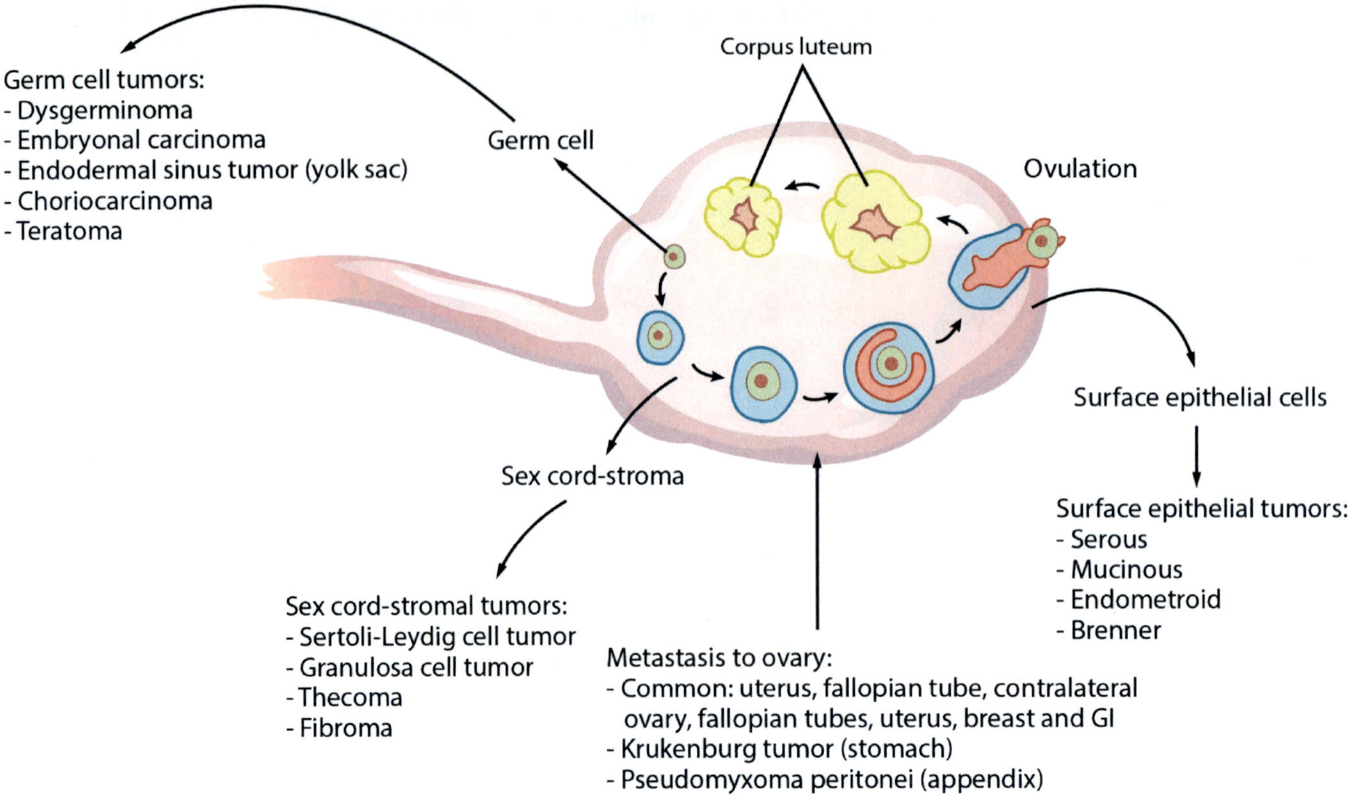

FIGURE 10.3.70 - Types of Ovarian Tumors

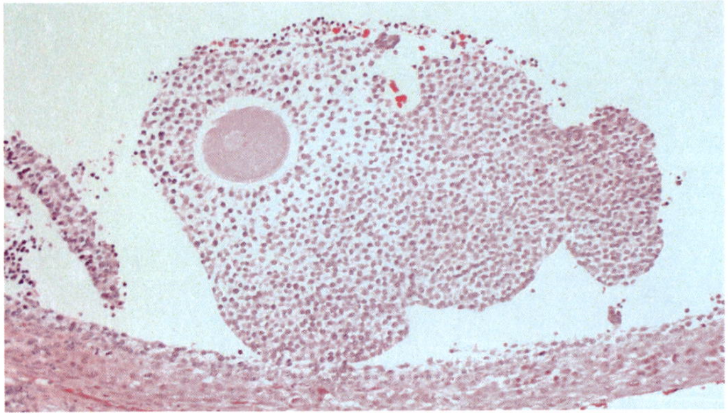

FIGURE 10.3.71 - Histological Image of Ovary

VI. Surface Epithelial Tumors
   A. Constitute about 70% of ovarian tumors
   B. Arise from coelomic epithelium
      1. Embryologic potential to form various tissues
         a) Serous lining in fallopian tubes
         b) Mucinous lining in endocervix
         c) Endometrial lining in uterus
         d) Linings of GI tract, lungs, and liver

Type	Characteristics	Classification
Serous	- Most common ovarian tumor - Bilateral - Secretes serous/watery fluid - Usually cystic, rarely solid - Lined by serous epithelium	- Benign: serous cystadenoma, ages 30-40 - Malignant: serous cystadenocarcinoma, ages 60-70, psammoma bodies - Borderline: metastatic potential
Mucinous	- Secretes thick, mucinous fluid - Cystic - Large mass - Lined by mucinous epithelium	- Benign: mucinous cystadenoma, ages 30-40, large and multiloculated - Malignant: mucinous cystadenocarcinoma, ages 60-70, secondary ovarian tumor, pseudomyxoma peritonei - Borderline: metastatic potential
Endometrioid	- Tubular glands that resemble endometrium - Can arise from endometriosis - 15% associated with endometrial carcinoma	- Malignant
Brenner	- Gross: solid, pale yellow-tan mass - Histologic: urothelium with coffee bean nuclei	- Benign

TABLE 10.3.7 - Surface Epithelial Tumors

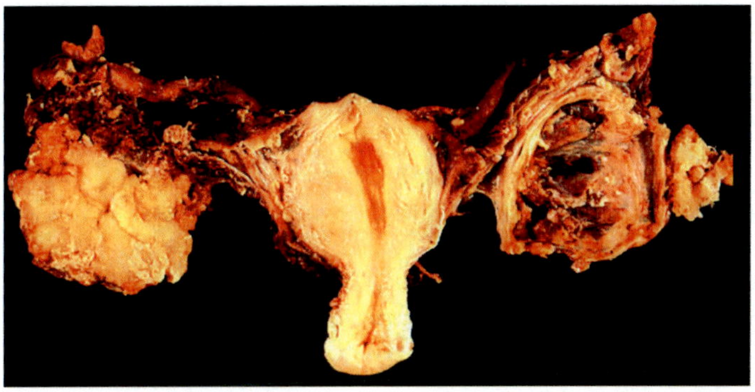

Photo Credit: Ed Uthman M.D. / Public domain

FIGURE 10.3.72 - Gross Image of Bilateral Ovarian Serous Carcinoma

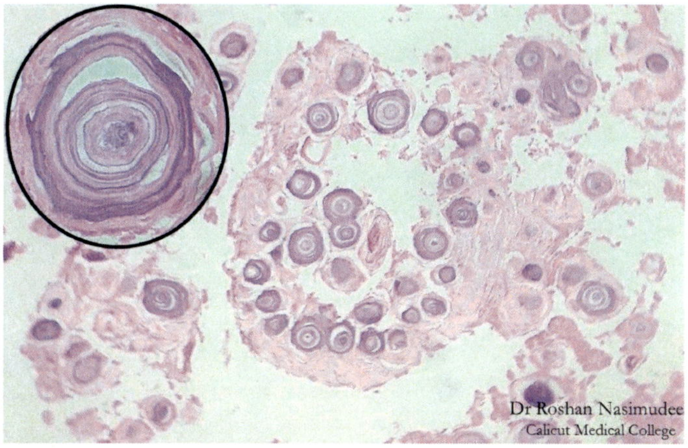

Photo Credit: Dr. Roshan Nasimudeen / CC BY-SA (https://creativecommons.org/licenses/by-sa/3.0)

FIGURE 10.3.74 - Histologic Image Showing Psammoma Bodies

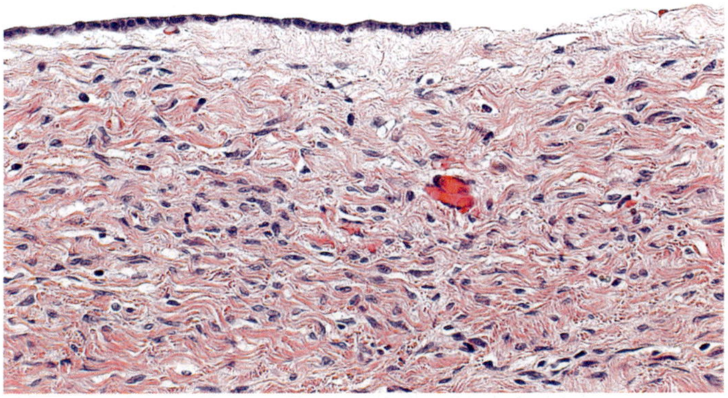

Photo Credit: Nephron / CC BY-SA (https://creativecommons.org/licenses/by-sa/3.0)

FIGURE 10.3.73 - Histologic Image of Serous Cystadenoma

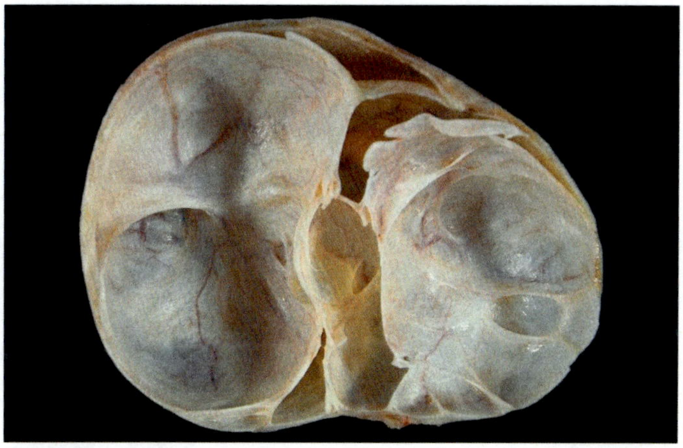

Photo Credit: Ed Uthman, MD. / Public domain

FIGURE 10.3.75 - Gross Image of Mucinous Cystadenoma

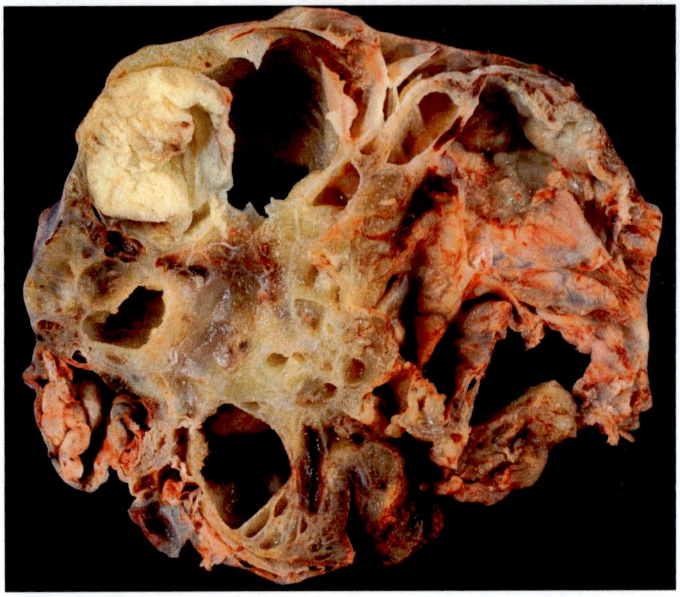

FIGURE 10.3.76 - Gross Image of Mucinous Cystadenocarcinoma

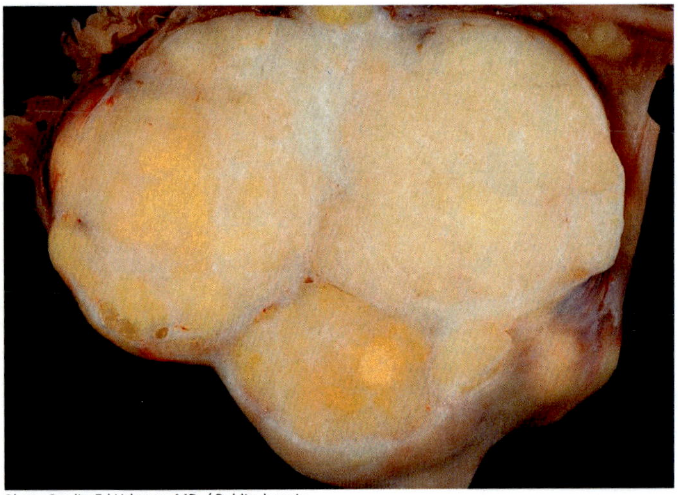

FIGURE 10.3.77 - Gross Image of Brenner Tumor

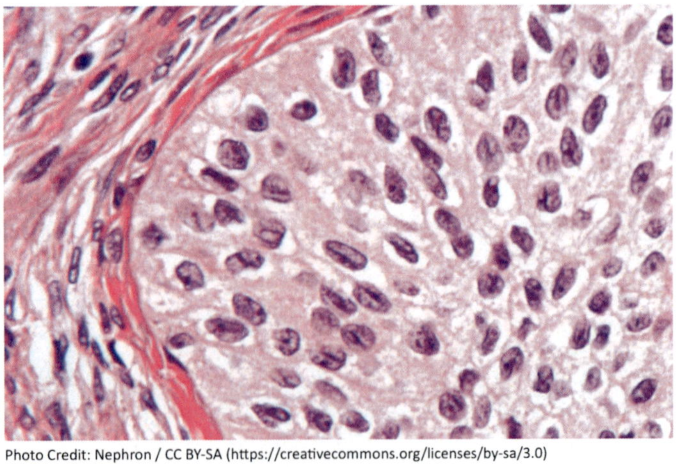

FIGURE 10.3.78 - Histological Image of Brenner Tumor

VII. Tumor Markers
   A. All surface epithelial ovarian tumors secrete CA-125
   B. Other conditions also secrete CA-125 (e.g. endometriosis)
   C. Not suitable for screening
   D. Aids with diagnosis, treatment, and recurrence monitoring

REVIEW QUESTIONS

1. A 31-year-old nulliparous woman with complaints of infertility, dysmenorrhea, and pelvic pain is undergoing workup for an ovarian tumor. Her past medical history is significant for endometriosis. Physical examination reveals no abnormal findings. Laparoscopic examination shows numerous yellow-brown “gunpowder” nodules over the peritoneal surface of the ovary and uterus. Histopathological examination of the ovary reveals tubular glands resembling the endometrium. Which type of ovarian tumor is most likely?

   A. Mucinous cystadenoma
   B. Brenner tumor
   C. Serous cystadenocarcinoma
   D. Endometrioid tumor

- **The answer is D.**
- This patient’s past medical history is significant for endometriosis, which is the presence of ectopic endometrial tissue.
- Her complaints are consistent with endometriosis because she has infertility, dysmenorrhea, and pelvic pain.
- Yellow-brown “gunpowder” nodules over the peritoneal surfaces point towards ectopically implanted endometrial tissue, a characteristic of endometriosis.
- Histopathological finding of tubular glands resembling the endometrium makes it clear that the tumor under discussion is endometrioid.
- Recall also from **TABLE 10.3.7 - Surface Epithelial Tumors** that endometrioid tumors are` characterized by tubular glands that resemble endometrium, and that they can arise from endometriosis.
- A is incorrect because, although mucinous tumors are the most common type of ovarian tumor, our histopathological finding is consistent with an endometrioid tumor.
- B is incorrect because Brenner tumors are quite rare and are marked by a bladder-like epithelium.
- C is incorrect because patients with *BRCA1* and *BRCA2* mutations are more likely to develop serous cystadenocarcinoma; this does not apply to patients with endometriosis. Moreover, histopathological finding is also inconsistent with serous cystadenocarcinoma.

Section XV - Other Ovarian Tumors

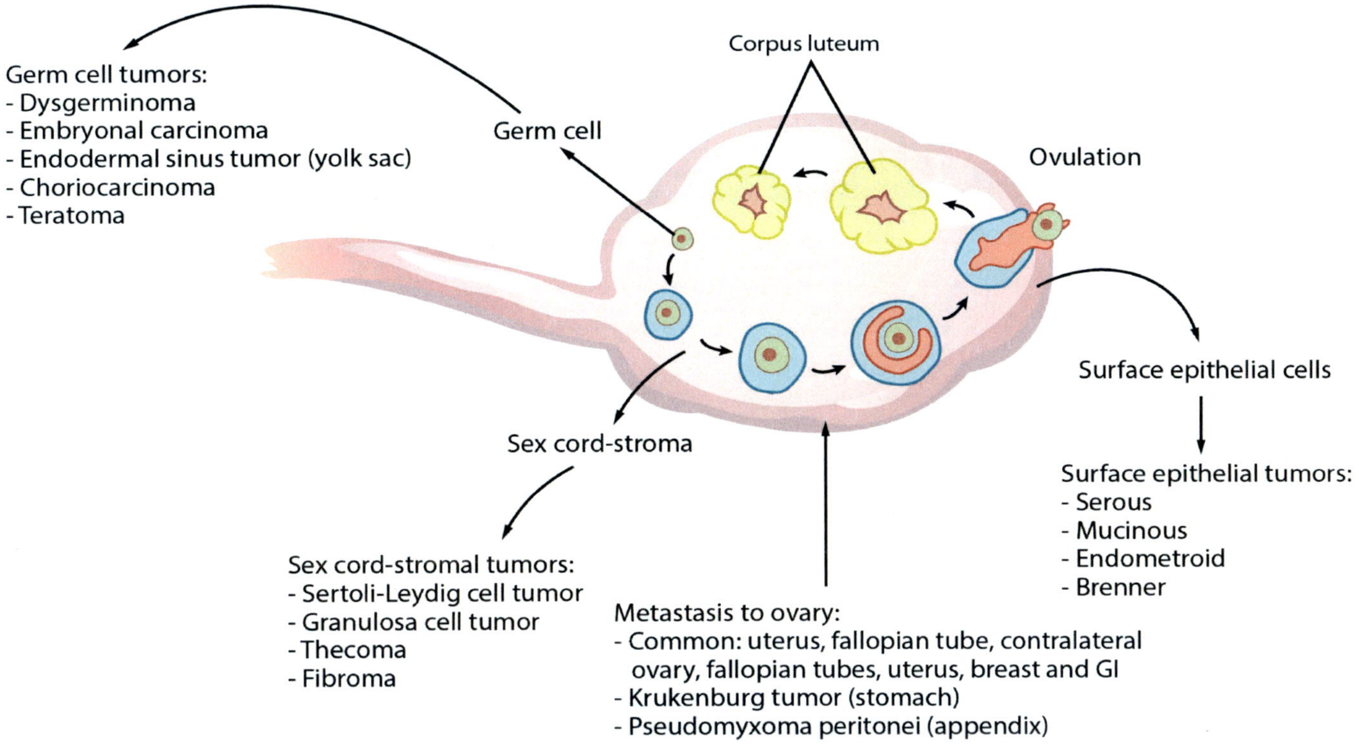

FIGURE 10.3.69 - Types of Ovarian Tumors

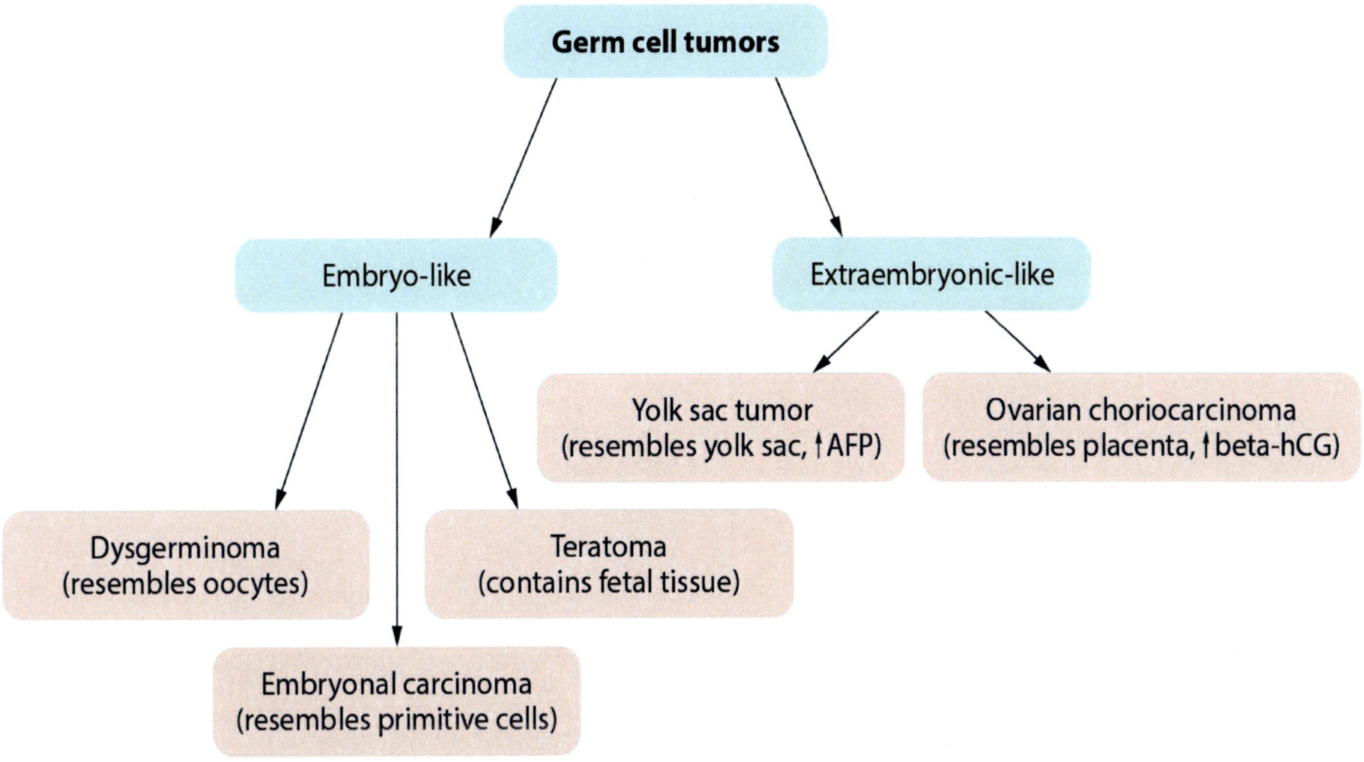

FIGURE 10.3.79 - Classifications of Germ Cell Tumors

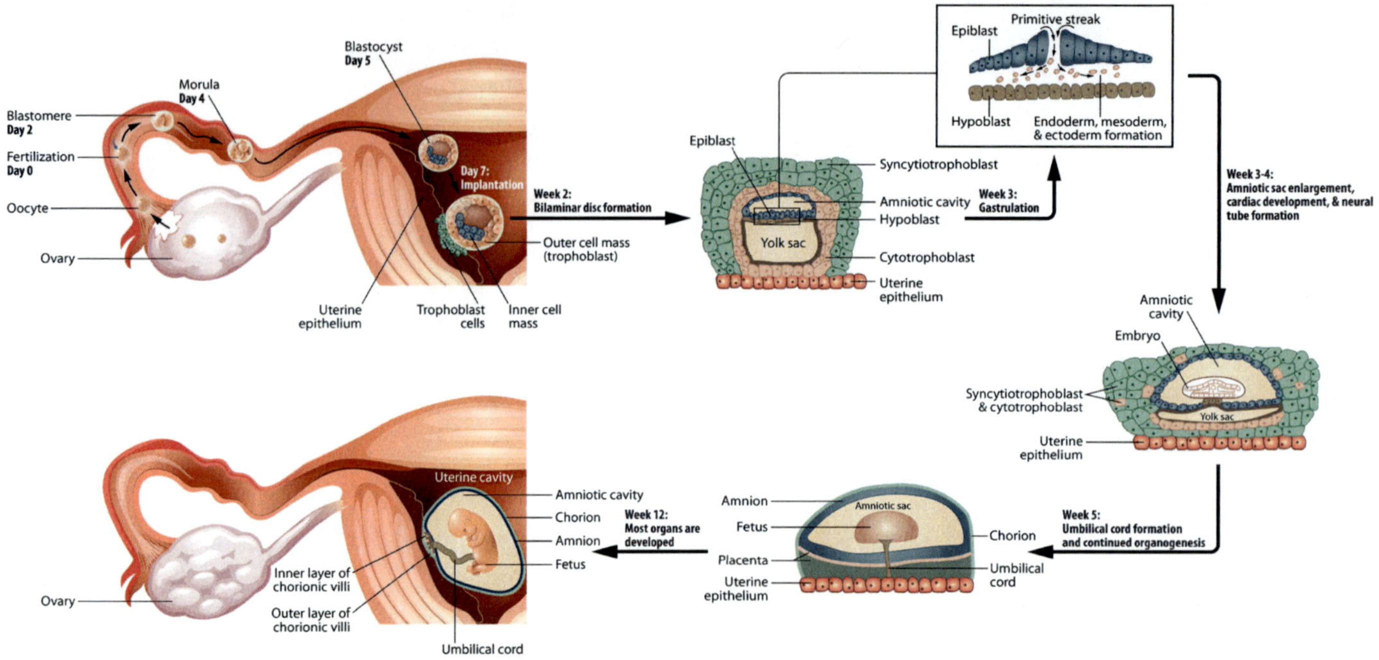

FIGURE 10.3.13 - Nonseminoma Tumor Marker Overview

Germ Cell Tumor	Features	Morphology	Tumor Markers and Treatment Response
Dysgerminoma	- Malignant - Adolescents (2nd-3rd decade) - Most common malignant germ cell tumor - Excellent prognosis - Testicular counterpart: seminoma	- Sheets or cords of uniform cells - "Fried-egg" cells	- Tumor markers: ↑ LDH, ↑ β-hCG - Sensitivie to radiotherapy
Embryonal carcinoma	- Rare - Highly malignant	- Primitive embryonal elements - Resembles embryonal carcinoma of testis	- Metastasizes early
Endodermal sinus (yolk sac) tumor	- Most common germ cell tumor in children - 2nd most common malignant germ cell tumor	- Resembles yolk sac - Schiller-Duval bodies	- Tumor marker: ↑ AFP - >80% survival rate
Ovarian choriocarcinoma	- Resembles placenta - Highly malignant - Usually mixed germ cell tumor	- Syncytiotrophoblasts and cytotrophoblasts	- Tumor marker: ↑ β-hCG - Hematogenous metastasis by the time of diagnosis is common (lungs, liver, bone)
Cystic teratoma	- Mature (benign): Also known as dermoid cyst and most common ovarian tumor in young females (10-30s) - Mature → squamous cell carcinoma - Immature (malignant): rare	- Mature: All 3 germ layers - Immature: immature tissue (neuroectoderm) - Struma ovarii (hyperthyroidism)	

TABLE 10.3.8 - Characteristics of Germ Cell Tumors

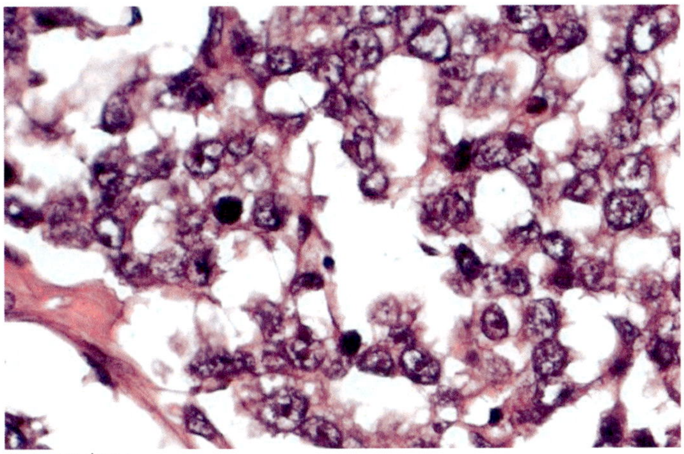

FIGURE 10.3.80 - Dysgerminoma Histology

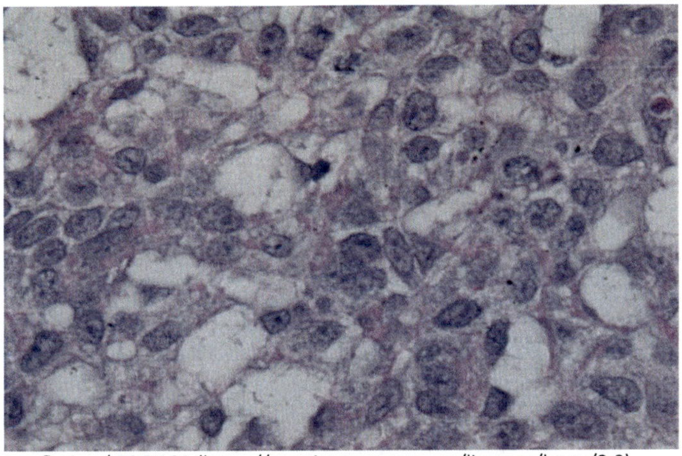

FIGURE 10.3.81 - Schiller-Duval Body in an Endodermal Sinus Tumor

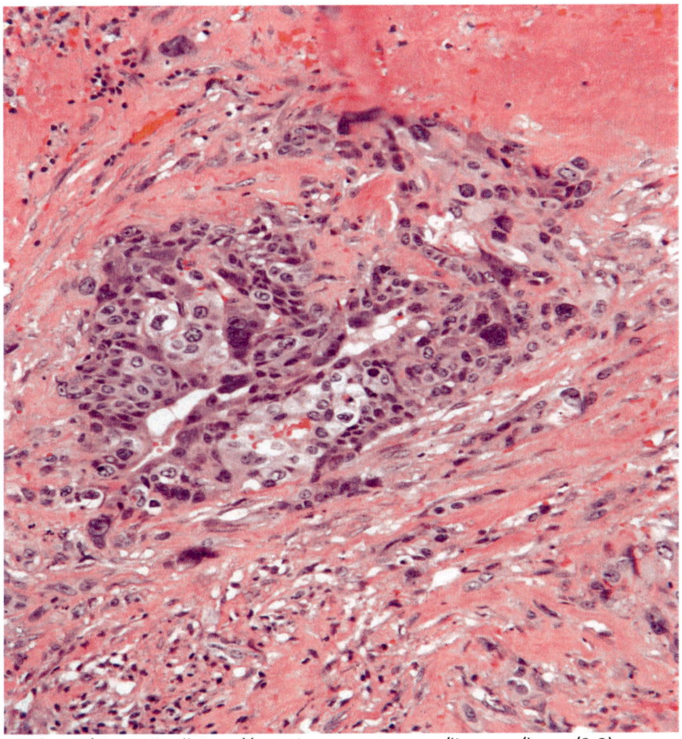

FIGURE 10.3.2 - Choriocarcinoma Histology

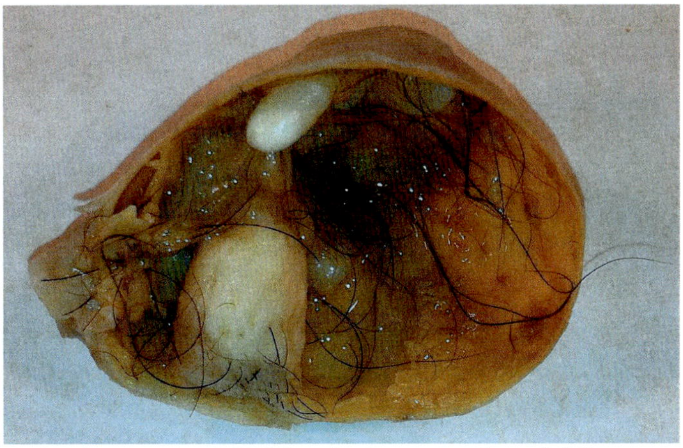

FIGURE 10.3.83 - Gross Image of Cystic Teratoma

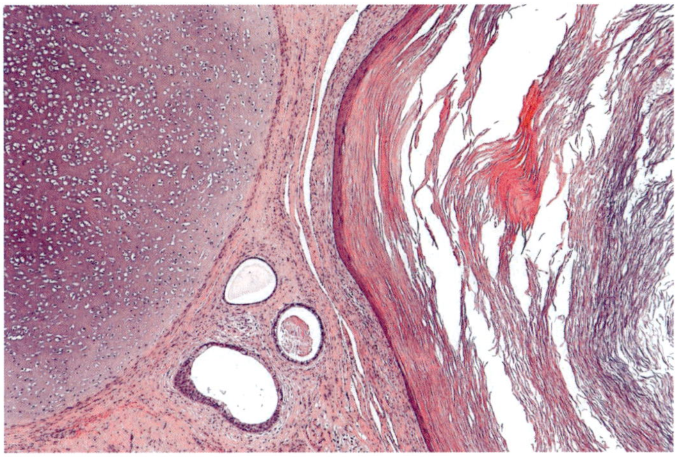

FIGURE 10.3.84 - Mature Cystic Teratoma Histology

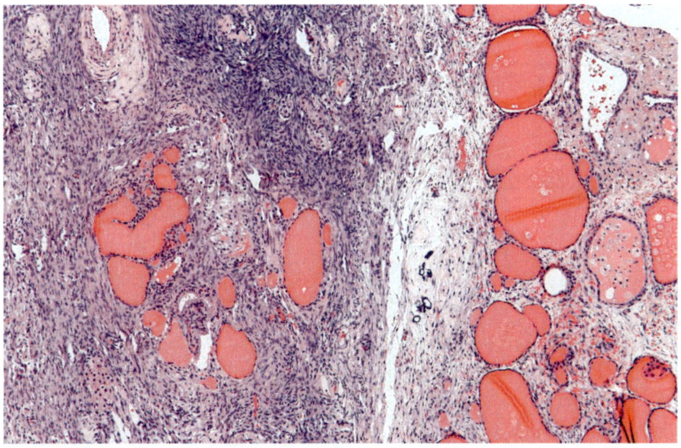

FIGURE 10.3.85 - Struma Ovarii Histology

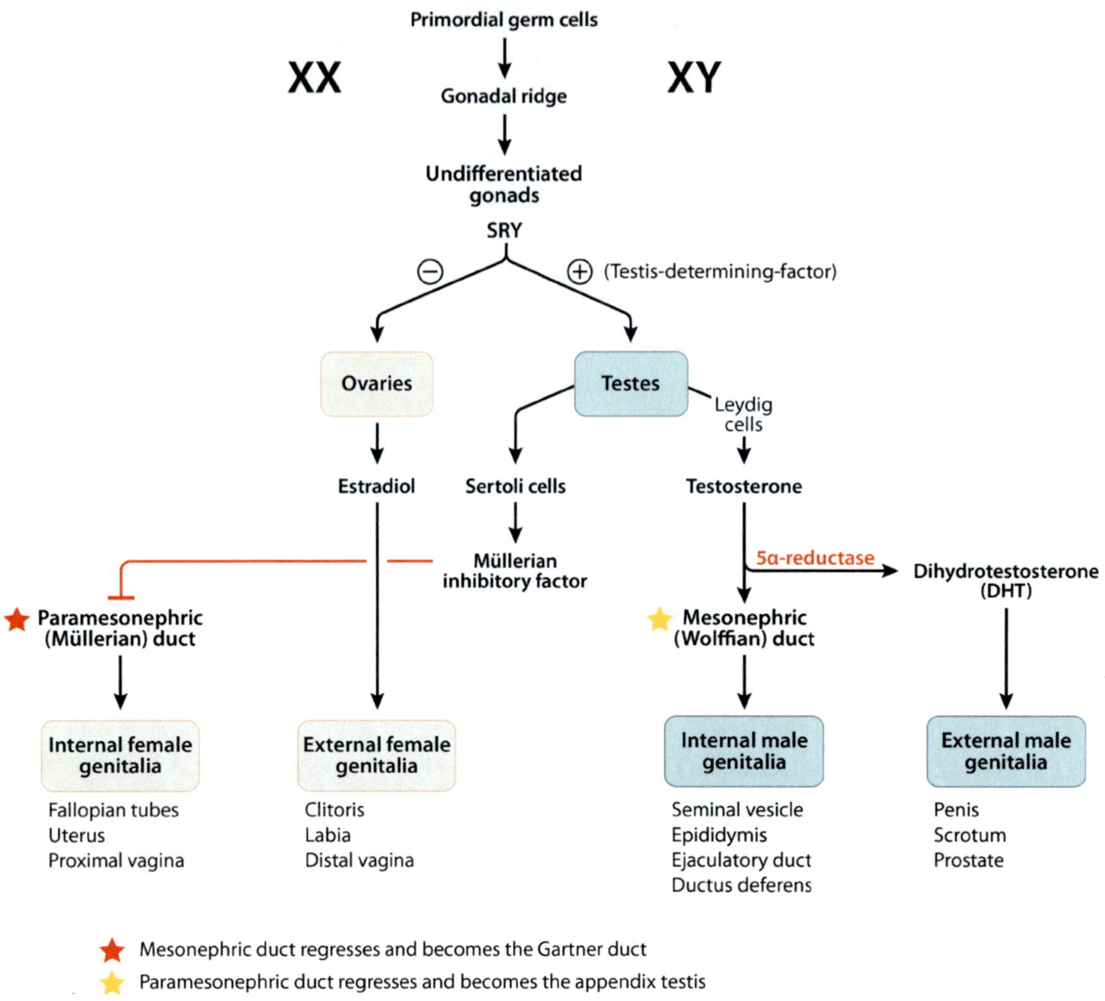

FIGURE 10.3.86 - Male and Female Differentiation

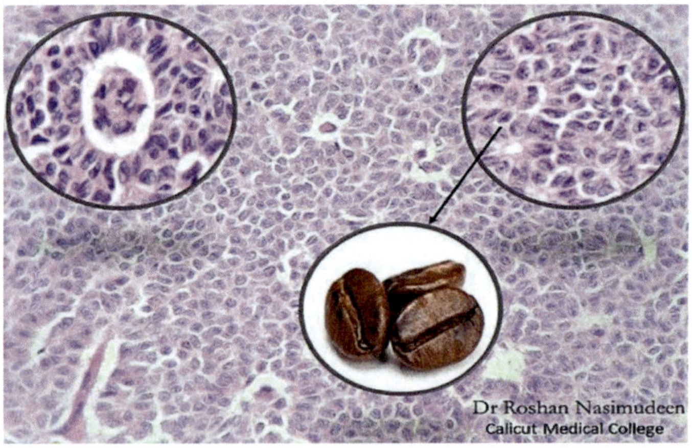

FIGURE 10.3.87 - Call-Exner bodies in a Granulosa Cell Tumor

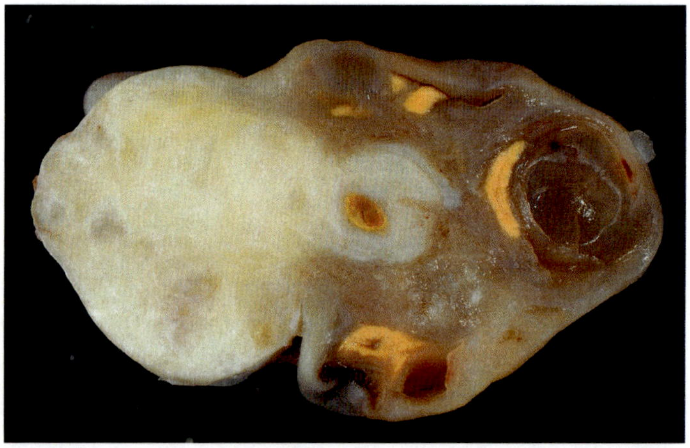

FIGURE 10.3.88 - Gross image of Ovarian Fibroma

I. Metastatic Tumors
   A. Common site of metastasis from the GI tract, breasts, uterus, Fallopian tubes, and the contralateral ovary
   B. Rare: Krukenberg tumor
      1. Gastric carcinoma involving both ovaries
      2. Hematogenous spread
      3. Signet-ring cells

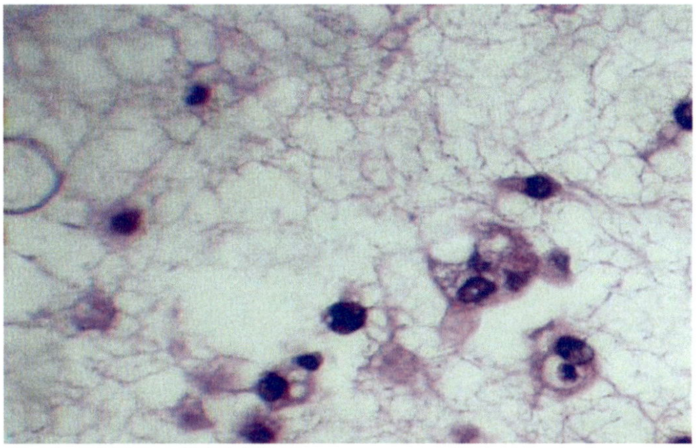

FIGURE 10.3.89 - Signet Ring Cells in a Krukenberg Tumor

REVIEW QUESTIONS

1. A histological slide of a 13-year-old female is being examined for a potential ovarian tumor. The histopathologist notes a structure that resembles the glomerulus. What is the most likely diagnosis?

   - **The most likely diagnosis is yolk sac tumor.**
   - You may recall that schiller duval bodies resemble glomeruli and these are characteristic of yolk sac tumors.
   - This is the most common germ cell tumor in children.

2. A 27-year-old woman presents with pelvic discomfort that she first noticed several months ago. On physical examination, a right adnexal mass is detected. The mass is resected laparoscopically. Gross examination reveals a 3.5 cm cystic mass. A histologic image of the mass is shown below. Which of the following is the most likely diagnosis?

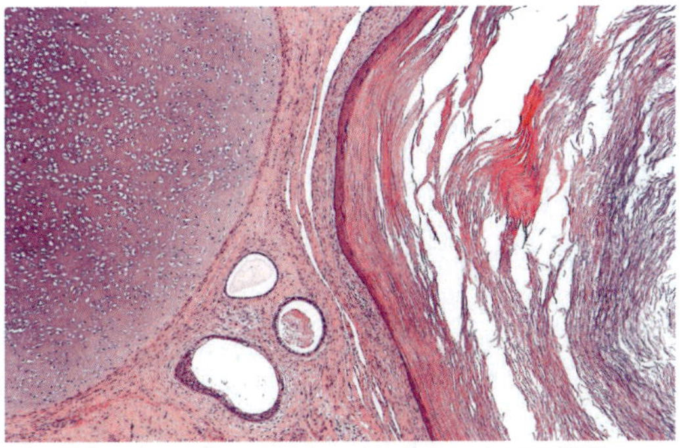

   A. Dysgerminoma
   B. Granulosa cell tumor
   C. Endodermal sinus tumor
   D. Benign cystic teratoma

- **The correct answer is D.**
- When you hear or read adnexal mass, the first thing that should come to your mind is the ovary. Adnexa technically refers to the fallopian tubes and ligaments that support the uterus, in addition to the ovaries. However, it's safe to think of an adnexal mass as being an ovarian mass.
- With that in mind, this histologic image is going to guide us to the likely type of ovarian mass.
- The image above shows elements from all 3 germ layers.
- We can see cartilage, gastrointestinal tissue, and epidermis.
- This tumor sounds like a benign cystic teratoma.
- Answer choice A is incorrect because this is a malignant germ cell tumor and is characterized by cords or sheets of uniform cells on histology.
- These cells are known as friend-egg cells.
- Answer choice B is incorrect because it is characterized by call exner bodies and coffee bean nuclei, unlike in this histological image.
- Answer choice C is incorrect because this has a classic "Schiller-Duval body" on histology.

Section XVI - Gestational Pathology

I. Miscarriage
  A. Pregnancy loss before 20 weeks gestational age
    1. Very common
  B. Most common cause is chromosomal abnormality (trisomies)
    1. Other causes are abnormally shaped uterus, antiphospholipid antibody syndrome, teratogens
  C. Symptoms are vaginal bleeding, uterine cramping
  D. Ultrasound findings
    1. Open cervix
    2. Empty uterus

II. Ectopic Pregnancy: Definition
  A. Pregnancy implantation outside of the uterus
    1. Most commonly located in the fallopian tube
    2. Other locations are rare

III. Ectopic Pregnancy: Symptoms and Risk Factors
  A. Symptoms
    1. Missed period
    2. Vaginal bleeding
    3. Abdominal pain
  B. Risk factors
    1. Pelvic inflammatory disease
    2. Previous ectopic pregnancy

IV. Ectopic Pregnancy: Diagnosis and Complications
  A. Diagnosis
    1. Serial hCG measurements with inadequate doubling every 48 hours
  B. Ultrasound
    1. Implantation outside uterus
  C. Complications
    1. hemorrhage with tube rupture
    2. Hemodynamic instability → death
    3. Surgical emergency

V. Placenta Previa
    1. The placenta covers the cervical os
    2. Vaginal bleeding
  A. Diagnosis
    1. Ultrasound, do NOT do a manual exam
  B. Complication
    1. Hemorrhage with rupture → fetal demise
  C. Treatment
    1. Cesarean section

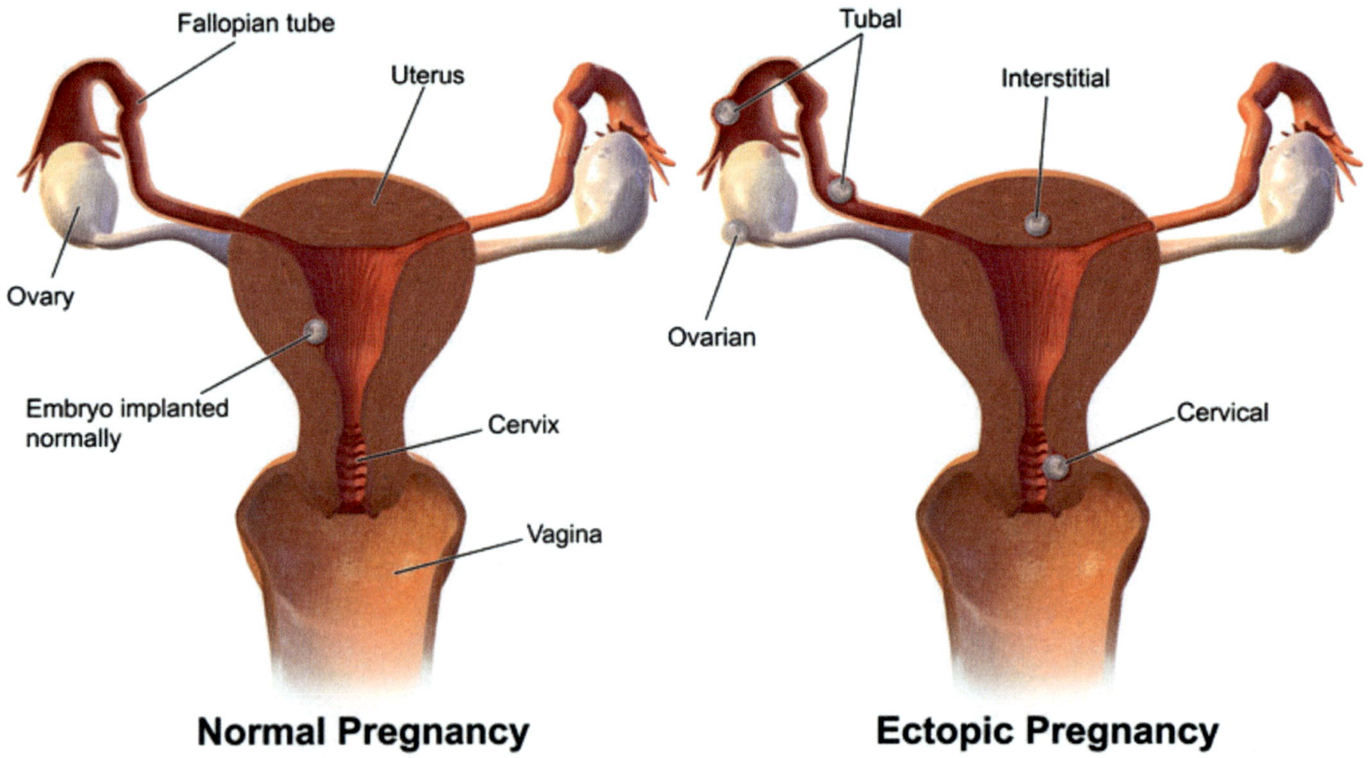

FIGURE 10.3.90 - Places of Ectopic Pregnancy

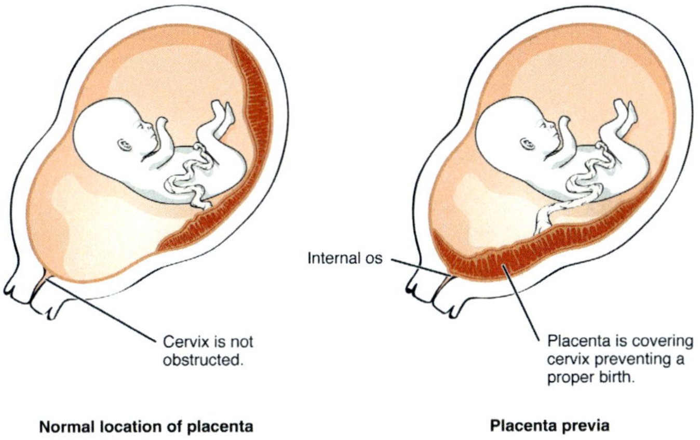

FIGURE 10.3.91 - Location of Placenta Previa

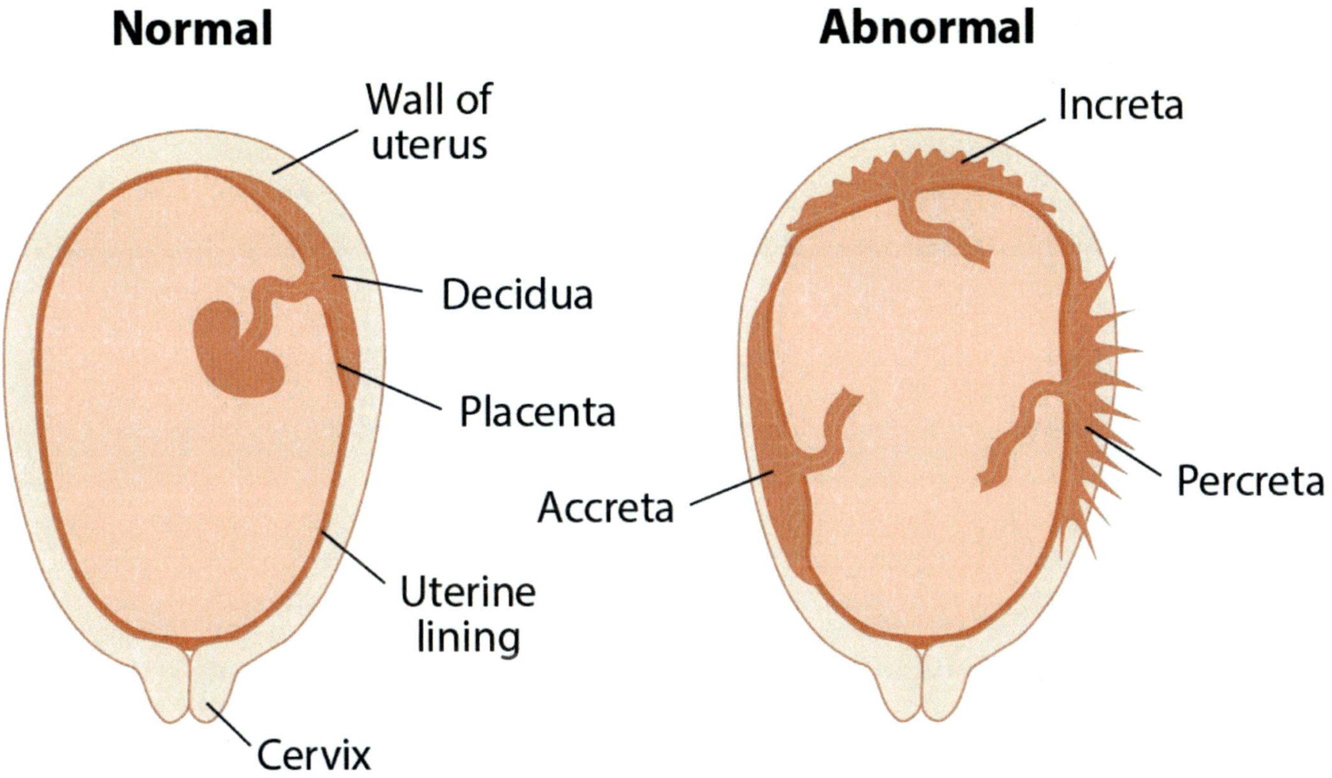

FIGURE 10.3.92 - Abnormal Implantation of Placenta

VI. Placenta Accreta/Increta/Percreta
   A. Defective decidua → pathologic attachment of placenta in uterus
   B. Accreta is when the placenta grows to myometrium, but not into it
   C. Increta is when the placenta grows into myometrium
   D. Percreta is when the placenta grows into, through and past myometrium
   E. Diagnosis
      1. Found on ultrasound
   F. Risks
      1. Incomplete delivery of placenta, continued bleeding, severe hemorrhage
   G. Treatment
      1. Hysterectomy

VII. Placental Abruption
   A. Placenta separates from the uterine wall before labor/delivery
      1. Vaginal bleeding (depends on location)
      2. Abdominal pain
   B. Risk factors
      1. Substance use: tobacco or cocaine
      2. Hypertension or preeclampsia
      3. Trauma
   C. Hemorrhage → fetal and/or maternal death

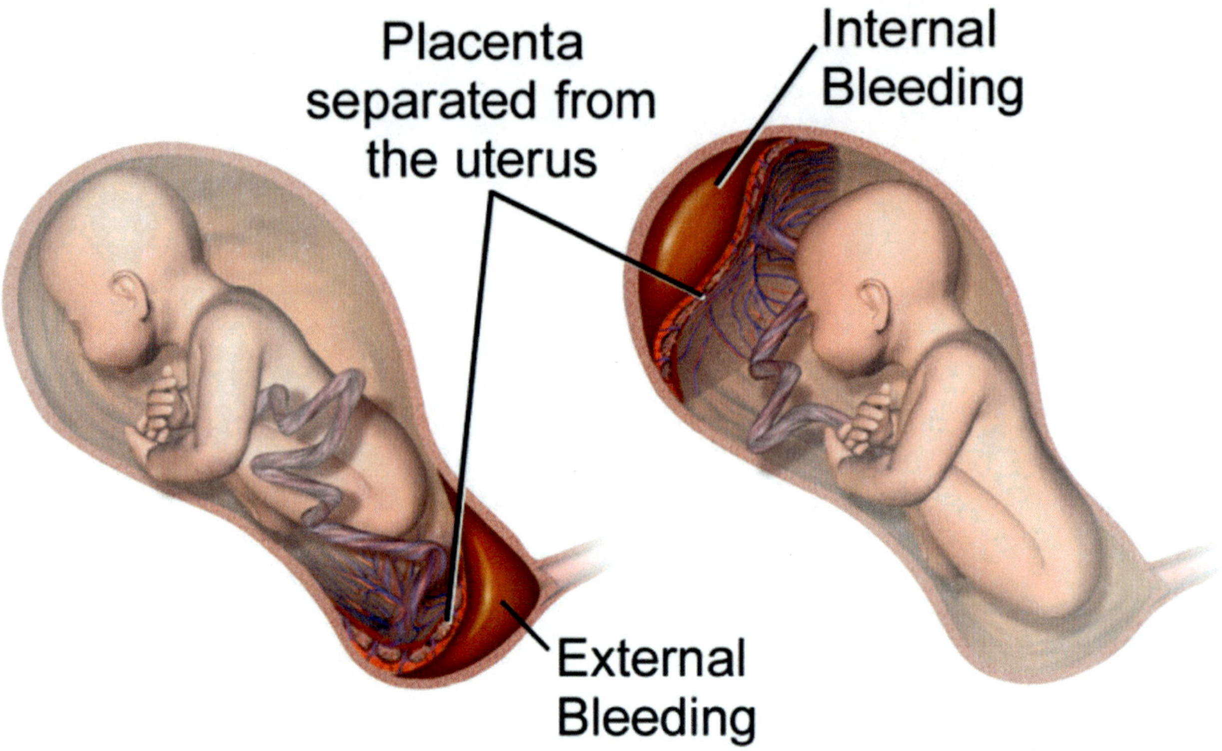

FIGURE 10.3.93 - Types of Placental Abruption

I. Molar Pregnancy: Definition
    A. AKA hydatidiform mole or gestational trophoblastic disease
    B. Pre-malignant, non-viable pregnancy
    C. Fertilized ovum with a relative excess of paternal genes
        1. Maternal genes have more control over fetal development
        2. Parental genes have more control over placental development → excessive proliferation of trophoblastic (placental) cells

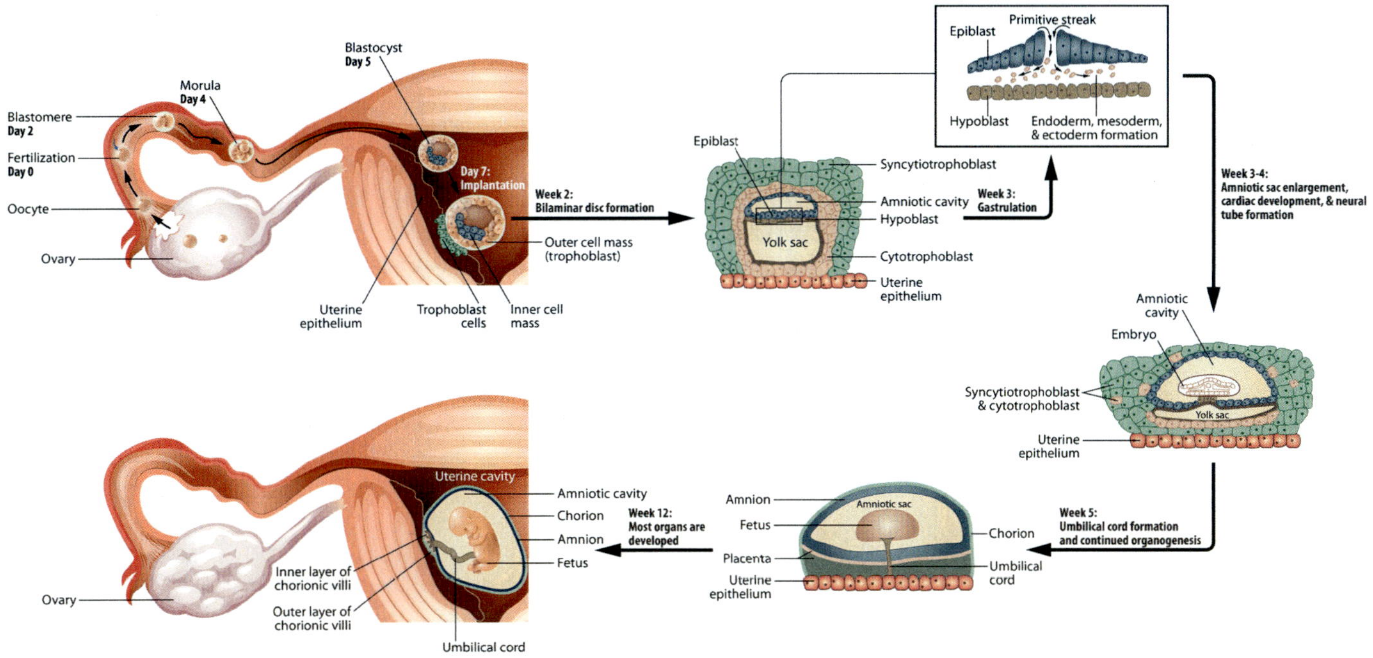

FIGURE 10.3.13 - Nonseminoma Tumor Marker Overview

I. Molar Pregnancy: Symptoms
   A. Vaginal bleeding
   B. Hyperemesis gravidarum
   C. Large uterus for gestational age

II. Molar Pregnancy: Types
   A. Complete mole: empty egg fertilized by one sperm that duplicates
      1. 46 chromosomes
      2. Partial mole: egg fertilized by two sperm
         a) 69 chromosomes
      3. Helpful tip: complete = completely trophoblast

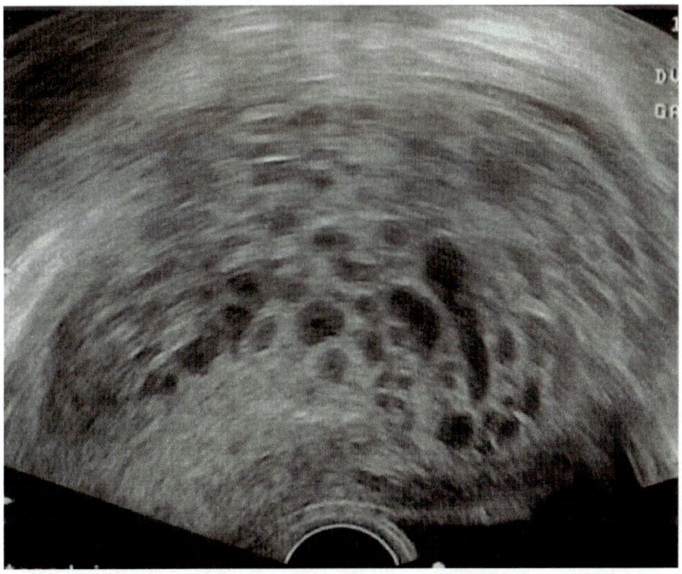

Häggström, Mikael (2014). "Medical gallery of Mikael Häggström 2014". WikiJournal of Medicine 1 (2). DOI:10.15347/wjm/2014.008. ISSN 2002-4436. Public Domain.orBy Mikael Häggström, used with permission. / CC0

FIGURE 10.3.94 - Ultrasound of "Snowstorm" Appearance of Molar Pregnancy

III. Molar Pregnancy: Diagnosis
   A. Ultrasound
   B. "Snowstorm" appearance in uterus

IV. Molar Pregnancy: Treatment
   A. Curettage or hysterectomy
   B. Surveillance: monitor hCG until undetectable
      1. Risk of progression to malignant choriocarcinoma (gestational trophoblastic neoplasia)
      2. Trophoblasts proliferate → mutations arise → cancer
   C. Birth control to prevent new pregnancy
      1. Pregnancy naturally increases hCG levels → obscured results

V. Preeclampsia
   A. New onset hypertension and proteinuria after 20 weeks gestation
   B. Systolic >140 OR diastolic > 90
   C. Other symptoms: pulmonary edema, headache, altered mental status, and vision changes
   D. Abnormal placenta → poor fetal perfusion → maternal inflammation
   E. Complications: stroke and placental abruption
      1. If complicated with seizures, it becomes eclampsia
   F. Eclampsia
      1. Preeclampsia with seizures
      2. Life threatening
   G. Preeclampsia and Eclampsia: Treatment
      1. Magnesium sulfate
      2. Deliver the fetus and placenta
   H. HELLP Syndrome
      1. Hemolysis, elevated liver enzymes, and low platelets
      2. Underlying cause is debated
      3. Often seen in patients with preeclampsia
      4. Treatment: immediate delivery

REVIEW QUESTIONS

1. A 21-year-old female presents to the emergency room complaining of severe lower right quadrant abdominal pain that started about 3 hours ago. She was treated for pelvic inflammatory disease 4 years ago. She is sexually active with her boyfriend of 2 years. She is not on birth control and does not use condoms. Her last menstrual period is unknown. What is the most likely diagnosis?

    A. Appendicitis
    B. Diverticulitis
    C. Ectopic pregnancy
    D. Molar pregnancy

- **The correct answer is C.**
- This is a 21-year-old female who is sexually active but does not use birth control or barrier contraception, and her last menstrual period is unknown.
- This should raise your concern for a pregnancy.
- With this potential pregnancy in the context of acute, severe right lower quadrant pain, this should raise your suspicion of an ectopic pregnancy.
- Her history of pelvic inflammatory disease, a known risk factor for ectopic pregnancy, further confirms the presentation of ectopic pregnancy.
- A is incorrect because, while right lower quadrant pain may be a sign of appendicitis, the information in the question stem is more consistent with ectopic pregnancy.
- They would also likely have physical exam signs such as a positive McBurney's sign.
- B is incorrect because while right lower quadrant pain may be a sign of diverticulitis, it is rare in a 21-year-old.
- D is incorrect because Molar pregnancy would likely present with hyperemesis gravidarum and a very large gestational age uterus, not severe abdominal pain and a history of PID.

NEUROPATHOLOGY

Section I - Meningitis

I. Anatomy
   A. The meninges are the protective layers that cover the brain and spinal cord
   B. Consist of dura, arachnoid, and pia mater

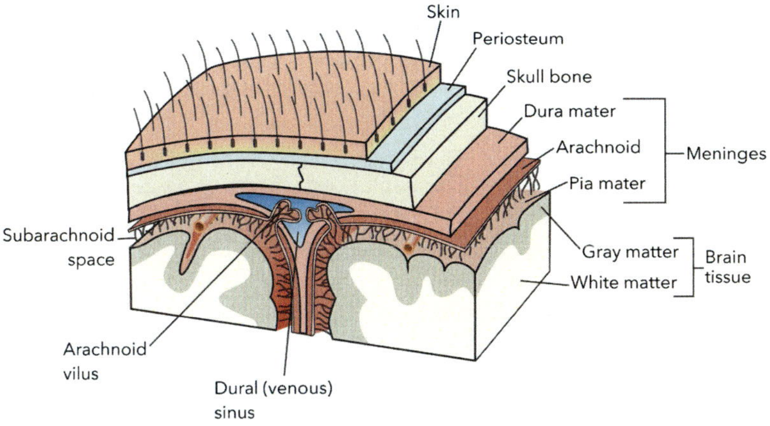

FIGURE 10.4.1 - Anatomy of the Meninges

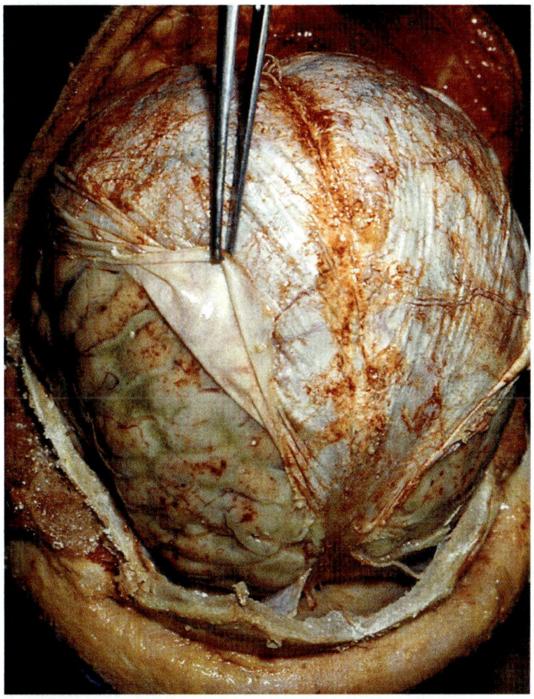

Photo Credit: Content Providers(s): CDC/ Dr. Edwin P. Ewing, Jr. / Public domain

FIGURE 10.4.2 - Brain Autopsy of Bacterial Meningitis

II. Etiology
   A. Inflammation of leptomeninges
   B. Most commonly due to an infectious agent
      1. Bacterial, viral, or fungal

Neonates	Children and teenagers	Adults	Elderly	Immunocompromised
- Group B *Streptococcus*	- *S. pneumoniae*	- *S. pneumoniae*	- *S. pneumoniae*	- *Cryptococcus neoformans*
- E. Coli	- *N. meningitidis*	- *N. meningitidis*	- *Listeria monocytogenes*	- CMV
- *Listeria monocytogenes*	- *H. influenzae*	- HSV		
	- Coxsackievirus			

TABLE 10.4.1 - Causative Agents in Meningitis

III. Symptoms
   A. Fever
   B. Headache
   C. Neck stiffness
   D. Photophobia
   E. Vomiting
   F. Altered mental status

IV. Clinical Features
   A. Diagnose via lumbar puncture
   B. Complications: death, seizure, and hydrocephalus

Etiology	Cell Type	Glucose	Protein
Bacterial	Neutrophils	Decreased	Increased
Viral	Lymphocytes	Normal	Slightly increased
Fungal	Lymphocytes	Decreased	Increased

TABLE 10.4.2 - Lumbar Puncture Findings in Meningitis

REVIEW QUESTIONS

1. A 70-year-old female with no past medical history presents to the physician with a fever, headache, and neck stiffness. A lumbar puncture confirms the etiology to be bacterial. What are the likely infectious causes of this patient's condition?
   - **The correct answer is S. *pneumoniae* and *Listeria monocytogenes.***
   - The patient is suffering from meningitis.
   - Fever, heachache, and neck stiffness are common symptoms that patients present with. A lumbar puncture is used to confirm the diagnosis.
   - The patient is over the age of 60, so the likely bacterial causes are *S.pneumoniae* and *listeria monocytogenes*.

2. A 29-year-old male with a medical history of HSV-1 presents with a fever, photophobia, and neck stiffness. The patient is thought to have meningitis. A lumbar puncture is performed and the etiology is confirmed to be viral. What will most likely be seen in this patient's CSF?
   - **The correct answer is lymphocytes, normal glucose levels, and slightly increased protein levels.**
   - The patient is suffering from meningitis.
   - Fever, photophobia, and neck stiffness are common symptoms of meningitis. The patient has a history of HSV-1 and the etiology is confirmed to be viral.
   - Viral CSF will have lymphocytes present, normal glucose levels, and slightly increased protein levels.

3. A 29-year-old female with no past medical history presents to the emergency department. The patient's current temperature is 40° C (104.0° F), blood pressure is 120/80 mmHg, heart rate is 110 beats/minute, and the respiratory rate is 24 breaths/minute. The patient vomited while in the waiting room and is complaining of neck stiffness. She states that these symptoms all came on within the last 24 hours. A lumbar puncture is performed and a bacterial etiology is confirmed. Which of the following cerebrospinal fluid characteristics would be seen in this patient's lumbar puncture?

   A. Lymphocytes present
   B. Decreased glucose
   C. Clear CSF
   D. Normal opening pressure

- **The correct answer is B.**
- The important thing to recognize here is that this patient is suffering from meningitis. The patient's rapid onset of fever, neck stiffness, and vomiting are indicative of meningitis. The patient is likely suffering from bacterial meningitis.
- A diagnosis of meningitis is made through a lumbar puncture. The cerebrospinal fluid (CSF) that is sampled will be analyzed. There are several key features that are used to aid in diagnosis. They include the cell type present, glucose levels, and protein levels within the CSF. Bacterial meningitis CSF will have neutrophils present, decreased glucose, and increased protein. Neutrophils phagocytose bacteria and glucose is utilized by bacteria. So it makes sense that in bacterial meningitis a CSF sample would show many neutrophils and the levels of glucose would be low.
- Viral meningitis CSF will have lymphocytes present, normal glucose, and slightly increased protein. Lymphocytes are the primary immune cell that deal with viruses so it makes sense the lymphocytes are present. Viruses also don't metabolize glucose so glucose levels are lonormal.
- Fungal meningitis CSF will have lymphocytes present, decreased glucose, and increased protein. Think of fungal meningitis as a combination of bacterial and viral as it will show elevated lymphocytes but decreased glucose. Again, just think of fungi metabolizing glucose for energy so this will be low.
- Finally, just remember that protein can be increased in all types.
- A is incorrect because lymphocytes are not seen in bacterial meningitis. Lymphocytes are seen in fungal and viral meningitis.
- C is incorrect because clear CSF is associated with viral meningitis. Viral meningitis in this age group may be due to HSV-1 or HSV-2; the patient does not have a history of either.
- D is incorrect because normal opening pressure is not associated with bacterial meningitis. Normal opening pressure is associated with viral meningitis.

Section II - Cerebrovascular Disease

I. Global Hypoperfusion
   A. Caused by low perfusion, chronic hypoxia, or hypoglycemia
   B. Mild global ischemia: brief confusion
   C. Moderate global ischemia: infarcts in watershed areas
      1. Cerebral cortex
      2. Hippocampus
      3. Cerebellum
   D. Severe global ischemia: necrosis and vegetative state

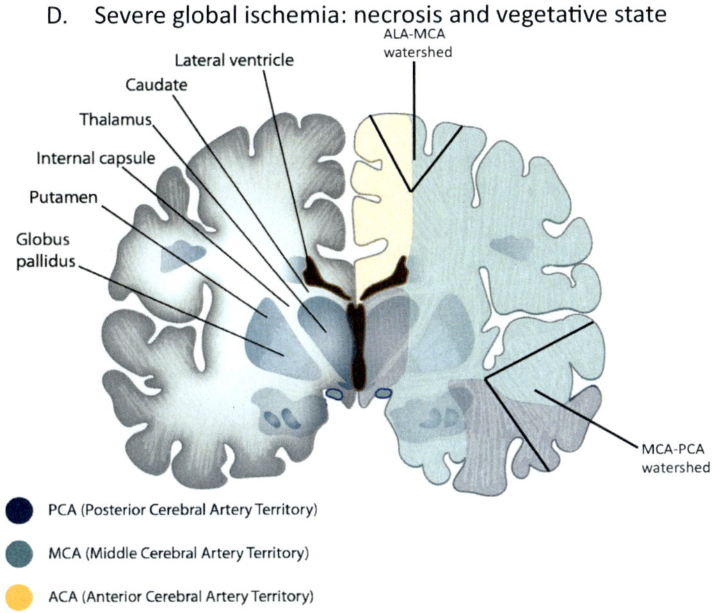

FIGURE 10.4.3 - Cerebrovascular Territories

II. Ischemic Strok
   A. Insufficient blood flow to meet metabolic demand
   B. Constitutes 85% of strokes
   C. Irreversible damage caused after 5 minutes
   D. Transient ischemic attack (TIA)
   E. Diagnosis
      1. CT (after 6 hours)
      2. MRI (within 30 minutes)

Time Since Stroke	Pathologic Features
12 - 24 hours	Eosinophilic cytoplasm and pyknotic nuclei (red neurons)
24 - 72 hours	Necrosis and neutrophils
3 - 5 days	Macrophages (microglia)
1-2 weeks	Reactive gliosis (astrocytes) and vascular proliferation
> 2 weeks	Glial scar (cyst surrounded by astrocyte processes)

TABLE 10.4.3 - Pathologic Changes in Ischemic Neural Tissue

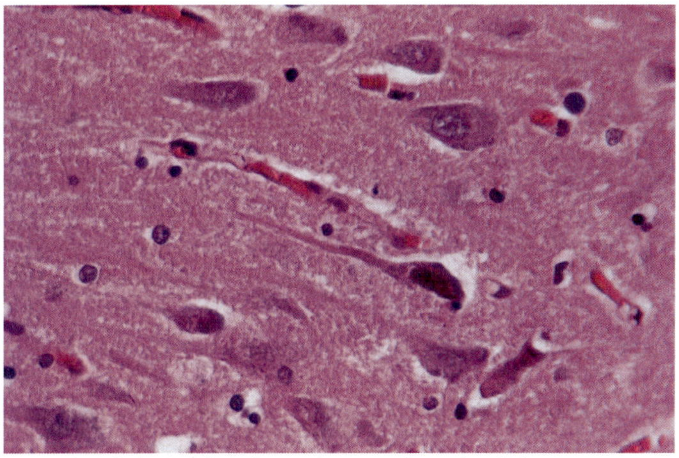

FIGURE 10.4.4 - Red Neurons

III. Ischemic Stroke: Thrombotic Stroke
   A. Clot formation at the site of infarction
   B. Ruptured atherosclerotic plaque
   C. Vessel branch points most common site
   D. Affects one territory
   E. Pale infarct at the periphery of the cortex

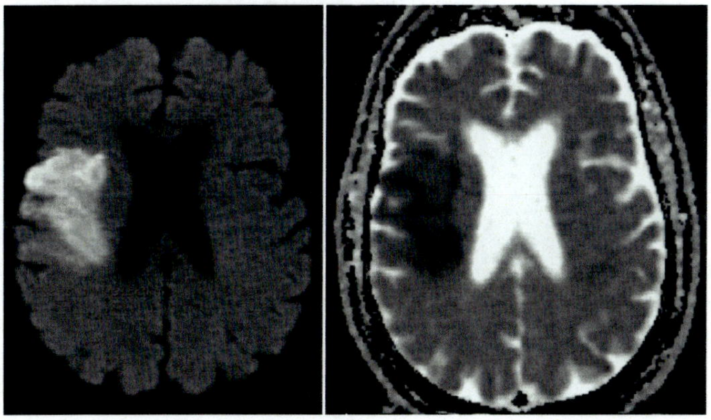

FIGURE 10.4.5 - Axial Brain MRI of Cerebral Infarction

IV. Ischemic Stroke: Embolic Stroke
   A. Clot from another part of the body
   B. Multiple vascular territories
   C. Common causes
      1. Atrial fibrillation
      2. Carotid artery stenosis
      3. DVT with patent foramen ovale
      4. Infective endocarditis

V. Ischemic Stroke: Lacunar Stroke
   A. Hyaline arteriosclerosis of smaller vessels
   B. Small, cystic areas of infarction
   C. Internal capsule: pure motor
   D. Thalamus: pure sensory

VI. Ischemic Brain Disease: Treatment
   A. tPA within 3 - 4.5 hours
   B. Thrombectomy

VII. Subarachnoid Hemorrhage: Findings
   A. Bleed in the subarachnoid space
   B. Saccular (berry) aneurysm
   C. Sudden, severe headache
   D. Lumbar puncture: xanthochromic CSF
   E. Associations: autosomal dominant polycystic kidney disease, Marfan syndrome, Ehlers-Danlos syndrome

VIII. Subarachnoid Hemorrhage: Complications
   A. Delayed vasospasm risk
      1. Several days after initial symptoms
      2. Vasoconstrictive factors
      3. Treat with nimodipine

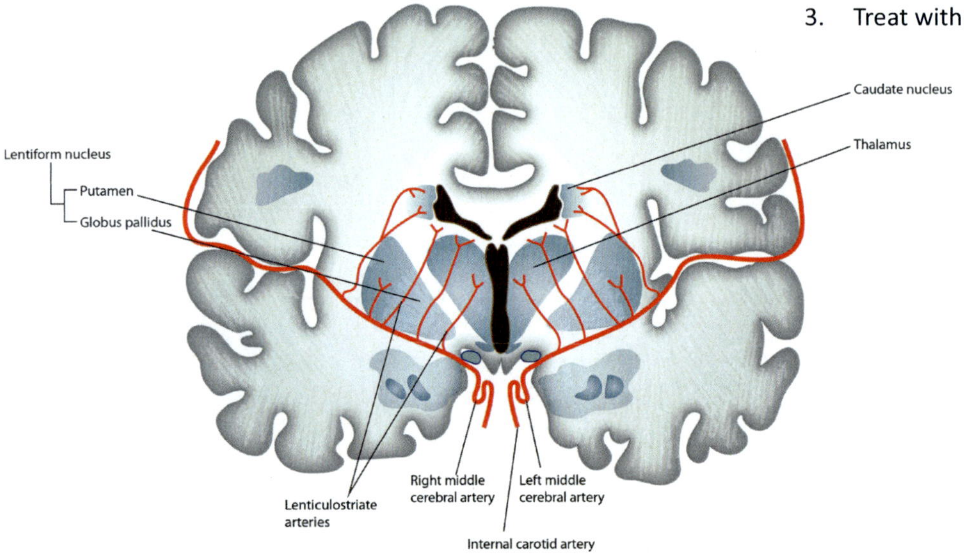

FIGURE 10.4.6 - Lenticulostriate Arteries

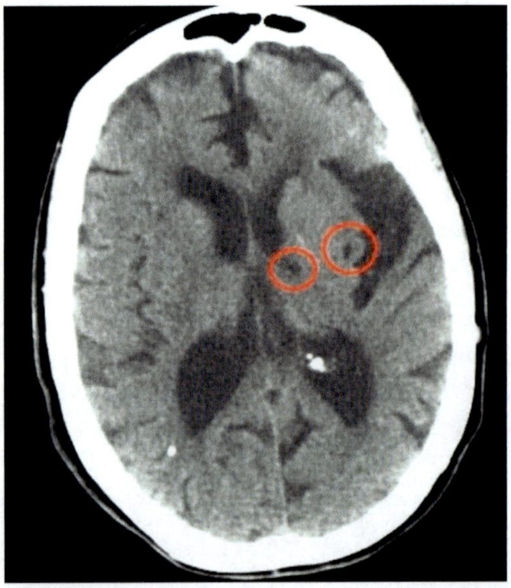

FIGURE 10.4.7 - Axial Brain MRI of Lacunar Stroke

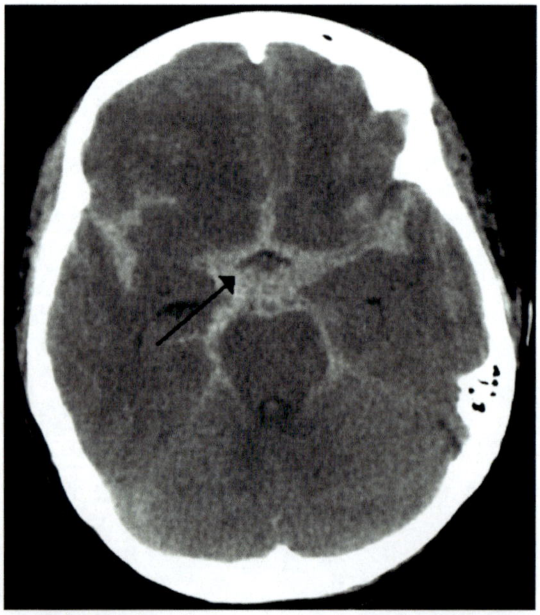

FIGURE 10.4.8 - Axial Head CT of Subarachnoid Hemorrhage

IX. Intraparenchymal Hemorrhage
   A. Bleed in brain parenchyma
   B. Lenticulostriate (Charcot-Bouchard) microaneurysm
   C. Basal ganglia
   D. Severe headache, nausea, vomiting, and coma
   E. Hypertension

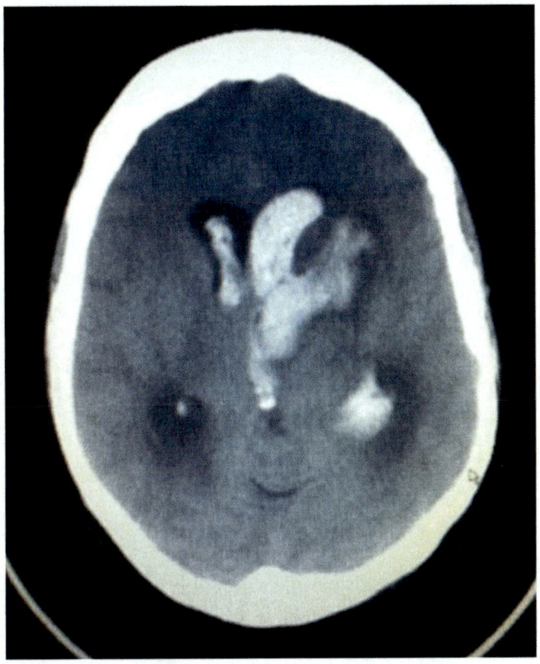

Photo Credit: Glitzy queen00 at English Wikipedia / Public domain

FIGURE 10.4.9 - Axial Head CT of Intraparenchymal Hemorrhage

REVIEW QUESTIONS

1. A 74-year-old man with hypertension, coronary artery disease, and obesity presents to the emergency department with 30 minutes of a severe crushing pressure in his chest. His blood pressure is 70/40 mmHg. He is immediately given vasopressor medications that cause his blood pressure to normalize. After his condition stabilizes, he is found to have some significant neurologic deficits. What aspects of cognition are most likely to have been affected in this patient?

- **This patient is most likely to have memory deficits, motor and balance problems, and/or man-in-a-barrel syndrome.**
- This is an acutely hypotensive patient in cardiogenic shock. Although his condition was promptly treated, he likely experienced global cerebral hypoperfusion, and as a result will have sustained some significant damage to his brain. The areas most likely to be affected by global hypoperfusion include the cerebral cortex, the hippocampus, and the cerebellum.

REVIEW QUESTIONS

- While damage to the cerebral cortex can cause a number of deficits, hypoperfusion of the hippocampus will likely cause memory deficits, and hypoperfusion of the cerebellum will likely cause difficulty with motor skills and balance.
- Man-in-a-barrel syndrome is likely due to the possibility of a watershed stroke, which would result in weakness in proximal limb muscles.

2. A 69-year-old male with a past medical history of hypertension presents to the clinic with an hour-long history of tingling and numbness on the left side of his face, his left arm, and his left leg. He has no other symptoms including motor weakness. A CT scan of the patient's brain shows no evidence of hemorrhage. Which of the following is the most likely cause of this patient's symptoms?

   A. Hyaline arteriosclerosis
   B. Embolism
   C. Thrombosis
   D. Hypoxia

- **The correct answer is A.**
- This patient's symptoms align with a pure sensory stroke consistent with a lacunar infarct affecting the thalamus. These types of strokes are almost always associated with hyaline arteriosclerosis, a consequence of hypertension.
- The thalamus is primarily supplied by lenticulostriate vessels. As these smaller vessels become narrowed by arteriosclerosis, the sensory function of the thalamus can be affected by the decreased blood supply.
- B is incorrect because embolic strokes tend to affect larger arteries such as the ACA, MCA, or PCA. Embolic strokes can also affect the posterior circulation, but it would be extremely uncommon for them to cause purely sensory symptoms.
- C is incorrect because, similar to embolic strokes, thrombotic strokes tend to cause symptoms in larger arteries. You would not expect a thrombotic stroke to cause purely sensory symptoms.
- D is incorrect because hypoxia and hypoperfusion tend to cause damage to the watershed regions of the brain: the cerebral cortex, the hippocampus, or the cerebellum. None of these would manifest with purely sensory symptoms.

Section III - Trauma

I. Epidural Hematoma
   A. Bleeding between the dura mater and the skull
   B. Occurs when temporal bone fracture tears middle meningeal artery

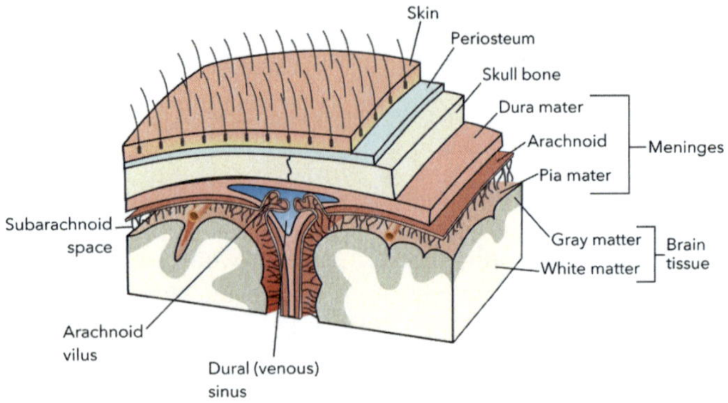

FIGURE 10.4.1 - Anatomy of the Meninges

II. Epidural Hematoma: Findings
   A. Lens-shaped lesions on CT
   B. Lucid interval
   C. Complication: herniation (lethal)

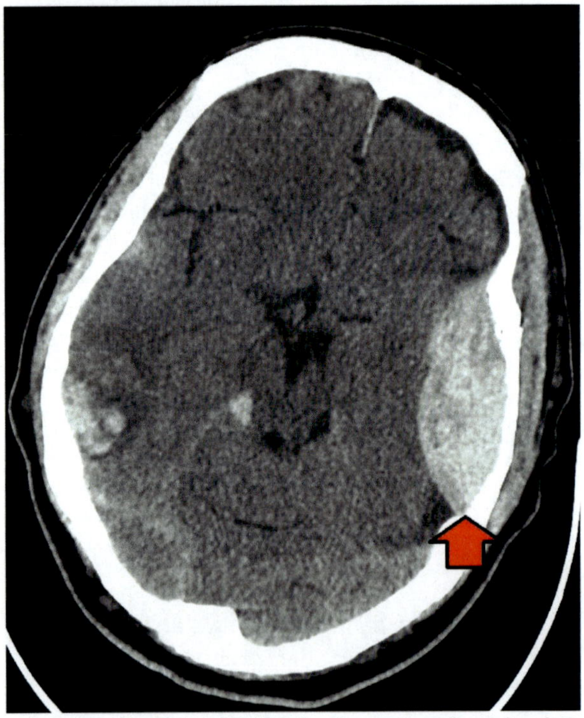

Photo Credit: James Heilman, MD / CC BY-SA (https://creativecommons.org/licenses/by-sa/4.0)

FIGURE 10.4.10 - Axial Head CT of Epidural Hematoma

III. Subdural Hematoma
   A. Bleeding between the brain and the dura mater
   B. Due to tears in bridging veins
      1. Associated with traumatic brain injury
      2. Located between the dura mater and arachnoid mater

IV. Subdural Hematoma: Findings
   A. Imaging: crescent-shaped lesion
   B. Progressive neurological signs
   C. Complication: herniation (lethal)

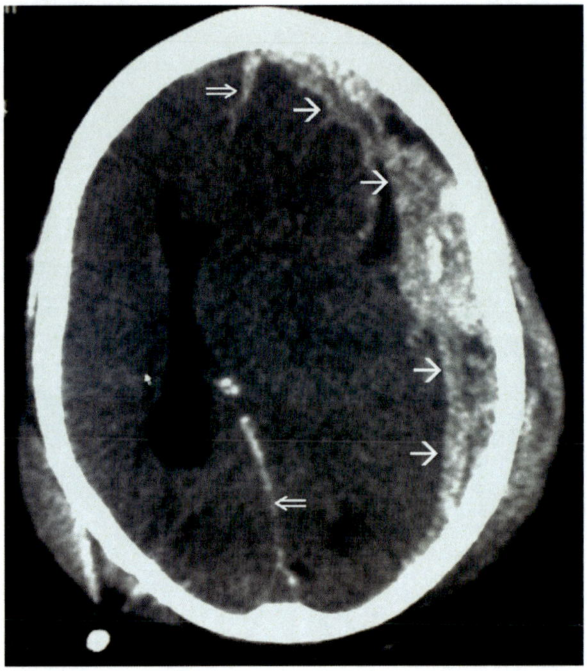

Photo Credit: 2007-06-24 17:16 Glitzy queen00 / Public domain

FIGURE 10.4.11 - Axial Head CT of Subdural Hematoma

V. Herniation
   A. Abnormal protrusion of brain tissue due to increased intracranial pressure
   B. Types of herniation
      1. Tonsillar herniation
      2. Subfalcine herniation
      3. Uncal herniation

VI. Tonsillar Herniation
   A. Protrusion of the cerebellar tonsils through the foramen magnum
      1. Compression of the brain stem → cardiopulmonary arrest

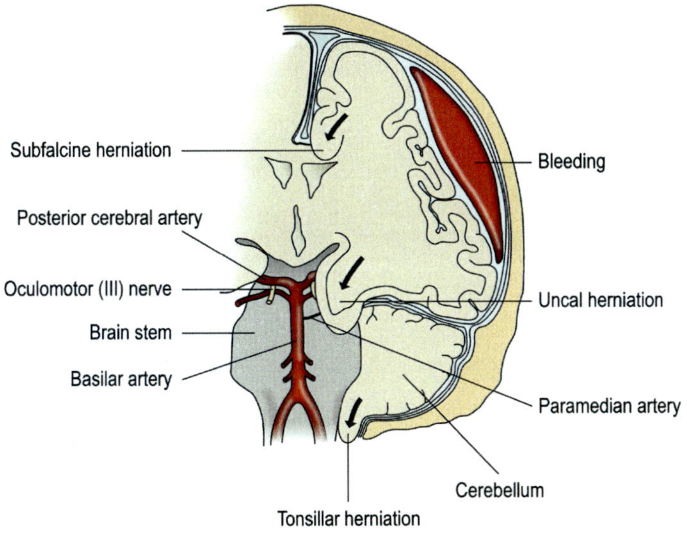

FIGURE 10.4.12 - Types of Brain Herniation

VII. Subfalcine Herniation

A. Protrusion of the cingulate gyrus under the falx cerebri

1. Compression of the anterior cerebral artery → infarction

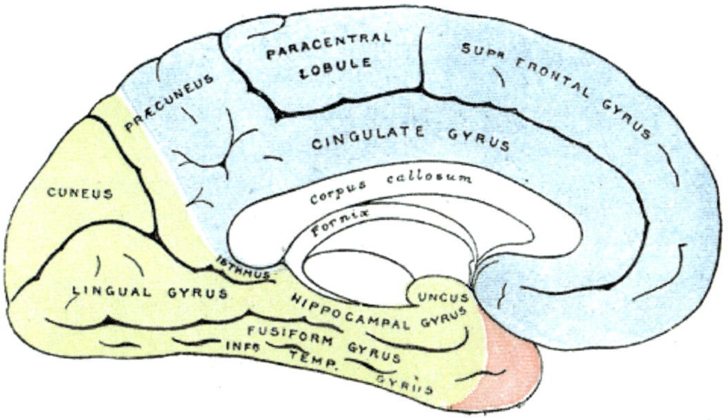

Photo Credit Henry Vandyke Carter / Public domain

FIGURE 10.4.13 - Anatomical Parts of the Brain

VIII. Uncal Herniation

A. Protrusion of the medial temporal lobe

1. Compression of CN III: "down and out" eyes with dilated pupils
2. Compression of PCA: contralateral homonymous hemianopia
3. Rupture of the paramedian artery: Duret hemorrhage

REVIEW QUESTIONS

1. A 34-year-old male presents to the emergency department after a motor vehicle accident. According to emergency medical services, the patient lost consciousness and recovered a few times before arriving at the emergency department. His head CT shows a lens-shaped lesion. Where is the blood accumulating in this patient?

    - **The correct answer is "between the dura mater and the skull."**
    - This is a 34-year-old man who lost consciousness and recovered a few times after a motor vehicle accident with a head CT showing a lens-shaped lesion.
    - Someone with a lucid interval after a head trauma, neurological signs, and head CT showing a lens-shaped lesion confirms the diagnosis of epidural hematoma. In someone with epidural hematoma, the blood accumulates in between the dura mater and the skull due to rupture of the middle meningeal artery.

2. A 62-year-old male with a past medical history of diabetes and hypertension presents with acute onset headache and weakness in his legs. Head CT scan shows a right temporal lobe hemorrhage and leftward shift of the cingulate gyrus under the falx cerebri. What artery is most likely to be compromised in this patient?

    A. Paramedian artery
    B. Middle cerebral artery
    C. Anterior cerebral artery
    D. Basilar artery

    - **The correct answer is C.**
    - This is a 62-year-old male presenting with acute onset headache and weakness in his legs. Head CT shows a right temporal lobe hemorrhage and leftward shift of the cingulate gyrus under the falx cerebri. Based on these findings, the patient is experiencing subfalcine herniation, in which the herniation of the cingulate gyrus compresses the anterior cerebral artery, resulting in the weakness in his legs.
    - A is wrong because the paramedian artery is located near the foramen magnum, and the rupture of the paramedian artery is associated with uncal herniations.
    - B is wrong because the middle cerebral artery supplies the lateral part of the cerebrum and is not associated with subfalcine herniations.
    - D is wrong because the basilar artery supplies the brainstem and the cerebellum and is not associated with subfalcine herniations.

Section IV - Demyelinating Disorders

I. Myelin
   A. Insulates axons and increases conduction velocity
   B. Oligodendrocytes synthesize myelin in CNS
   C. Schwann cells synthesize myelin in PNS

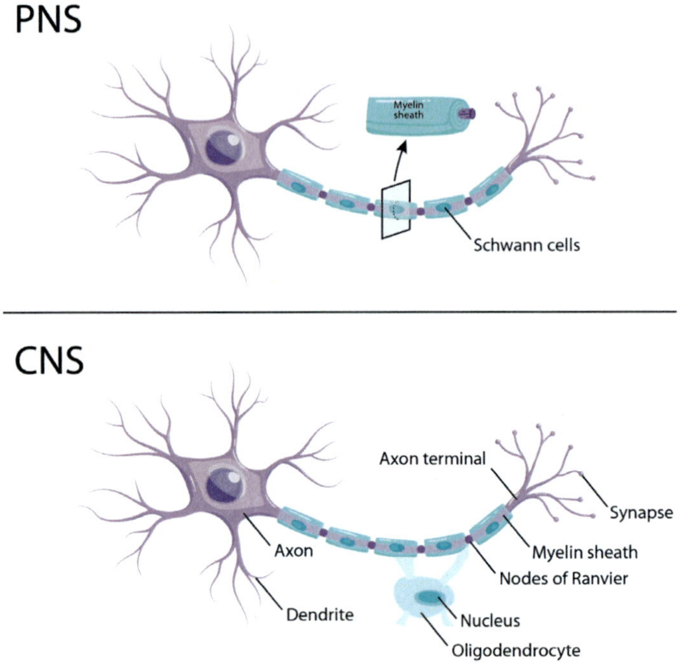

FIGURE 10.4.14 - Parts of a Neuron

II. Multiple Sclerosis: Etiology
   A. Autoimmune demyelination of CNS neurons
   B. T-cell-mediated destruction of oligodendrocytes

III. Multiple Sclerosis: Epidemiology
   A. Increased incidence in women between 20 and 30 years of age
   B. Increased incidence in colder temperatures
   C. Associated with HLA-DRB1

IV. Multiple Sclerosis: Symptoms
   A. Symptoms are relapsing and remitting
   B. Optic neuritis
   C. Internuclear ophthalmoplegia
   D. Bladder and bowel incontinence
   E. Spasticity and hemiparesis symptoms
   F. Scanning speech

V. Multiple Sclerosis: Findings and Treatment
   A. MRI shows periventricular plaques
   B. Lumbar puncture shows increased IgG, oligoclonal bands, myelin basic protein, and lymphocytes
   C. Treat acute attacks with intravenous steroids
   D. Treat chronically with interferon beta

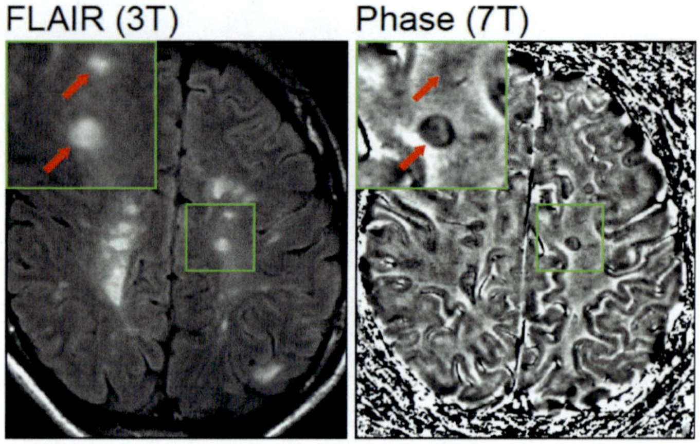

FIGURE 10.4.15 - Periventricular Plaques in Multiple Sclerosis

VI. Guillain-Barré Syndrome
   A. A group of disorders resulting in progressive muscle weakness
   B. Most common form is acute inflammatory demyelinating polyradiculoneuropathy (AIDP)
      1. Autoimmune destruction of Schwann cells
      2. Often occurs following infection (e.g. *Campylobacter jejuni*)
      3. Ascending paralysis → absent deep tendon reflexes → respiratory failure
      4. Treat with respiratory support, plasma exchange, and IVIG

VII. Acute Disseminated Encephalomyelitis
   A. Autoimmune demyelinating condition of the CNS
   B. Occurs following vaccination or infection
   C. Presents with multifocal neurological symptoms (eg, motor deficits) and encephalopathy (e.g. altered mental status)

VIII. Charcot-Marie-Tooth Disease
   A. Group of genetic disorders
   B. Defect of myelin or peripheral nerve proteins
   C. Most common type is CMT1A (PMP22 gene duplication)
   D. Sensory deficits, lower extremity weakness, and foot abnormalities (e.g. pes cavus)

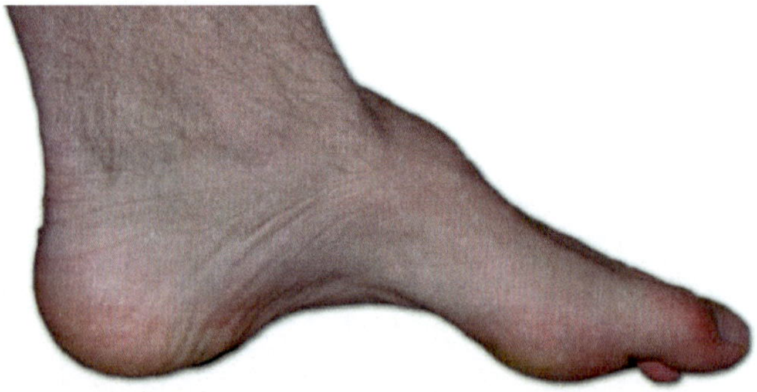

FIGURE 10.4.16 - Pes Cavus

IX. Central Pontine Myelinolysis: Etiology
   A. Iatrogenic
   B. Rapid correction of hyponatremia

X. Central Pontine Myelinolysis: Pathophysiology
   A. Rapid elevation in sodium levels leads to excess water being pulled from neurons
   B. Pontine demyelination

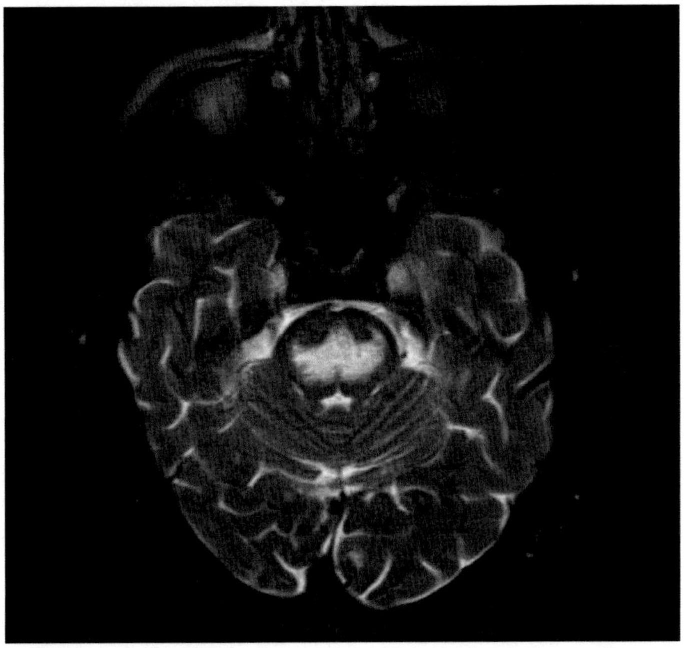

FIGURE 10.4.17 - Axial Brain MRI of Central Pontine Myelinolysis

XI. Central Pontine Myelinolysis: Clinical Features
   A. Locked-in syndrome

XII. Other Disorders
   A. Lysosomal storage diseases
      1. Krabbe disease
      2. Adrenoleukodystrophy
      3. Metachromatic leukodystrophy
   B. Subacute sclerosing panencephalitis - measles
   C. Progressive multifocal leukoencephalopathy
      1. JC virus

REVIEW QUESTIONS

1. A 29-year-old female with no past medical history presents to the physician with sudden painful vision loss. The patient states she had an episode of similar vision loss 9 months ago. The patient lives in Florida. What will most likely be seen on MRI in this patient?

- **An MRI will show periventricular plaques.**
- The patient is suffering from multiple sclerosis. Sudden painful vision loss, also known as optic neuritis, is a classic symptom with multiple sclerosis. Incidences of multiple sclerosis are increased in women between the ages of 20 and 30. There is also an increased incidence in warm climates.

REVIEW QUESTIONS

2. A 22-year-old female with no past medical history is brought to the emergency department after collapsing at a marathon. The patient's current temperature is 38 °C (100.4 °F), blood pressure is 110/80 mmHg, heart rate is 95 beats/minute, and the respiratory rate is 19 breaths/minute. The patient appears lethargic and is arousable to pain. Her friend states that she was drinking a lot of water and sweating profusely during the race. While the physician performs a physical exam, the patient begins to have a seizure. Serum sodium levels are 110 mmol/L (normal: 135 - 145 mmol/L). Which of the following is a likely consequence of the rapid correction of this patient's electrolyte disturbance?

   A. Pontine demyelination
   B. Increased ventricular pressure
   C. Brain herniation
   D. Cardiac arrhythmias

- **The correct answer is A.**
- The important thing to recognize here is that this patient is suffering from hyponatremia. The patient was running a marathon, drinking a lot of water, and sweating profusely. This caused her sodium levels to drop to dangerous levels. Rapid correction of low sodium level can lead to central pontine myelinolysis. This can lead to pontine demyelination and ultimately cause locked-in syndrome.
- The pathophysiology of central pontine myelinolysis is due to the rapid correction of hyponatremia. Rapid elevation of sodium levels leads to excess water being pulled from neurons. This leads to demyelination that occurs in the pons.
- B is incorrect because increased ventricular pressure is not involved with central pontine myelinolysis. Normal pressure hydrocephalus is caused by increased ventricular pressure.
- C is incorrect because brain herniation is associated with rapid correction of hypernatremia.
- D is incorrect because cardiac arrhythmias are not associated with hyponatremia. Potassium disturbances can cause cardiac arrhythmias.

Section V - Dementia and Degenerative Disorders

I. Alzheimer Disease: Epidemiology
   A. The most common cause of dementia
   B. Increased risk with Down syndrome
   C. Late onset: sporadic form most commonly seen in the elderly
   D. Early onset: familial forms associated with presenilin-1 and presenilin-2 mutations
   E. APOE-4 gene increases the risk
   F. APOE-2 gene decreases the risk

II. Alzheimer Disease: Morphologic Features
   A. Degeneration and atrophy of cortex
   B. Narrowing of sulci and widening of gyri
   C. Beta-amyloid plaques
   D. Neurofibrillary tangles
   E. Altered nucleus basalis of Meynert

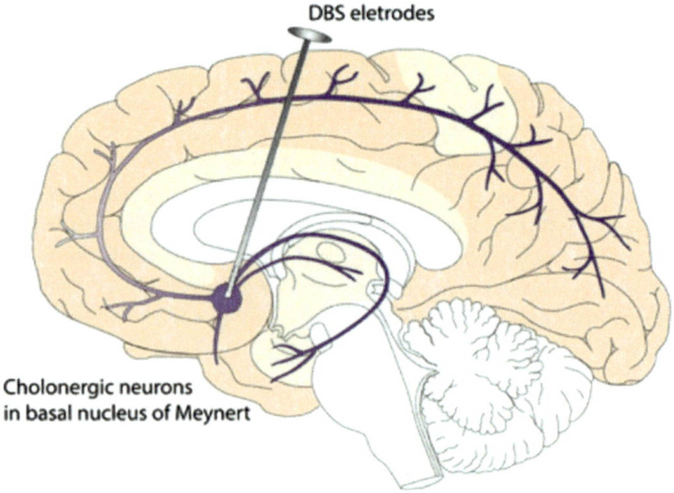

Photo Credit: Zhang Q, Kim Y-C and Narayanan NS / CC BY (https://creativecommons.org/licenses/by/4.0), edited bt Physeo

FIGURE 10.4.18 - Anatomical Location of Nucleus Basalis of Meynert

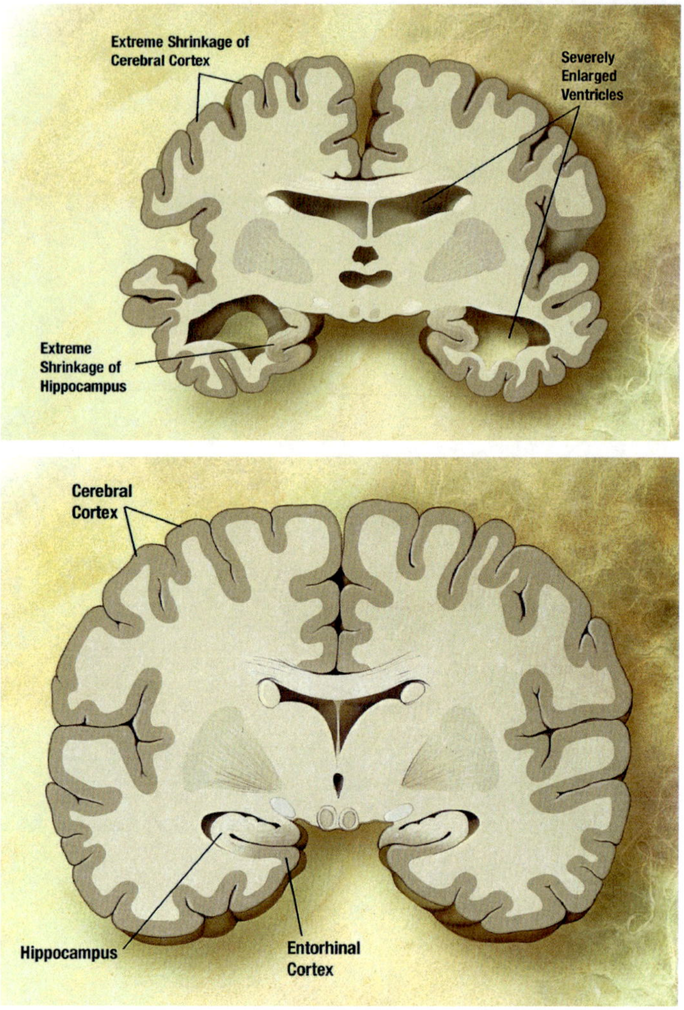

Photo Credit: ADEAR: "Alzheimer's Disease Education and Referral Center, a service of the National Institute on Aging." / Public domain

FIGURE 10.4.19 - Gross Pathological Changes in Alzheimer Disease (Top) vs. Normal Brain (Bottom)

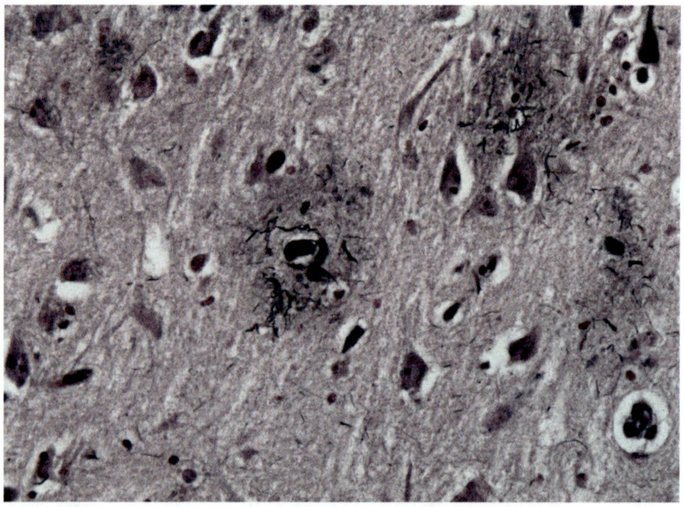

Photo Credit: Jensflorian / CC BY-SA (https://creativecommons.org/licenses/by-sa/3.0)

FIGURE 10.4.20 - Beta-Amyloid Plaques

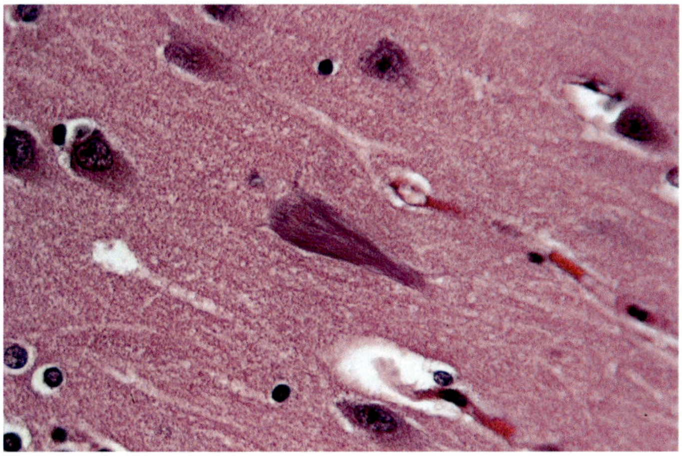

FIGURE 10.4.21 - Neurofibrillary Tangles

III. Alzheimer Disease: Clinical Features
   A. Diagnosis is presumed clinically
   B. Confirmatory diagnosis is made postmortem histologically
   C. Slowly progressive memory loss
   D. Behavioral and psychological impairment
   E. Visuospatial and language defects

IV. Vascular Dementia
   A. Caused by numerous arterial infarcts
   B. Stepwise decline in cognition
   C. The second most common cause of dementia

V. Pick Disease
   A. Also known as frontotemporal dementia
   B. Neurodegeneration of the frontal and temporal regions
   C. Behavioral and personality changes
   D. Pick bodies seen histologically

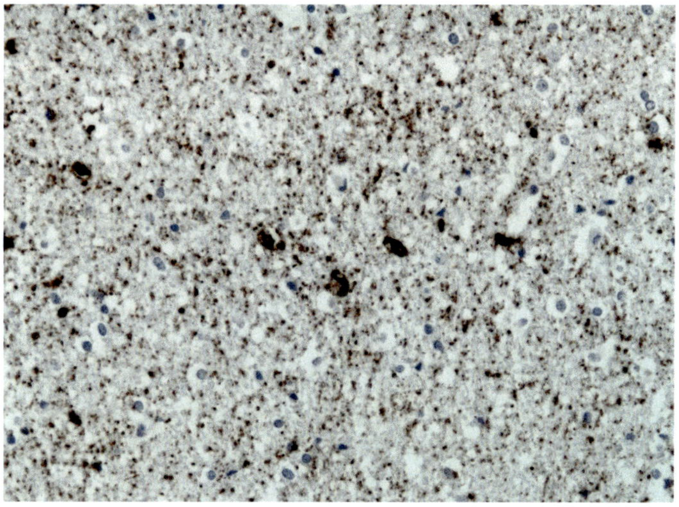

FIGURE 10.4.22 - Pick Bodies

VI. Huntingtin Disease: Etiology
   A. Autosomal dominant
   B. CAG trinucleotide repeat expansion in huntington gene
   C. Chromosome 4
   D. Genetic anticipation

VII. Huntington Disease: Pathophysiology
   A. Degeneration of caudate nucleus and putamen in basal ganglia
   B. Increased dopamine
   C. Decreased GABA and acetylcholine

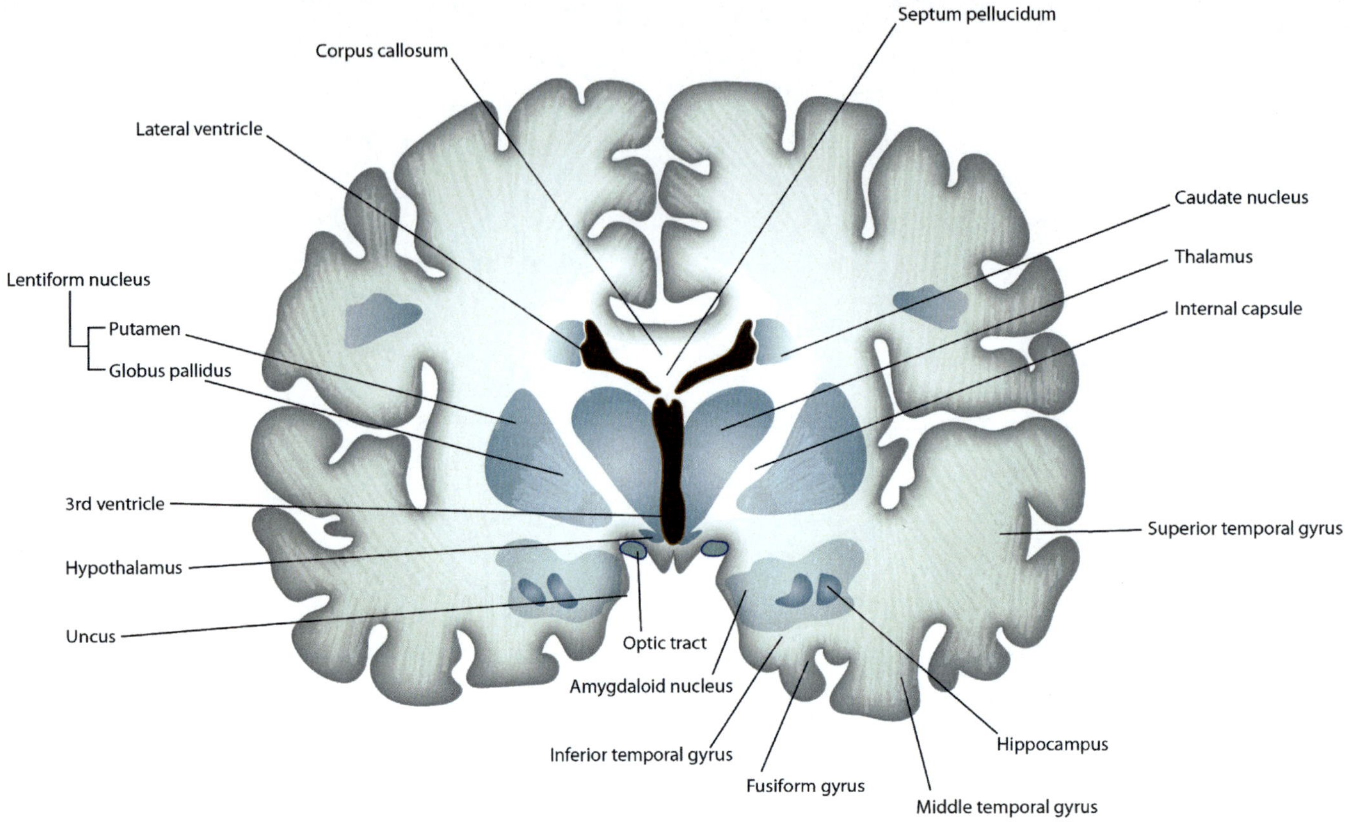

FIGURE 10.4.23 - Anatomy of the Brain

VIII. Huntingtin Disease: Clinical Features
- A. Choreiform movements
- B. Dementia
- C. Depression
- D. Common cause of death: suicide

IX. Parkinson Disease
- A. Unknown etiology
- B. MPTP is toxic to substantia nigra
- C. Loss of dopaminergic neurons in the substantia nigra pars compacta in the basal ganglia
- D. Disruption of nigrostriatal pathway
- E. Lewy bodies seen histologically

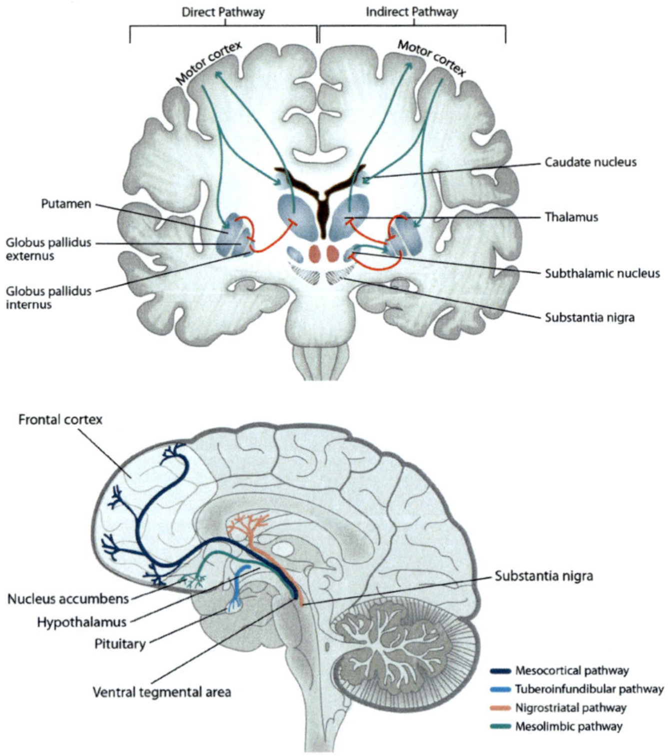

FIGURE 10.4.24 - Coronal Section (Top) and Sagittal Section (Bottom) of the Brain

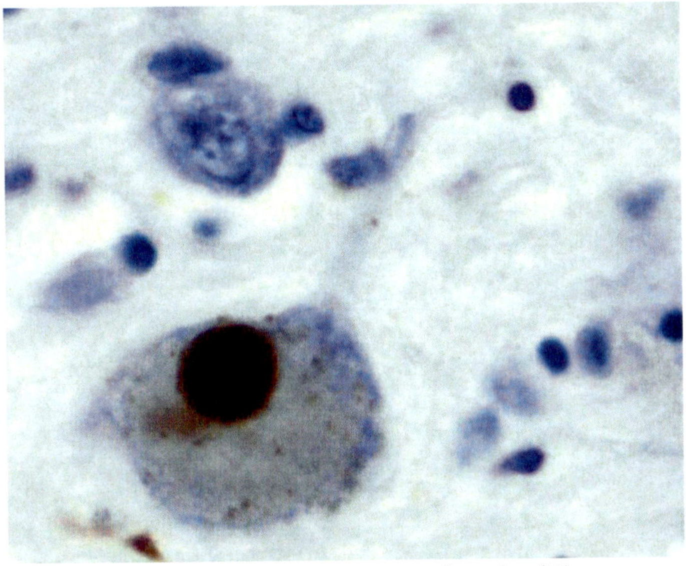

FIGURE 10.4.25 - Lewy Body

X. Parkinson Disease: Clinical Features
   A. Pill-rolling tremor
   B. Cogwheel rigidity
   C. Akinesia or bradykinesia
   D. Postural instability
   E. Shuffling gait
   F. Late-onset dementia

XI. Spongiform Encephalopathy: Etiology
   A. Prion protein disorder
   B. Most commonly sporadic
   C. Exposure to prion-infected cattle or human tissue
   D. Fatal familial insomnia

XII. Spongiform Encephalopathy: Pathophysiology
   A. Prion proteins are normally in an alpha-helical (PrP^{C}) formation
   B. Prion conversion to beta-pleated (PrP^{sc}) formation results in disease
   C. Beta-pleated formation is resistant to proteases
   D. Accumulation leads to cytoplasmic vacuoles and neuronal death

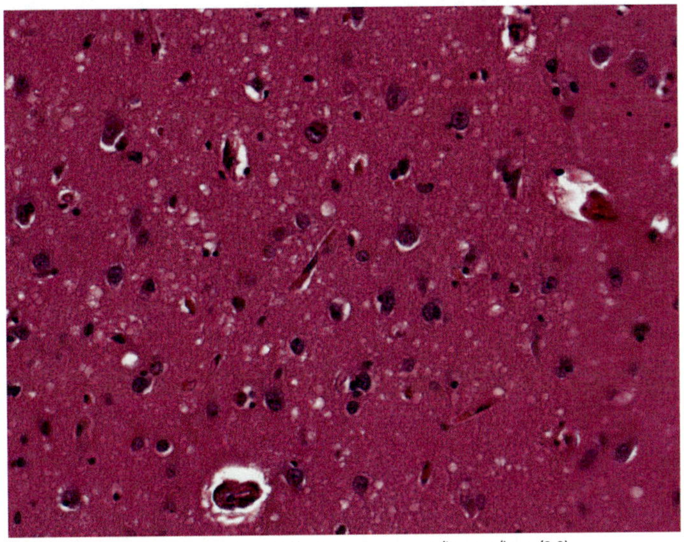

FIGURE 10.4.26 - Cytoplasmic Vacuoles

XIII. Spongiform Encephalopathy: Clinical Features
   A. Rapidly progressive dementia
   B. Myoclonus
   C. Death within a year
   D. Periodic sharp waves on EEG
   E. 14-3-3 protein in CSF

XIV. Normal Pressure Hydrocephalus: Etiology
   A. Idiopathic
   B. Most commonly seen in elderly

XV. Normal Pressure Hydrocephalus: Pathophysiology
   A. Increased cerebrospinal fluid
   B. Dilation of ventricles
   C. Stretching of corona radiata
   D. Urinary incontinence
   E. Gait and cognitive impairment
   F. Symptoms may be relieved with lumbar puncture
   G. Treat with ventriculoperitoneal shunt

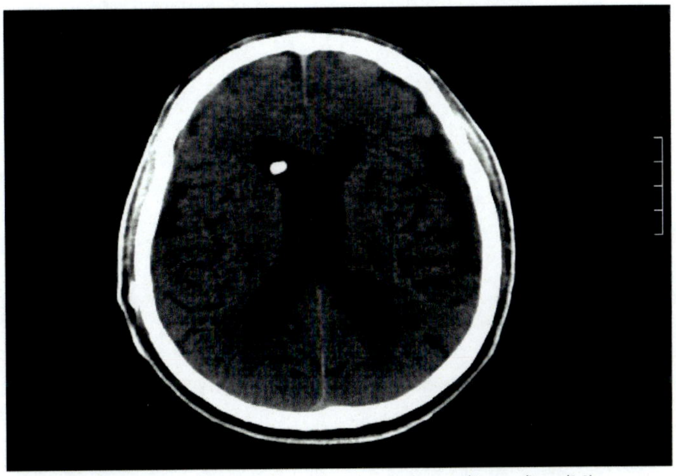

FIGURE 10.4.27 - Axial Brain MRI of Normal Pressure Hydrocephalus

REVIEW QUESTIONS

1. A 72-year-old male with a past medical history of hypertension and type 2 diabetes mellitus is brought to the physician by his wife due to concerns about his memory. The patient admits he has had trouble with his short term memory over the past few years and thinks it is worsening. The patient denies any hallucinations or bradykinesia. Which histological features are seen in this patient's condition?

   - **Histology will show beta-amyloid plaques and neurofibrillary tangles.**
   - The patient is suffering from Alzheimer disease. This is the most common cause of dementia and typically affects the elderly.
   - Beta-amyloid plaques are seen histologically. A dysfunction in amyloid precursor protein cleavage results in the overproduction of beta-amyloid.
   - Another histological finding is neurofibrillary tangles. These are caused by the accumulation of hyperphosphorylated tau protein.

2. A 69-year-old female with no past medical history presents to the physician due to concerns of uncontrollable hand movement. The patient appears to have rigid movements on physical exam and a resting tremor of the hand is noted. What is the anatomical location of this patient's brain abnormality that is responsible for her current symptoms?

   - **The correct answer is the substantia nigra pars compacta.**
   - The patient is suffering from Parkinson disease.
   - A pill-rolling tremor and cogwheel rigidity are symptoms of Parkinson disease. This is due to a loss of dopaminergic neurons in the substantia nigra pars compacta.

3. A 45-year-old female with no past medical history presents to the physician for her annual physical examination. The patient's current temperature is 36.89 °C (98.4 °F), blood pressure is 128/80 mmHg, heart rate is 69 beats/minute, and the respiratory rate is 13 breaths/minute. The patient states she has felt depressed over the last year. Further questioning reveals her father committed suicide in his early 50s. On physical examination, the patient is noted to have jerky, writhing, uncontrollable movements in her arms and legs. Which of the following is most likely seen in this patient's condition?

   A. Elevated levels of dopamine
   B. Loss of dopaminergic neurons
   C. Accumulation of cytoplasmic vacuoles
   D. Narrowing of sulci and widening of gyri

   - **The correct answer is A.**
   - The important thing to recognize here is that the patient is experiencing depression and choreiform movements. Therefore, the patient is suffering from Huntington's disease. Another clue to her disorder is her father committing suicide at an early age. Huntington's disease is an autosomal dominant disorder and suicide is a common cause of death.
   - The disease leads to the degeneration of the caudate nucleus and putamen in the basal ganglia. This causes an increase in dopamine and a decrease in GABA and acetylcholine. Elevated dopamine levels activate the nigrostriatal pathway, which results in choreiform movements. Elevated dopamine levels also activate the mesolimbic, which results in psychotic symptoms.
   - B is incorrect because this refers to Parkinson disease. Loss of dopaminergic neurons results in a constellation of symptoms including a pill-rolling tremor, cogwheel rigidity and dementia.
   - C is incorrect because the accumulation of cytoplasmic vacuoles is seen in spongiform encephalopathy, which leads to neurodegeneration and rapidly progressive dementia. Death usually occurs within a year.
   - D is incorrect because narrowing of sulci and widening of gyri is associated with Alzheimer disease and is the result of cerebral atrophy.

Section VI - Brain Tumors

I. Brain Tumors
   A. Metastatic
      1. Multiple tumors with well-demarcated margins
      2. Common sources: lung and breast
   B. Primary
      1. Classified according to origin of cells
      2. Locally destructive but rarely metastasize
      3. Usually supratentorial in adults and infratentorial in children

II. Glioblastoma Multiforme
   A. Fast-growing, malignant tumor that develops from astrocytes
   B. Most common primary malignant CNS tumor in adults
   C. Found in cerebral hemisphere
   D. Can cross corpus callosum ("butterfly" lesion)
   E. Histology: pleomorphic tumor cells surrounding the central areas of necrosis (pseudopalisading)

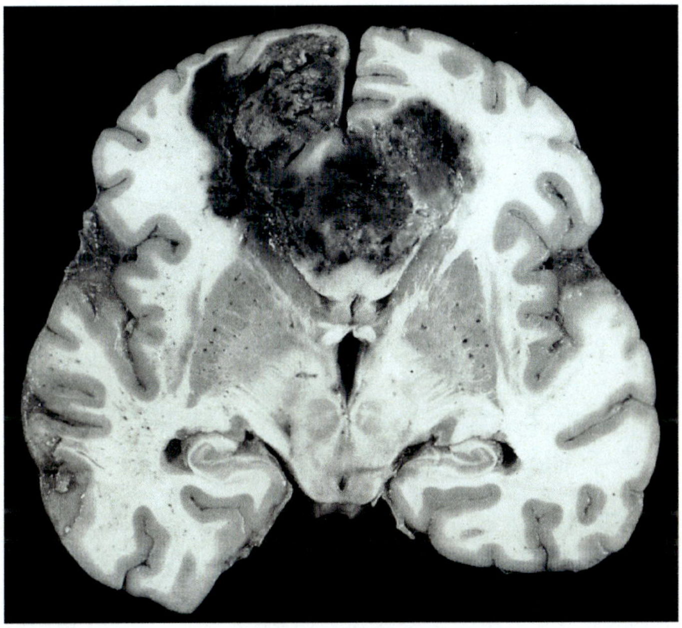

FIGURE 10.4.28 - Gross Pathology of Glioblastoma Multiforme

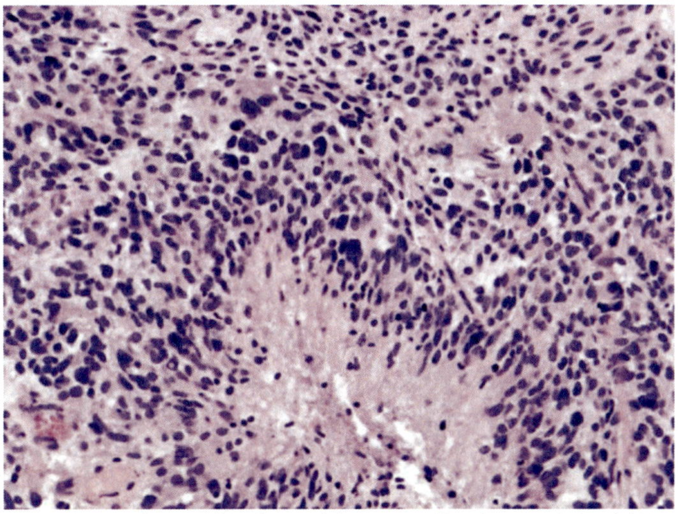

FIGURE 10.4.29 - Pseudopalisading Pattern

III. Meningioma
   A. Benign tumor of arachnoid cells
   B. Most common primary benign CNS tumor in adults
      1. More common in females
   C. May present with seizures or focal neurologic signs
   D. Tumor compresses but does not invade the cortex
   E. Imaging: round mass attached to dura mater
   F. Histology: whorled pattern; psammoma bodies

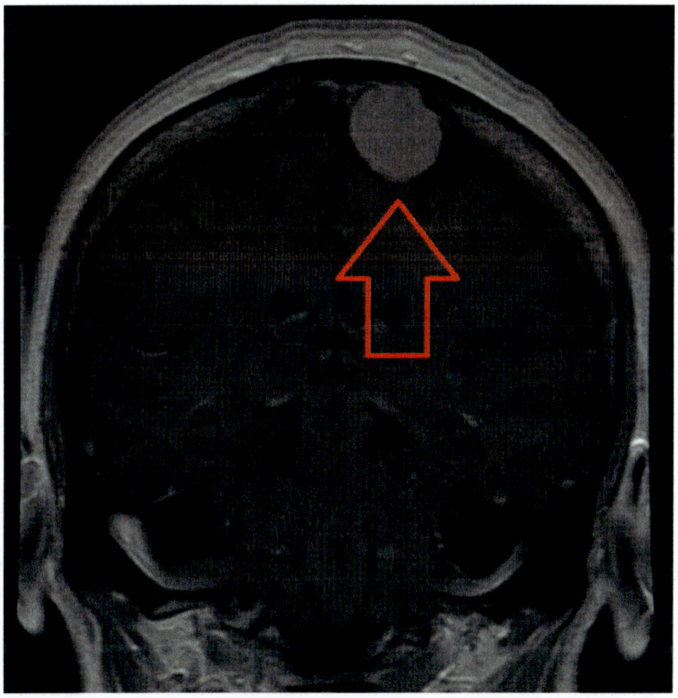

FIGURE 10.4.30 - Coronal Brain MRI of Meningioma

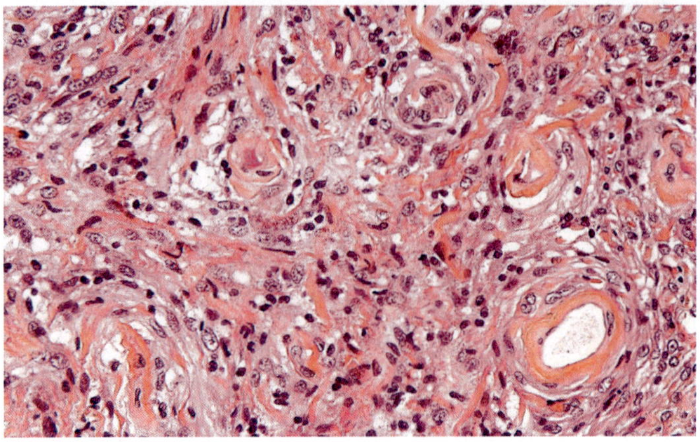

FIGURE 10.4.31 - Whorled Pattern in Meningioma

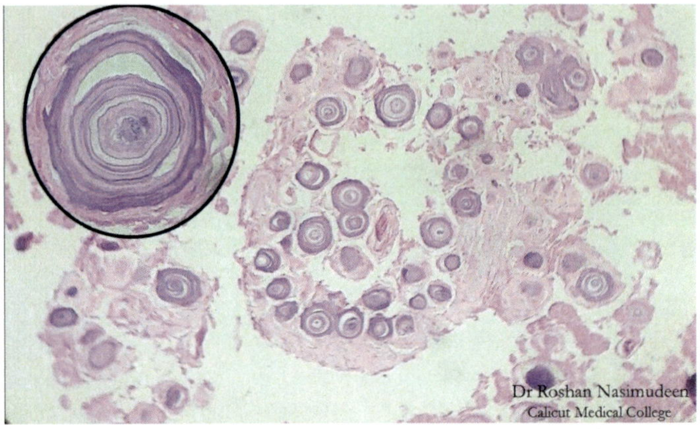

FIGURE 10.4.32 - Psammoma Bodies

IV. Schwannoma
   A. Benign tumor of Schwann cells
   B. Can be along any peripheral nerves
      1. Often localized to CN VIII at cerebellopontine angle (presents as hearing loss and tinnitus)
   C. Tumor cells are S-100 positive
   D. Bilateral tumors found in neurofibromatosis type 2

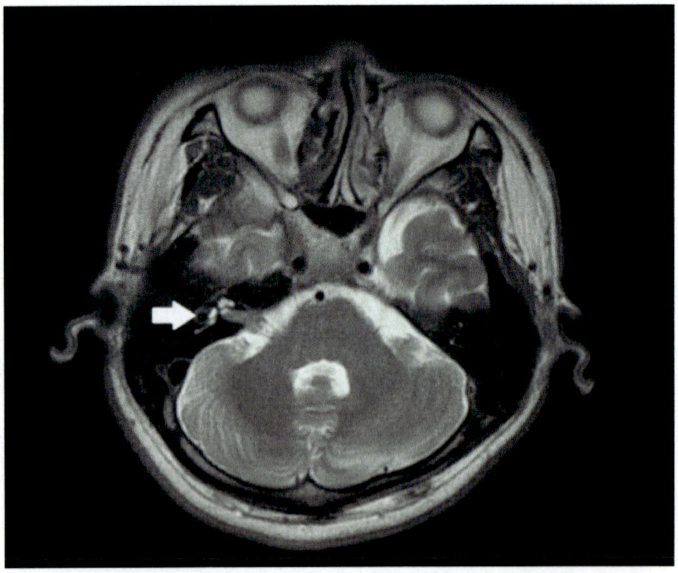

FIGURE 10.4.33 - Axial Head MRI of Schwannoma

V. Oligodendroglioma
   A. Malignant tumor of oligodendrocytes
   B. Imaging: calcified tumor in frontal lobe
   C. Presents with seizures
   D. Histology: "fried-egg" cells (round nuclei with clear cytoplasm)

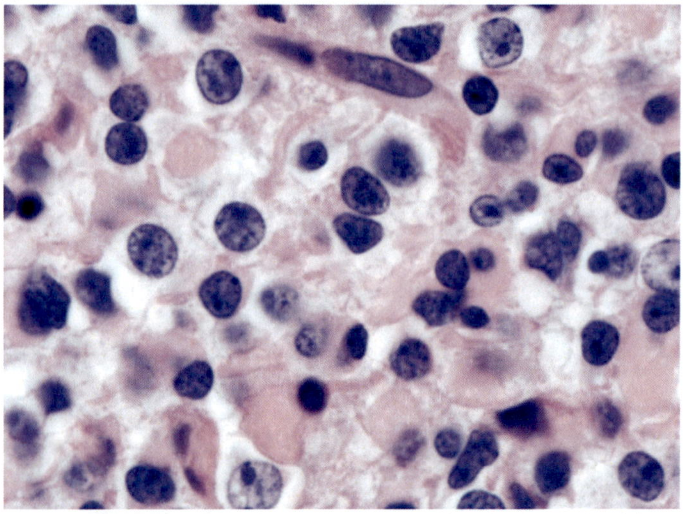

FIGURE 10.4.34 - 'Fried-Egg' Appearance in Oligodendroglioma

VI. Pilocytic Astrocytoma
   A. Benign tumor of astrocytes
   B. Most common primary CNS tumor in childhood
   C. Commonly involves the cerebellum
   D. Tumor cells are GFAP positive
   E. Imaging: a large cystic lesion with a brightly enhancing mural nodule
   F. Histology: Rosenthal fibers (thick eosinophilic corkscrew fibers)

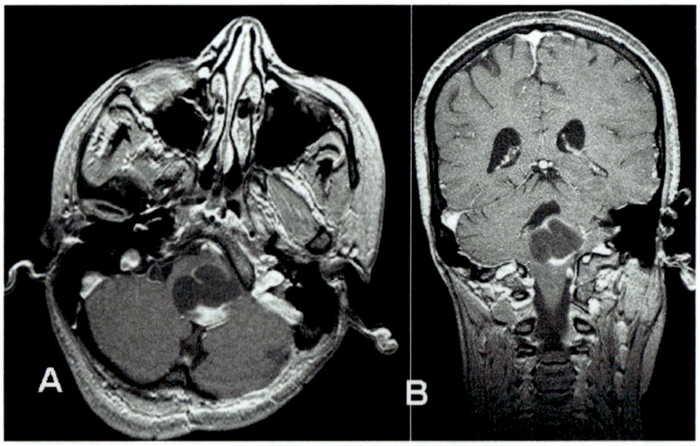

FIGURE 10.4.35 - Axial (Left) and Coronal (Right) Brain MRI of Pilocytic Astrocytoma

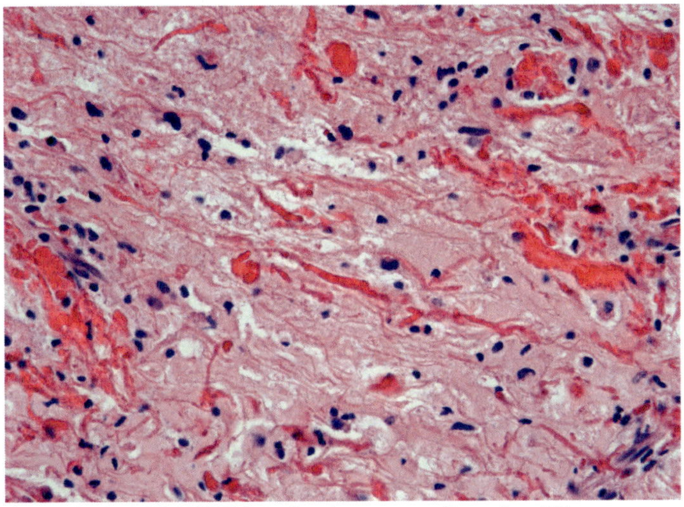

Photo Credit: Marvin 101 / CC BY-SA (https://creativecommons.org/licenses/by-sa/3.0)

FIGURE 10.4.36 - Rosenthal Fibers

VII. Medulloblastoma
    A. Most common malignant tumor in childhood
    B. Derived from granule cells of the cerebellum
    C. Tumor cells are synaptophysin positive
    D. Histology: small blue cells, Homer-Wright rosettes
    E. Poor prognosis: tumor rapidly spreads via CSF
        1. Metastasis to the cauda equina (drop metastasis)

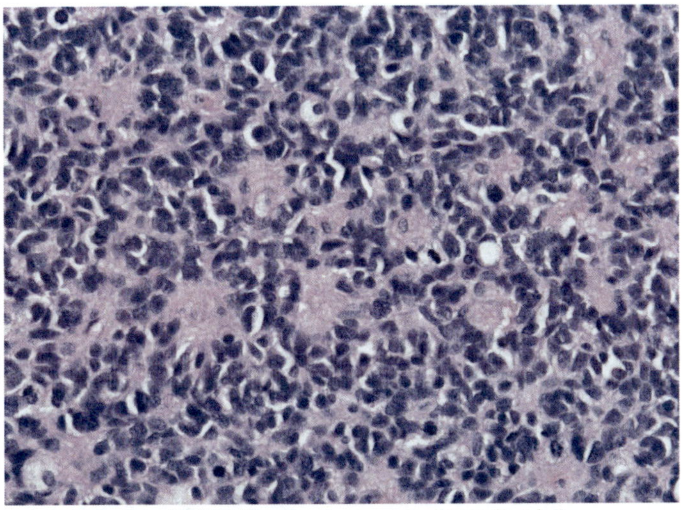

Photo Credit: Jensflorian / CC BY-SA (https://creativecommons.org/licenses/by-sa/3.0)

FIGURE 10.4.37 - Homer-Wright Rosette

VIII. Ependymoma
    A. Malignant tumor of ependymal cells
    B. Seen in children
    C. Most commonly found in 4th ventricle
        1. Obstruction of 4th ventricle → hydrocephalus
    D. Present with hydrocephalus
    E. Histology: perivascular pseudorosettes

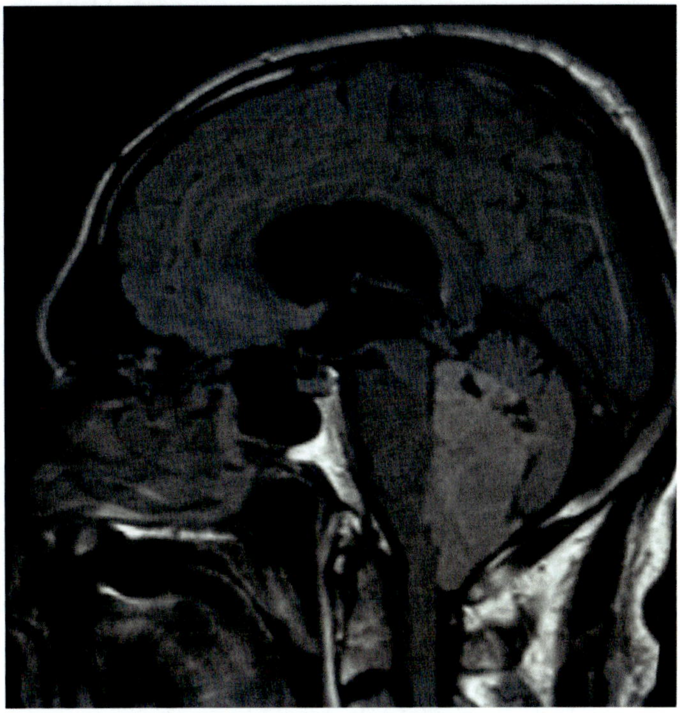

Photo Credit: Hellerhoff / CC BY-SA (https://creativecommons.org/licenses/by-sa/3.0)

FIGURE 10.4.38 - Sagittal Brain MRI of Ependymoma

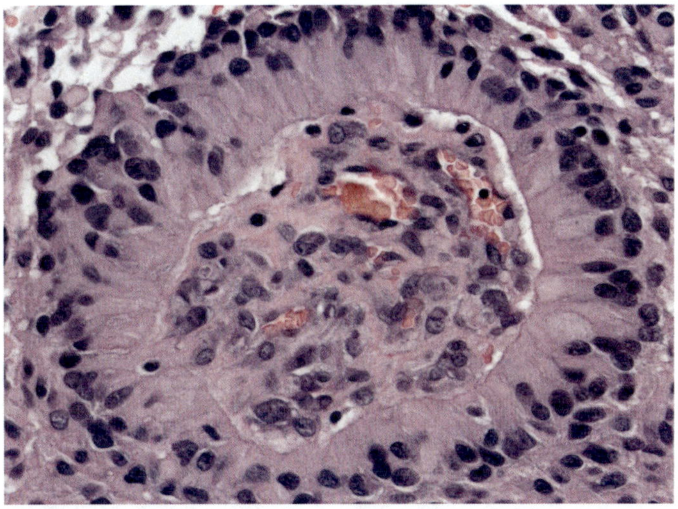

Photo Credit: Jensflorian / CC BY-SA (https://creativecommons.org/licenses/by-sa/3.0)

FIGURE 10.4.39 - Perivascular Pseudorosettes

IX. Craniopharyngioma
    A. Tumor derived from remnants of Rathke's pouch
        1. Invagination of ectoderm from roof of mouth
    B. Most common supratentorial tumor in childhood
    C. Compresses optic chiasm → bitemporal hemianopsia
    D. Imaging: calcifications

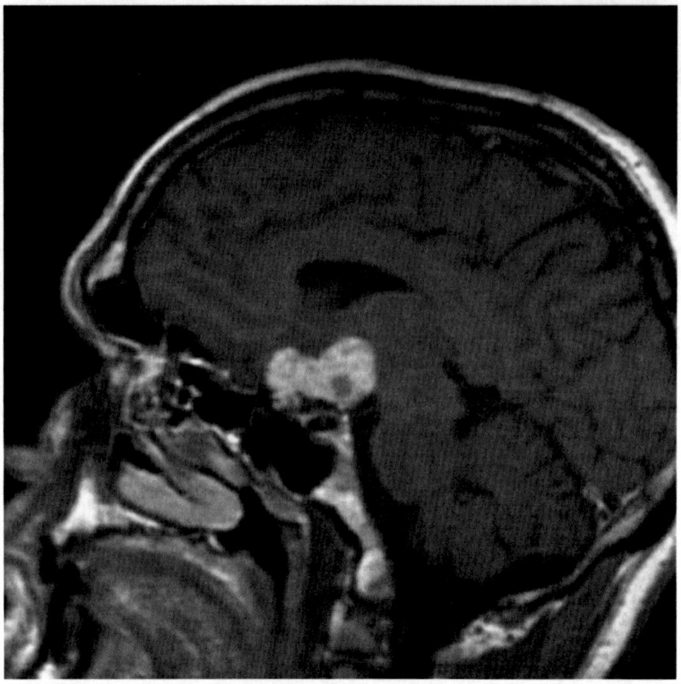

FIGURE 10.4.40 - Sagittal Brain MRI of Craniopharyngioma

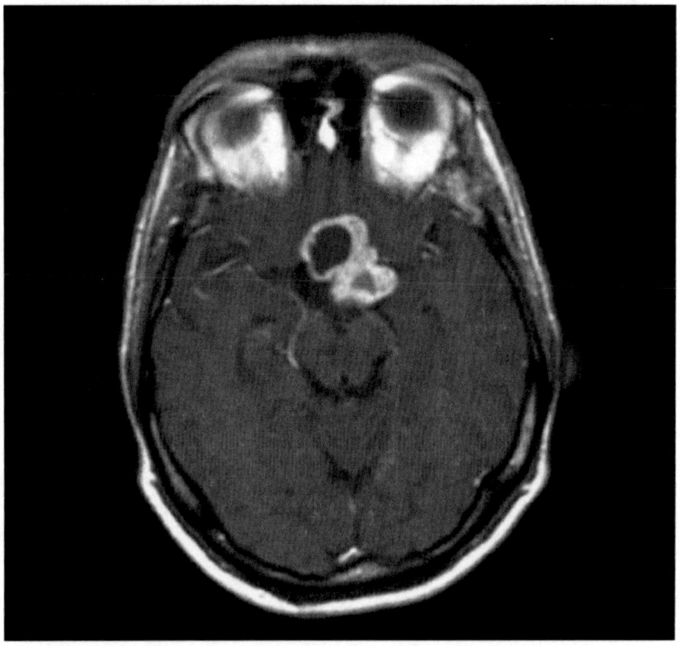

FIGURE 10.4.41 - Axial Brain MRI of Craniopharyngioma

REVIEW QUESTIONS

1. A 51-year-old woman with a past medical history of hypertension and diabetes presents to the emergency department after a seizure. An MRI of the brain shows a round mass attached to the dura mater. The physician notices the tumor compresses, but does not invade, the left cortex. What histopathological findings may be present in this patient?

REVIEW QUESTIONS

- **The correct answer is a whorled pattern of cells with psammoma bodies.**
- This is a 51-year-old woman presenting with a seizure. The MRI shows a round mass attached to the dura mater that compresses but does not invade the cortex. These presentations clearly indicate the diagnosis of meningioma. The histopathological findings would show a whorled pattern of cells with psammoma bodies.

2. A 5-year-old boy presents with his mother to the emergency department for a severe headache and vomiting. The boy has no significant past medical history. An MRI of the brain shows a cerebellar cystic mass with mural nodules. What is the cellular origin of these tumor cells?

- **The correct answer is astrocytes.**
- This is a 5-year-old boy presenting with a severe headache and vomiting. The MRI shows a cerebellar cystic mass with mural nodules. These presentations indicate the diagnosis of pilocytic astrocytoma. Pilocytic astrocytoma is a benign tumor of astrocytes.

3. A 6-year-old girl presents with her mother to the emergency department with a progressively worsening headache. Physical examination shows papilledema. An MRI of the brain demonstrates a mass in the fourth ventricle. What characteristic histological finding may be present on a biopsy of this mass?

    A. Homer-Wright rosettes
    B. Rosenthal fibers
    C. Perivascular pseudorosettes
    D. Fried-egg appearance of cells

- **The correct answer is C.**
- This is a 6-year-old girl presenting with a progressively worsening headache. Physical exam shows papilledema and the MRI of the brain demonstrates a mass in the 4th ventricle. These findings indicate the diagnosis of ependymoma. Perivascular pseudorosettes are a characteristic finding on histology.
- A is incorrect because Homer-Wright rosettes are characteristically seen in patients with medulloblastoma.
- B is incorrect because Rosenthal fibers are characteristically seen in patients with pilocytic astrocytoma.
- D is incorrect because cells with a fried-egg appearance are characteristically seen in patients with oligodendroglioma.

Section VII - Headaches

I. Basic Principles
   A. Headache: pain due to irritation of structures
      1. Dura mater
      2. Cranial nerves
      3. Extracranial structures
   B. More common in females, except cluster headaches

II. Cluster Headache
   A. Unilateral
   B. 15 minutes - 3 hours, recurrent
   C. Intense periorbital pain with nasal discharge and tearing eyes
   D. May present with Horner syndrome
   E. Men > women

III. Cluster Headache: Treatment
   A. Acute treatment
      1. 100% oxygen
      2. Sumatriptan
   B. Prophylactic treatment
      1. Verapamil

IV. Migraine Headache
   A. Unilateral
   B. 4-72 hours
   C. Throbbing and pulsating pain
   D. Nausea
   E. Sensitivity to light and sound
   F. May have "aura" before or with headache
   G. Due to irritation of CN V, releasing vasoactive neuropeptides

V. Migraine Headache: Treatment
   A. Acute treatment: NSAIDs, sumatriptan, and dihydroergotamine
   B. Prophylactic treatment
      1. Lifestyle changes
      2. Beta blockers
      3. Amitriptyline
      4. Botulinum toxin
      5. Anti-CGRP monoclonal antibodies

VI. Tension Headache
   A. Bilateral
   B. 4-6 hours
   C. Steady, "band-like" pain
   D. No aura
   E. No sensitivity to light and sound

VII. Tension Headache: Treatment
   A. Acute treatment
      1. NSAIDs
      2. Acetaminophen
   B. Prophylactic treatment
      1. Amitriptyline
      2. Behavioral therapy

VIII. Other Causes of Headache
   A. Subarachnoid hemorrhage
   B. Hydrocephalus
   C. Meningitis
   D. Trigeminal neuralgia
   E. Giant cell (temporal) arteritis

REVIEW QUESTIONS

1. A 35-year-old woman presents with a throbbing headache affecting the left side of her head. She reports that her headache is accompanied by nausea and a tingling sensation on the left side of her face. Her past medical history is unremarkable. What is the most likely cause of her headache?
   - **The correct answer is irritation of trigeminal nerve.**
   - This is a 35-year-old woman presenting with a left-sided throbbing headache along with nausea and a tingling sensation on the left side of her face. A unilateral throbbing headache with nausea and aura indicates migraine headache.
   - Migraine headache is due to irritation of trigeminal nerve (CN V), the nerve that supplies sensation to the head and the face. Activation of the trigeminal nerve causes release of vasoactive neuropeptides such as serotonin and calcitonin gene-related peptide (CGRP), both of which cause blood vessels in the brain to swell.

2. A 32-year-old man presents with excruciating right-sided periorbital pain. He reports that the headache occurs once or twice a week, often lasting about 30 minutes. During his headache episodes, he often experiences a runny nose and tearing eyes. What other symptoms could this patient experience in a future episode?

   A. Flashes of light
   B. Sensitivity to sound
   C. Drooping of the eyelid
   D. Difficulty speaking

   - **The correct answer is C.**
   - This is a 32-year-old man presenting with an excruciating right-sided periorbital pain. The pain is recurrent in nature and lasts for 30 minutes, during which the patient experiences a runny nose and tearing eyes. These findings indicate the diagnosis of cluster headache. Someone with cluster headache may also present with Horner syndrome, which presents with a triad of ptosis, miosis, and anhidrosis. Therefore, drooping of the eyelid (ptosis) is the correct answer.
   - A and D are incorrect because flashes of light and difficulty speaking are part of the sensory disturbances known as "aura" that are associated with migraine headache.
   - B is incorrect because sensitivity to sound is also associated with migraine headache, not cluster headache.

Section VIII - Seizures

I. Basic Principles
   A. Abnormal electrical activity of the brain due to neuron hyperexcitability
   B. Partial or generalized
   C. Causes: genetic defects, structural abnormalities, metabolic abnormalities, tumors, infection, trauma, and stroke
   D. Symptoms depend on location of abnormal activity
   E. Provoked by lack of sleep, stress, and alcohol

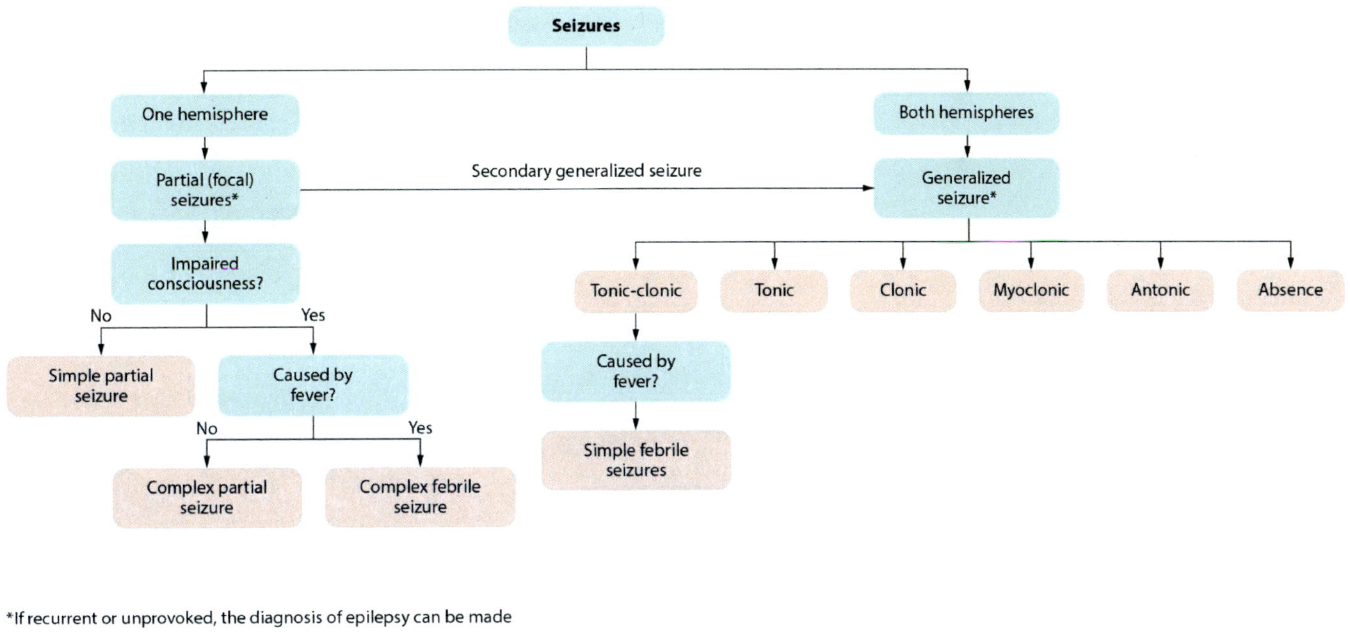

FIGURE 10.4.42 - Classification of Seizures

II. Partial Seizures: Definition
   A. Affect a single area of the brain or confined to only one side of the brain
   B. Also called focal seizures

III. Partial Seizures: Overview
   A. Most commonly due to a structural brain abnormality
      1. Temporal lobe (most common)
   B. May experience an aura
   C. Symptoms present contralateral to affected side of brain
   D. Types: simple or complex

IV. Partial Seizures: Simple Partial
   A. Focal seizures where consciousness remains intact
   B. Symptoms vary depending on affected region
      1. Motor: repetitive muscle movements or Jacksonian march
      2. Sensory: vertigo, olfactory, or tingling
      3. Autonomic: Sweating or flushing
      4. Psychic: fear or hallucinations
   C. Partial Seizures: Complex Partial
      1. Focal seizures where consciousness is impaired
      2. Automatisms: lip smacking, chewing, or swallowing
   D. Partial Seizures: Complex Febrile
      1. Similar to a complex partial seizure but the cause is due to a fever

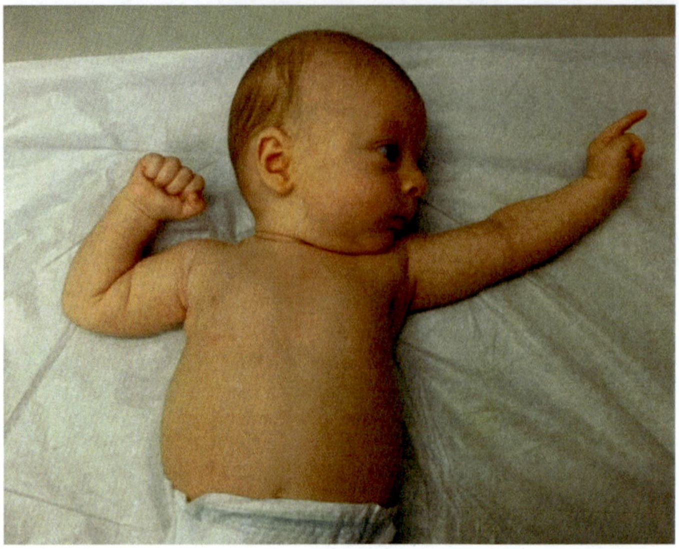

Mjissner/CC0

FIGURE 10.4.43 - Asymmetrical Limb Involvement "Fencing Position" of a Partial Seizure

V. Generalized Seizures: Types
   A. Tonic-clonic: most common; altering tonic (stiffening) and clonic (uncontrolled, repetitive muscle movements) phases
   B. Myoclonic: Rapid, repetitive, and arrhythmic muscle jerks
   C. Atonic: loss of muscle tone; drop to floor; can lead to falls and injuries; often confused with fainting
   D. Absence: brief episodes of blank stares; no aura or postictal state; occur many times throughout the day; most common in children; classic 3Hz spike-and-wave complexes on EEG; ethosuximide

VI. Generalized Seizures: Simple Febrile
   A. A generalized seizure caused by a fever
   B. Most commonly tonic-clonic in nature

I. Epilepsy
   A. Disorder of chronic, recurrent, and unprovoked seizures
   B. Status Epilepticus: single seizure lasting 5+ minutes or the presence of recurrent seizures without regaining consciousness in between
      1. Emergency
      2. Treatment: IV benzodiazepines

	Fever	Hyperthermia
Pathophysiology	- Hypothalamus responds to cytokines by increasing basal body temperature	- Increase in temperature that exceeds body's ability to dissipate heat
Etiology	- Infection - Inflammation	- External: heat stroke - Internal: medications (serotonin syndrome) and metabolic diseases
Body Temperature	- <40 °C (< 104 °F)	- <40 °C (< 104 °F)
Treatment	- Antipyretics: NSAIDs and acetaminophen - Treat underlying cause (e.g. antibiotics for infection)	- Rapid reduction of body temperature via physical means: cool bath, rehydration, no cooling blankets (excess vasoconstriction → decrease heat loss) - Antipyretics do not help
Prognosis	- Usually self-limited - Resolves by treating underlying cause	- Rapidly fatal if not treated promptly
Complications	- Febrile seizures (children)	- Respiratory dysfunction (ARDS), arrhythmia/cardiac dysfunction, neurologic dysfunction, organ failure

TABLE 10.4.4 - Fever Vs. Hyperthermia

REVIEW QUESTIONS

1. A 10-year-old girl is brought to the emergency department by her mother, who witnessed her undergo an episode of upper right arm jerking. The mother adds that during the episode, her daughter was unresponsive. The episode lasted for about 2 minutes, after which she was confused and sleepy. When asked about the event, she had no recollection of it. Her temperature is 37 C (98.6 F). What is the most likely type of seizure that this patient experienced?

- **The correct answer is a complex partial seizure.**
- This is a 10-year-old who was witnessed by her mother having a seizure, her arm was jerking.
- We see that only her right upper arm was affected, so only one side of the body had abnormal activity.
- This indicates that she had a partial seizure.
- According to her mother, the girl was not responsive during the episode, and the girl does not recall having the episode.
- This indicates a complex seizure, since consciousness was impaired.
- This all points towards the most likely type of seizure, being a complex partial seizure.
- Remember that complex partial seizures are focal seizures where the consciousness is impaired.

2. A 9-year-old boy is brought to the physician by his parents due to inattention. His parents complain that he does not listen to them and is frequently found staring into the distance. They have also received various phone calls from his teachers due to his declining academic grades. They do not report any abnormal body movements or loss of consciousness. His medical history is significant for a mild upper respiratory tract infection that resolved on its own three weeks ago. On physical examination, the boy is alert, answers questions appropriately, and is playful. What is the most likely diagnosis?

   A. Simple partial seizure
   B. Partial complex seizure
   C. Absence seizure
   D. Generalized myoclonic Seizure

- **The correct answer is C.**
- From the question stem, you notice that this child is frequently found staring into the distance. He also is inattentive and has declining academic performance.
- Collectively, this is consistent with an absence seizure.
- Recall that absence seizures are a form of generalized seizures that present with brief episodes of blank stares.
- All other choices are incorrect as they do not classify present frequent staring episodes, which is typical for absence seizures.
- For example, choice A can present with motor symptoms, such as repetitive muscle jerks or other sensory or autonomic abnormalities, which has not occurred in this case.
- Option B is wrong because these are commonly associated with automatisms, such as lip smacking or chewing.
- Option D is incorrect because generalized myoclonic seizures present with rapid, repetitive muscle jerks.

Section IV - Neurocutaneous Disorders

I. Basic Principles
   A. Inherited disease that primarily affect central nervous system and skin
   B. Commonly autosomal dominant (except Sturge-Weber)
   C. Mutations in tumor suppressor genes (except Sturge-Weber)

II. Sturge-Weber Syndrome: Overview
   a. Nonhereditary anomaly of neural crest derivatives
   b. Somatic mosaicis mutation in *GNAQ* gene
   c. Capillary-venous malformations in skin, eyes, and brain

III. Sturge-Weber Syndrome: Presentation
   A. Port-wine stain capillary malformation of face
      1. V1/V2 distribution of trigeminal nerve
   B. Leptomeningeal angioma [arrow] ipsilateral to port-wine stain
      1. Intellectual disability and seizures/epilepsy
   C. Episcleral hemangioma
      1. Increased intraocular pressure and glaucoma

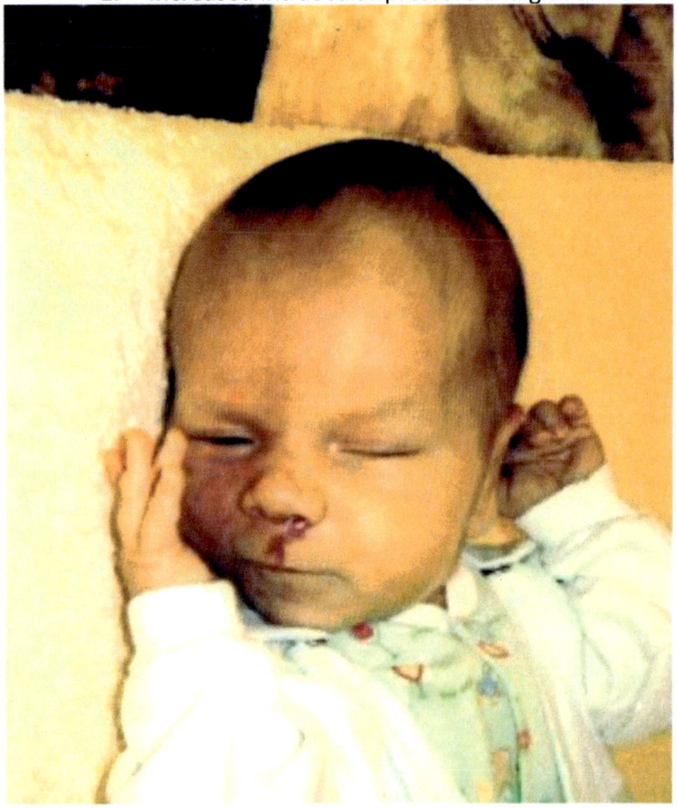

FIGURE 10.4.44 - Infant with Port-Wine Stain

IV. Von Hippel-Lindau Syndrome: Overview
   A. Autosomal dominant
   B. Deletion of *VHL* gene on chromosome 3
   C. Benign and malignant tumors

V. Von Hippel-Lindau Syndrome: Presentation
   A. Hemangioblastomas
      1. Most commonly in retina, cerebellum, and spinal cord
   B. Bilateral renal cell carcinoma
   C. Pheochromocytoma
   D. Cysts in various organs
      1. Kidneys, pancreas, liver

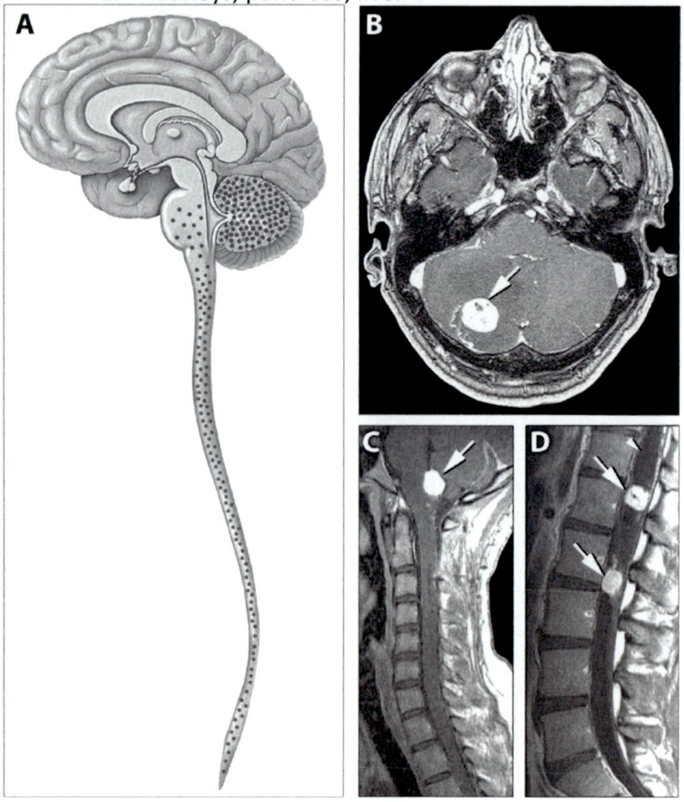

https://commons.wikimedia.org/wiki/File:Hippel_Lindau.gif

FIGURE 10.4.45 - Typical Distribution Sites of Hemangioblastomas

VI. Tuberous Sclerosis: Overview
   A. Autosomal dominant
   B. Mutation in either
      1. *TSC1* on chromosome 9 (hamartin)
      2. *TSC2* on chromosome 16 (tuberin)
   C. Hamartomas, other benign tumors, and specific cutaneous manifestations

VII. Tuberous Sclerosis: Presentation
   A. Cortical hamartomas ("tubers")
      1. Intellectual disability, seizures
   B. Cardiac rhabdomyoma
   C. Renal angiomyolipoma
   D. Cutaneous manifestations
      1. Adenoma sebaceum, ash-leaf spots, shagreen patches, periungual fibromas

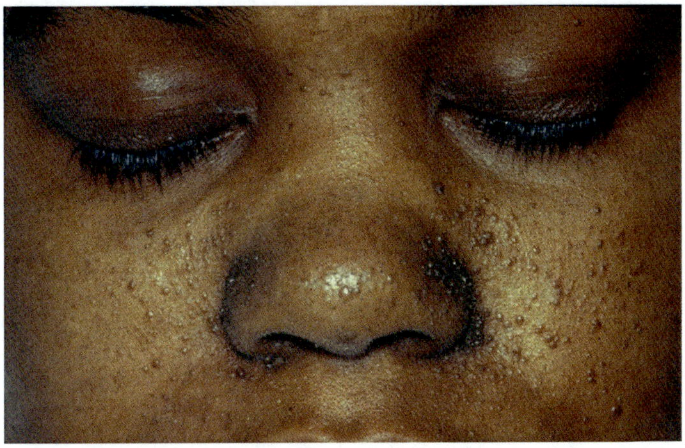

Herbert L. Fred, MD and Hendrik A. van Dijk / CC BY-SA

FIGURE 10.4.46 - Skin Findings of Tuberous Sclerosis

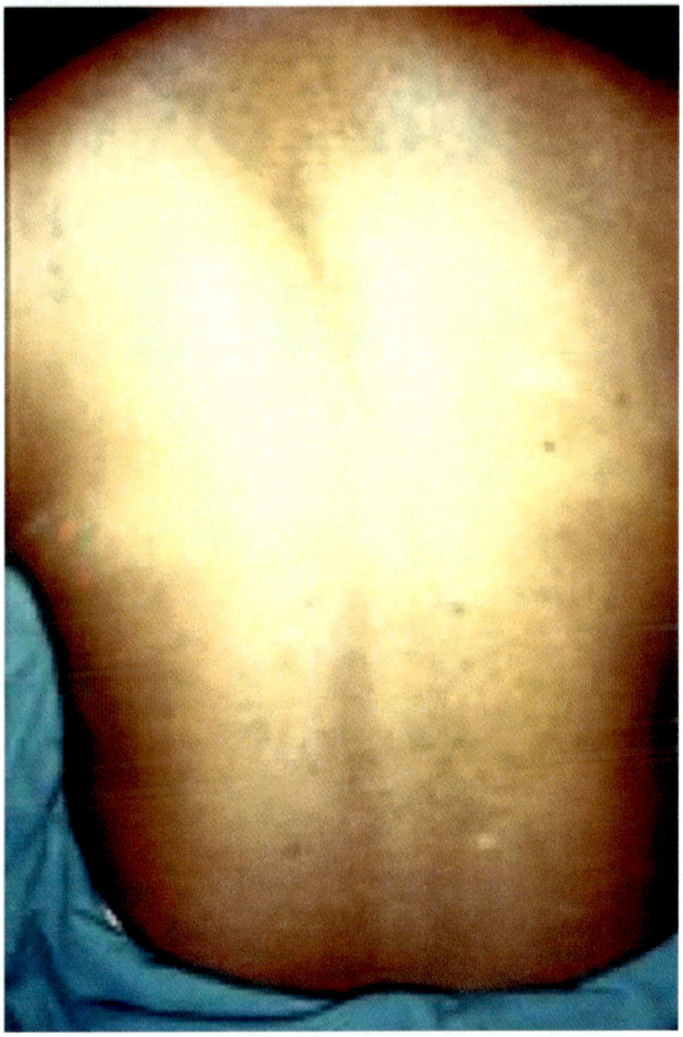

Herbert L. Fred, MD, Hendrik A. van Dijk / CC BY (https://creativecommons.org/licenses/by/2.0)

FIGURE 10.4.47 - Ash-Leaf Spots

VIII. Neurofibromatosis Type I: Introduction
- A. Most common type of neurofibromatosis
  - 1. Also known as von Recklinghausen disease
- B. Autosomal dominant
- *C.* *NF1* on chromosome 17 (neurofibromin)
- D. Variable presentation but characteristic neurofibromas and cutaneous manifestations

IX. Neurofibromatosis Type I: Presentation
- A. Neurofibromas - nodules on or under the skin
  - 1. Intellectual disability or seizures when in CNS
- B. Eye involvement
  - 1. Lisch nodules and optic gliomas
- C. Pheochromocytoma
- D. Cutaneous manifestations
  - 1. Café-au-lait spots
  - 2. Axillary and inguinal freckling

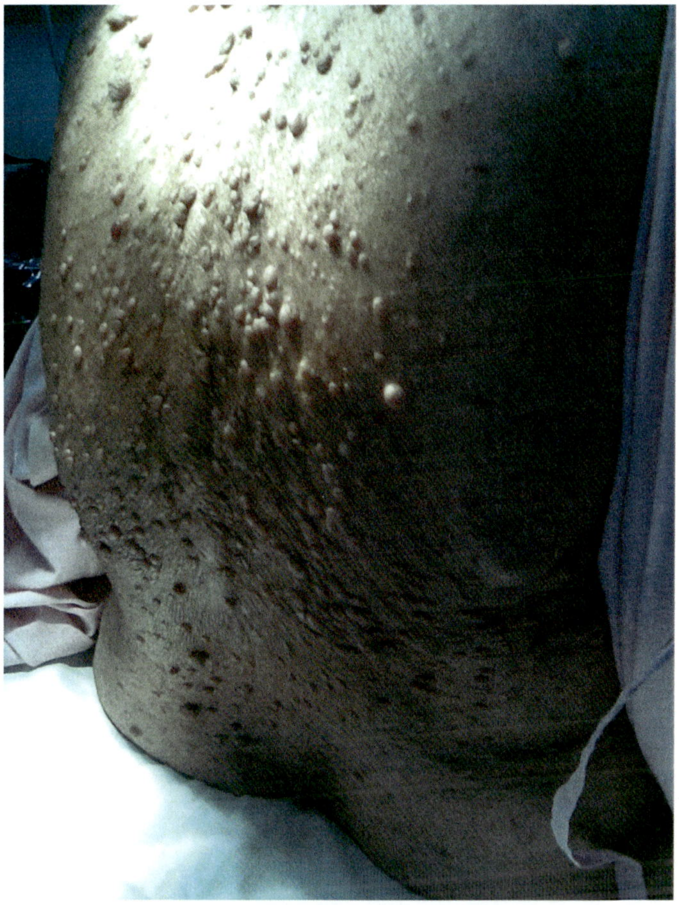

Almazi / Public Domain

FIGURE 10.4.48 - Neurofibromas

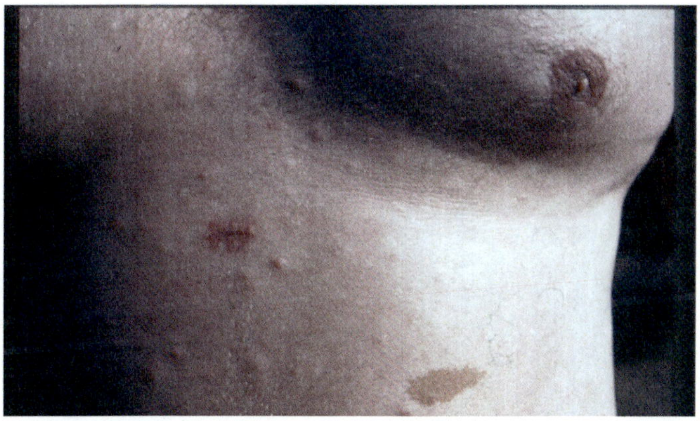

Haymanj / Public Domain

FIGURE 10.4.49 - Café-Au-Lait Spot

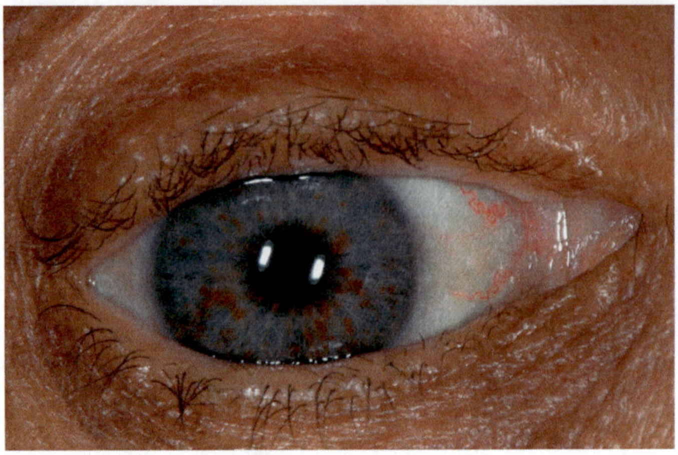

FIGURE 10.4.50 - Lisch Nodule

X. Neurofibromatosis Type II: Overview
   A. Autosomal dominant
   B. *NF2* on chromosome 22 (merlin)
   C. Affects both eyes and ears
   D. "*NF2* on chromosome 22 affects 2 eyes and 2 ears"

XI. Neurofibromatosis Type II: Presentation
   A. Bilateral vestibular schwannomas ("acoustic neuromas")
      1. Tinnitus, hearing loss, vertigo
   B. Juvenile cataracts
   C. Meningiomas
   D. Ependymomas

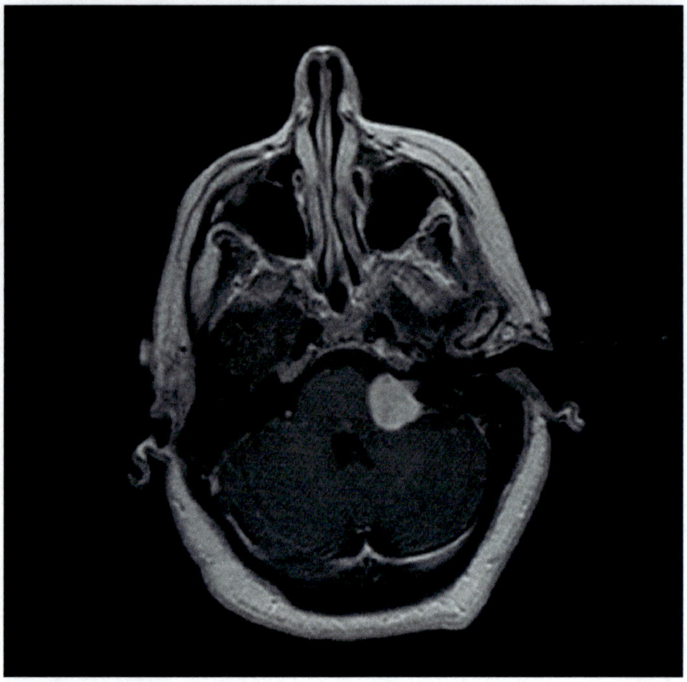

FIGURE 10.4.51 - Head CT Showing Bilateral Vestibular Schwannomas

REVIEW QUESTIONS

1. A 23-year-old female presents to the emergency department complaining of headaches, blurred vision, sweating, and "a racing heart." Upon admission, her blood pressure is 165/98 mmHg, and her heart rate is 109 beats/minutes. She has no significant past medical history, but her father was seen for similar symptoms around her age and was eventually diagnosed with renal cell carcinoma. A 24-hour urine test shows increased levels of metanephrines. A mutation in which chromosome would be expected in this patient?

- **The correct answer is chromosome 3.**
- This patient has symptoms indicative of sympathetic hyperactive activity: Headaches, blurred vision, sweating, palpitations, hypertensions, and tachycardia.
- Furthermore, she has increased levels of metanephrines in her urine, indicating a possible pheochromocytoma.
- Her father's past medical history of similar symptoms, leading to renal cell carcinoma, provides evidence that this disorder is inherited.
- An inherited disorder is indicative of Von Hippel-Lindau Syndrome and this syndrome occurs due to a mutation due to a *VHL* gene of chromosome 3.

2. A 24-year-old Caucasian man presents for a routine visit to his primary care physician. He does not have any current complaints. Vital signs are within normal limits. On physical exam, he has numerous firm, rubbery nodules of varying sizes on his back. He also has small, pigmented spots on his irises and a hyperpigmented macular lesion on his left lateral thigh. What other cutaneous findings could be present as a result of this patient's condition?

- **The correct answer is neurofibromatosis type 1. The other skin findings that could be found in this patience is axillary and inguinal freckling.**
- This patience clearly has neurofibromas, as suggested by the numerous, firm rubbery nodules of varying sizes on his back.
- He also has lisch nodules, the small, pigmented spots on his irises as well as a cafe-au-lait spot, which is the hyperpigmented macular lesion on his left lateral thigh.

3. 3. A 5-month-old infant is brought to the emergency department after suffering a seizure at daycare. His daycare provider said she was holding him in her lap when he had a strong, bilateral symmetric jerk of his torso, extremities, and head. This occurred about eight times in quick succession. He is afebrile and all vitals are within normal limits. Developmentally, he does not roll or grasp at objects, but he does orient toward sound. He has multiple pink papules on his nasolabial folds and cheeks, and a coarse plaque on the lumbosacral region. Renal ultrasound is most likely to reveal which of the following?

   A. Angiomyolipoma
   B. Renal Cell Carcinoma
   C. Wilms Tumor
   D. Multiple Cysts

- **The correct answer is A.**
- This patient is presenting with afebrile convulsive seizure, developmental delay, and cutaneous findings.
- Multiple plink papules on his nasolabial folds and cheeks is indictivative of adenoma sebaceum.
- A coarse plaque in the lumbosacral region is describing a shagreen patch.
- Therefore, the patient likely has tuberous sclerosis, which commonly presents with renal angiomyolipoma.
- Patients with tuberous sclerosis can present with many symptoms, including intellectual disability, seizures, angiomyolipoma, adenoma sebaceum, and shagreen patches.
- B is incorrect because while renal cell carcinoma can occur in patients with tuberous sclerosis, it is a very small percentage and angiomyolipomas are much more common.
- C is incorrect because Wilms tumor is a kidney tumor that primarily affects children, but is not associated with tuberous sclerosis.
- D is incorrect because the presents of multiple cysts is associated with polycystic kidney disease.

CARDIAC PATHOLOGY

Section I - Hyperlipidemia Signs

I. Xanthomas
  A. Localized deposits of lipids that may manifest as nodules, plaques, or papules
  B. Inflammatory cells engulf lipids, resulting in a broad range of histological findings (e.g. foam cells, lipid-laden histiocytes)

II. Xanthelasma
  A. Xanthomas that occur on the eyelid

III. Tendinous Xanthoma
  A. Xanthomas that occur over tendons or ligaments
  B. Achilles tendon frequently affected

IV. Corneal Arcus
  A. Lipid deposition within the cornea, resulting in a circumferential gray or white ring
  B. Common in the elderly

V. Management
  A. Fasting lipid profile
  B. Detailed family history
  C. Genetic testing

REVIEW QUESTIONS ?

1. A 28-year-old previously healthy female presents to the clinic due to a cosmetic abnormality on her left eyelid that she first noticed several weeks ago. Physical examination reveals a yellow plaque on the surface of the left eyelid. What is the next best step in the management of this patient?

    A. EKG
    B. Prescribe antibiotics
    C. Fasting lipid profile
    D. Incision and drainage

- **The correct answer is C.**
- The patient has a yellow plaque on the surface of the left eyelid, which is consistent with a xanthelasma and is indicative of hyperlipidemia. A fasting lipid profile will allow us to determine if the patient has hyperlipidemia and provide appropriate management, such as administration of a lipid-lowering agent.
- A is incorrect because this would be indicated only if ischemic heart disease were suspected. While hyperlipidemia is a risk factor for developing ischemic heart disease, this patient has no signs or symptoms consistent with this diagnosis.
- B and D are incorrect because these are referring to a stye, which is a bacterial infection of the eyelid. A stye would present with a red, swollen, and painful eyelid, which this patient does not have. Therefore these treatments are not appropriate.

Section II - Hypertension

I. Hypertension
   A. Elevated blood pressure (> 130/80)
   B. Determined by cardiac output and systemic vascular resistance
   C. Based on equation BP = CO X SVR
   D. Major factors that influence blood pressure
      1. Sympathetic nervous system
      2. Plasma volume
      3. Renin-angiotensin-aldosterone system

II. Primary (Essential) Hypertension
   A. Exact pathogenesis poorly understood
   B. Likely due to environmental and genetic changes that affect cardiovascular and renal function
   C. Most common cause of hypertension (90%)
   D. Risk factors are many including age, obesity, family history, race (African American), high sodium diet, and inactivity

III. Secondary Hypertension
   A. An underlying medical condition that is responsible for the elevated blood pressure
   B. Examples include renal artery stenosis, fibromuscular dysplasia, pheochromocytoma, Cushing's syndrome, and obstructive sleep apnea
   C. Uncommon cause of hypertension (< 10%)

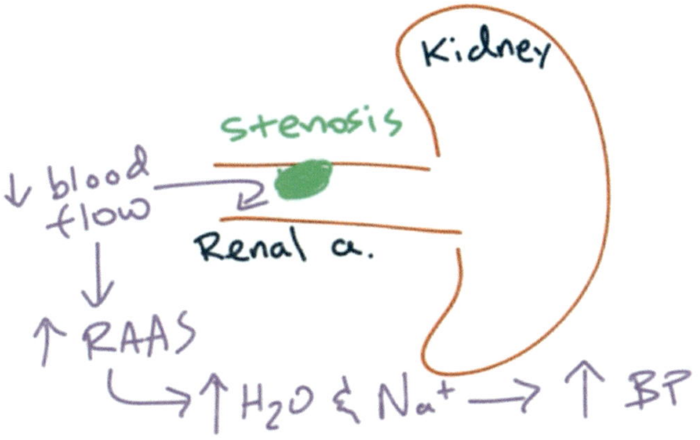

FIGURE 10.5.1 - Renal Artery Stenosis Causing Elevated BP

IV. White Coat h=Hypertension
   A. Blood pressure that is elevated during office visits but is normal in other settings

V. Hypertensive Urgency
   A. Severe hypertension (≥ 180 mmHg systolic or ≥ 120 mmHg diastolic) without evidence of acute end-organ damage (e.g. retinopathy, left ventricular hypertrophy, ischemic cardiovascular disease, stroke, kidney disease)

VI. Hypertensive Emergency
   A. Severe hypertension (≥ 180 mmHg systolic or ≥ 120 mmHg diastolic) with evidence of acute end-organ damage

REVIEW QUESTIONS ?

1. A 64-year-old obese male presents to the clinic due to worsening fatigue over the past several weeks. He states that he always feels tired despite sleeping 9 hours a night. His blood pressure is 172/98 mmHg. His current medications include lisinopril, amlodipine, and hydrochlorothiazide. What is the most likely diagnosis?

   A. Primary hypertension
   B. Hypertensive urgency
   C. Hypertensive emergency
   D. Secondary hypertension

- **The correct answer is D.**
- The patient is obese, has worsening fatigue and a blood pressure of 172/98, and is currently on three antihypertensive medications. We should consider a diagnosis of obstructive sleep apnea, which is common in obese patients and is associated with loud snoring and excessive daytime sleepiness. Sleep apnea is a known cause of secondary hypertension in patients like this one, who is on three antihypertensive medications but still has a blood pressure of 172/98.
- A is incorrect because his hypertension can best be explained by an underlying medical condition.
- B and C are incorrect because this patient does not have a blood pressure of 180/120 or greater.

Section III - Arteriosclerosis

I. Arteriosclerosis
   A. Hardened and thickened arteries
   B. Three types
      1. Atherosclerosis
      2. Arteriosclerosis
      3. Mönckeberg medial sclerosis

II. Atherosclerosis
   A. Definition: fibrous plaque that obstructs blood flow in the large and medium-sized arteries

III. Atherosclerosis: Risk Factors
   A. Dyslipidemia
   B. Diabetes mellitus
   C. Obesity
   D. Hypertension
   E. Smoking

IV. Atherosclerosis: Complications
   A. > 70% stenosis → symptomatic ischemia
   B. Aneurysm
   C. Thrombosis
   D. Embolization

V. Arteriolosclerosis
   A. Occlusion of the small arteries (arterioles)
   B. Two types
      1. Hyperplastic
      2. Hyaline

VI. Hyperplastic Arteriolosclerosis
   A. Smooth muscle cell hyperplasia → occlusion of lumen
   B. Caused by severe hypertension
   C. "Onion-skin" appearance seen on histology

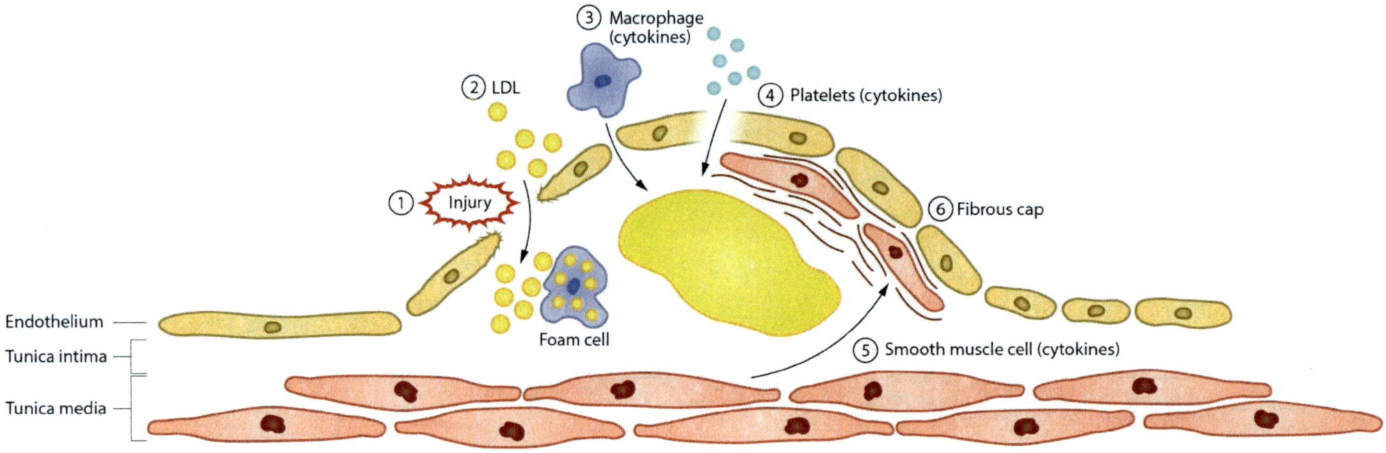

FIGURE 10.5.2 - Pathophysiology of Atherosclerosis

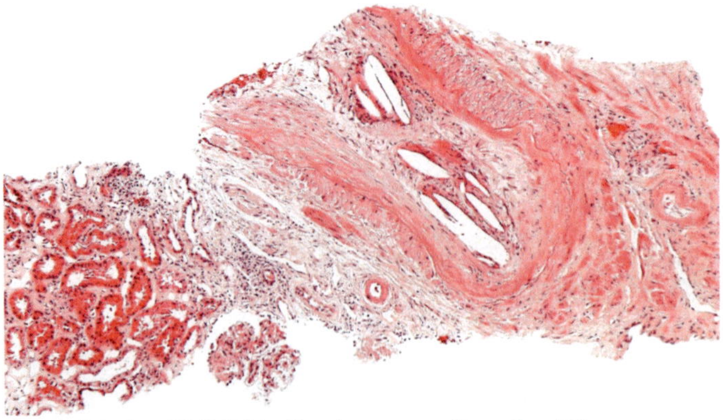

FIGURE 10.5.3 - Embolus in a Medium-Sized Artery in the Kidney

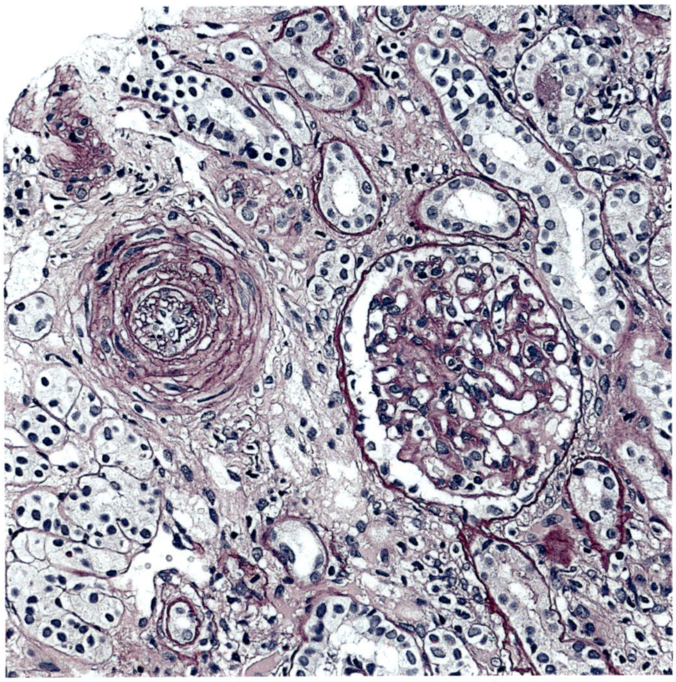

FIGURE 10.5.4 - Hyperplastic Arteriolosclerosis in the Kidney

VII. Hyaline Arteriolosclerosis
  A. Protein deposited in the vessel wall → occlusion of lumen
  B. Caused by uncontrolled hypertension and diabetes
  C. Eosinophilic hyaline thickening seen on histology
  D. Complications include ischemia, atrophy, and scarring (e.g. arteriolonephrosclerosis)

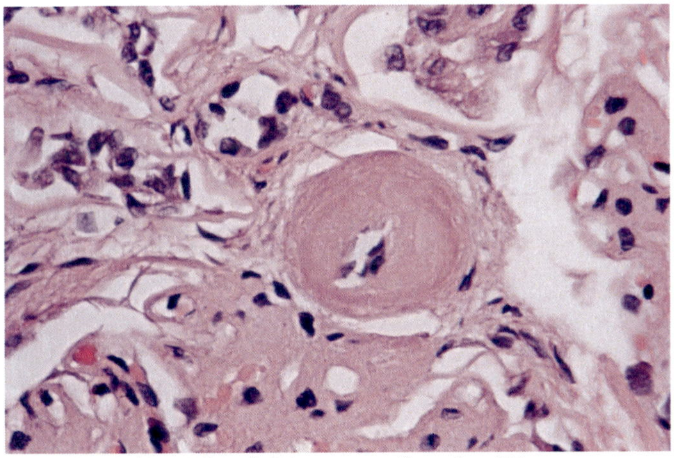

FIGURE 10.5.5 - Hyaline Arteriolosclerosis in the Kidney

VIII. Mönckeberg Medial Sclerosis
  A. Non-obstructive calcification of the tunica media within medium-sized arteries
  B. Clinically insignificant
  C. May be seen on mammography or X-ray as an incidental finding
  D. "Pipestem" appearance on X-ray

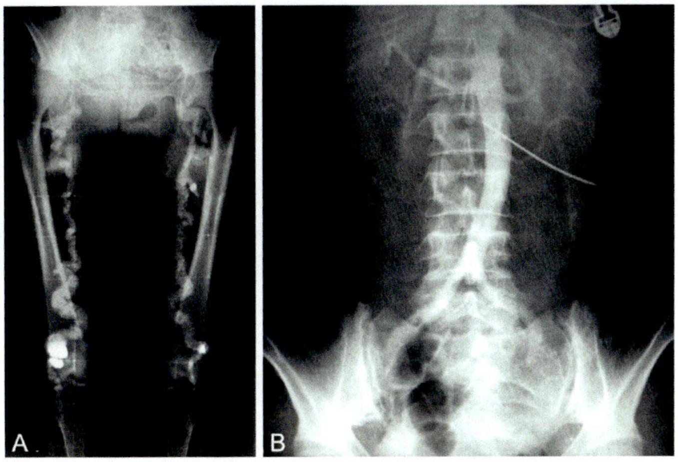

FIGURE 10.5.6 - X-ray of Lower Extremities Showing Calcification of Femoral Arteries

REVIEW QUESTIONS

1. A 59-year-old male presents to the emergency department due to sudden-onset chest pain that began 30 minutes ago. He is diaphoretic and short of breath. Despite aggressive intervention, the patient dies suddenly. An autopsy reveals the presence of atherosclerosis throughout the coronary arteries. The pathological process most likely began many years prior to this patient's death beginning with injury to the vascular endothelium. What pathological process occurred directly following injury to the vascular endothelium?

    A. Foam cell formation
    B. Extracellular matrix deposition
    C. Entry of LDL through the injured site
    D. Smooth muscle cell hyperplasia

- **The correct answer is C.**
- The patient had a myocardial infarction and atherosclerosis was present at autopsy. The process that occurred directly following injury to the vascular endothelium was entry of LDL through the injured site.
- A, B, and D are all incorrect because these steps happen later and do not directly follow injury to the vascular endothelium.

Section IV - Aortic Dissection and Aneurysm

I. Aortic Dissection
   A. A tear in the tunica intima extends into the tunica media, which can then dissect proximally or distally through the aorta
   B. Pre-existing weakness in the tunica media → intimal tears can extend into the tunica media → dissection

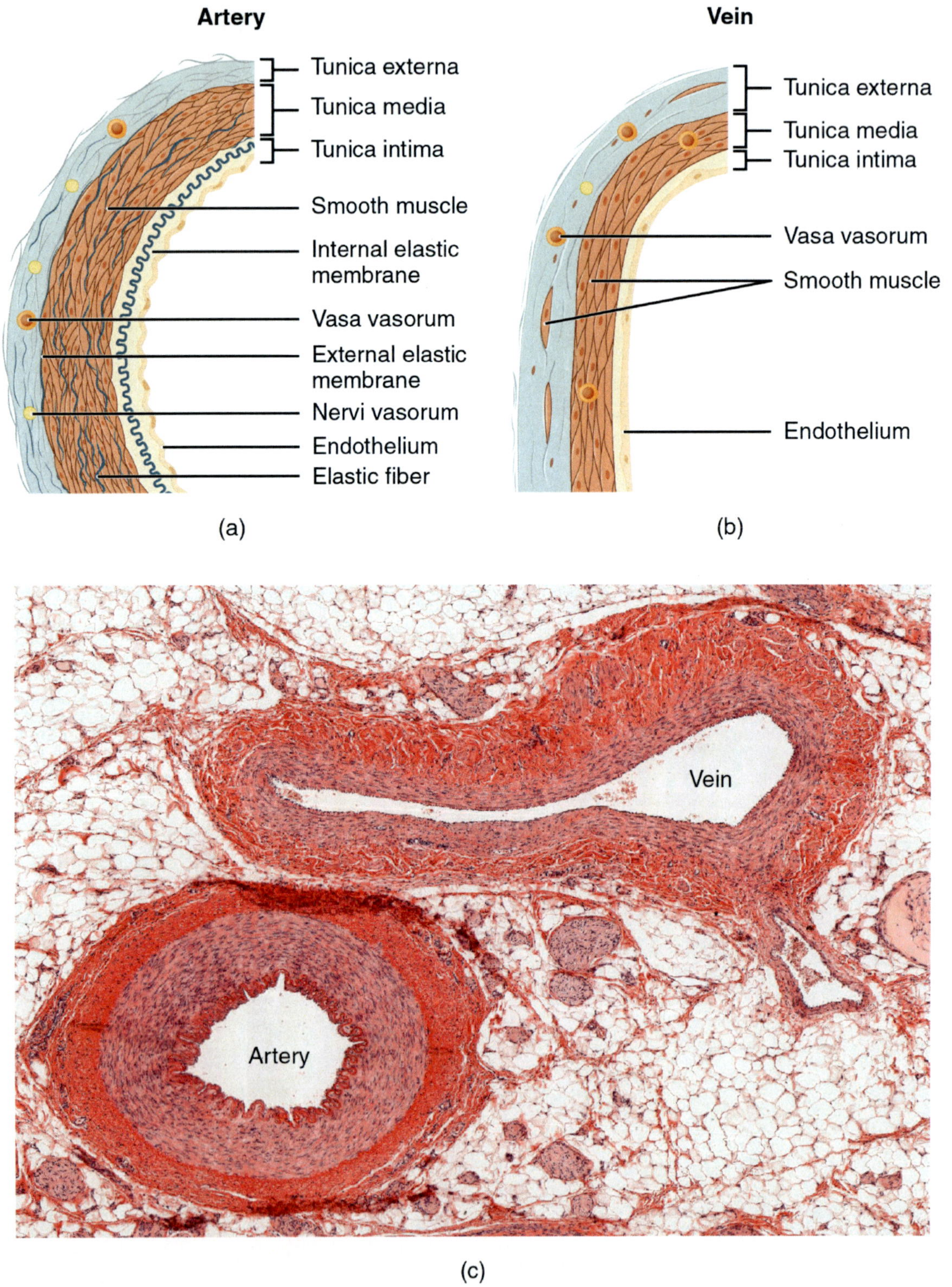

Photo Credit OpenStax College / Anatomy & Physiology, Connexions Website (http://cnx.org/content/col11496/1.6/)

FIGURE 10.5.7 - Histology of Blood Vessels

II. Aortic Dissection: Types
   A. Proximal dissection (Stanford type A)
      1. Involves ascending aorta and may extend to involve the heart (e.g. cardiac tamponade, aortic regurgitation)
      2. May also involve the descending aorta *in addition* to the ascending aorta
   B. Distal dissection (Stanford type B)
      1. Involves *only* the descending aorta

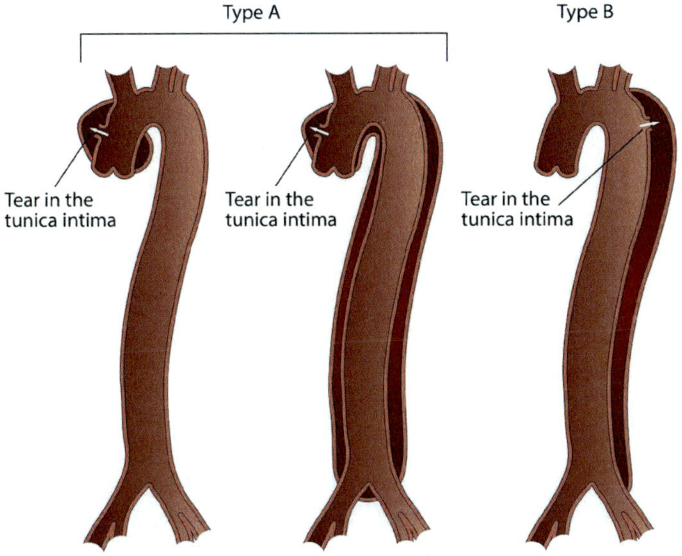

FIGURE 10.5.8 - Stanford Classification of Aortic Dissection

III. Aortic Dissection: Risk Factors
   A. Hypertension (most common)
      1. Hyaline arteriosclerosis of the vasa vasorum → smooth muscle atrophy → weakening of the tunica media
   B. Age
      1. ↑ age → disruption of collagen, smooth muscle, and elastin in the tunica media → replaced with a mucoid extracellular matrix → weakening of the tunica media
   C. Genetic defects
      1. Disruption of the extracellular matrix (e.g. fibrillin-1 defect) → fragmentation of elastic tissue in the tunica media → weakening of the tunica media

IV. Aortic Dissection: Presentation
   A. Sharp sudden-onset chest pain that radiates to the back
   B. Widened mediastinum may be seen on chest X-ray
   C. Double lumen seen on CT

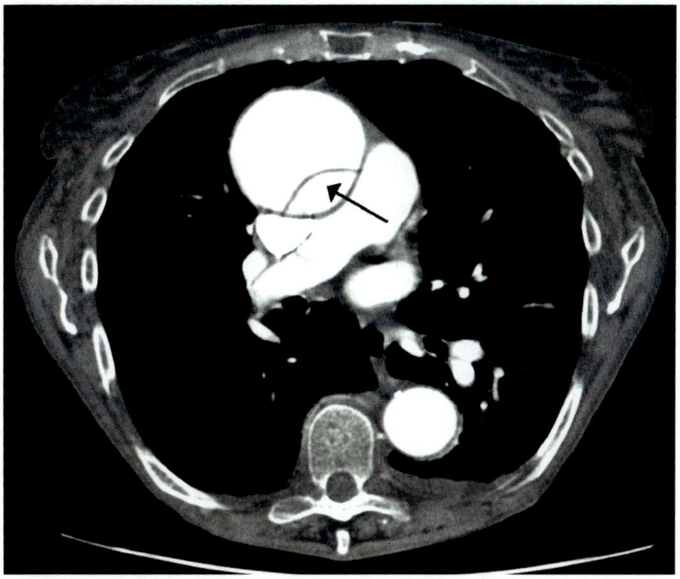

FIGURE 10.5.9 - Axial Chest CT of Aortic Dissection

V. Aortic Dissection: Histology
   A. Cystic medial degeneration
   B. Fragmentation of elastic tissue

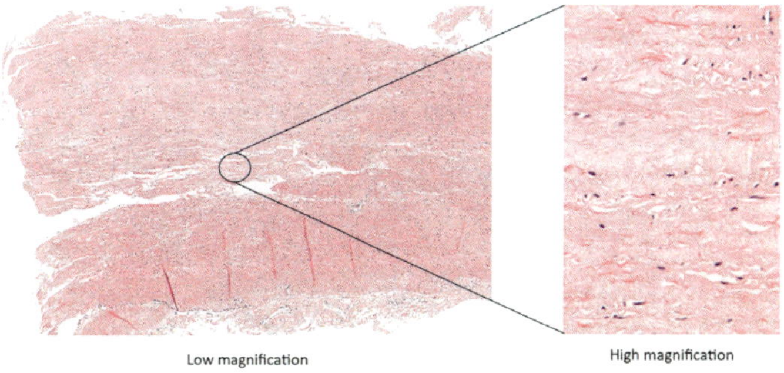

FIGURE 10.5.10 - Cystic Medial Degeneration of the Aorta

VI. Traumatic Aortic Rupture
   A. A tear through the entire wall of the aorta (from the tunica intima to the adventitia)
   B. Most commonly occurs following a motor vehicle accident
   C. Usually at the isthmus of the aorta just distal to the left subclavian artery
   D. Mediastinal widening seen with imaging

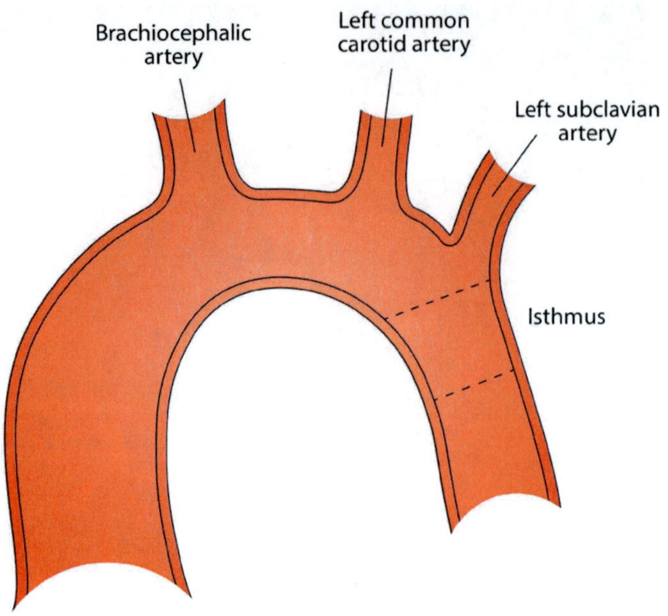

FIGURE 10.5.11 - Anatomy of the Arch of the Aorta

VII. Aortic Aneurysm
   A. Stress-related dilation of the aortic wall
   B. A true aneurysm involves all three histological layers (from the tunica intima to the adventitia)
   C. Two types
      1. Abdominal aortic aneurysm (AAA)
      2. Thoracic aortic aneurysm (TAA)

VIII. AAA: Pathogenesis
   A. Highly associated with atherosclerosis
   B. This and other risk factors (e.g. age > 60, male sex, smoking, hypertension) lead to chronic transmural inflammation of the aortic wall
   C. Inflammatory cells release enzymes (e.g. metalloproteinases) that degrade elastin → weakening of wall → aneurysm development
   D. Atherosclerosis → decreased perfusion of tunica media → atrophy

IX. AAA: Presentation
   A. Most are asymptomatic
   B. When symptomatic it is usually associated with abdominal, back, or flank pain
   C. Classic triad of rupture includes acute pain, hypotension, and a pulsatile abdominal mass
   D. Risk of rupture is significant when > 5.5 cm

X. TAA: Pathogenesis
   A. Nonatherosclerotic in nature (most are idiopathic or sporadic)
   B. Associated with connective tissue-related genetic defects (eg, Marfan syndrome, Ehlers-Danlos syndrome)
      1. Degeneration of tunica media → weakening of aortic wall → aneurysm
   C. Less frequently associated with infections (e.g. tertiary syphilis) or inflammatory disorders (e.g. Takayasu arteritis)
      1. Inflammation of vasa vasorum → ischemia → aortic wall atrophy → aneurysm

XI. TAA: Presentation
   A. Dilation near the aortic root → aortic regurgitation
   B. Expansion of the aneurysm can compress structures causing hoarseness, dysphagia, and/or pain
   C. Rupture/dissection presents with hemodynamic collapse and severe sudden-onset chest pain or back pain
   D. Mediastinal widening seen with imaging

XII. TAA: Histology
   A. Degeneration of the tunica media with a cystic appearance

REVIEW QUESTIONS ?

1. A 67-year-old male presents to the emergency department due to sudden-onset chest pain that began approximately 30 minutes ago. He states that the pain is 10/10 and radiates to his back. A chest X-ray reveals a widened mediastinum. An EKG is normal. A D-dimer is normal. Which of the following is most likely associated with this patient's condition?
   A. Ventricular pseudoaneurysm
   B. Aortic regurgitation
   C. Pericarditis
   D. A swollen calf

- **The correct answer is B.**
- This patient has a classic presentation of aortic dissection including sudden-onset chest pain that radiates to the back and a widened mediastinum on CXR.
- A and C are wrong as these are both complications of a myocardial infarction. This patient's EKG is normal and there was no mention of troponin enzymes or other features that would lead us to believe that this patient is having a heart attack.
- D is a reference to a pulmonary embolism. However, this is unlikely considering that the D-dimer was normal.

Section V - Angina

I. Basic Principles
   A. Ischemic heart disease: an imbalance of oxygen supply from the coronary vessels and oxygen demand of the myocardium
   B. Encompasses a group of syndromes related to myocardial ischemia
      1. Angina pectoris
      2. Acute MI
      3. Chronic ischemic heart disease
      4. Sudden cardiac death
      5. Coronary steal syndrome

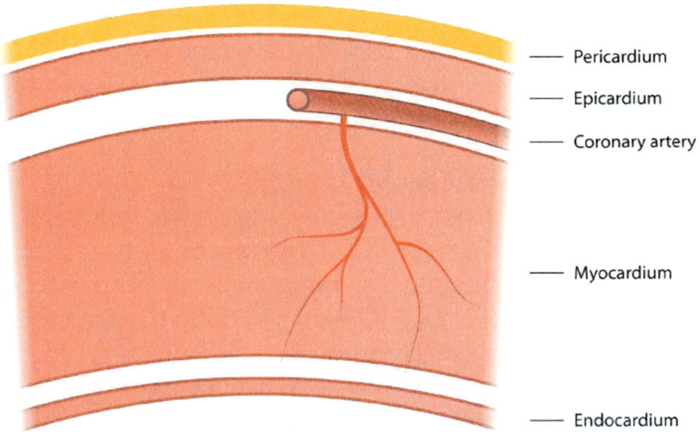

FIGURE 10.5.12 - Coronary Vascular Supply of the Layers of the Heart

II. Stable Angina: Causes
   A. Most commonly caused by atherosclerosis
   B. Stenosis of > 70% of a coronary artery
   C. Other causes include left ventricular hypertrophy and cocaine use

III. Stable Angina: Findings
   A. Chest pain lasting < 20 minutes, accompanied by diaphoresis, SOB, and radiating pain
   B. EKG is usually normal, but a stress test will show ST segment depression (subendocardial ischemia)
   C. Reversible injury to the myocytes
   D. Gradual occlusion of vessels promotes release of growth factors (VEGF) → improved blood flow despite near-total occlusion of arteries

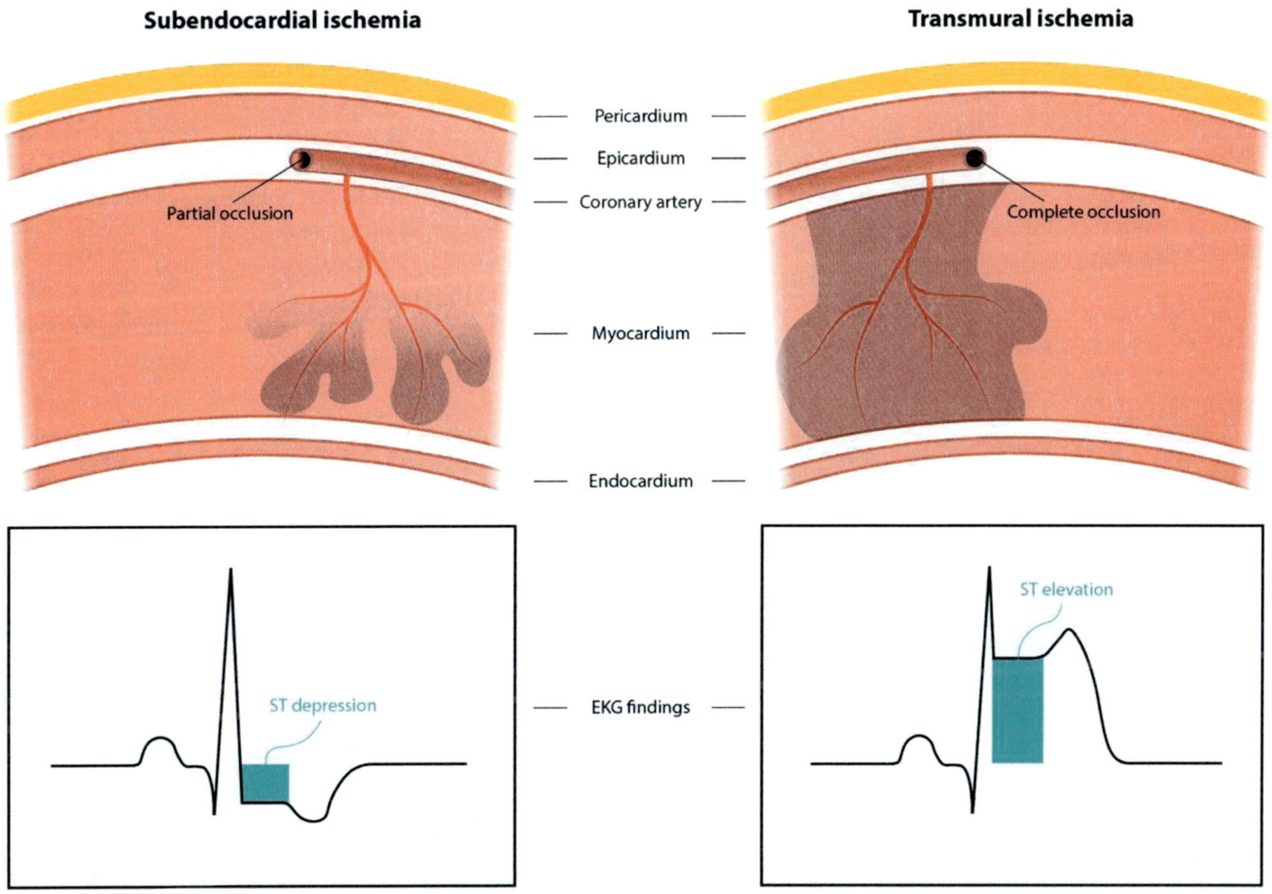

FIGURE 10.5.13 - Subendocardial Ischemia vs. Transmural Ischemia

IV. Stable Angina: Treatment
  A. Beta blockers are preferred
    1. ↓ HR and contractility → decreased O_2 myocardial demand
  B. Calcium channel blockers alternatively used
    1. ↑ coronary/peripheral vasodilation and ↓ contractility → decreased myocardial O_2 demand
  C. Nitroglycerin used for acute symptoms
    1. ↑ venodilation → decreased preload → decreased O_2 myocardial demand

V. Unstable Angina: Causes
  A. Severe atherosclerotic disease that has enlarged
  B. Plaque rupture
  C. Thrombosis
  D. Hemorrhage
  E. Still incomplete occlusion of a coronary artery

VI. Unstable Angina: Findings
  A. Chest pain that occurs at rest and lasts > 20 minutes; pain is more frequent and/or occurs with less exertion compared to previous episodes (presents similarly to MI)EKG may show ST segment depression at rest (subendocardial ischemia)
  B. Reversible injury to the myocytes

VII. Unstable Angina: Treatment
  A. Similar to myocardial infarction ("MONA BASH T")
    1. Morphine (reserved for patients with severe pain)
    2. Oxygen (when O_2 saturation < 90%)
    3. Nitroglycerin
    4. Aspirin
    5. Beta blockers (if hemodynamically stable)
    6. ACE inhibitor (not part of immediate treatment)
    7. Statin
    8. Heparin (anticoagulant)
    9. Ticagrelor (ADP receptor inhibitor)

VIII. Prinzmetal Angina: Cause
  A. Coronary artery vasospasm

IX. Prinzmetal Angina: Findings
  A. Episodic chest pain that occurs sporadically and is not necessarily related to exertion
  B. A stress test may show ST segment elevation (transmural ischemia)
  C. Reversible injury to the myocytes

X. Prinzmetal Angina: Treatment
  A. Calcium channel blockers
  B. Nitroglycerin
  C. Avoid beta blockers and sumatriptan

REVIEW QUESTIONS ?

1. A 71-year-old male presents to the emergency department due to sudden onset chest pain that began approximately 30 minutes ago. He states that the pain began while he was sitting in a chair at home and watching television. An EKG shows ST-segment depression in multiple leads. Labs are repeated multiple times and troponin enzymes are consistently within a normal reference range. This patient's immediate presentation is best characterized by which of the following?
   A. Gradual occlusion of a coronary artery
   B. Plaque rupture
   C. Complete occlusion of a coronary artery
   D. Vasospasm

- **The correct answer is B.**
- The pain began 30 minutes ago while sitting in a chair, an EKG shows ST-segment depression in the ED, and troponin enzymes are within a normal reference range. Collectively, these clues point us towards a diagnosis of unstable angina.
- Recall that with unstable angina the chest pain typically lasts longer than 20 minutes, occurs at rest, and is accompanied by ST segment depression.
- A is wrong because this is describing stable angina. Stable angina typically presents with chest pain that lasts less than 20 minutes and occurs with activity, not at rest. An EKG will be normal.
- C is wrong because this is describing myocardial infarction. An MI would present with elevated troponin enzymes, which is not the case. Remember, stable angina and unstable angina are characterized by incomplete occlusion of a coronary artery.
- D is wrong because this is describing Prinzmetal angina. This would show ST segment elevation.

Section VI - Myocardial Infarction

I. Definition
   A. Necrosis of the myocardium

II. Causes
   A. Atherosclerotic plaque rupture (most common)
      1. Necrotic material and subendothelial collagen exposed → coagulation cascade activated → thrombus formation
   B. Less common causes include cocaine use, vasculitis, coronary artery dissection, prolonged vasospasm (e.g. Prinzmetal angina), and thrombotic syndromes (e.g. antithrombin III deficiency)

III. Types
   A. STEMI
   B. NSTEMI

IV. STEMI
   A. Most commonly due to complete occlusion of a coronary artery, leading to transmural infarction of the myocardium
   B. EKG will show ST-segment elevation
   C. Cardiac enzymes (troponin) will be elevated

V. NSTEMI
   A. Most commonly due to partial occlusion of a coronary artery, leading to subendocardial infarction of the myocardium
   B. EKG will show ST segment depression
   C. Cardiac enzymes (troponin) will be elevated

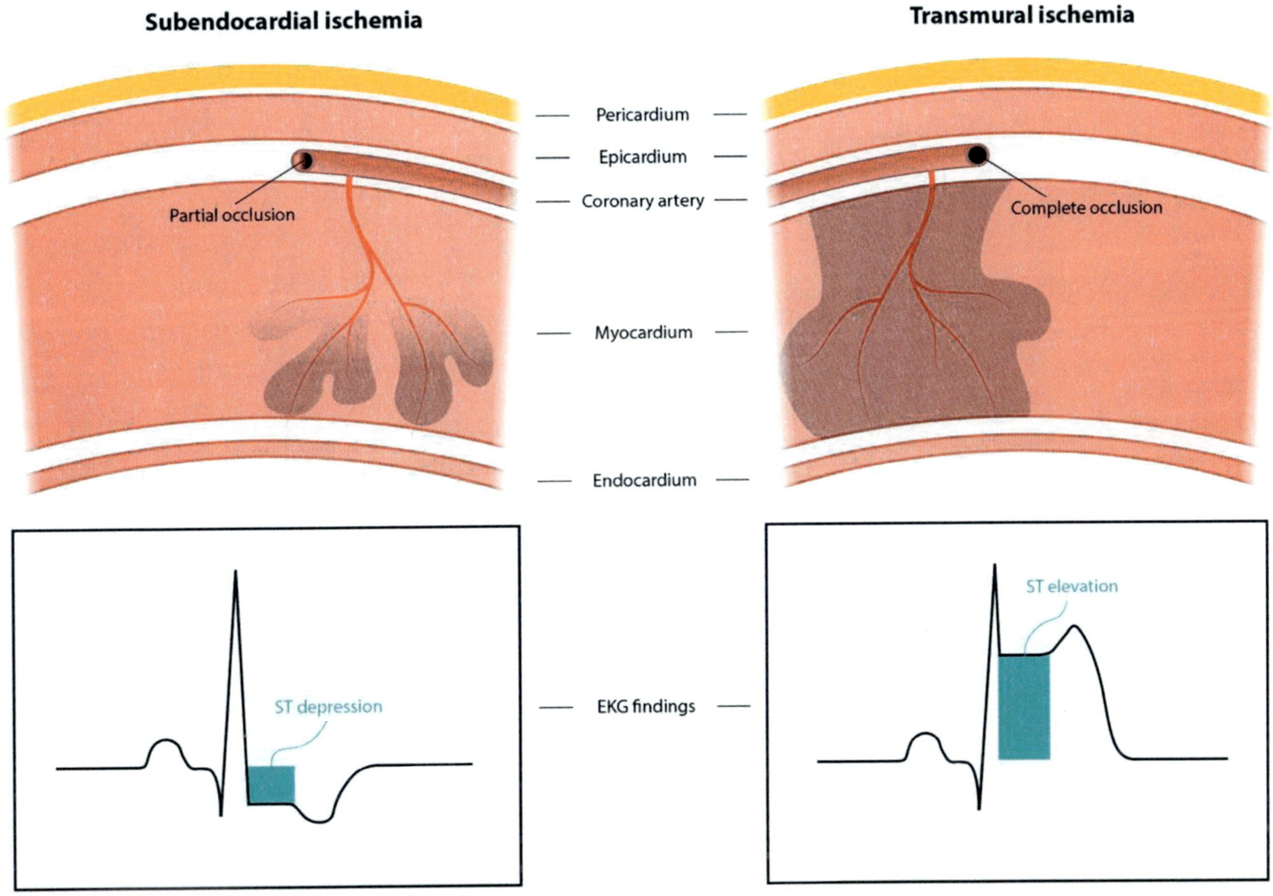

FIGURE 10.5.13 - Subendocardial Ischemia vs. Transmural Ischemia

Time Since Event	Gross Changes	Microscopic Changes	Complications
< 4 hours	None	None	- Transient mitral regurgitation - Arrhythmia
< 1 day	Dark tissue	Coagulative necrosis	- Arrhythmia
< 1 week	Yellow pallor	Inflammation (neutrophils followed by macrophages)	- Peri-infarction pericarditis - Permanent mitral regurgitation - Interventricular rupture → VSD - Ventricular free wall rupture → tamponade / pseudoaneurysm
> 1 week	Hyperemic border	Healing (granulation tissue)	
> 1 month	White scar	Healing (fibrosis)	- Aneurysm - Mural thrombus - Dressler syndrome

TABLE 10.5.1 - Evolution of Myocardial Infarction

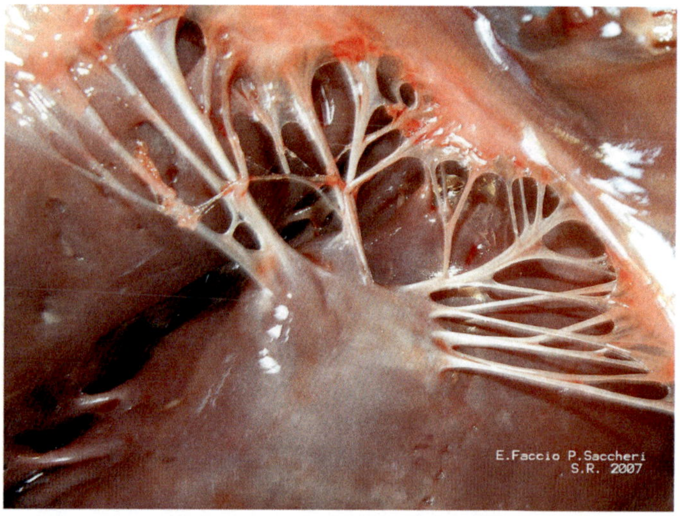

FIGURE - 10.5.14 - Papillary Muscle

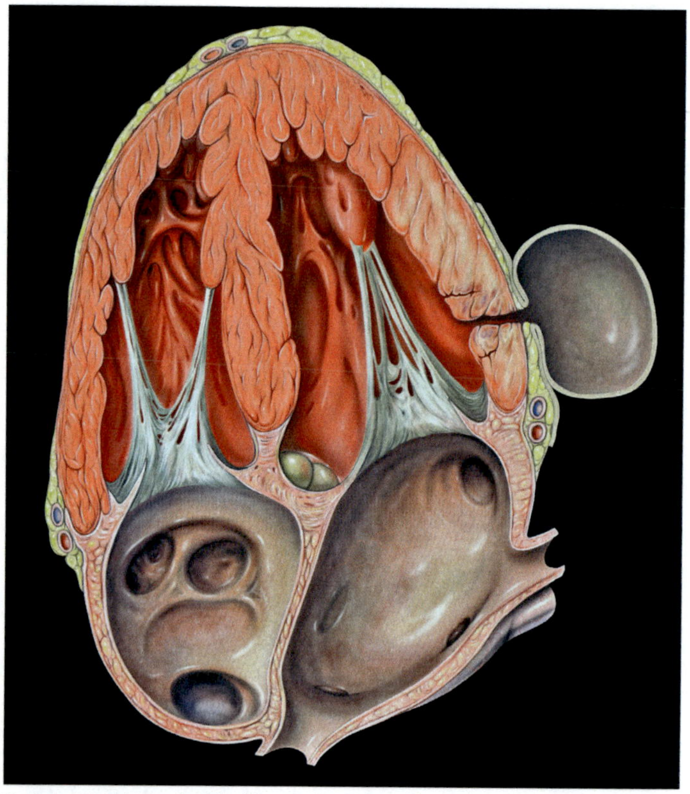

FIGURE - 10.5.15 - Pseudoaneurysm

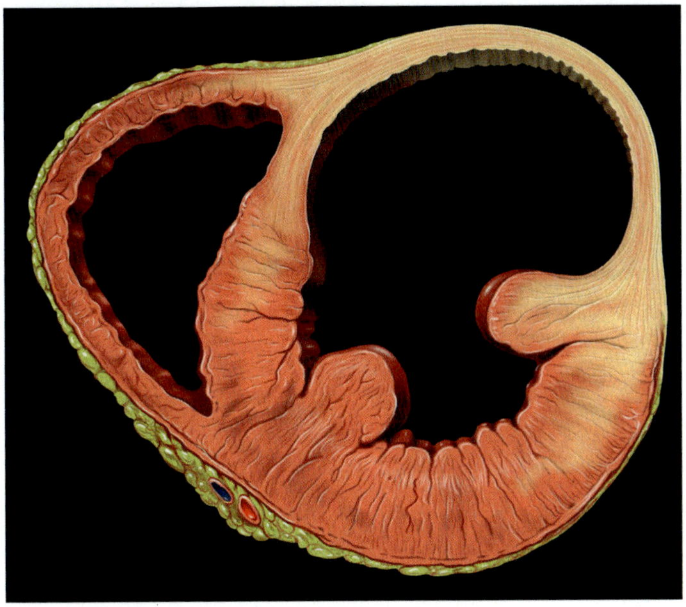

FIGURE 10.5.16 - True Ventricular Aneurysm

VI. Other Complications
   A. Left ventricular failure leading to pulmonary edema
   B. ↓ LV output → increased LA volume → increased volume in pulmonary veins

VII. Treatment: NSTEMI and Unstable Angina
   A. "MONA BASH T"
      1. Morphine (reserved for patients with severe pain)
      2. Oxygen (when O_2 saturation < 90%)
      3. Nitroglycerin
      4. Aspirin
      5. Beta blockers (if hemodynamically stable)
      6. ACE inhibitor (not part of immediate treatment)
      7. Statin
      8. Heparin (anticoagulant)
      9. Ticagrelor (ADP receptor inhibitor)

VIII. Treatment: STEMI
   A. Reperfusion therapy in addition to "MONA BASH T"
   B. Percutaneous coronary intervention (PCI) preferred
   C. Fibrinolysis in those unable to receive PCI

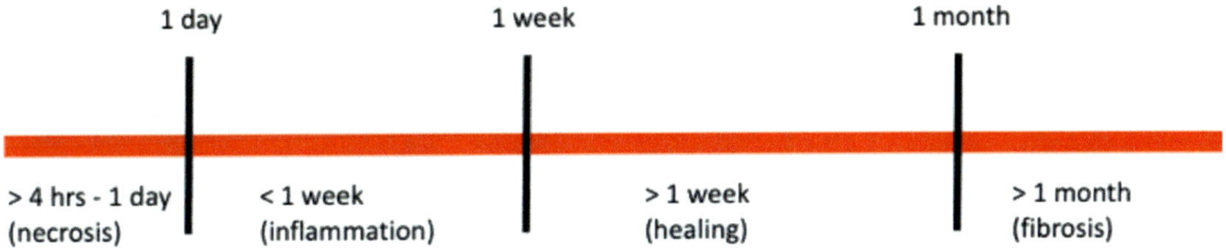

FIGURE 10.5.17 - Timeline of a Myocardial Infarction

REVIEW QUESTIONS

1. A 63-year-old male presents to the emergency department due to sudden-onset chest pain. The pain started 30 minutes ago and radiates to his shoulder. An EKG reveals ST segment depression in leads V_1-V_4. Does this patient have a myocardial infarction?

- **The answer to the question is we don't know yet.**
- The patient has acute chest pain and an EKG reveals ST segment depression. You may be tempted to immediately say "no" because there is no ST segment elevation. However, we don't have enough information to distinguish between unstable angina and an NSTEMI because both can present almost identically to one another.
- Troponin enzymes must be ordered in order to make a diagnosis of an MI or unstable angina, which we were not given in the question stem. If they're not elevated, then we can give a diagnosis of unstable angina. If they are elevated then the patient is having an NSTEMI.

2. An autopsy is performed on a 64-year-old male who died suddenly. Gross examination of the myocardium reveals dark tissue. Microscopy of the same region reveals coagulative necrosis. After additional testing it is confirmed that this individual died as a complication of a myocardial infarction. The patient most likely died how many days following the infarction?

   A. 1
   B. 7
   C. 14
   D. 32

- **The correct answer is A.**
- This patient died after a myocardial infarction. Gross examination of the myocardium reveals dark tissue and microscopy reveals coagulative necrosis, which is consistent with the MI occurring 1 day before death.
- B and C are incorrect because by this point, the heart is healing and would show a hyperemic border along with granulation tissue. Recall that healing occurs after 1 week and continues until about 1 month.
- D is incorrect because after 1 month the tissue would be replaced with a fibrotic scar.

Section VII - Other Ischemic Heart Diseases

I. Chronic Ischemic Heart Disease
   A. Gradual CHF related to persistent ischemic injury to the myocardium
   B. Normal tissue is replaced with noncontractile scar tissue

II. Sudden Cardiac Death
   A. Cardiac-related death within one hour of symptom onset
   B. Lethal arrhythmia (e.g. ventricular fibrillation) caused by coronary artery disease is the most common cause
   C. Other causes include hypertrophic dilated cardiomyopathy and hereditary ion channelopathies

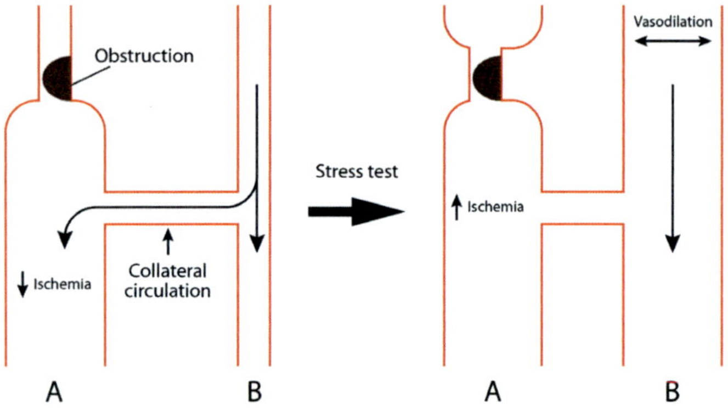

FIGURE 10.5.18 - Coronary Steal Syndrome

III. Coronary Steal Syndrome
   A. Gradual occlusion of a coronary artery promotes collateral circulation to the ischemic region
   B. Vasodilation of the ischemic region facilitates blood flow
   C. Administration of vasodilators (e.g. dipyridamole) dilates unobstructed coronary vessels → loss of pressure gradient → shunts blood away from the ischemic region
   D. The basis for pharmacologic stress test in patients with CAD

REVIEW QUESTIONS ?

1. A 68-year-old male presents to the emergency department due to sudden-onset chest pain that began approximately 45 minutes ago. An EKG is obtained and reveals ST segment elevation in multiple leads. After 30 minutes the patient dies despite aggressive intervention. What is the most likely diagnosis?

   A. Chronic ischemic heart disease
   B. Coronary steal syndrome
   C. Sudden cardiac death
   D. None of the above

- **The correct answer is D.**
- From the question stem, we learn that this patient had chest pain that began 45 minutes before entering the ED. The patient then dies 30 minutes after entering the ED.
- Collectively, it has been 1 hour and 15 minutes since the patient began having symptoms.
- Option C is incorrect because in sudden cardiac death, the death must occur within one hour of symptom onset.
- Option A is unlikely as the patient does not present with symptoms of congestive heart failure.
- Option B is incorrect as it is unrelated to the question stem. This has more to do with pharmacologic stress tests, as discussed above.

Section VIII - Lead EKG Introduction

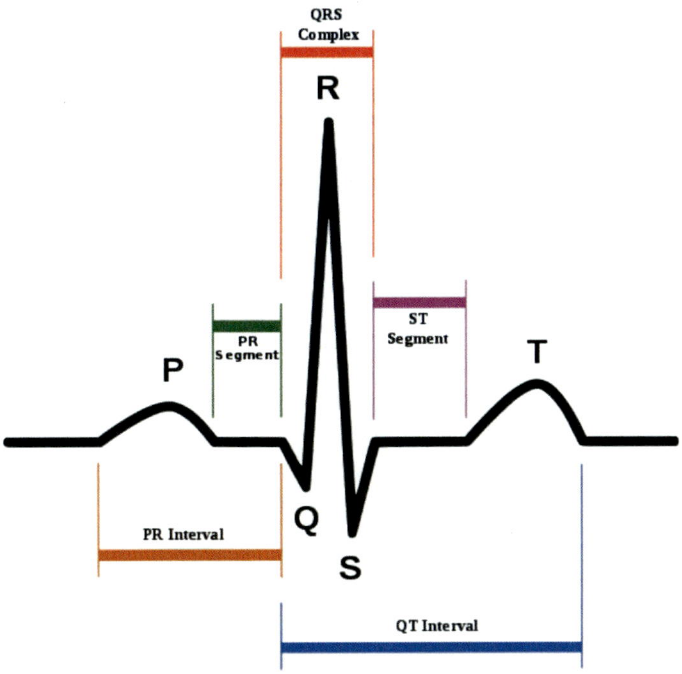

Photo Credit: Agateller [Public domain]

FIGURE 10.5.19 - Normal EKG

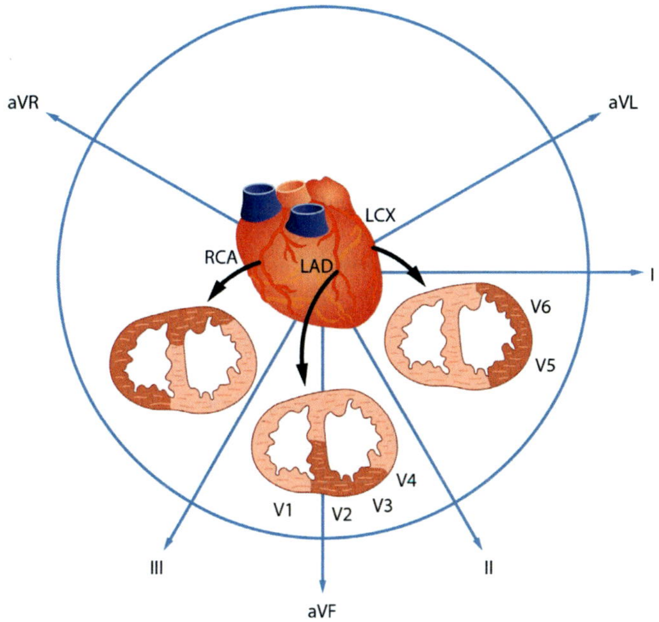

FIGURE 10.5.21 - Heart with Corresponding EKG Leads

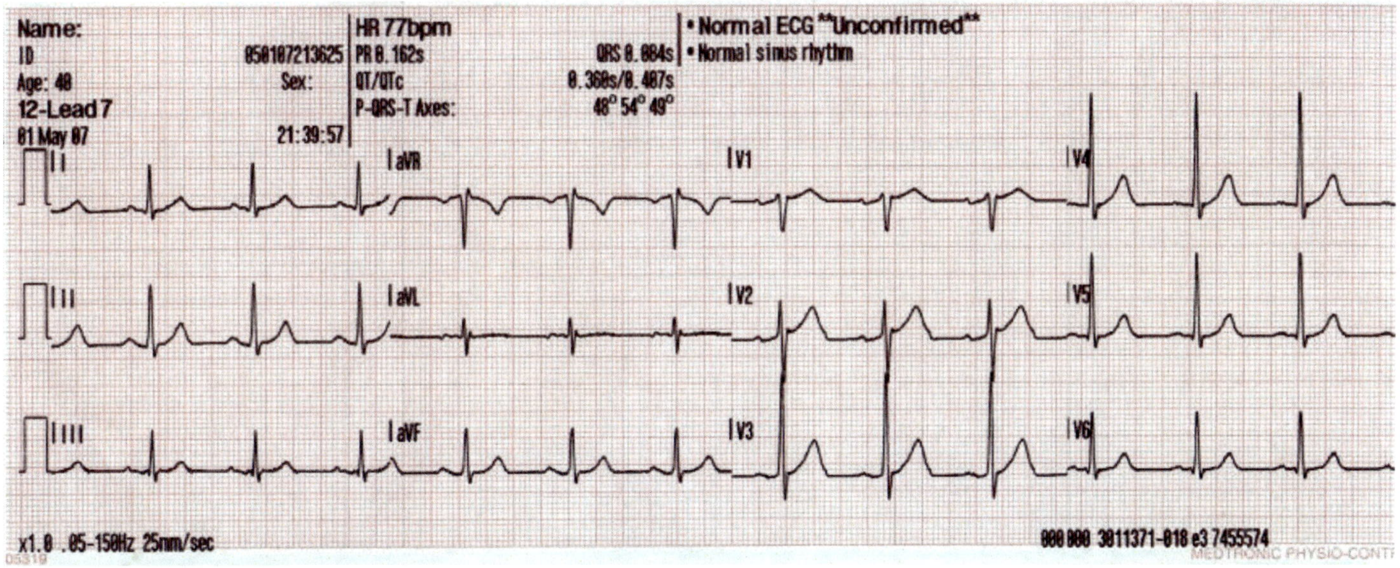

Photo Credit: Glenlarson [Public domain]

FIGURE 10.5.20 - Normal 12-Lead EKG

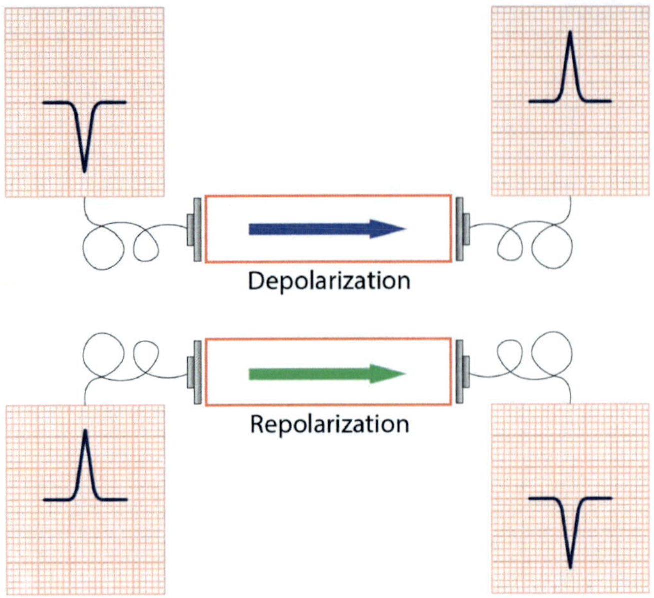

FIGURE 10.5.22 - Pattern of Depolarization and Repolarization

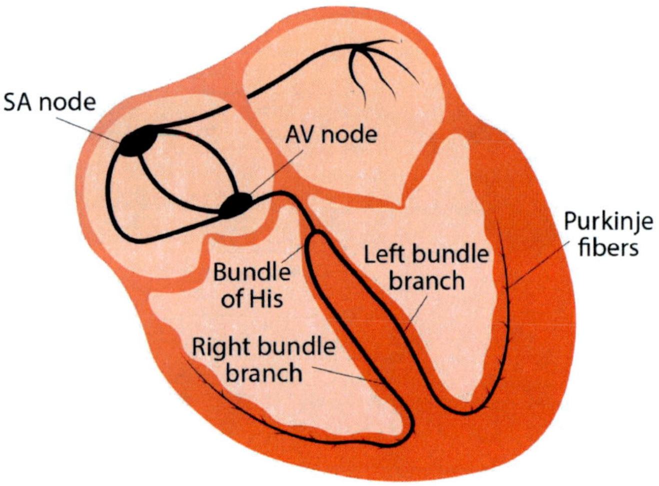

FIGURE 10.5.23 - Path of Electrical Activity in the Heart

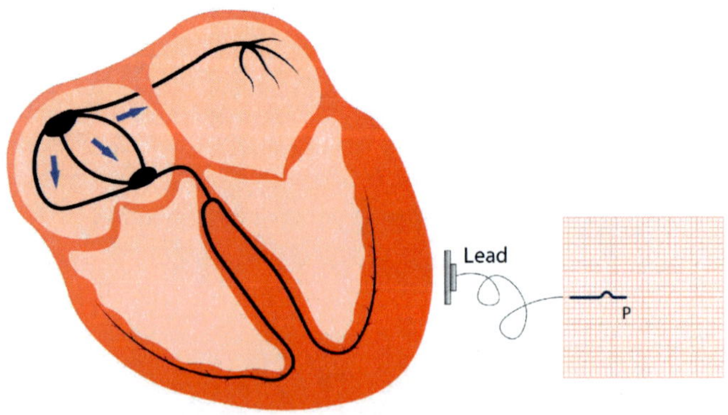

FIGURE 10.5.24 - SA Node Depolarization and EKG Interpretation

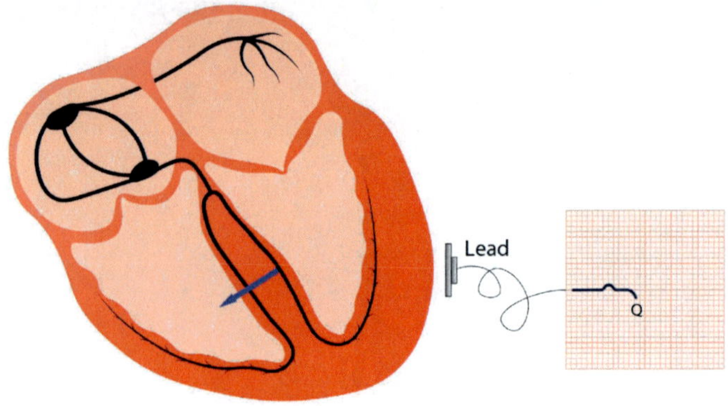

FIGURE 10.5.25 - Septal Depolarization and EKG Interpretation

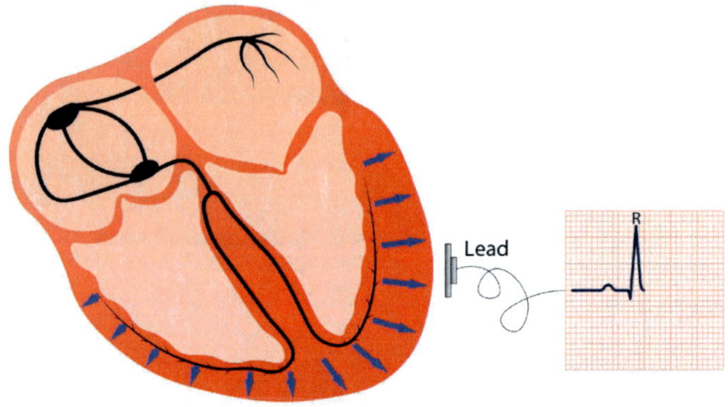

FIGURE 10.5.26 - Ventricular Depolarization and EKG Interpretation

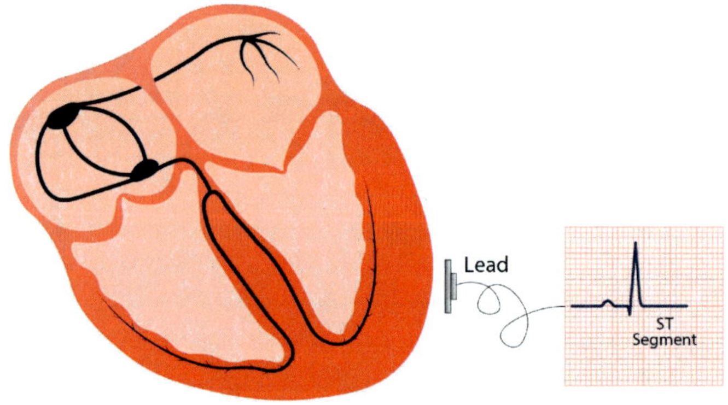

FIGURE 10.5.27 - Isoelectric Line on EKG Immediately Following Ventricular Depolarization

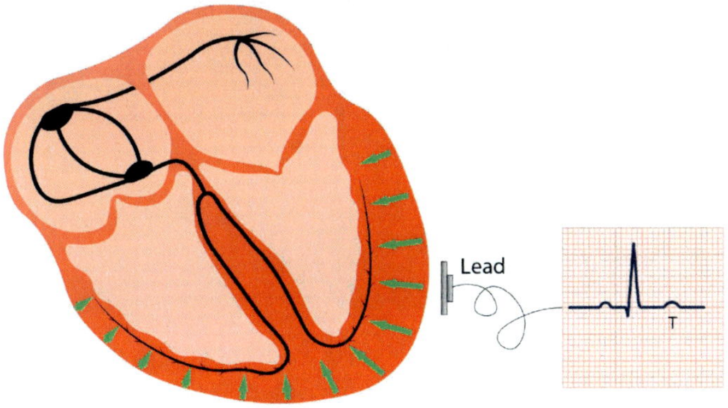

FIGURE 10.5.28 - Repolarization of Ventricles and EKG Interpretation

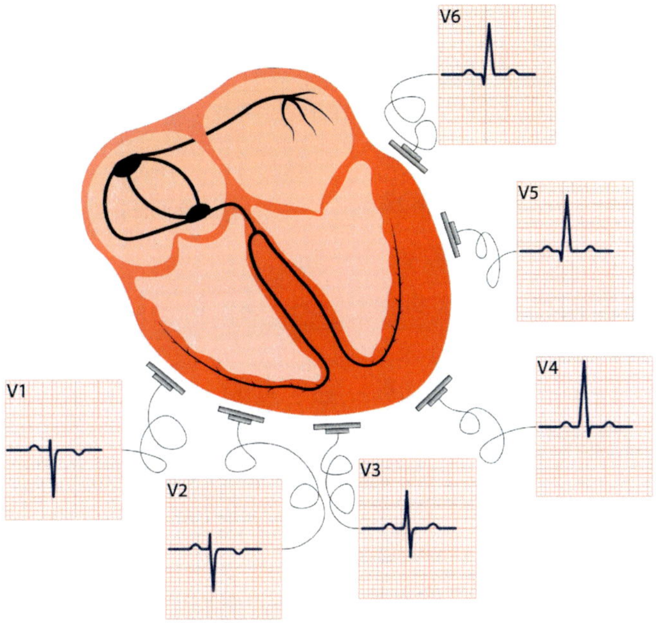

FIGURE 10.5.29 - EKG During a Normal Electric Cycle

REVIEW QUESTIONS

1. A 66-year-old male presents to the emergency department with sudden-onset chest pain that began 20 minutes ago. The physician orders an EKG as part of the workup for myocardial infarction. Abnormalities are seen in leads V5 and V6. Which artery is most likely involved?

    A. Left anterior descending artery
    B. Right coronary artery
    C. Posterior coronary artery
    D. Left circumflex artery

- **The correct answer is D.**
- There are abnormalities in leads V5 and V6, which assess the left lateral ventricle. The left lateral ventricle receives blood from the left circumflex artery.
- A, B, and C are incorrect as these supply other regions of the heart and would be unlikely to cause abnormalities in leads V5 and V6.

Section IX - Basic EKG Interpretation

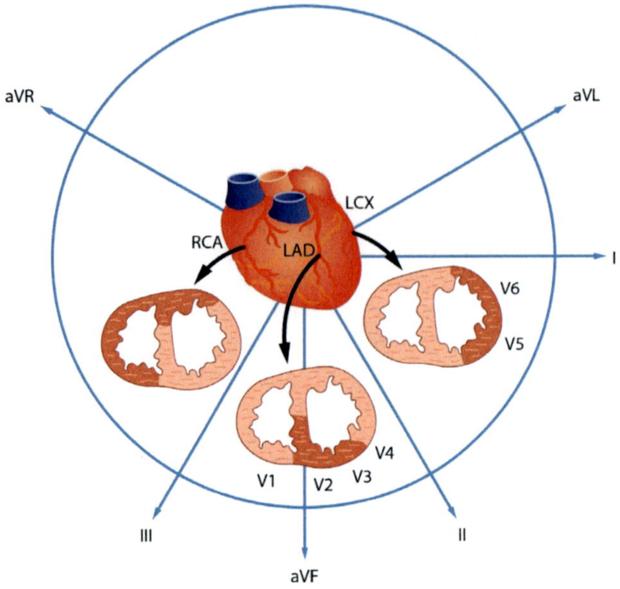

FIGURE 10.5.30 - Placement of EKG Leads

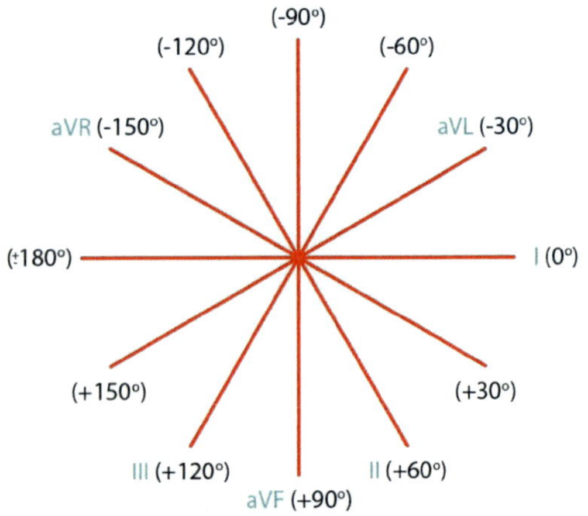

FIGURE 10.5.31 - Electrical Axis of the Heart

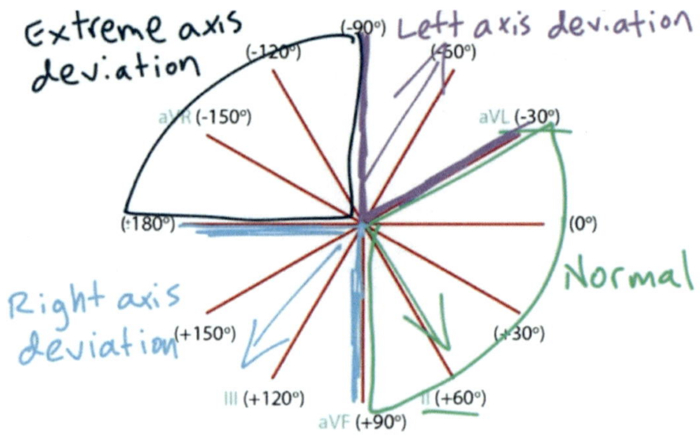

FIGURE 10.5.32 - Heart Axis Deviation

I. QRS Axis
   A. Locate the isoelectric limb lead
   B. The vector will be moving perpendicular to this lead
   C. Positive deflection → moving towards lead
   D. Negative deflection → moving away from lead

II. Rate
   A. Normal heart rate in adults is 60-100 bpm
   B. > 100 bpm = tachycardia
   C. < 60 bpm = bradycardia
   D. Heart rate = 300 divided by the number of large boxes between two R waves

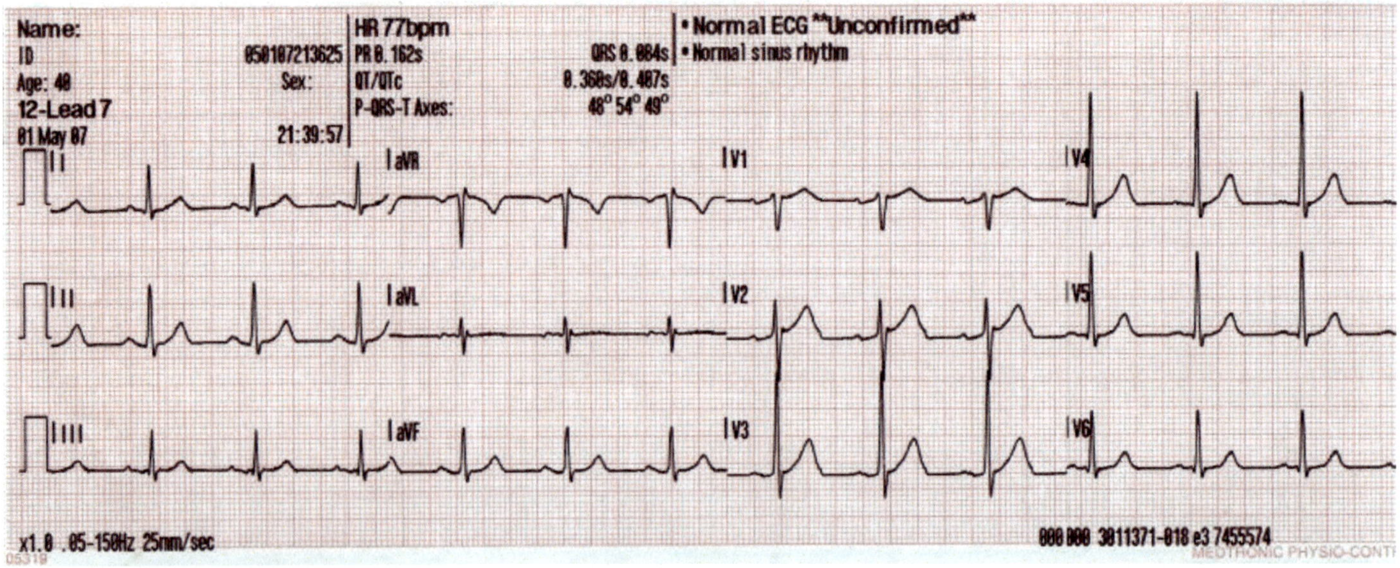

Photo Credit: Glenlarson [Public domain]

FIGURE 10.5.20 - Normal 12-Lead EKG

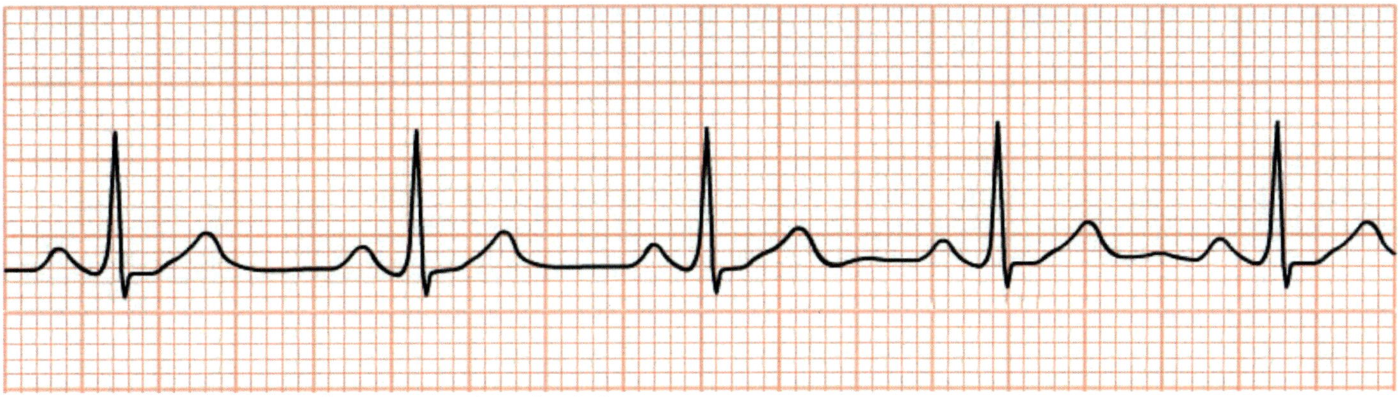

FIGURE 10.5.33 - EKG Lead II

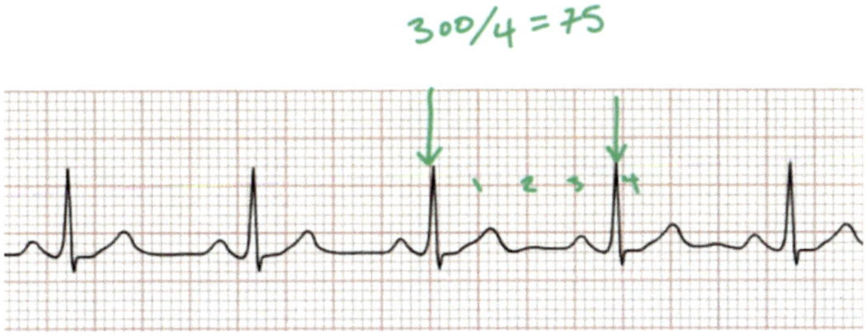

FIGURE 10.5.34 - Rate Calculation using EKG

III. Rhythm
   A. Is the electrical activity beginning in the SA node and traveling normally through the rest of the electrical system?
      1. Are P waves present and upright in lead II?
      2. Is every P wave followed by a QRS complex?
      3. Is the PR interval constant?

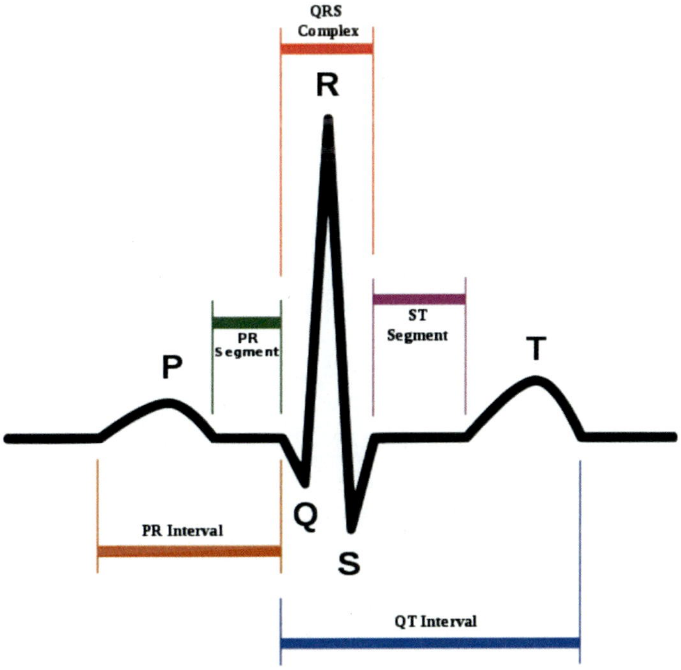

FIGURE 10.5.35 - Normal EKG Parts

IV. Segments and Intervals
   A. EKGs are recorded on graph paper with 1 mm^2 boxes
   B. EKG paper speed is typically 25 mm/s
   C. 1 small box = 40 ms
   D. 1 large box = 200 ms (5 small boxes)
   E. PR interval should be < 200 ms
   F. QRS complex should be < 120 ms
   G. QT interval should be < ½ RR interval
   H. Elevations or depressions in the ST segment

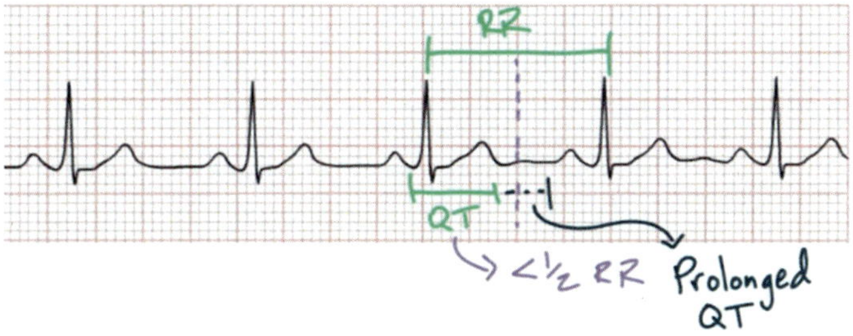

FIGURE 10.5.36 - EKG Showing Prolonged QT Interval

REVIEW QUESTIONS

1. What is the diagnosis?

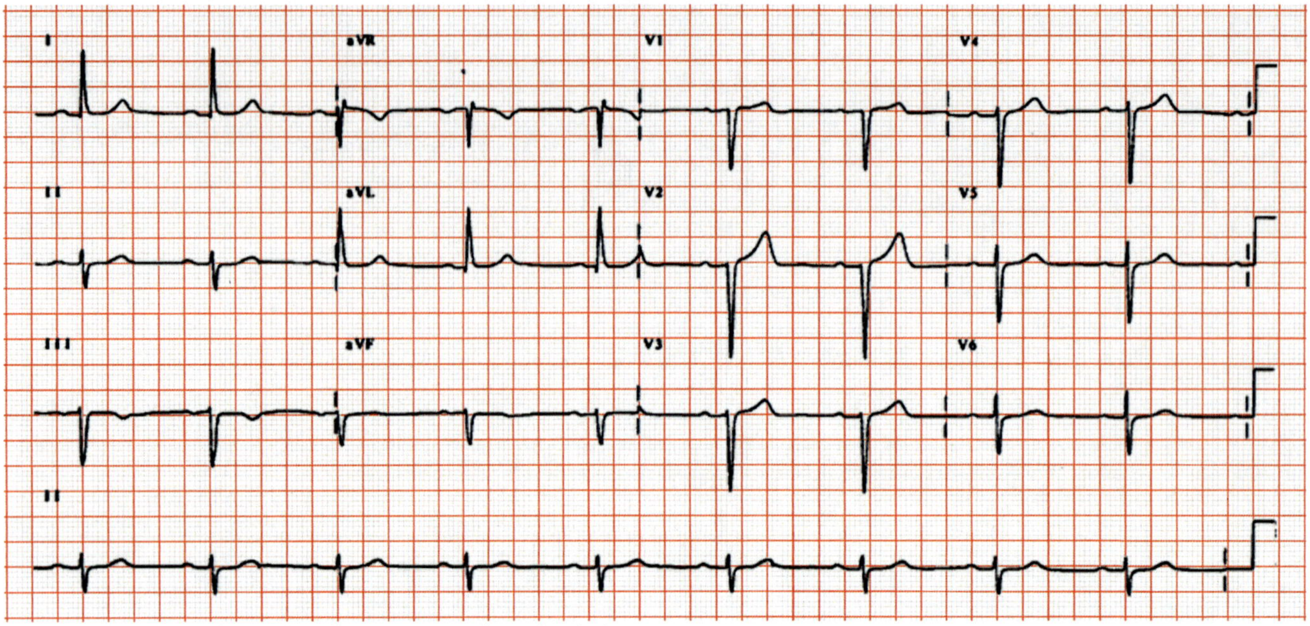

Photo Credit: Andrewmeyerson / CC BY-SA (https://creativecommons.org/licenses/by-sa/3.0)

- **The diagnosis is 1st degree heart block.**
- It looks like limb lead II is isoelectric. The lead perpendicular to this is aVL.
- aVL has a positive QRS complex. The axis is about -30 degrees. Negative 30 to positive 90 degrees is normal, so this EKG represents a normal QRS axis.
- The next thing to look at is rate. If we look at the rhythm strip down at the bottom we can see several QRS complexes that begin near a large box. If we look at the first one and count the number of boxes until the next one it is 5.
- 300 divided by 5 is 60. 60 to 100 is normal, so the rate is normal.
- The following thing to note is rhythm. The P waves appear to be upright in lead II. Every P wave is followed by a QRS complex.
- The PR interval appears to be constant. There are approximately 5.5 to 6 small boxes for the PR interval and this persists across the rhythm strip.
- However, anything over 5 small boxes is too long. Recall that a PR interval greater than 5 small boxes, or 200 ms, is called 1st degree heart block.
- This is benign and asymptomatic.
- If we look at the other segments and intervals, including the QRS complex, the QT interval, and the ST segment, they are normal.

Section X - Ischemic EKG Changes

I. Ischemic Changes
   A. ST elevation
   B. ST depression
   C. Peaked T waves
   D. Inverted T waves
   E. Pathologic Q waves
   F. Poor R wave progression
   G. New bundle branch block

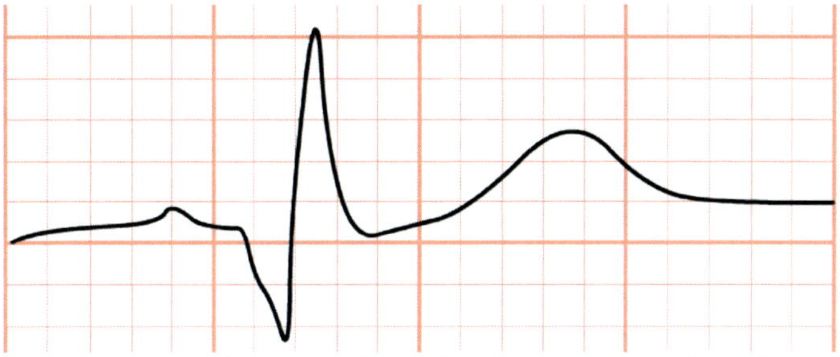

Photo Credit: CardioNetworks: Googletrans [CC BY-SA (https://creativecommons.org/licenses/by-sa/3.0)]

FIGURE 10.5.37 - Pathological Q Wave

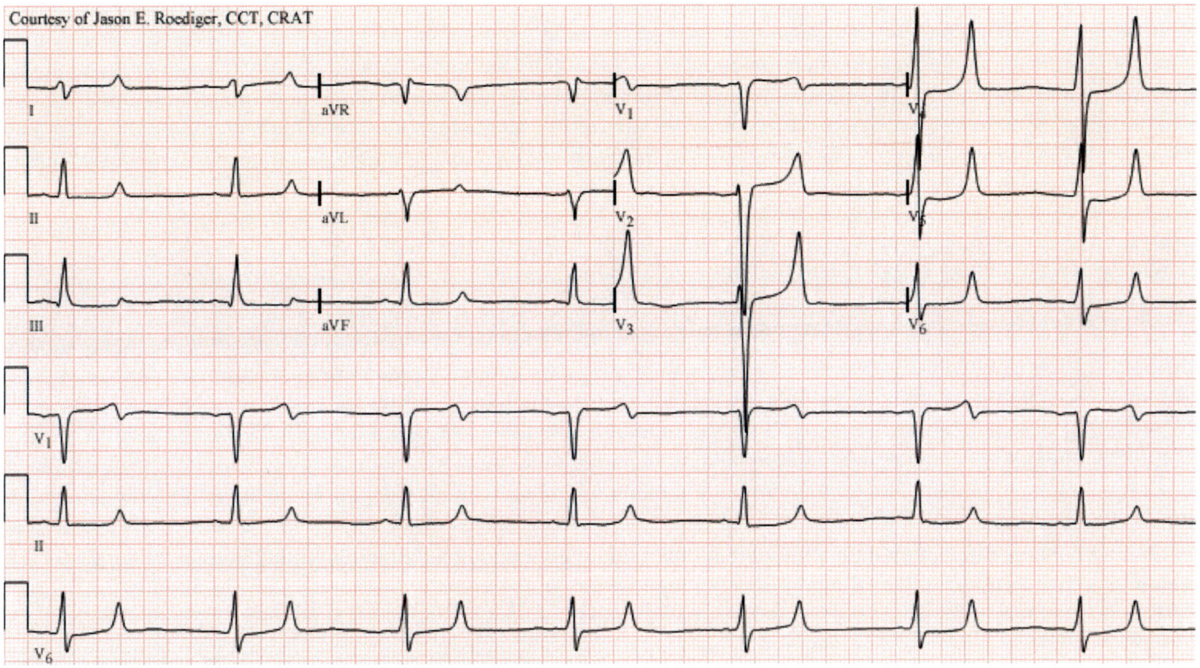

Photo Credit: Jer5150 [CC BY-SA (https://creativecommons.org/licenses/by-sa/3.0)]

FIGURE 10.5.38 - Peaked T Waves in Leads V4 and V5

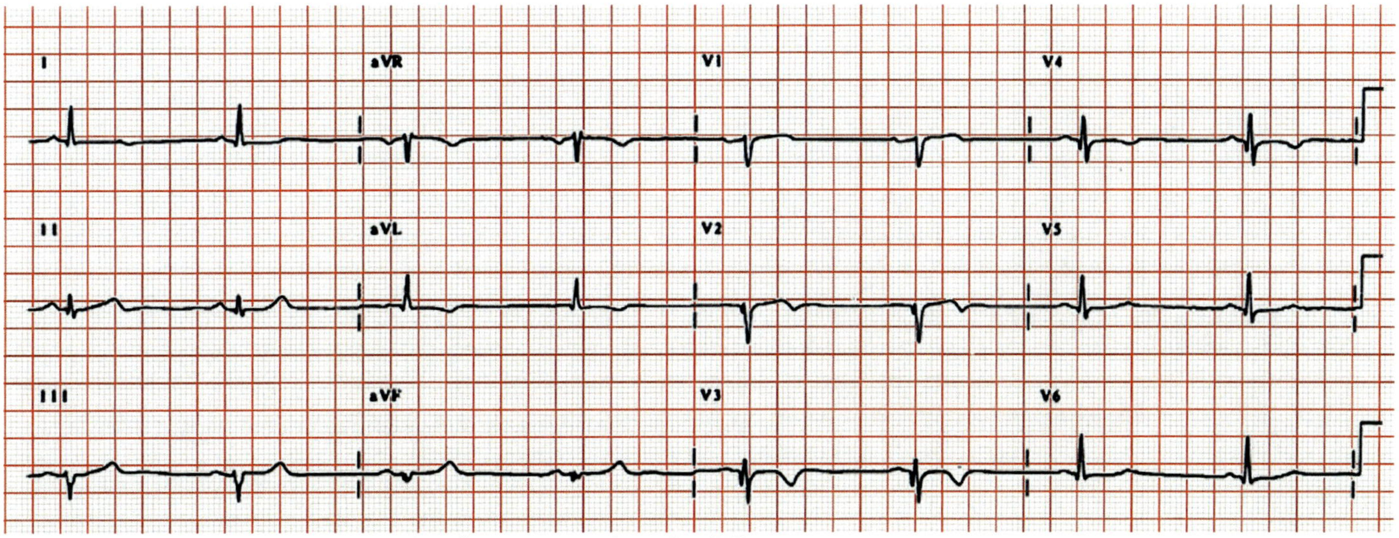

Photo Credit: Michael Rosengarten BEng, MD.McGill [CC BY-SA (https://creativecommons.org/licenses/by-sa/3.0)]

FIGURE 10.5.39 - Inverted T Waves in Leads V1 Through V4

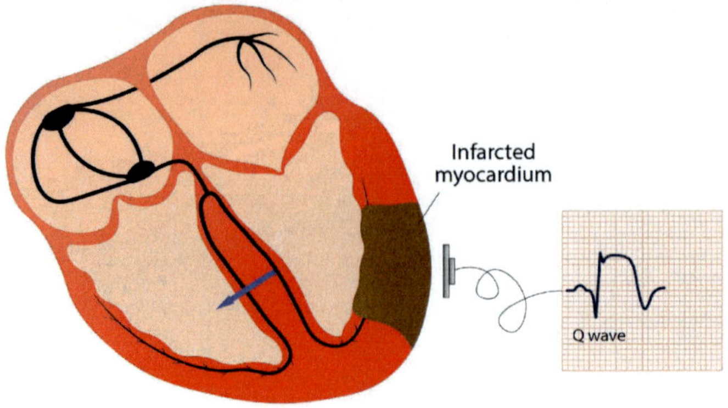

FIGURE 10.5.40 - Infarcted Myocardium Resulting in Pathological Q Wave

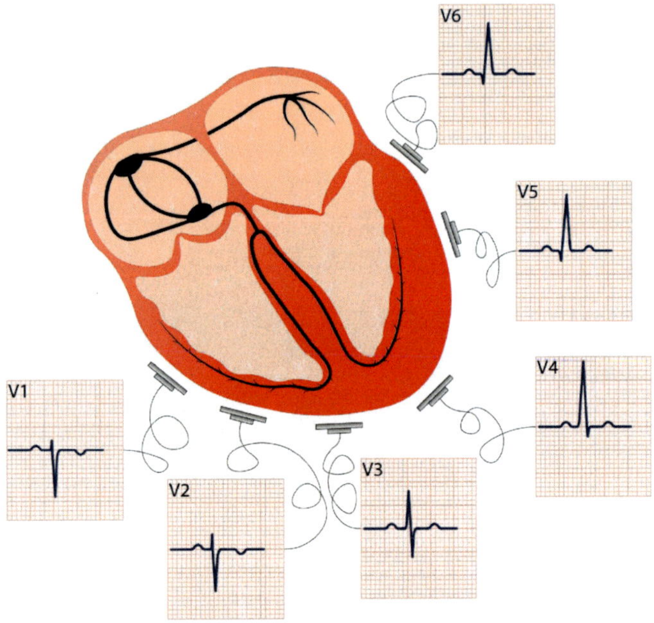

FIGURE 10.5.41 - Poor R Wave Progression

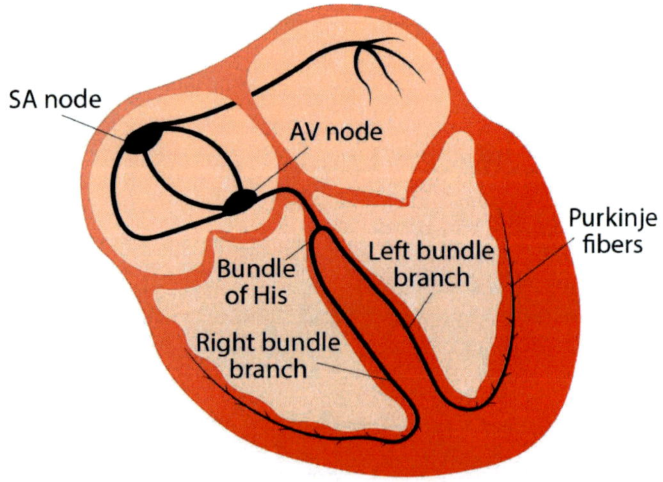

FIGURE 10.5.42 - New Bundle Branch Block

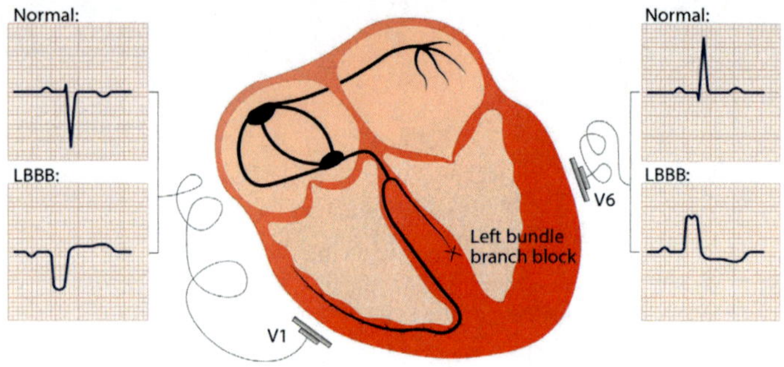

FIGURE 10.5.43 - Changes After a Left Bundle Branch Block

II. Left Bundle Branch Block
   A. Wide QRS complex
   B. Absence of Q waves in the left chest leads
   C. Deep S waves in right chest leads

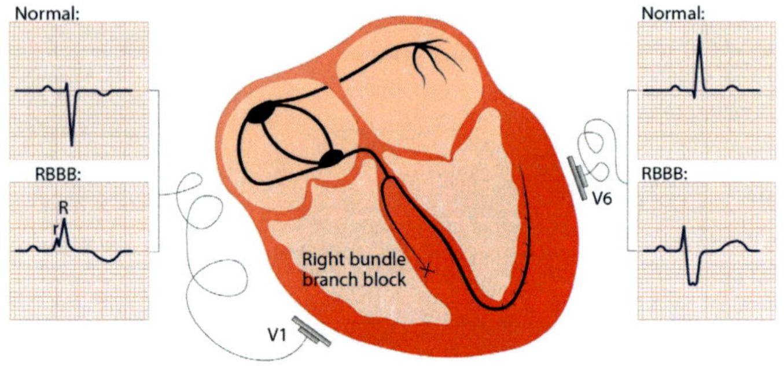

FIGURE 10.5.44 - Changes After a Right Bundle Branch Block

III. Right Bundle Branch Block
   A. Wide QRS complex
   B. Overall positive QRS complex in lead V1 (e.g. rSR pattern)

REVIEW QUESTIONS

1. What is the diagnosis?

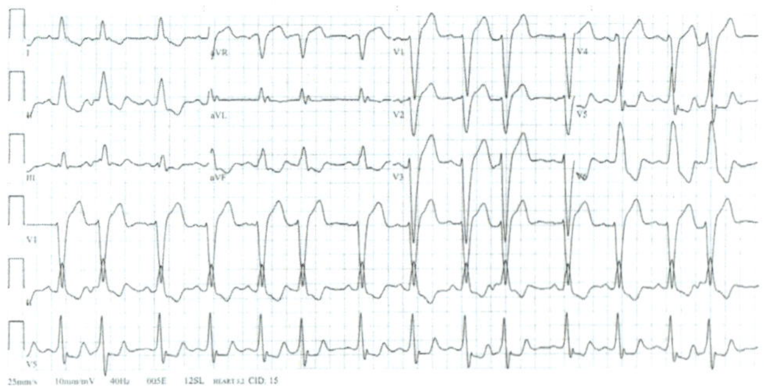

Photo Credit: Steven Fruitsmaak [CC BY-SA (https://creativecommons.org/licenses/by-sa/3.0)]

- **The correct diagnosis is a left bundle branch block.**
- Look at the QRS complex, rate, rhythm, segments and intervals. The QRS complexes are wider than normal. In leads V1 through V4 there are strong negative deflections, and there is an absence of Q waves in V5 and V6.

Section XI - EKG Localization of Myocardial Infarction

Infarcted Artery	Leads with Diagnostic Changes
LAD	$V_1 - V_4$
LCX or LAD	$V_5 - V_6$
LCX	I, aVL
RCA	II, III, aVF
PDA	$V_1 - V_3$ (ST depression and tall R waves)

TABLE 10.5.2 - Location of Infarction Based on EKG

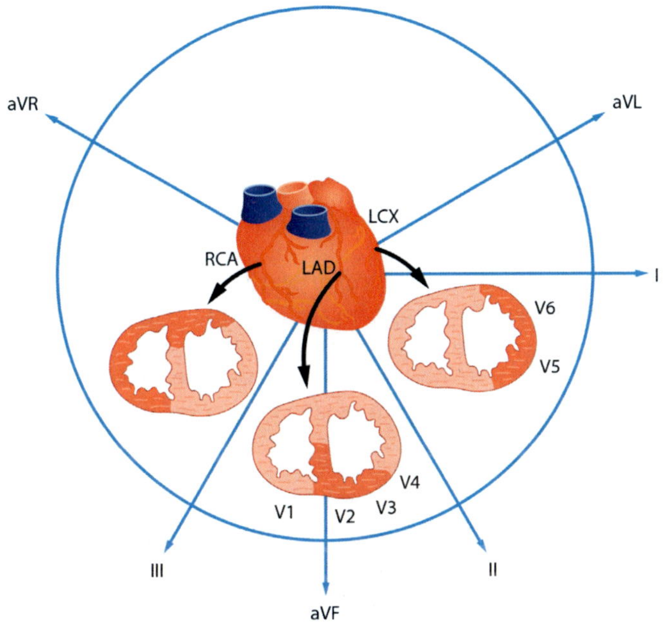

FIGURE 10.5.45 - Placement of EKG Leads

REVIEW QUESTIONS

1. A 70-year-old female presents to the emergency department with sudden-onset chest pain that began 25 minutes ago. An EKG is ordered and reveals ST segment elevation in leads V1, V2, V3, and V4. An infarction involving which artery is the most likely cause of this patient's condition?

   A. Left anterior descending artery
   B. Right coronary artery
   C. Posterior coronary artery
   D. Left circumflex artery

- **The correct answer is A.**
- The question states that ST segment elevation is present in leads V1 through V4.
- Recall that leads V1 through V4 correspond to the LAD. Hence, we can deduce that the infarcted artery must be the left anterior descending.
- Options B, C, and D are incorrect as these supply other regions of the heart and would be unlikely to cause ST segment elevation in leads V1 through V4.

Section XII - Cardiomyopathy

I. Cardiomyopathy
   A. Group of diseases that result in myocardial dysfunction
   B. Typically presents as heart failure or sudden death

II. Overview
   A. Dilated cardiomyopathy
   B. Hypertrophic cardiomyopathy
   C. Restrictive cardiomyopathy
   D. Stress-induced (Takotsubo) cardiomyopathy

III. Dilated Cardiomyopathy: Etiology
   A. Most common type of cardiomyopathy
   B. Global dilation of the heart
   C. Most often idiopathic or due to coronary artery disease
   D. Other causes include genetic mutations of the TTN gene (encodes the titin protein), postpartum state, infection, and drugs (cocaine, alcohol, doxorubicin)

IV. Dilated Cardiomyopathy: Pathophysiology
   A. Myocardial insult → decreased contractility → dilation

V. Dilated Cardiomyopathy: Findings
   A. Eccentric hypertrophy
   B. ↑ compliance
   C. ↑ EDV (diastolic function preserved)
   D. ↓ EF (systolic dysfunction)
   E. Heart failure
   F. Mitral and tricuspid valve regurgitation
   G. Arrhythmia

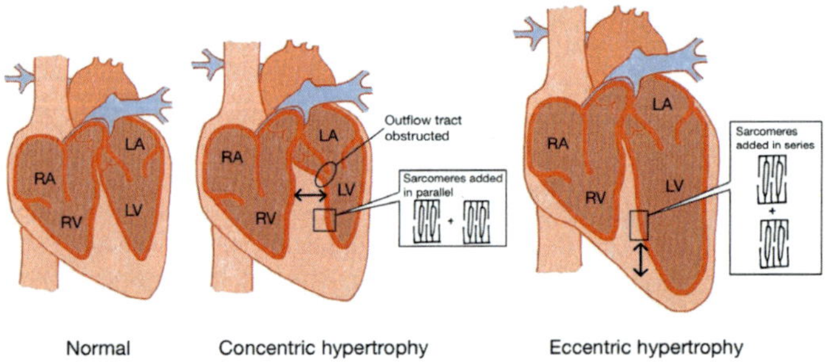

FIGURE 10.5.46 - Difference Between Concentric and Eccentric Hypertrophy

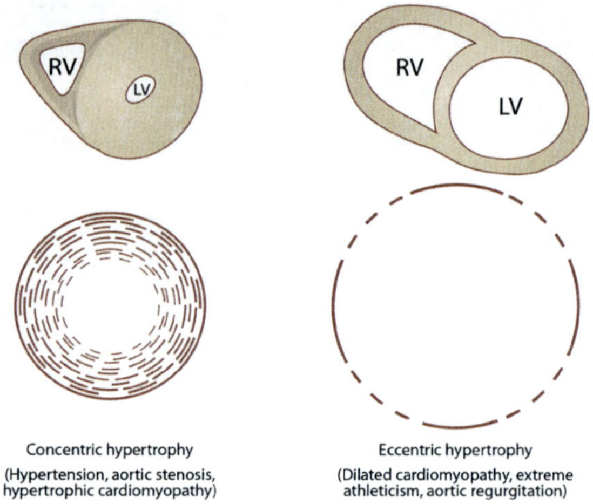

FIGURE 10.5.47 - Difference Between Concentric and Eccentric Hypertrophy

VI. Dilated Cardiomyopathy: Treatment
   A. Early administration of ACEi may slow disease progression
   B. ICD for arrhythmia
   C. Heart failure symptoms are treated similarly to heart failure (e.g. diuretics, beta blockers, spironolactone, sodium restriction)
   D. Transplant is definitive

VII. Hypertrophic Cardiomyopathy: Etiology
   A. Asymmetric interventricular septal hypertrophy
   B. Nondilated hypertrophic left ventricle
   C. Mutation involving sarcomere genes, which encode for contractile proteins (e.g. beta-myosin heavy chain and myosin binding protein-C)

VIII. Hypertrophic Cardiomyopathy: Pathophysiology
   A. Genetic mutations → hypertrophy
   B. Mitral valve leaflet and thickened interventricular septum can obstruct left ventricular outflow → syncope

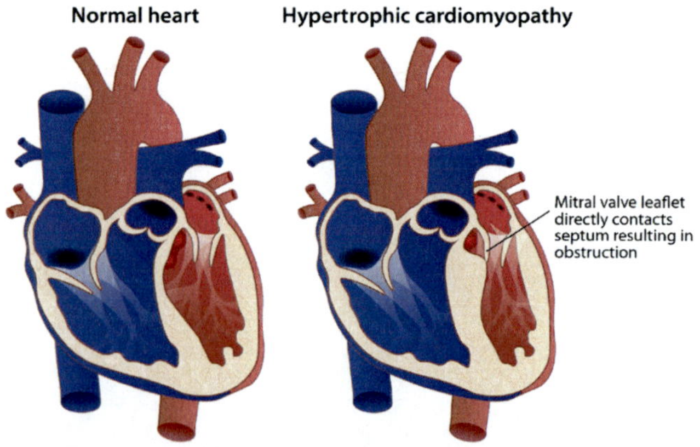

FIGURE 10.5.48 - Difference Between Normal Heart and Hypertrophic Cardiomyopathy

IX. Hypertrophic Cardiomyopathy: Findings
- A. Microscopy reveals myofiber disarray with interstitial fibrosis
- B. Aberrant myofibers in conduction system → arrhythmia
- C. Often presents as a young athlete who has a syncopal episode and dies suddenly
- D. Impaired closure of mitral valve → mitral regurgitation
- E. Concentric enlargement
- F. Diastolic dysfunction (normal EF)

X. Hypertrophic Cardiomyopathy: Treatment
- A. Avoidance of high-intensity activity
- B. Beta blockers
- C. Non-dihydropyridine calcium channel blockers (e.g. verapamil)
- D. ICD

XI. Restrictive Cardiomyopathy
- A. Ventricular wall stiffness resulting in restricted filling during diastole
- B. Causes include amyloidosis, sarcoidosis, hemochromatosis, postradiation fibrosis, Loeffler endocarditis, and endocardial fibroelastosis
- C. Low voltage EKG

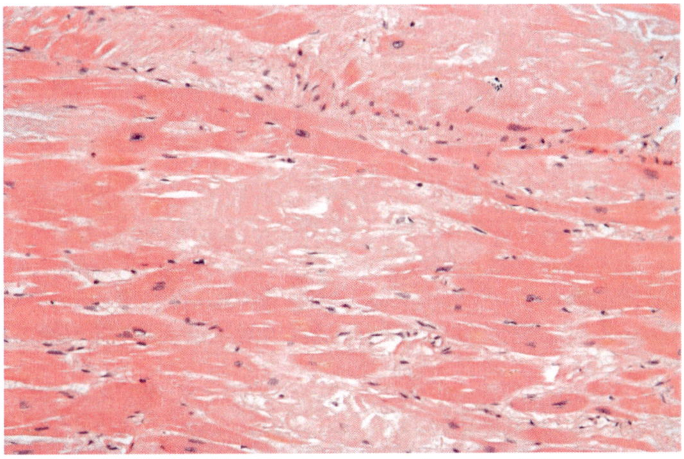

FIGURE 10.5.49 - Histological Image of Amyloidosis in Cardiac Myocytes

XII. Stress-Induced (Takotsubo) Cardiomyopathy
- A. Physical/emotional stress → catecholamine surge → vascular spasm → ischemia → myocardial dysfunction of the LV
- B. Apical hypokinesis + basal hyperkinesis → LV resembles a Japanese octopus trap ("takotsubo")
- C. Systolic dysfunction with reduced EF
- D. Typically self-resolving within several weeks

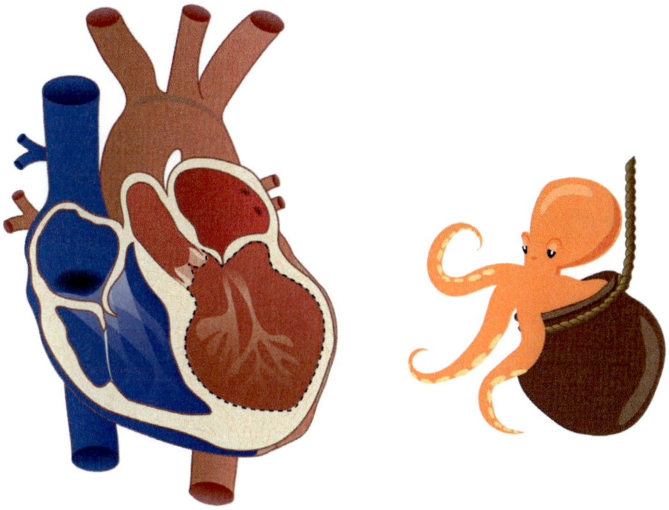

FIGURE 10.5.50 - Stress-Induced (Takotsubo) Cardiomyopathy

REVIEW QUESTIONS

1. A 17-year-old male is brought to the emergency department immediately following a syncopal episode. His father reports that he collapsed suddenly while competing in a high school basketball game. Additional workup reveals a mutation involving sarcomere genes, which encode contractile proteins in the heart. This patient's heart will be most similar to a patient with which of the following conditions?
   - A. Aortic regurgitation
   - B. Hypertension
   - C. Extreme athleticism
   - D. Chagas disease

- **The correct answer is B.**
- The patient is 17-years-old and had a syncopal episode due to a mutation involving sarcomere genes which encode for contractile proteins in the heart. These clues lead to a diagnosis of hypertrophic cardiomyopathy. Hypertrophic cardiomyopathy causes concentric hypertrophy of the heart, which is also seen in hypertension.
- A, C, and D are all incorrect because they all cause eccentric hypertrophy.

Section XIII - Heart Failure

I. Definition
   A. Clinical syndrome in which the heart fails to produce sufficient cardiac output to keep up with the body's demand

II. Left-Sided Heart Failure
   A. Orthopnea
   B. Paroxysmal nocturnal dyspnea.
   C. Pulmonary edema
   D. CXR findings
   E. HFrEF (systolic heart failure): reduced ejection fraction (< 50%)
   F. HFpEF (diastolic heart failure): preserved ejection fraction (50-75%)

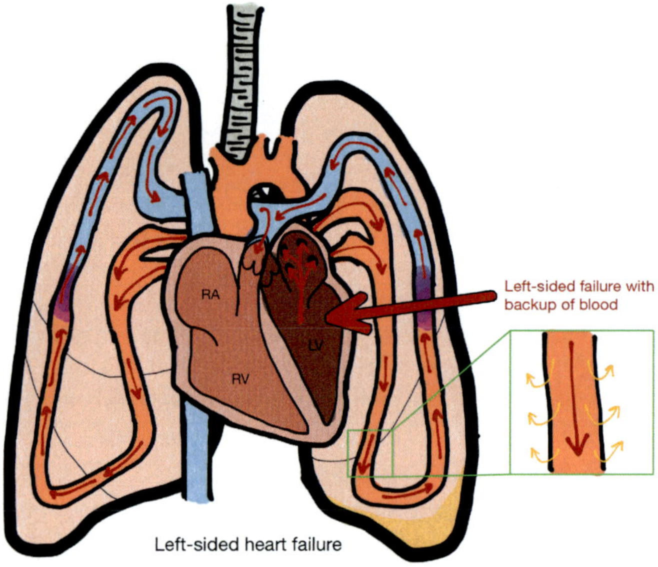

FIGURE 10.5.51 - Left-Sided Heart Failure

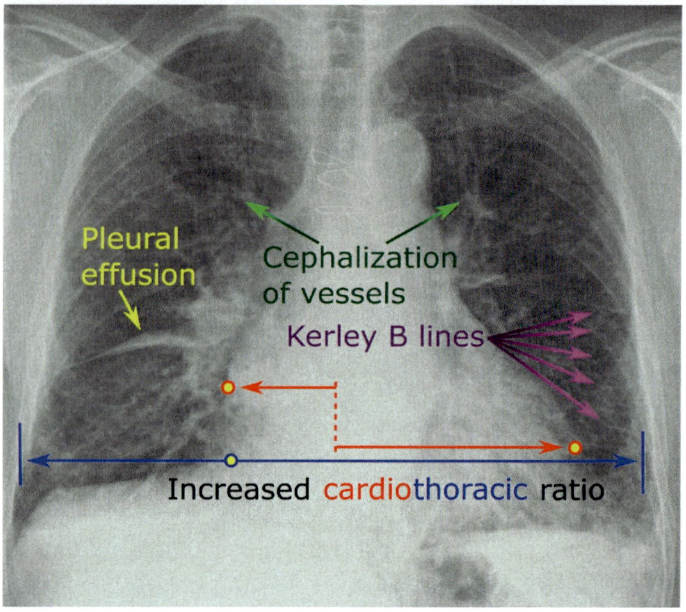

Photo Credit: Mikael Häggström, M.D. / CC BY-SA (https://creativecommons.org/licenses/by-sa/1.0)

FIGURE 10.5.53 - Left-Sided Heart Failure CXR Findings

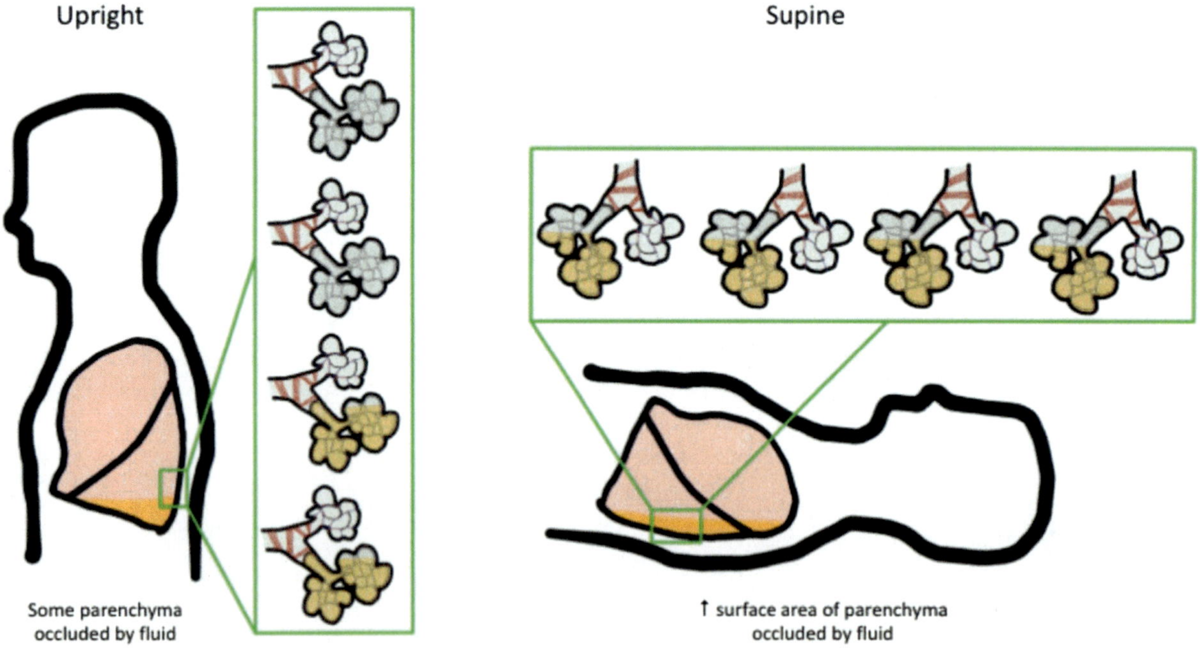

FIGURE 10.5.52 - Orthopnea and Paroxysmal Nocturnal Dyspnea

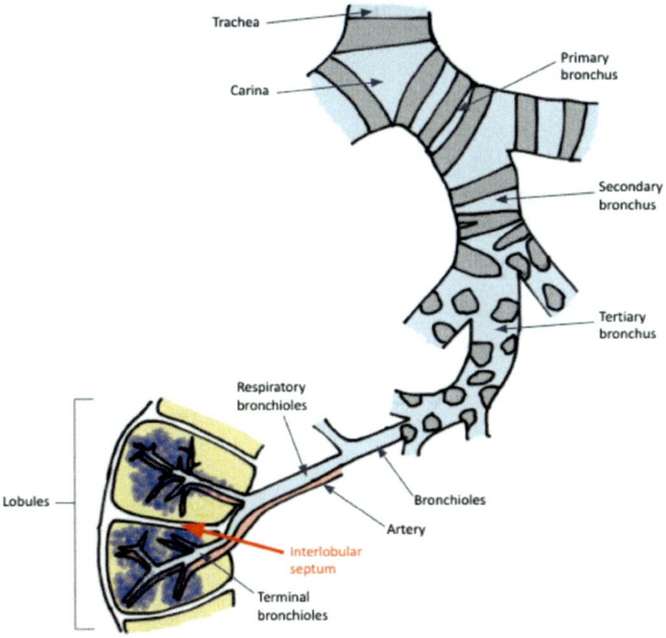

FIGURE 10.5.54 - Kerley B Lines

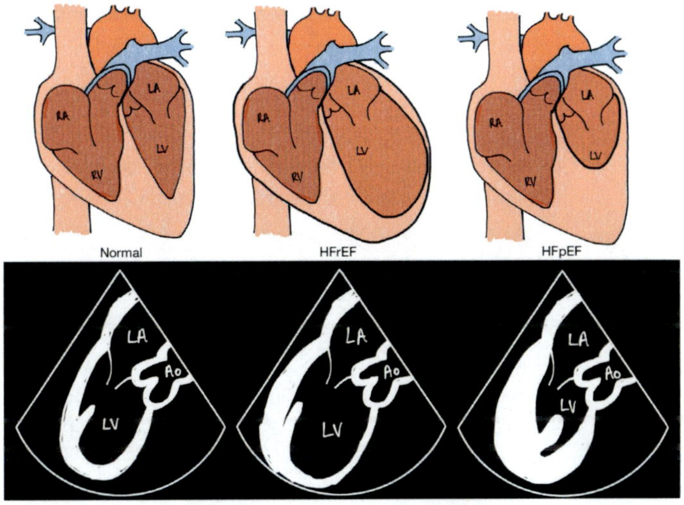

FIGURE 10.5.55 - Anatomical Representation (Top) and Sonographic Findings (Bottom) of Heart Failure

III. Right-Sided Heart Failure
   A. Secondary to left-sided heart failure vs. cor pulmonale
   B. Findings
      1. JVD
      2. Peripheral edema
      3. Hepatomegaly (nutmeg liver)

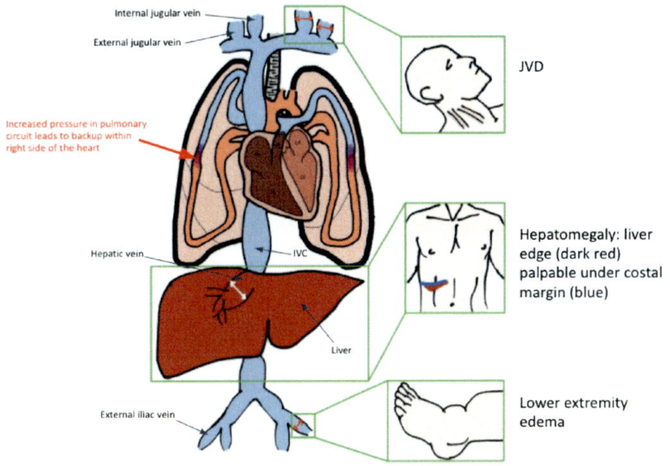

FIGURE 10.5.56 - Right-Sided Heart Failure

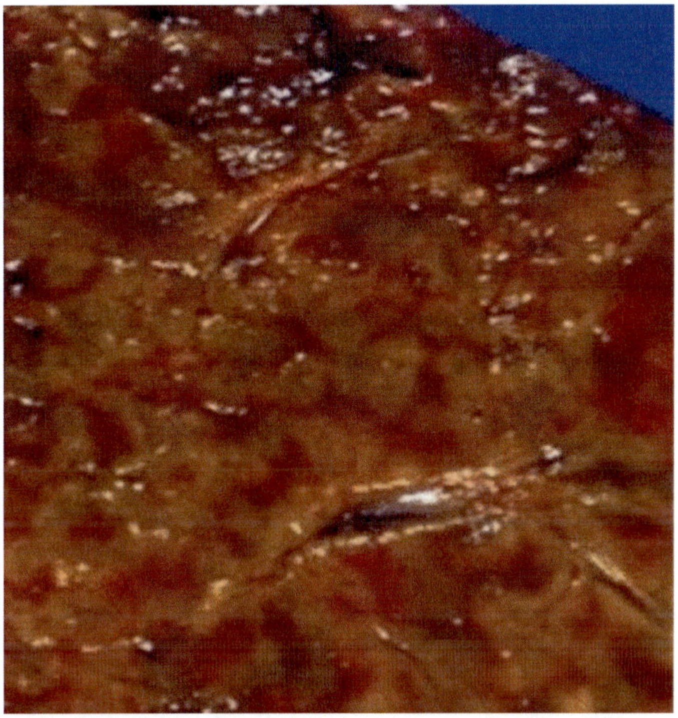

FIGURE 10.5.57 - Nutmeg Liver

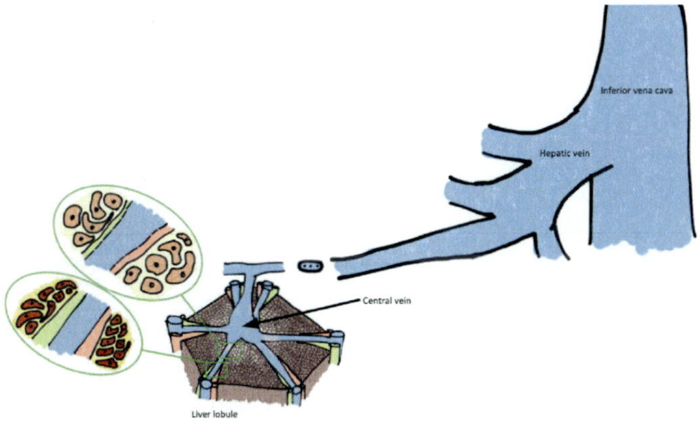

FIGURE 10.5.58 - Pathophysiology of Nutmeg Liver Secondary to Right-Sided Heart Failure

IV. Cor Pulmonale
  A. Pulmonary hypertension
    1. Normal mean pulmonary artery pressure: 10 - 14 mmHg
    2. Pulmonary hypertension: ≥ 25 mmHg at rest
  B. Obstructive and restrictive lung diseases
    1. Obstructive: chronic hypoxic pulmonary vasoconstriction
    2. Restrictive: mechanical compression of pulmonary vasculature

V. Pressure-Volume (P-V) Loops
  A. HFrEF has decreased contractility (rightward shift of P-V loop)
  B. HFpEF has decreased compliance

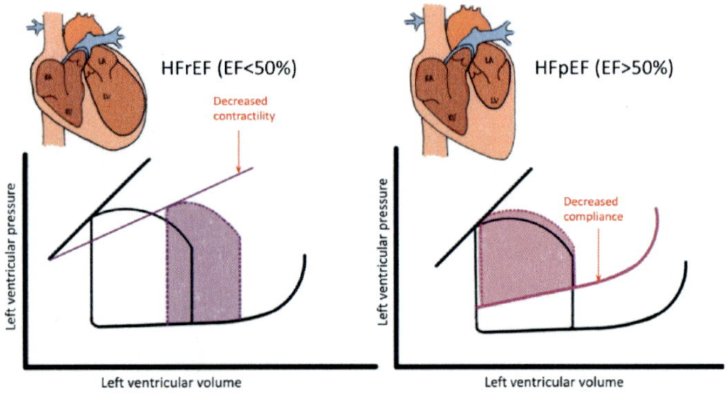

FIGURE 10.5.59 - Pressure-Volume Loops

VI. Treatments
  A. Life-prolonging
  B. ACEi/ARB (angiotensin converting enzyme inhibitors/ angiotensin receptor blockers)
  C. Beta-blockers (bisoprolol, carvedilol, metoprolol)
  D. Potassium-sparing diuretics
  E. Hydralazine and nitrates (AA patients)
  F. Symptomatic relief
    1. Loop/thiazide diuretics
    2. Digoxin

REVIEW QUESTIONS

1. A 58-year-old male with a past medical history of COPD and tinnitus presents with shortness of breath and episodes of waking up gasping for air in the middle of the night. He states that his breathing is worse when lying down. He is afebrile but is slightly tachycardic with a pulse rate of 109 beats/min. Physical examination reveals coarse crackles in the lower lung lobes bilaterally but is otherwise unremarkable. An echocardiogram shows an ejection fraction of 45%. How would this patient's pressure-volume loop be different from that of a healthy individual?

   A. Rightward shift
   B. Leftward shift
   C. Widening
   D. No change

- **The correct answer is A.**
- Though this question mentions COPD history, his clinical presentation with orthopnea, paroxysmal dyspnea, and no mention of peripheral edema suggest left-sided heart failure. Furthermore, his echocardiographic findings indicate a reduced ejection fraction.
- Thus, the diagnosis is left-sided heart failure with reduced ejection fraction.
- In heart failure with reduced ejection fraction, there is decreased contractility. When plotting heart failure with reduced ejection fraction on a P-V loop, rightward shift indicates decreased contractility.
- B is incorrect because a leftward shift of the P-V loop indicates increased contractility.
- C is wrong because widening of the loop would indicate an increased stroke volume -- something that would not be found in a P-V loop of heart failure with reduced ejection fraction.
- Finally, we absolutely do expect a change in the P-V loop for this patient, so D is wrong.

Section XIV - Shock

I. Shock
   A. Critical state of insufficient organ perfusion
   B. Life-threatening

II. Stages
   A. Initial/compensatory: body responds to diminished tissue perfusion
      1. Hyperlactatemia sign of early shock
   B. Progressive: compensatory mechanisms fail
   C. Irreversible: profound hypotension, hypoxemia, and organ failure; poor prognosis

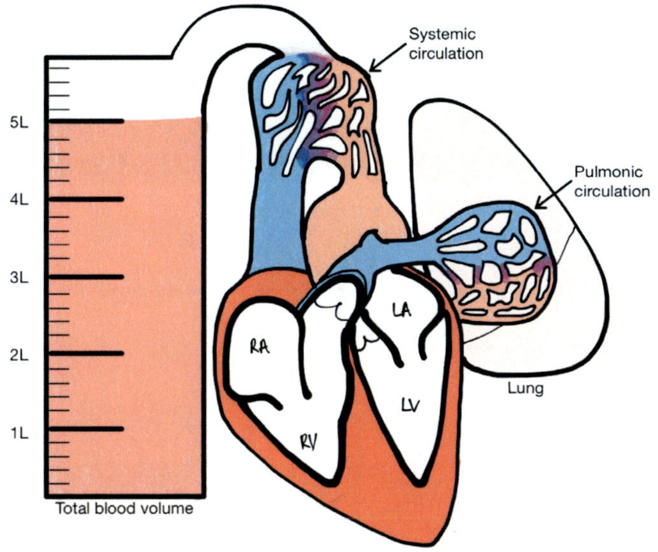

FIGURE 10.5.60 - Types of Shock

Type	Cause	CO	SVR (afterload)	PCWP (preload)	Extremities	Treatment
Cardiogenic	- **LV dysfunction** (MI, HF, arrhythmia)	↓↓	↑	↑	- Cold - Clammy	- Inotropes - Diuresis
	- **RV dysfunction** (HF, MI)			↓		
Obstructive	- **Pulmonary vascular** (pulmonary embolism, pulmonary hypertension) - **Mechanical** (tension pneumothorax, pericardial tamponade)	↓↓	↑	↓/↑ (Tamponade)	- Cold - Clammy	- Relieve obstruction
Hypovolemic	- **Hemorrhagic** (bleeding) - **Non-hemorrhagic** (severe dehydration)	↓	↑	↓↓	- Cold - Clammy	- IV fluids
Distributive	- **Septic**	↑	↓↓	↓	- Warm - Flushed	- IV fluids - Vasopressors
	- **Anaphylactic** - **Neurogenic** (trauma)	↓			- Warm - Itchy - Warm -Dry	

TABLE 10.5.3 - Types of Shock

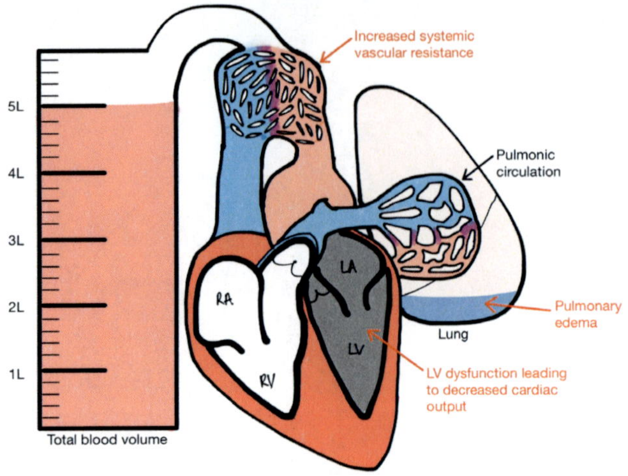

FIGURE 10.5.61 - Cardiogenic Shock (LV Dysfunction)

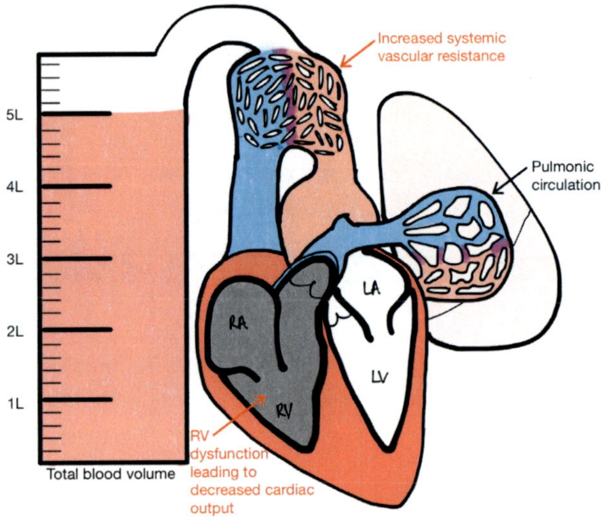

FIGURE 10.5.62 - Cardiogenic Shock (RV Dysfunction)

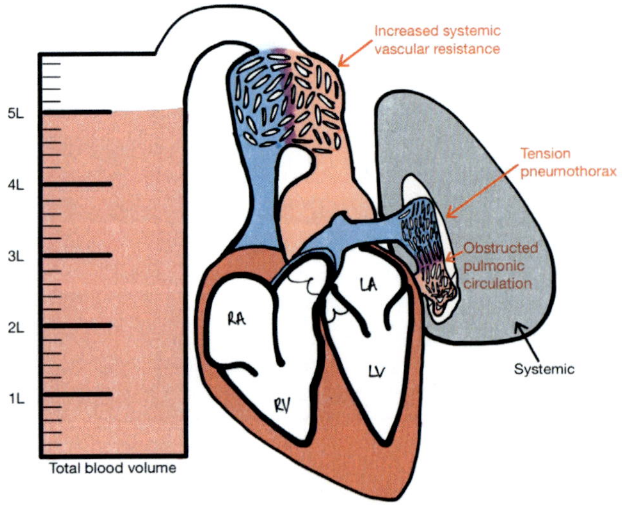

FIGURE 10.5.63 - Obstructive Shock (Tension Pneumothorax)

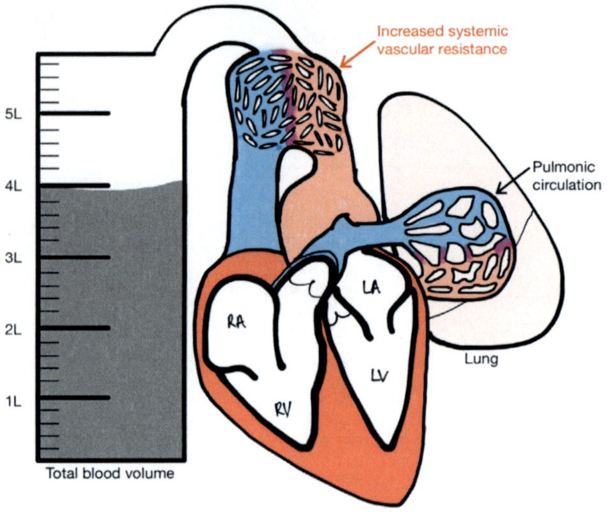

FIGURE 10.5.64 - Hypovolemic Shock

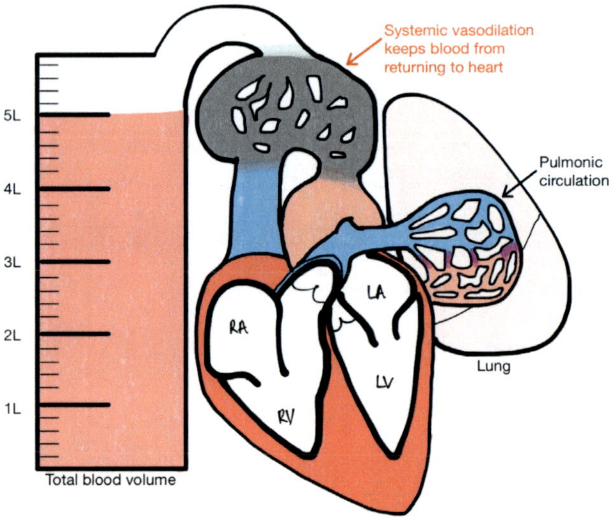

FIGURE 10.5.65 - Distributive Shock (Septic Shock)

III. Distributive shock
   A. Neurogenic
      1. Spinal trauma → loss of sympathetic nervous stimulation
      2. Classic triad: bradycardia, hemodynamic instability, massive vasodilation
   B. Anaphylaxis
      1. Systemic allergic reaction leading to hemodynamic instability
      2. Massive histamine release

IV. Complications
   A. Systemic hypotension→ inadequate perfusion → tissue hypoxia → inability to meet metabolic demands → vital organ dysfunction
   B. Brain
      1. Regions with high metabolic demand and watershed areas
      2. Hippocampus, cerebellar Purkinje cells, cerebral convexities
   C. GI
      1. Splenic flexure, rectosigmoid junction

REVIEW QUESTIONS

1. An 85-year-old man is brought to the emergency department from his nursing home with an altered mental status. According to his nurse, he has been disoriented and belligerent for the past 2 days. During this time he has had diarrhea, loss of appetite, and increased frequency of urination with an unpleasant odor. His temperature is 37.6 °C (99.7° F), blood pressure is 85/60 and pulse is 110/min. His extremities are warm and appear flushed. He has a weak pulse but no other cardiac findings. Which of the following hemodynamic changes will be evident in this patient?
    A. Decreased CO, decreased PCWP, decreased SVR
    B. Decreased CO, increased PCWP, decreased SVR
    C. Increased CO, decreased PCWP, decreased SVR
    D. Increased CO, increased PCWP, decreased SVR

- **The correct answer is C.**
- Hopefully from this question, you noticed that this patient is suffering a distributive shock. More specifically, septic shock.
- He has an altered mental status, fever, hypotension, and cloudy urine, possibly due to a urinary tract infection.
- Septic shock occurs due to pathogens causing the release of vasodilatory substances like nitric oxide and histamine, which results in a very low systemic vascular resistance (SVR). This is compensated by the increase in HR to increase cardiac output.
- In this type of shock, the increased blood delivery to the periphery causes the extremities to be warm, as seen in this patient.
- Option A is incorrect because in distributive septic shock, there's increased cardiac output due to the increase in heart rate.
- Option B is incorrect because in septic shock the cardiac output is increased and the pulmonary capillary wedge pressure (PCWP) is decreased.
- Option D is incorrect because in septic shock, pulmonary capillary wedge pressure (PCWP) is decreased. This occurs because the profound vasodilation in this type of shock decreases the venous return (VR).

Section XV - Cardiac Tamponade

I. Basic Principles
   A. Fluid compresses the heart
   B. Caused by infections, drugs, malignancy, or connective tissue disease
   C. Pericardial disorder → pericardial effusion → mechanical compression of heart → decreased venous return, CO, and ROM

II. Clinical Features
   A. Dyspnea, tachypnea, fatigue, lightheadedness/ dizziness, chest discomfort
   B. Clear lungs
   C. Beck's triad
   D. Pulsus paradoxus

III. Beck's Triad
   A. Jugular venous distention (JVD)
   B. Hypotension
   C. Distant heart sounds

IV. Pulsus Paradoxus
   A. Drop in systolic BP > 10 mmHg during inspiration
   B. Bowing of the interventricular septum towards the left ventricle
   C. Collapse of the right atrium and ventricle
   D. Occurs in patients with asthma, COPD, and constrictive pericarditis

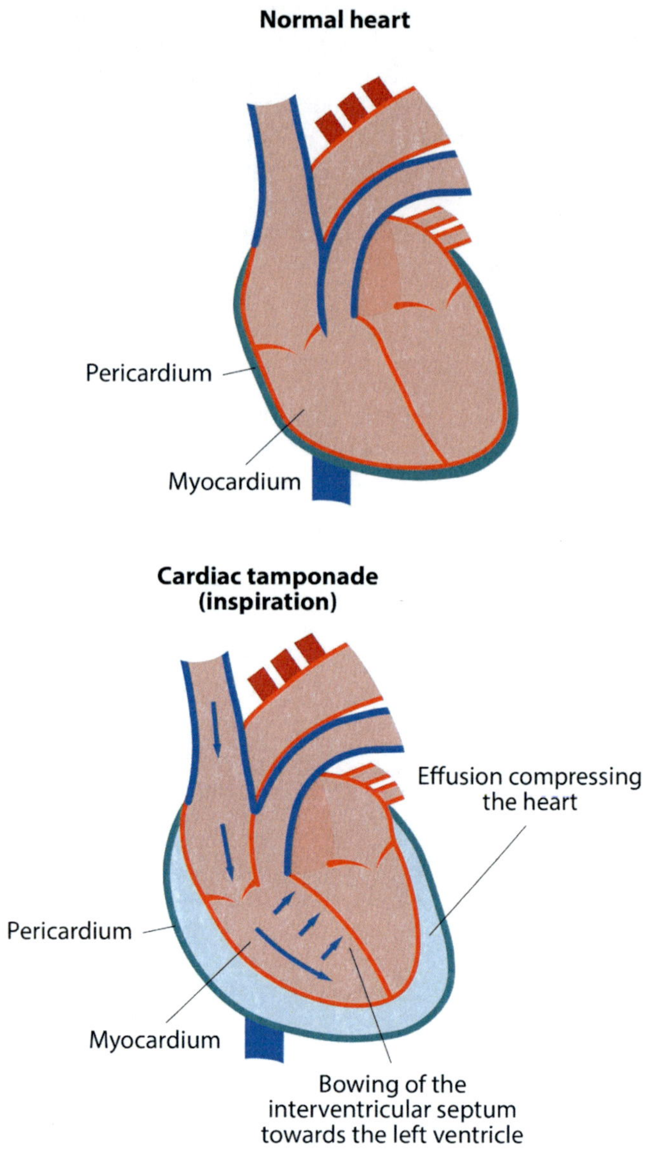

FIGURE 10.5.66 - Normal Heart at Rest, and a Heart with Cardiac Tamponade During Inspiration

V. Diagnosis
   A. Primarily diagnosed through ECG and chest X-ray
   B. Low-voltage QRS complexes
   C. Electrical alternans
   D. Enlarged, water bottle-shaped heart

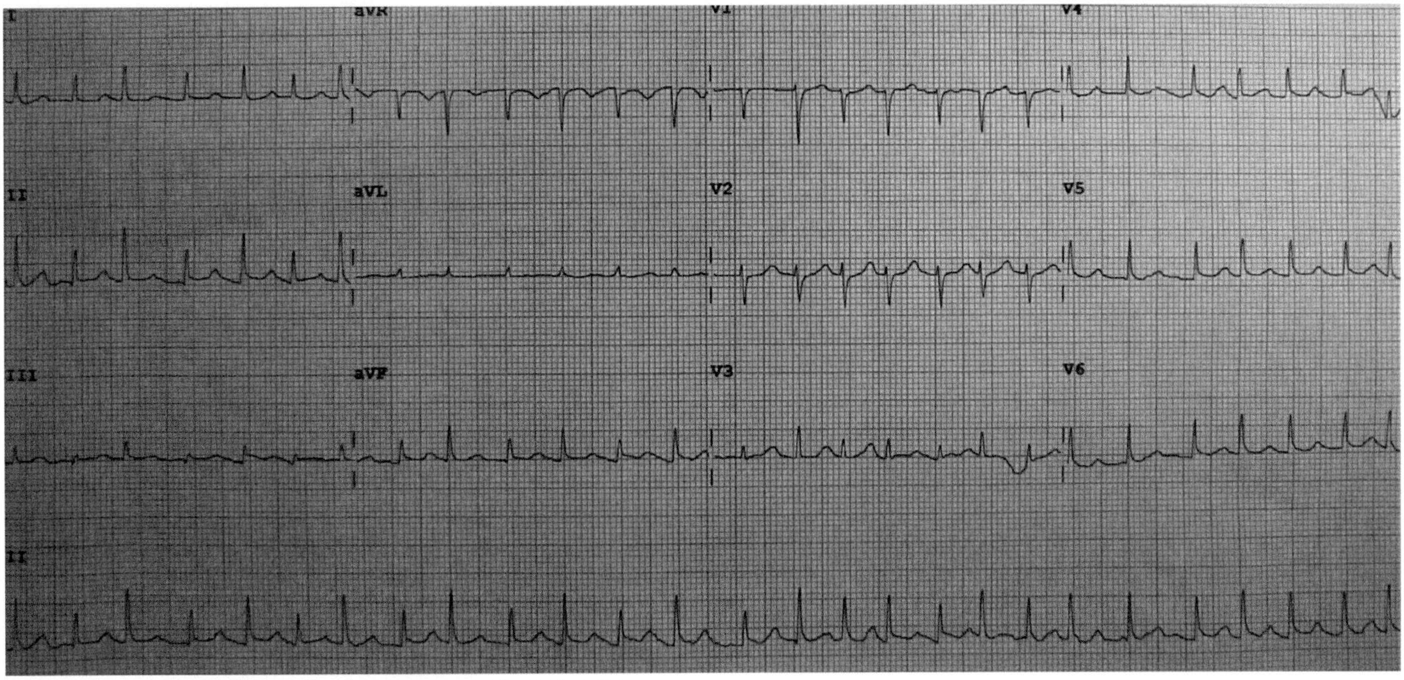

Photo Credit: James Heilman, MD / CC BY-SA (https://creativecommons.org/licenses/by-sa/3.0)

FIGURE 10.5.67 - ECG of Electrical Alternans

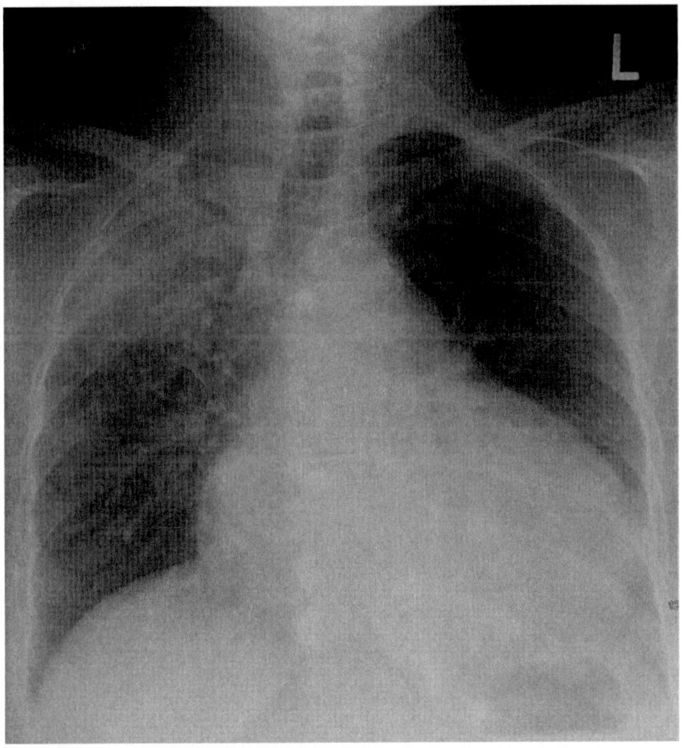

Photo Credit: James Heilman, MD / CC BY-SA (https://creativecommons.org/licenses/by-sa/3.0)

FIGURE 10.5.68 - Chest X-Ray of Cardiac Tamponade

VI. Treatment
   A. Perform a pericardiocentesis
   B. Treat the underlying cause
   C. Inotropic drug (e.g. dobutamine) administration to increase blood pressure and improve heart function

REVIEW QUESTIONS

1. A 34-year-old male presents with severe dyspnea and lightheadedness. He recently had an upper respiratory infection that resolved after a few days. Temperature is 37 °C (98.6 °F), pulse is 114/min, and blood pressure is 80/40 mmHg. His lungs are clear to auscultation bilaterally, but jugular venous distension is present and there is a noticeable drop in pulse amplitude during inspiration. Which of the following will most likely be seen on the physical exam?

    A. Hepatomegaly
    B. Loud S2
    C. Bounding pulses with head bobbing
    D. Diminished heart sounds
    E. Rales and rhonchi

- **The correct answer is D.**
- Cardiac tamponade can classically follow a viral infection, which predisposes a patient to buildup of fluid within the pericardial space and eventual compression of the heart. Cardiac tamponade can be diagnosed with Beck's triad. The components of Beck's triad are jugular venous distension, hypotension, and distant heart sounds.
- This patient has hypotension with a blood pressure of 80/40 and JVD. The finding of pulsus paradoxus, or the drop in pulse amplitude during inspiration, is an important finding for diagnosing cardiac tamponade.
- A is incorrect because hepatomegaly is strongly tied to right heart failure due to systemic fluid overload.
- B is incorrect because a loud S2 component is most commonly seen in pulmonary hypertension. Furthermore, Beck's triad includes muffled heart sounds, so a loud S2 would not be possible.
- C is incorrect because bounding pulses with head bobbing describes aortic regurgitation and is not part of the clinical presentation of cardiac tamponade.
- E is incorrect because in cardiac tamponade, the lungs will be clear to auscultation. Rales and rhonchi, or crackles and wheezes, can be seen in cases of pulmonary edema.

Section XVI - Endocarditis

I. Endocarditis
   A. Inflammation of the endocardium (the inner lining of the heart chambers and valves)

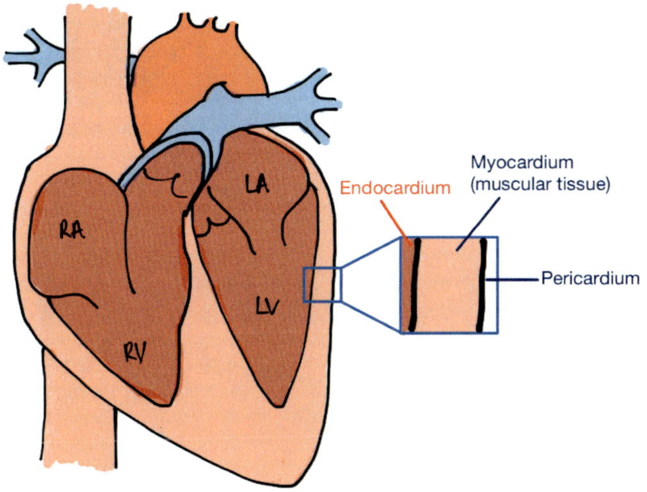

FIGURE 10.5.69 - Endocardium

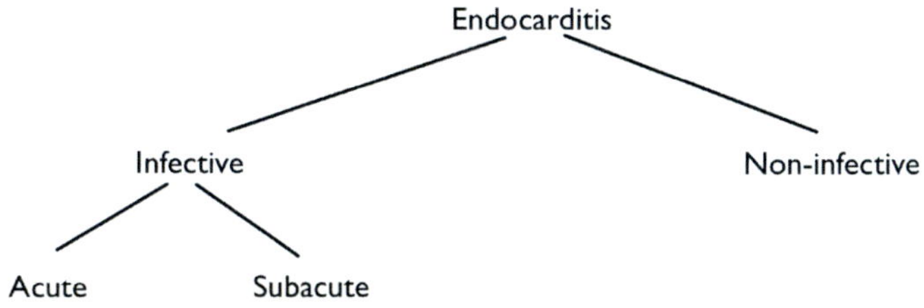

FIGURE 10.5.70 - Classification of Endocarditis

II. Non-Infective Endocarditis
   A. SLE (Libman-Sacks), advanced malignancy, or hypercoagulable state
   B. Sterile vegetations
   C. Pathophysiology
      1. SLE → immune complex deposition→ inflammation and vegetations on both sides of the mitral valve → mitral regurgitation
      2. Malignancy, hypercoagulable state → fibrin vegetations on mitral valve along lines of closure → mitral regurgitation

III. Infective Endocarditis
   A. Most commonly due to a bacterial infection
   B. Non-sterile vegetations
   C. Bacteremia → adherence to valves → damage

IV. Acute Endocarditis
   A. Abrupt onset and rapid course (days to weeks)
   B. On a previously normal valve
   C. Destroys normal valve
   D. Most commonly tricuspid valve (IV drug users)
   E. *Staphylococcus aureus*

V. Subacute Endocarditis
   A. Gradual course (weeks to months)
   B. On abnormal or diseased valves (e.g. rheumatic heart disease, mitral valve prolapse) or sequela of dental procedures
   C. Does not destroy the valve
   D. Most commonly mitral valve
   E. Viridans streptococci

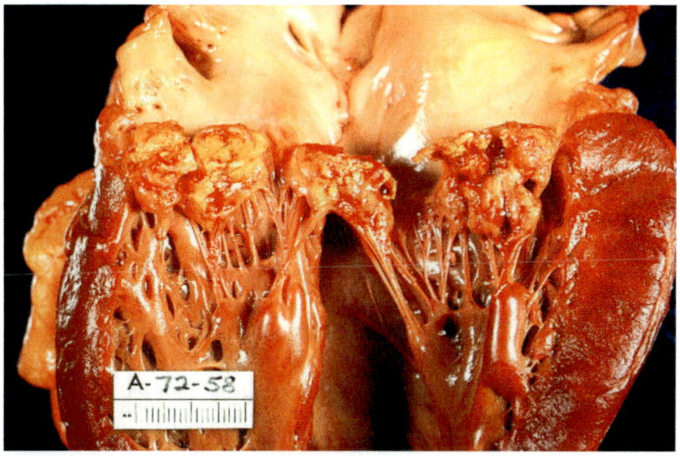

Photo Credit: https://commons.wikimedia.org/wiki/File:Haemophilus_parainfluenzae_Endocarditis_PHIL_851_lores.jpg

FIGURE 10.5.71 - Infective Bacterial Endocarditis of the Mitral Valve

Agent(s)	Association(s)
- *S. aureus*	- IV drug users
- *S. epidermidis*	- Prosthetic valves - IV catheter
- *S. bovis (gallolyticus)*	- Underlying colorectal carcinoma
- HACEK	- Native valve
- *Coxiella burnetii* - *Bartonella spp.*	- Culture negative

TABLE 10.5.4 - Causes of Infective Endocarditis

VI. Symptoms
   A. Variable depending on the underlying cause (infective, non-infective)
   B. Nonspecific symptoms are common (fatigue, fever, or chills)
   C. New-onset heart murmur

D. Mnemonic: FROM JANE
1. Fever
    a) Due to the bacteremia
2. Roth spots
    a) Retinal hemorrhages with small, clear centers
    b) Due to antigen-antibody complex deposits in eyes
3. Osler nodes
    a) Painful, raised lesions on the finger or toe pads (Ouch, Ouch, Osler)
    b) Due to antibody complex deposits in pads of digits
4. Murmur
    a) Due to turbulent blood flow past the damaged heart valve
5. Janeway lesions
    a) Erythematous, small, flat, painless
    b) Due to emboli to skin vessels
6. Anemia (of chronic disease)
7. Nail-bed hemorrhage (splinter hemorrhage)
    a) Splinter hemorrhages
    b) Due to deposition of emboli
8. Emboli
    a) Vegetations detach from the valve
    b) Deposit elsewhere (e.g. nail beds, kidneys, spleen, central nervous system)

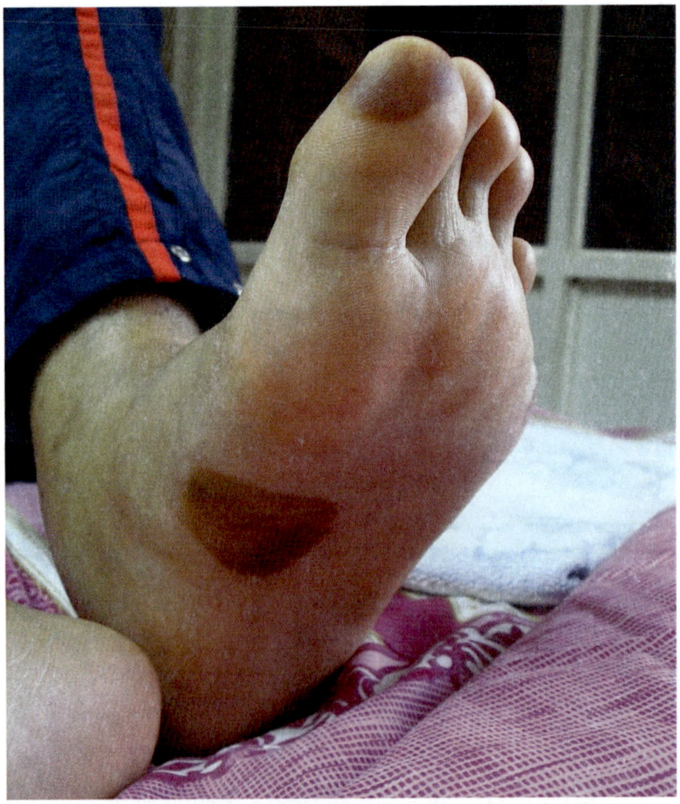

Photo Credit: Roberto J. Galindo / CC BY-SA (https://creativecommons.org/licenses/by-sa/4.0)

FIGURE 10.5.72 - Osler's Nodes

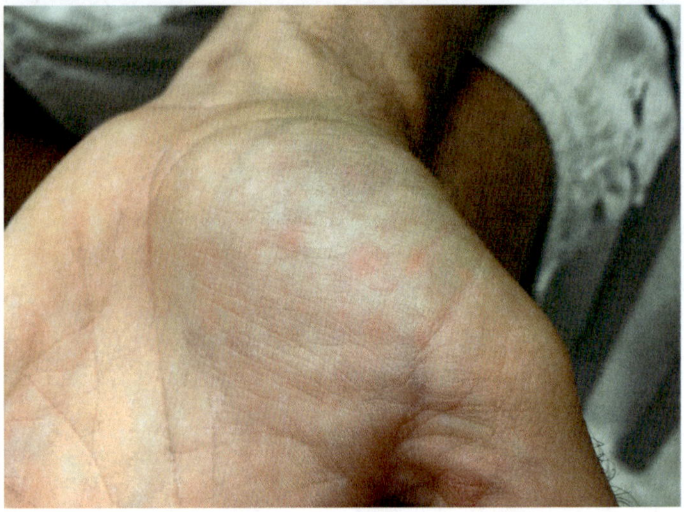

Photo Credit: Warfieldian / CC BY-SA (https://creativecommons.org/licenses/by-sa/4.0)

FIGURE 10.5.73 - Janeway Lesions (Palm)

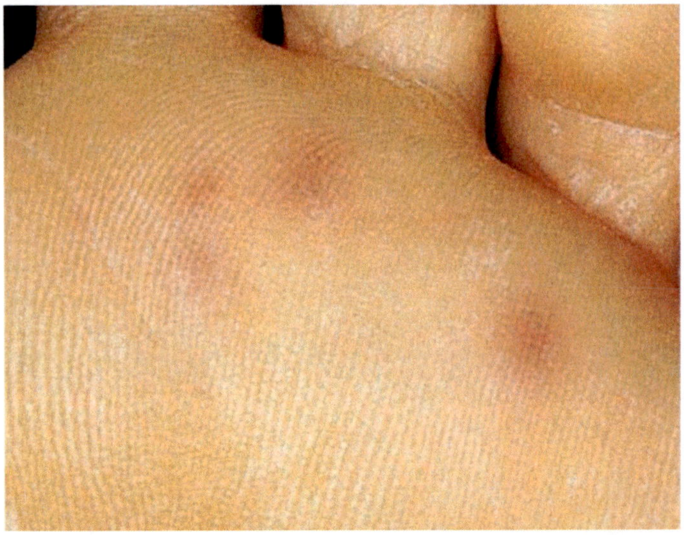

Photo Credit: https://flickr.com/photos/58146070@N07/8621673442/in/photolist-e8SkaN-e8Sk97-e8Skaj-e8LG5i

FIGURE 10.5.74 - Janeway Lesions (Foot)

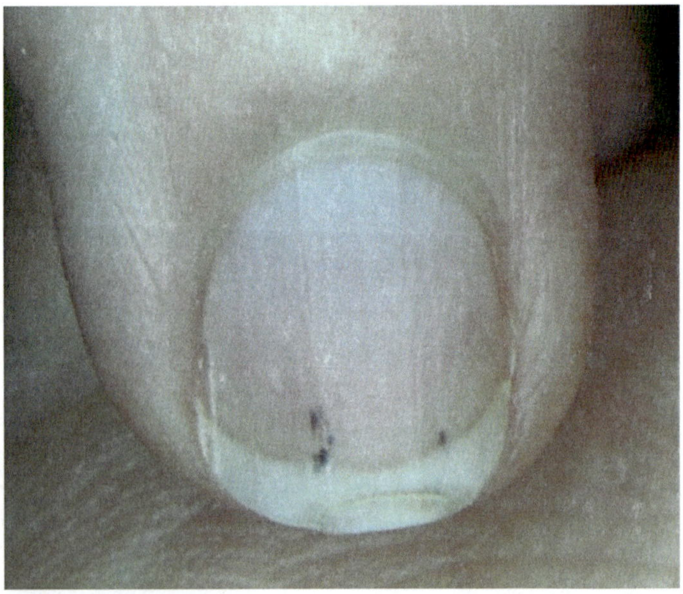

Photo Credit: Splarka / Public domain

FIGURE 10.5.75 - Splinter Hemorrhages

VII. Lab Findings
   A. Blood cultures
   B. Anemia of chronic disease: ↓ Hb, ↓ MCV, ↑ ferritin, ↓ TIBC, ↓ serum iron, and ↓ % saturation
   C. Transesophageal echocardiogram is useful for detecting lesions on valves
   D. History

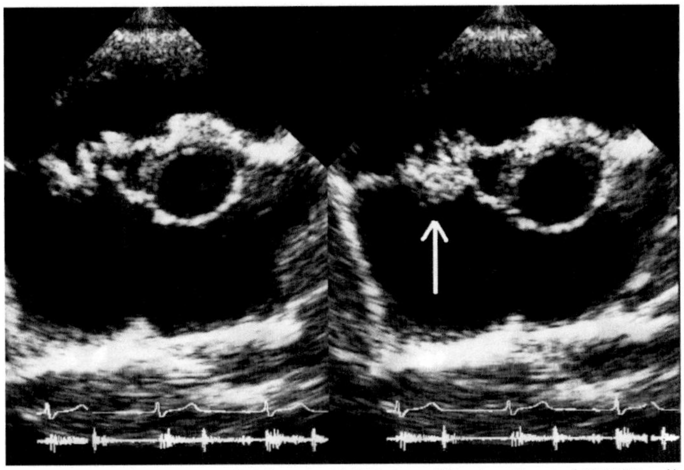

FIGURE 10.5.76 - Echocardiogram Showing Vegetations on the Tricuspid Valve

REVIEW QUESTIONS

1. A 45-year-old man is evaluated for progressive weakness, fatigue, and a low-grade fever that has persisted for the past 5 weeks. He immigrated from China 20 years ago. He has a history of heart disease but is otherwise healthy. A 2/6 diastolic murmur is heard on chest auscultation. Physical exam reveals poor dentition and an erythematous, flat lesion on his palm. The lesion is not painful on palpation. What is the pathophysiological mechanism of this lesion?
   A. Immune complex deposition within the skin vessels
   B. Emboli causing occlusion of small vessels of the skin
   C. Superficial infection of the skin
   D. Itching and dryness of the skin

- **The correct answer is B.**
- Hopefully from the question, you noted that this man's symptoms are due to infective subacute endocarditis.
- The lesion is described as erythematous, flat, and painless, which is consistent with a Janeway lesion. These occur due to heart vegetations' embolization to the skin.
- This man's endocarditis is evident by weakness, fatigue, low-grade fever, and a heart murmur.
- The patient's immigration from China and his history of heart disease point towards rheumatic heart disease causing damage to the heart valves and predisposing the patient to subacute endocarditis.
- Option A is incorrect because it refers to the immunological phenomenon that results in Osler's nodes, where the lesion would be painful and raised.
- C and D are both wrong because they don't account for the weakness, fatigue, or heart murmur evident in this patient.

Section XVII - Rheumatic Fever

I. Basic Principles
   A. A serious complication of group A beta-hemolytic streptococcal infection
   B. Can cause rheumatic heart disease leading to valvular damage
   C. Inadequate treatment of group A beta-hemolytic streptococcal infection

II. Pathophysiology
   A. Inappropriate immune system reaction to group A streptococcal infection
   B. Type II hypersensitivity reaction
   C. Molecular mimicry results in M proteins cross-reacting with self-antigens

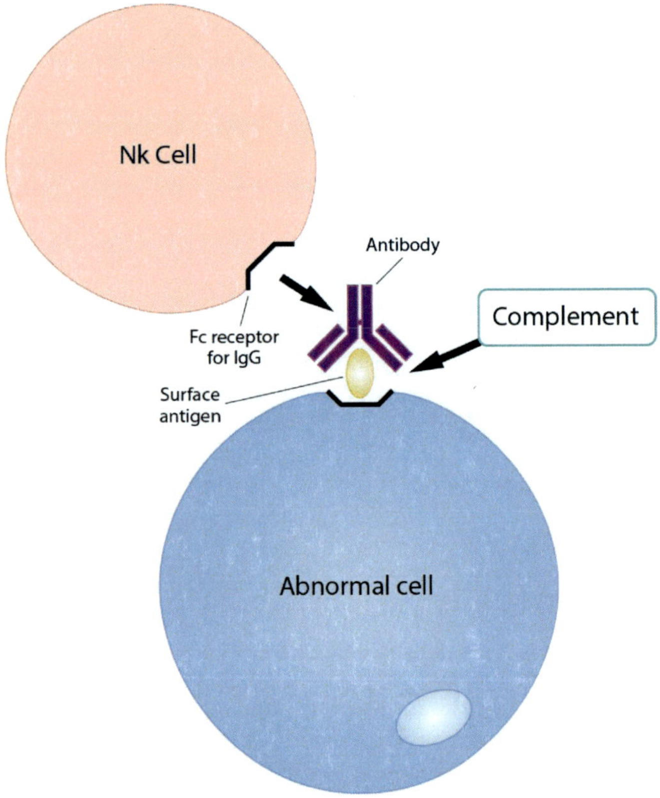

FIGURE 10.5.77 - Type II Hypersensitivity Reaction

III. Histopathology
   A. Aschoff bodies are granulomas with giant cells
   B. Anitschkow cells are enlarged macrophages inside of Aschoff bodies

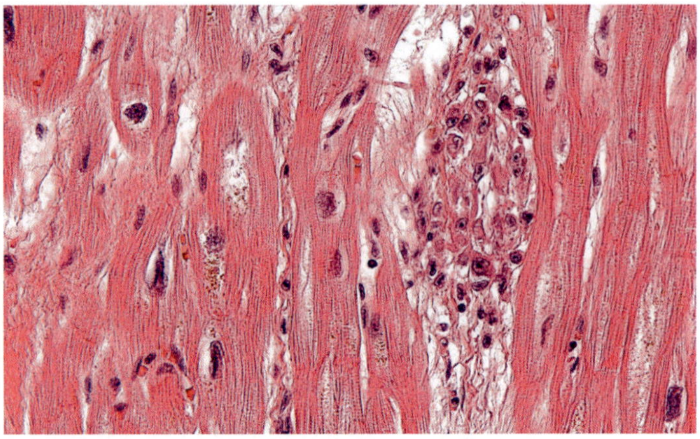

FIGURE 10.5.78 - Anitschkow Cells within an Aschoff Body

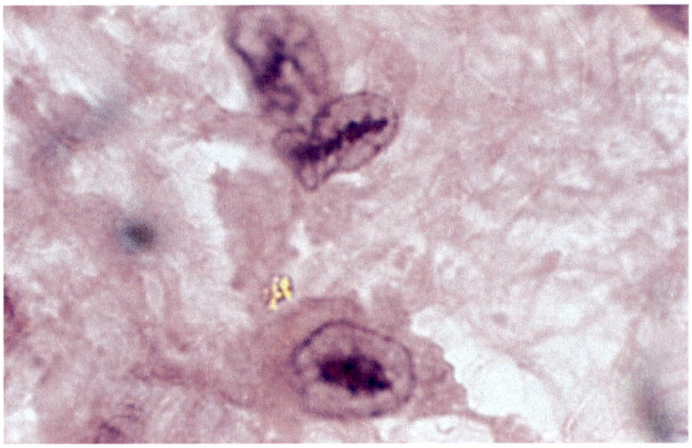

FIGURE 10.5.79 - Anitschkow Cell

IV. Findings
   A. Symptoms include migratory joint pain, fever, chest pain, dyspnea
   B. The physical exam may show a new cardiac murmur, subcutaneous nodules, erythema marginatum, and Sydenham chorea

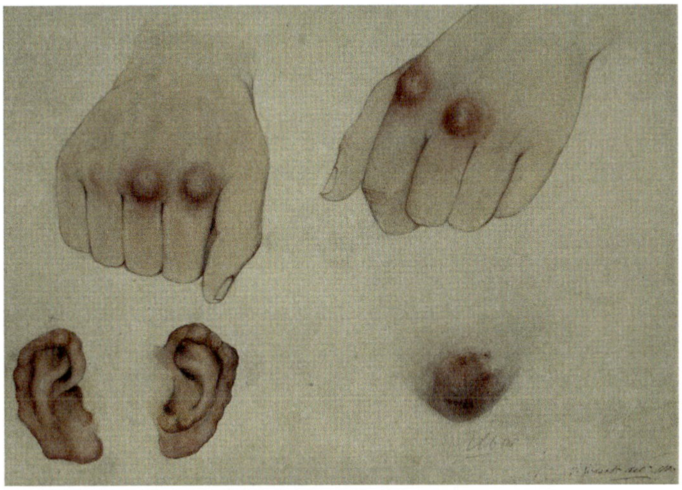

Photo Credit: [CC BY (https://creativecommons.org/licenses/by/4.0)]

FIGURE 10.5.80 - Subcutaneous Nodules

   C. Labs may show increased anti-streptolysin O and anti-deoxyribonuclease B titers
   D. Prolonged PR interval on EKG
   E. A positive throat culture or rapid strep test

V. Diagnosis
   A. Diagnosis is based on the clinical presentation, previous group A streptococcal infection, and the Jones criteria
   B. Patients must have either 2 major Jones criteria or 2 minor and 1 major

Criteria	Features
Major criteria (JONES)	- Migratory arthritis - Carditis - Subcutaneous nodules - Erythema marginatum - Sydenham chorea
Minor criteria	- Arthralgias - Previous group A streptococcal infection - Fever - First-degree heart block - Increased erythrocyte sedimentation rate - Increased C-reactive protein

TABLE 10.5.5 - Jones Criteria

VI. Physical exam
   A. Cardiac abnormalities
      1. The mitral valve is the most commonly affected
      2. Patients may present with mitral stenosis or regurgitation

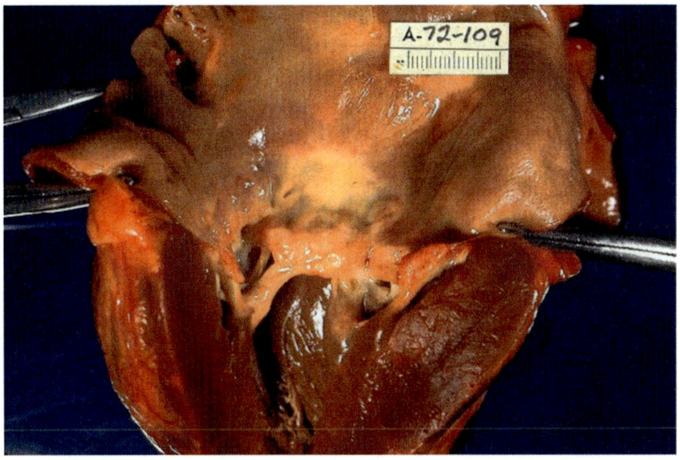

Photo Credit: Public Health Image Library (PHIL) ID#: 847

FIGURE 10.5.81 - Rheumatic Heart Disease with Thickened Mitral Valve

   B. Dermatologic abnormalities
      1. Painless subcutaneous nodules may appear
      2. Erythema marginatum (circular macular or papular rash

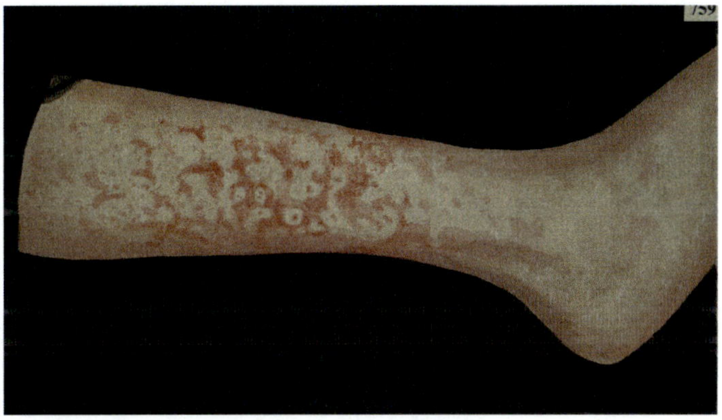

Photo Credit: [CC BY (https://creativecommons.org/licenses/by/4.0)]

FIGURE 10.5.82 - Erythema Marginatum

   C. Neurological abnormalities
      1. Sydenham chorea (involuntary jerky movement)
      2. This is caused by antibodies that bind to dopamine receptors

VII. Treatment
   A. Penicillin
   B. Macrolides
   C. Non-steroidal anti-inflammatory drugs

REVIEW QUESTIONS

1. A 12-year-old boy with no significant past medical history is brought to the local pediatrician by his parents due to concerns about what they describe as abnormal movements. The boy states he is unable to control these movements and they come and go. The patient's parents state he has been healthy and has not had any injuries other than a sore throat 2 months ago. During the physical examination, there are uncontrollable jerky movements in the patient's face and arms. Which of the following is a potential complication of this patient's condition?

    A. Mitral stenosis
    B. Hepatocellular carcinoma
    C. Huntington disease
    D. Complex seizure disorder

- **The correct answer is A.**
- The important things to recognize in this question are the patient's history of a recent sore throat combined with jerky maneuvers, which are suspicious for Sydenham chorea.
- Valvular disease is a potential complication of rheumatic fever, and the mitral valve is most commonly affected.
- B is incorrect because hepatocellular carcinoma is not a complication of rheumatic fever.
- Hepatocellular carcinoma can arise from a number of etiologies, such as hemochromatosis. This is a hereditary disease that leads to an iron overloaded state. It does not usually affect children.
- C is incorrect because rheumatic fever does not have an association with Huntington disease.
- Huntington disease does have a characteristic choreiform movement, but this disorder presents between the ages of 30 and 50. Patients will present with dementia, depression, and an ataxic gait.
- D is incorrect because complex seizure disorders do not occur in rheumatic fever.
- Complex seizure disorders may present with lip-smacking or involuntary limb movements and will have impaired consciousness.

Section XVIII - Pericarditis

I. Basic Principles
   A. Pericardium: fluid-filled sac around heart
   B. Pericarditis: inflammation of pericardium

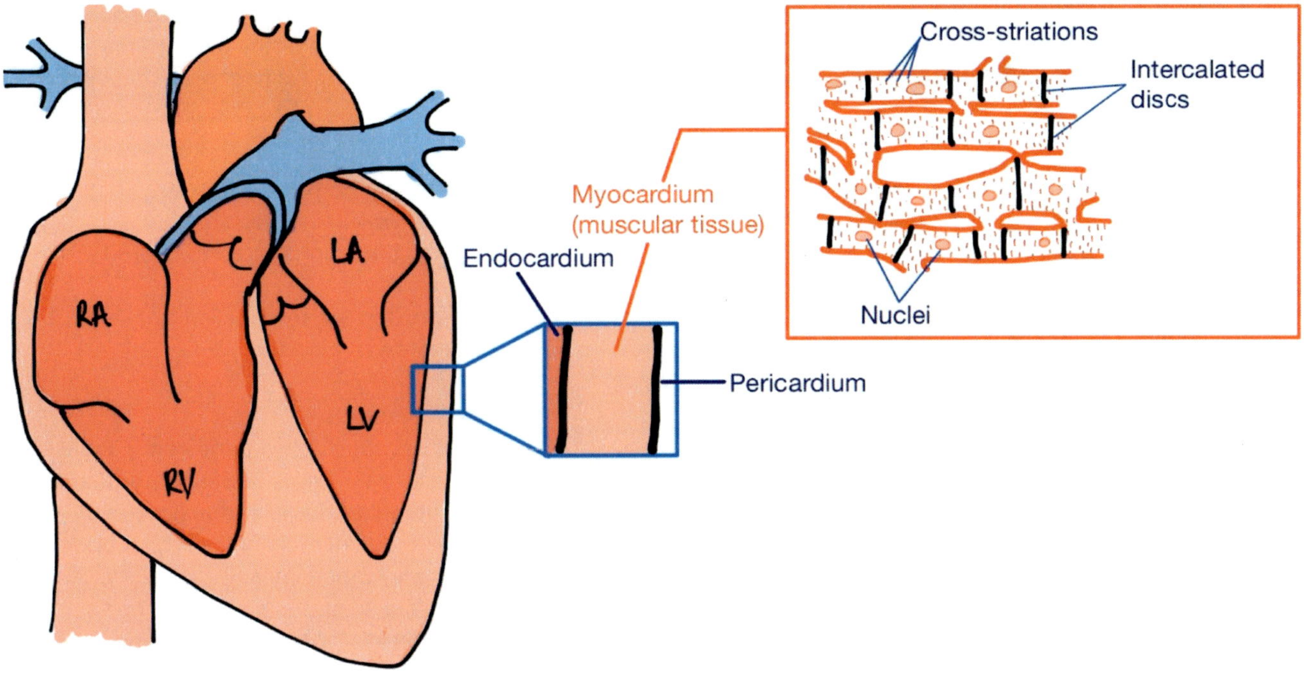

FIGURE 10.5.83 - Layers of Heart Wall

II. Etiology
   A. Viral (most common cause)
   B. Post-MI (2-4 days after)
   C. Dressler syndrome (week to months after MI)
   D. Uremia
   E. SLE
   F. Neoplasm

III. Clinical Findings
   A. Chest pain (pleuritic and positional)
   B. Diffuse ST elevation and/or PR depression on EKG
   C. Friction rub on physical exam
   D. Pericardial effusion on echocardiogram

IV. Complications
   A. Pericardial effusion
   B. Cardiac tamponade
   C. Constrictive pericarditis

V. Constrictive Pericarditis
   A. Increasingly rigid pericardial tissue → restricted ventricular filling → decreased cardiac output
   B. Kussmaul's sign: ↑ jugular venous pressure on inspiration
   C. Pulsus paradoxus: > 10 mmHg drop in systolic BP on inspiration
   D. Pericardial knock: high-pitched early diastolic sound

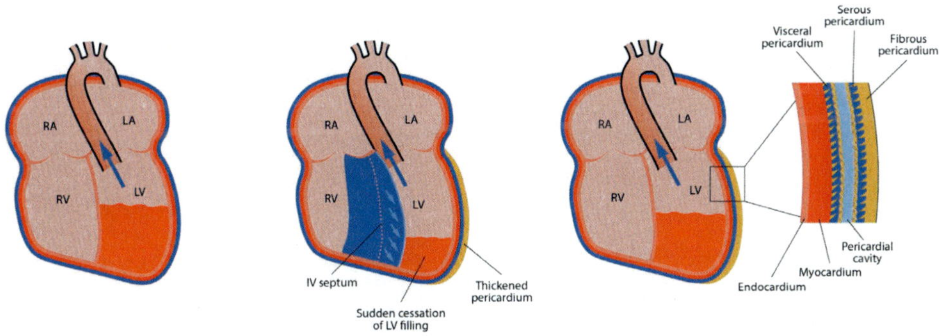

FIGURE 10.5.85 - Constrictive Pericarditis

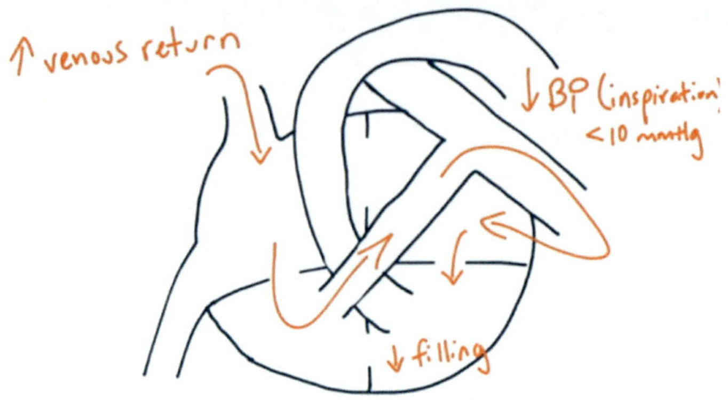

FIGURE 10.5.85 - BP Changes in Normal Inspiration

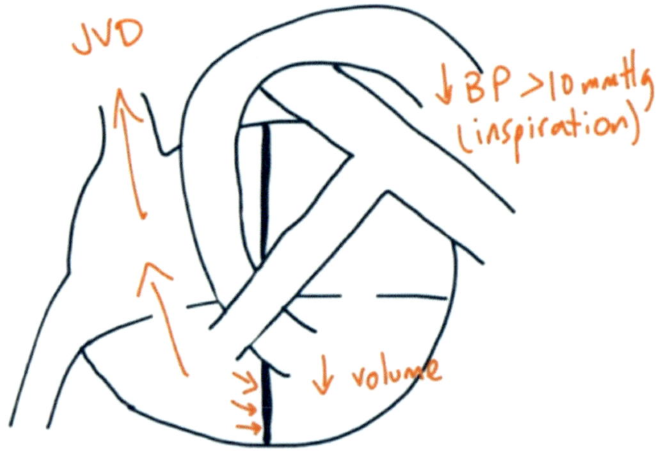

FIGURE 10.5.86 - BP Changes in Inspiration with Constrictive Pericarditis

VI. Treatment
   A. Non-steroidal anti-inflammatory drugs (NSAIDs) and colchicine
   B. Steroids (not preferred)
   C. If constrictive pericarditis → pericardiectomy

REVIEW QUESTIONS ?

1. A 34-year-old female is brought to the emergency department for chest pain. She was recently in the emergency department for a similar episode a few days ago. An echocardiogram is performed and shows increased thickness of the pericardium. Which of the following physiological findings is most likely not present?

   A. Distended neck veins on inspiration
   B. BP changing from 140/80 to 140/50 upon inspiration
   C. BP changing from 150/80 to 130/80 upon inspiration
   D. High-pitched diastolic murmur heard best at the left lower sternal border

- **The correct answer is B.**
- The patient has constrictive pericarditis, as shown by the increased thickness of the pericardium. We can assume that this is a complication of acute pericarditis since she had a similar episode a few days ago. Among our several findings would be Kussmaul's sign, pulsus paradoxus, and a pericardial knock.
- Choice B is correct because it is describing a decrease in diastolic pressure upon inspiration, which is not describing pulsus paradoxus. In constrictive pericarditis, we'd see a decrease in only systolic pressures, not diastolic.
- A is incorrect because this is describing Kussmaul's sign, which we would see in acute pericarditis. Constrictive pericarditis causes decreased filling into the right ventricle, resulting in fluid backup similar to that seen in right-sided heart failure. As a result, we'd see jugular venous distension on inspiration in what is known as Kussmaul's sign.
- C is incorrect because it is describing a decrease in systolic pressure upon inspiration. In constrictive pericarditis, we would see pulsus paradoxus, which is a > 10 mmHg decrease in systolic blood pressure upon inspiration.
- D is incorrect because it is referring to a pericardial knock, which we are likely to hear in constrictive pericarditis. Recall that it is due to a sudden pause in filling of the ventricles.

Section XIX - Myocarditis

I. Myocarditis: Definition
   A. Inflammation of the myocardial tissue layer

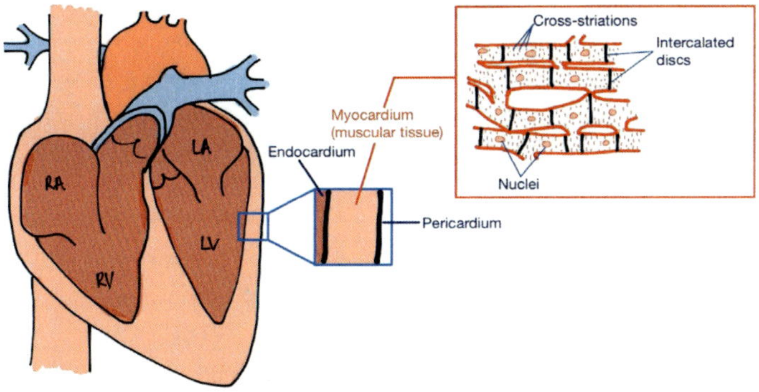

FIGURE 10.5.80 - Layers of Heart Wall

II. Myocarditis: Etiology
   A. Infectious (most common)
   B. Non-infectious

III. Infectious Myocarditis: Etiology
   A. North America: Coxsackie B virus
   B. Worldwide: Chagas disease (*T. cruzi*; transmitted by reduviid or "kissing" bugs)

Type of Pathogen	Infectious Etiologies
Viruses	Coxsackie B (most common cause in US), parvovirus B19, echovirus, HIV, HHV-6, adenovirus, Epstein-Barr virus, influenza, CMV, hepatitis A and B, poliovirus, RSV, rubella, vaccinia, VZV, etc.
Bacteria	*Borrelia burgdorferi* (i.e. Lyme disease), *Mycoplasma pneumoniae, Treponema pallidum* (i.e. syphilis), *Corynebacterium diphtheriae*, group A strep, *S. aureus, Leptospira spp., Rickettsia spp., Salmonella spp.*, etc.
Fungi	*Candida spp., Aspergillus spp., Histoplasma spp., Blastomyces spp., Cryptococcus spp., Coccidiomycosis spp.*
Parasites	*Trypanosoma cruzi* (most common cause worldwide), *Toxoplasma spp., Schistosoma spp., Trichinella spp.*

TABLE 10.5.6 - Infectious Causes of Myocarditis

IV. Non-Infectious Myocarditis: Etiology
   A. Rheumatic fever (J♥NES)
   B. Autoimmune (e.g. SLE, Kawasaki disease)
   C. Toxin/drug (e.g. arsenic, carbon monoxide, cocaine)
   D. Idiopathic (e.g. giant cell myocarditis, sarcoidosis)

V. Myocarditis: Pathophysiology
   A. Damage to myocardium and immune response
   B. Dilated cardiomyopathy
   C. Signs and symptoms of heart failure
   D. Arrhythmias

VI. Myocarditis: Histopathology
   A. Myofibrillary necrosis (always)
   B. Mononuclear cell infiltrates
      1. Lymphocytes: viral
      2. Neutrophils: bacterial
      3. Eosinophils: hypersensitivity
   C. Granulomas: sarcoidosis or giant cell myocarditis
   D. Parasites

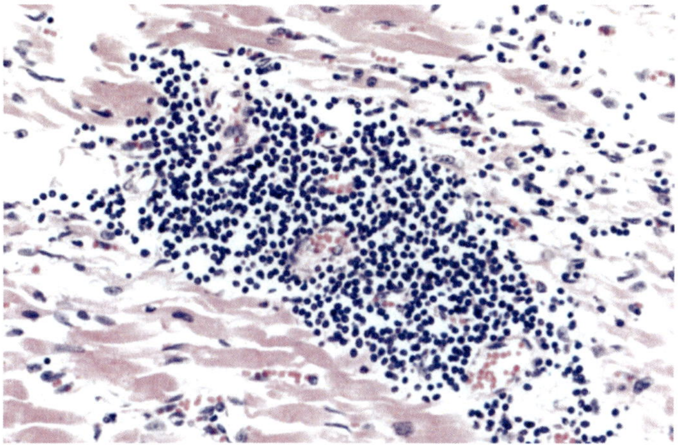

FIGURE 10.5.87 - Histopathology of Myocarditis

VII. Myocarditis: Clinical Findings
   A. Highly variable (dyspnea, chest pain, fever, arrhythmia)
   B. Persistent tachycardia out of proportion to fever
   C. Prodromal viral illness
   D. Dilated cardiomyopathy leading to heart failure
   E. Sudden cardiac death < 40 years of age

VIII. Myocarditis: Treatment
   A. Supportive
   B. Treat underlying cause
   C. Exercise restriction

REVIEW QUESTIONS

1. A 5-year-old boy with a family history of asthma presents to his pediatrician with a flu-like illness that has been ongoing for 3 days. He complains of myalgias involving his entire body. His temperature is 38.9 °C (102 °F), respiratory rate is 24/min, and heart rate is 148/min. A week later, he returns to his pediatrician with progressive dyspnea and chest pain. His temperature is now 37.6 °C (99.7 °F), respiratory rate is 32/min, and heart rate is 146/min. Physical examination reveals rhonchi over the lung bases bilaterally. An EKG shows sinus tachycardia. A cardiac biopsy reveals myofibrillary necrosis and lymphocytic infiltrates. What is the most likely cause of his illness?

    A. Allergic reactive airway disease
    B. A virus similar to the one that causes hand, foot, and mouth disease
    C. *T. cruzi* infection
    D. Autoimmune disease secondary to molecular mimicry

- **The correct answer is B.**
- The tachycardia is out of proportion and persists beyond the course of the fever. There is also heart failure after viral illness, myofibrillary necrosis and lymphocytic infiltrates. Additionally, dyspnea and rhonchi or crackles suggest heart failure. All these findings lead us to consider viral myocarditis. Since no risk factors such as recent travel, sick contact, or underlying disease are mentioned, we should think of Coxsackie B myocarditis because it is the most common cause of myocarditis in the U.S. B is the correct answer, since Coxsackie A virus is the one that causes hand, foot, and mouth disease.
- A is incorrect because it is talking about asthma. Asthma can present with dyspnea and chest pain secondary to cough; however, it does not explain the persistent tachycardia out of proportion to fever or the apparent heart failure. Furthermore, the histology described implies viral myocarditis.
- C is incorrect because T. cruzi is a non-viral cause of myocarditis, while the question stem mentioned a prodromal viral illness and lymphocytic infiltrates, making viral etiology fairly clear. There was no discussion of travel or if the patient was a recent immigrant, so Chagas disease is less likely than Coxsackie B; therefore, C is wrong.
- D is incorrect because of the boy's history of flu-like illness rather than a Group A strep infection leading to rheumatic fever. There is no description of pharyngeal exudate, sore throat, and tender anterior cervical adenopathy in addition to his fever. There are also no features of rheumatic fever being described. Furthermore, rheumatic fever presents 2-4 weeks after sore throat, not 1 week after illness as in the case of this patient's myocarditis.

Section XX - Vasculitis

I. Basic Principles
   A. Inflammation of blood vessel wall
      1. 3 layers of the arterial wall: endothelial tunica intima, smooth muscle tunica media, connective tissue tunica adventitia
   B. Unknown etiology (usually not infectious)
   C. General clinical features
      1. Nonspecific: fever, fatigue, weight loss, myalgias
      2. Organ ischemia due to luminal narrowing or thrombosis

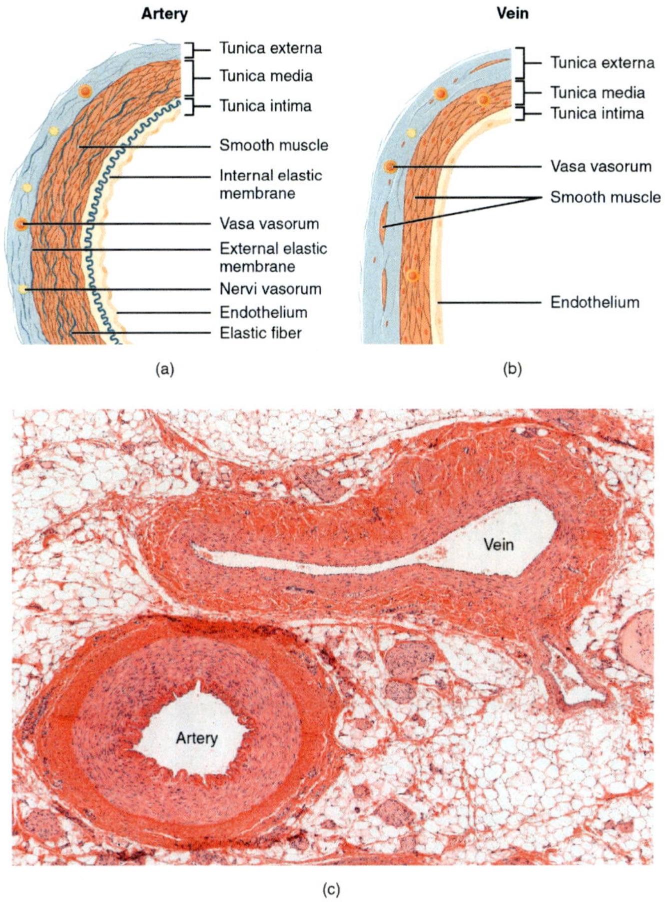

FIGURE 10.5.88 - Normal Artery

Disease	Definition and Epidemiology	Presentation	Lab/Biopsy Findings	Treatment
Temporal (giant cell) arteritis	- Granulomatous vasculitis involving branches of carotid artery - Most common vasculitis in females > 50yrs	- Headache (temporal a.) - Visual disturbance (ophthalmic a.) - Jaw claudication - Polymyalgia rheumatica	- Elevated ESR and CRP - Inflamed vessel wall with granulomatous multinucleated giant cells and intimal fibrosis - Segmental lesions	- Corticosteroids - Start treatment immediately to prevent blindness
Takayasu arteritis	- Granulomatous vasculitis involving aortic arch and its branches - Young Asian females	- Visual or neurologic symptoms - Weak/absent pulse in upper extremity ("pulseless disease") - Claudication - Bruits	- Elevated ESR and CRP - Granulomatous inflammation of tunica media - Transmural fibrous thickening - Luminal narrowing	- Corticosteroids

TABLE 10.5.7 - Types of Large Vessel Vasculitis

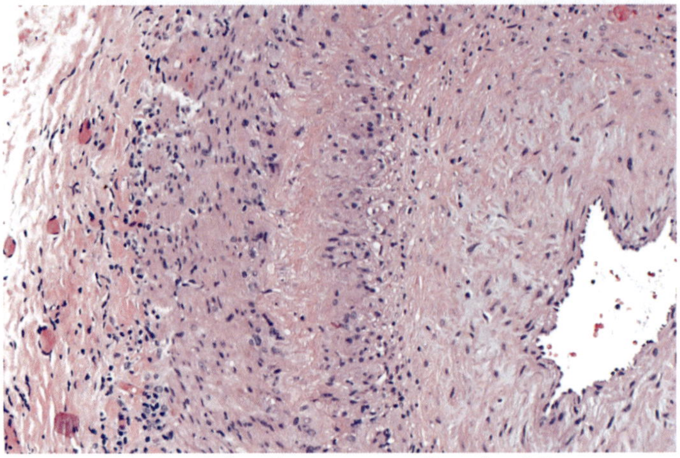

Photo Credit: Nephron / CC BY-SA (https://creativecommons.org/licenses/by-sa/3.0)

FIGURE 10.5.89 - Biopsy of Temporal Arteritis

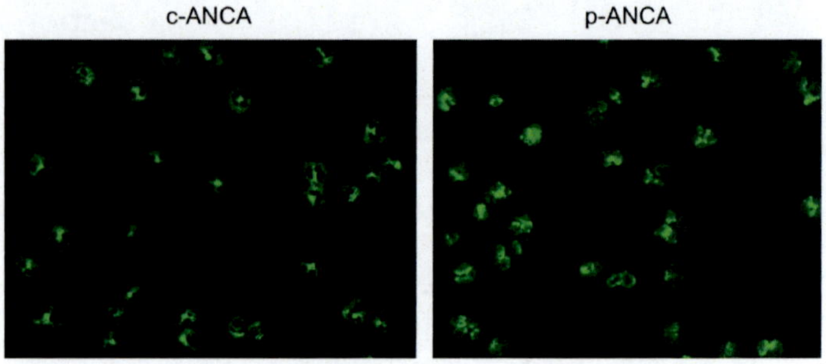

Photo Credit: Simon Caulton / CC BY-SA (https://creativecommons.org/licenses/by-sa/3.0)

FIGURE 10.5.90 - Immunofluorescence Showing Cytoplasmic Anti-Neutrophil Cytoplasmic Antibodies (c-ANCA) and Perinuclear Anti-Neutrophil Cytoplasmic Antibodies (p-ANCA)

Disease	Definition and Epidemiology	Presentation	Lab/Biopsy Findings	Treatment
Polyarteritis nodosa	- Necrotizing vasculitis - Lungs spared - Young adults	- Hypertension (renal a.) - Abdominal pain and melena (mesenteric a.) - Headache - Seizure - Skin nodules - Myalgias and arthritis	- Serum HBsAg - Nongranulomatous lesions of varying stages - Early: transmural inflammation, fibrinoid necrosis - Late: fibrosis, "string of pearls"	- Corticosteroids - Cyclophosphamide - Fatal if untreated
Kawasaki disease	- Coronary artery - Asian children < 4yrs	- Fever - Bilateral conjunctivitis - Rash on palms and soles - Cervical LAD - Upper extremity edema - Strawberry tongue - MI and coronary artery thrombosis	- Elevated ESR and CRP	- Aspirin - IVIG
Buerger disease	- Necrotizing vasculitis of digits - Smokers - Males < 45yrs	- Digital ulceration - Gangrene - Autoamputation of digits - Raynaud phenomenon	- Inflammatory intraluminal thrombi - Vessel wall spared - Extension into adjacent veins and nerves	- Smoking cessation

TABLE 10.5.8 - Types of Medium Vessel Vasculitis

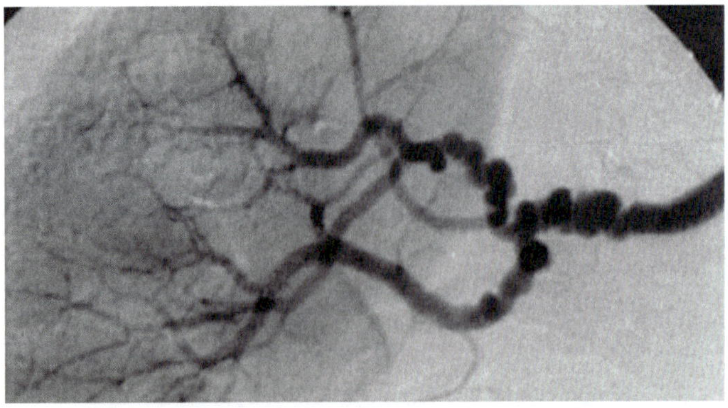

Photo Credit: Pierre-Fran9

FIGURE 10.5.90 - "String of Pearls" Appearance

Disease	Definition and Dpidemiology	Presentation	Lab/Biopsy Findings	Treatment
Granulomatosis with polyangiitis	- Necrotizing granulomatous vasculitis - Nasopharynx, lungs, kidneys - Granulomatosis with polyangiitis (formerly known as Wegener granulomatosis) - Middle-aged males	- Sinusitis - Nasopharyngeal ulceration - Hemoptysis - Bilateral nodular lung infiltrates - Hematuria (RPGN)	- Serum c-ANCA - Necrotizing granulomas and vasculitis	- Corticosteroids - Cyclophosphamide - Relapse common
Microscopic polyangiitis	- Necrotizing vasculitis - Lung and kidney	- Hemoptysis - Bilateral nodular lung infiltrates - Hematuria	- Serum p-ANCA	- Corticosteroids - Cyclophosphamide - Relapse common
Eosinophilic granulomatosis with polyangiitis	- Granulomatous necrotizing vasculitis with eosinophils - "Churg-Strauss syndrome" - Lungs most affected	- Late-onset asthma - Rinosinusitis - Pulmonary infiltrates - Mononeuritis multiplex - Skin nodules	- Eosinophilia - Serum p-ANCA - Eosinophils on biopsy	- Corticosteroids
IgA vasculitis	- IgA immune complex deposition - "Henoch-Schönlein purpura" - Most common vasculitis in children (boys 2-10 yrs)	- Follows URI - Palpable purpura - Abdominal pain and bleeding - Hematuria (IgA nephropathy)	- IgA immune complex deposition in affected organs	- Corticosteroids - Self-limiting

TABLE 10.5.9- Types of Small Vessel Vasculitis

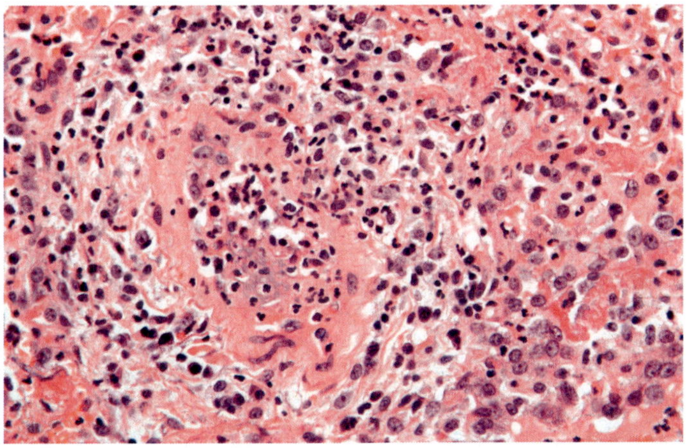

Photo Credit: Nephron / CC BY-SA (https://creativecommons.org/licenses/by-sa/3.0)

FIGURE 10.5.92 - Biopsy of Granulomatosis with Polyangiitis

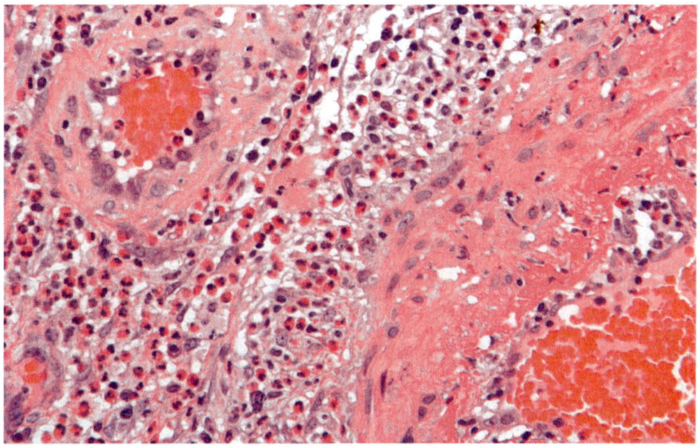

Photo Credit: Nephron / CC BY-SA (https://creativecommons.org/licenses/by-sa/3.0)

FIGURE 10.5.93 - Biopsy of Eosinophilic Granulomatosis with Polyangiitis

REVIEW QUESTIONS

1. A 68-year-old female complains of trouble chewing. She has noticed difficulty chewing tough foods, like steak, for the past 2 months. She has also experienced intermittent loss of vision in her left eye. No gross abnormalities are noted on physical exam; however, she has unintentionally lost 15 pounds since her last visit 3 months ago. An arterial biopsy is ordered. What histological feature will most likely be observed upon biopsy of the causative lesion?

    - **The correct answer is segmental inflammation of the vessel wall with granulomatous multinucleated giant cells and intimal fibrosis.**
    - Here we have a 68-year-old female with difficulty chewing tough foods — a sign of jaw claudication. She also complains of loss of vision and has unintentional weight loss.
    - Together, these findings suggest a diagnosis of temporal arteritis.
    - On biopsy, you would expect to see an inflamed vessel wall with granulomatous multinucleated giant cells and intimal fibrosis.
    - These lesions are segmental, so a large portion of the artery must be sampled.

2. A 3-year-old boy of Asian descent presents with a fever and "pink eye." His mom says he has had these symptoms for the past 3 days. On physical exam, bilateral conjunctival injection, an enlarged red tongue, and erythema on the palms and soles are noted. How should this patient be treated?

    - **The correct answer is aspirin and IVIG.**
    - Here we have a 3-year-old Asian boy with a fever, bilateral conjunctial injection, an enlarged red "strawberry tongue," and a rash on the palms and soles.
    - This is all consistent with Kawasaki disease.
    - Kawasaki disease is treated with aspirin and IVIG.

3. A 49-year-old man presents with frequent "nosebleeds" and a bloody cough. Past medical history is significant for recurrent gross hematuria and hemoptysis. Physical examination reveals ulceration of the nasal mucosa. A chest X-ray shows bilateral nodular lung infiltrates. Which of the following is an expected serum lab finding in this patient?

    A. c-ANCA
    B. p-ANCA
    C. Hepatitis B surface antigen
    D. Eosinophilia

    - **The correct answer is A.**
    - The patient in the vignette is a middle-aged male suffering from nasopharyngeal ulceration, hemoptysis, and hematuria.
    - This is all consistent with a diagnosis of granulomatosis with polyangiitis. It is a necrotizing granulomatous vasculitis involving the nasopharynx, lungs, and kidneys.
    - The main lab finding in granulomatosis with polyangiitis is a positive serum c-ANCA.
    - B is incorrect, as p-ANCA is characteristic of both microscopic polyangiitis and eosinophilic granulomatosis with polyangiitis.
    - C is incorrect, as hepatitis B surface antigen is characteristic of polyarteritis nodosa.
    - D is incorrect, as eosinophilia is characteristic of eosinophilic granulomatosis with polyangiitis.

Section XXI - Cardiac Tumors

I. Myxoma
   A. Benign tumor of mesenchymal origin
      1. Most common adult primary cardiac tumor
   B. Gelatinous, pedunculated mass
      1. Histology: pink ground substance
   C. Arises in left atrium
      1. Obstruction of mitral valve → syncope, dyspnea
      2. Early diastolic tumor "plop" on auscultation

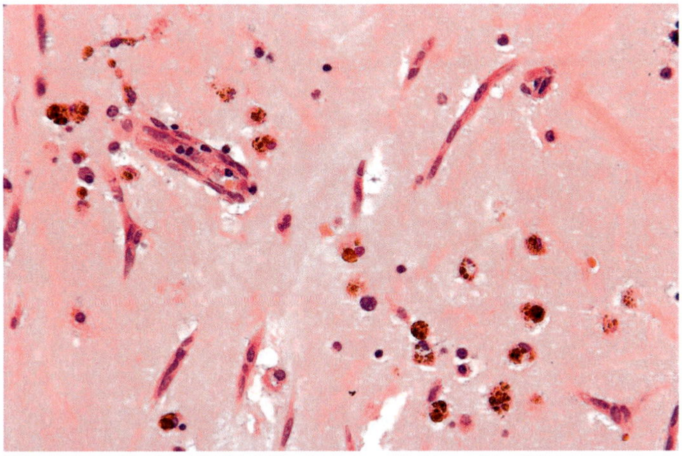

FIGURE 10.5.94 - Globular Myxoma Cells and Hemosiderin-Laden Macrophages in Myxoma

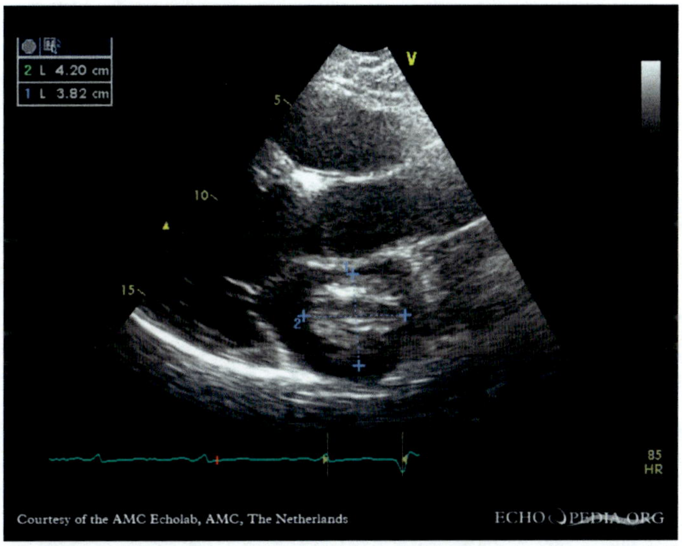

FIGURE 10.5.95 - Echocardiogram of Myxoma

II. Rhabdomyoma
   A. Benign cardiac hamartoma
      1. Most common pediatric primary cardiac tumor
      2. Tuberous sclerosis
   B. Arises in ventricles → outflow obstruction

III. Metastasis
   A. More common than primary cardiac tumors
   B. From breast or lung carcinoma, melanoma, lymphoma
   C. Metastasize to pericardium → pericardial effusion

REVIEW QUESTIONS ?

1. A 27-year-old man with no significant past medical history presents with worsening dizziness and shortness of breath. He does not use tobacco, alcohol, or illicit drugs. Lungs are clear to auscultation. On cardiac auscultation, a faint early diastolic sound is heard at the apex. Echocardiography demonstrates a 3 cm cardiac mass. Which of the following is the likely location of this mass?

   A. Pericardium
   B. Left atrium
   C. Right atrium
   D. Left ventricle

- **The correct answer is B.**
- Here we have an adult male with syncope and dyspnea. He also has an early diastolic tumor "plop" on cardiac auscultation. These signs and symptoms are all consistent with a myxoma. Echocardiography confirms the presence of a cardiac mass, but the question asks for the likely location of this mass. Recall that myxomas most commonly arise from the left atrium.
- A is incorrect because the history and physical exam support a diagnosis of myxoma, which is a primary cardiac tumor. The pericardium is the most common location of metastases to the heart, which can present with signs of pericardial effusion.
- C is incorrect because it is more common for myxomas to arise in the left atrium than the right atrium.
- D is incorrect because rhabdomyomas commonly present in children and arise in the ventricles, causing an outflow obstruction.

Section I - Rhinosinusitis

I. Definition
   A. Symptomatic inflammation of the nasal cavity and paranasal sinuses

II. Etiology

Pathogen Type	Common Examples
Viruses	Rhinovirus, influenza virus, and parainfluenza virus
Bacteria	*Steptococcus pneumoniae, Haemophilus influenzae,* and *Moraxella catarrhalis*
Fungi	*Aspergillus, Mucor,* and *Rhizopus* species

Table 10.6.1 - Most Common Infectious Etiologies of Rhinosinusitis

III. Pathophysiology
   A. Viral
      1. Infection via direct contact with conjunctiva or nasal mucosa
      2. Spreads to paranasal sinuses by systemic or direct routes
   B. Bacterial
      1. Most often due to secondary complication of viral infection
      2. Conditions that obstruct nose or impair immune function
   C. Fungal
      1. Involves patients with immunosuppression

IV. Anatomy
   A. Major sinuses involved are maxillary, frontal, sphenoid and ethmoid
   B. Rhinosinusitis most commonly affects the maxillary sinuses
      1. Ostia that connect the maxillary sinuses and middle meatus are located superomedially
      2. Prone to congestion as maxillary sinuses have to drain against gravity into the middle meatus

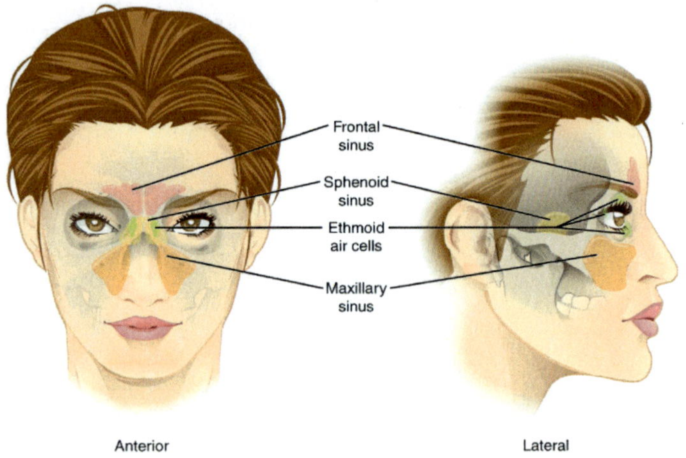

FIGURE 10.6.1 - Major Sinuses

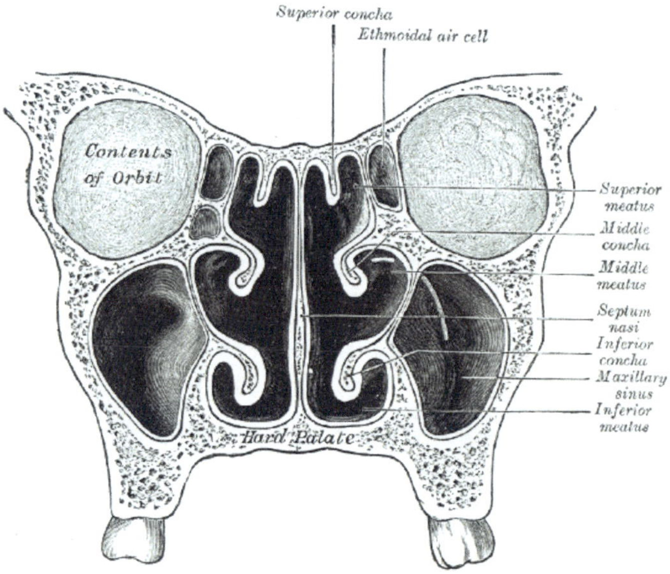

FIGURE 10.6.2 - Maxillary Sinuses in Relation to Middle Meatus

V. Clinical Findings
   A. Nonspecific (e.g. fever, fatigue, headache, cough)
   B. Nasal congestion, purulent nasal drainage, facial pressure and pain, and hyposmia (diminished sense of smell)
   C. Erythema or edema over involved cheekbone or periorbital area
   D. Tenderness with percussion of upper teeth
   E. Opacity on transillumination of sinuses (maxillary and frontal)

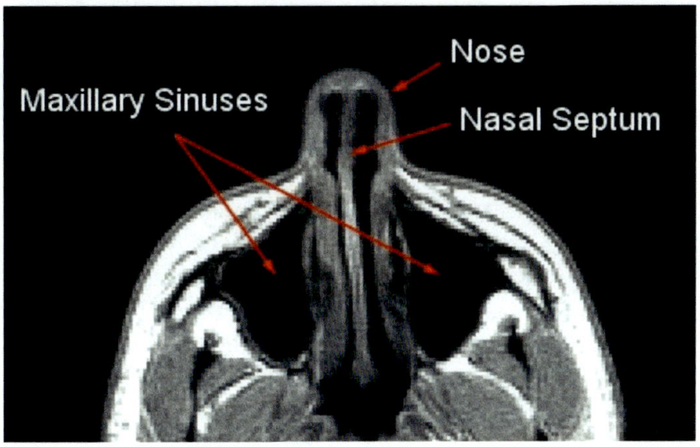

Photo Credit: Markhamilton / Public domain

FIGURE 10.6.3 - CT of Healthy Maxillary Sinuses

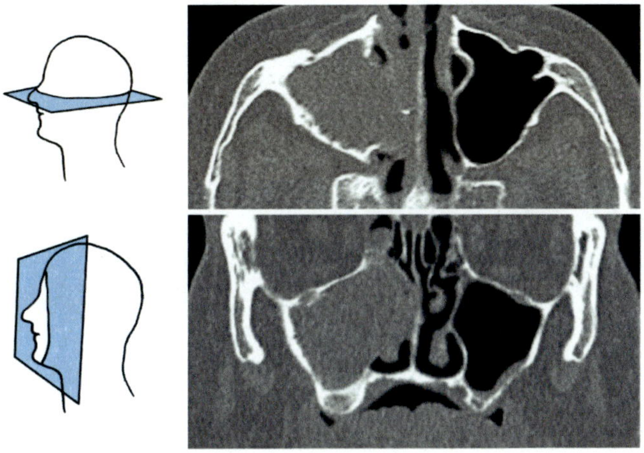

Photo Credit: Mikael Häggström, M.D. - Author info - Reusing images Written informed consent was obtained from the individual, including online publication. / CC0

FIGURE 10.6.4 - CT of Inflamed Right Maxillary Sinus

VI. Complications
   A. Mainly seen in bacterial rhinosinusitis
   B. Local spread (e.g. orbit, CNS)
   C. Periorbital cellulitis, orbital cellulitis, meningitis, cavernous sinus syndrome, intracranial abscess, osteomyelitis

REVIEW QUESTIONS

1. A 4-year-old male with a one-week history of bacterial sinusitis presents to the emergency department complaining of severe right eye pain. On physical examination, he also has notable swelling, erythema, discharge and proptosis. Vital signs include a temperature of 38.9 °C (102 °F). The pain is most severe when he tries to track objects. Ocular movement is noticeably decreased. Fundoscopic examination is unremarkable and visual acuity is unaffected. What is the most likely diagnosis?
   A. Periorbital cellulitis
   B. Bacterial conjunctivitis
   C. Orbital cellulitis
   D. Orbital fracture
   E. Viral conjunctivitis

- **The correct answer is C.**
- The patient was recently diagnosed with acute bacterial sinusitis, and the complaint is unilateral and painful, particularly when trying to move the eye. He has proptosis and his ocular movement is decreased. Therefore, this patient has orbital cellulitis.
- A is incorrect because although periorbital cellulitis also presents with swelling, erythema and pain (usually mild), there is no pain with eye movement, decreased eye movement, or proptosis. lPeriorbital cellulitis is a superficial infection of tissue surrounding the eye, whereas orbital cellulitis involves orbital fat and ocular muscles.
- B is incorrect because bacterial conjunctivitis more characteristically presents with a minimally painful eye that is red with purulent discharge. Vision and ocular movement are not affected.
- D is incorrect because orbital fracture commonly presents with pain in the eye after a traumatic event. Physical examination may show periorbital edema and bruising. The most common locations of orbital fractures are the inferior orbital wall and the medial orbital wall ("blowout fractures").
- E is incorrect because viral conjunctivitis presents similarly to bacterial conjunctivitis. You would also see minimally painful eyes that are red with a watery discharge. Vision, again, is not affected.

Section II - Epistaxis

I. Basic Principles
   A. Nosebleed
   B. Most are benign and self-limiting, but can be life-threatening

II. Types of Epistaxis
   A. Anterior epistaxis: most common
   B. Posterior epistaxis: more severe

III. Anterior Epistaxis
   A. Bleeding from the anterior segment of nostril
   B. Often occurs in children and young adults
   C. Involves the Kiesselbach plexus (Little's area)

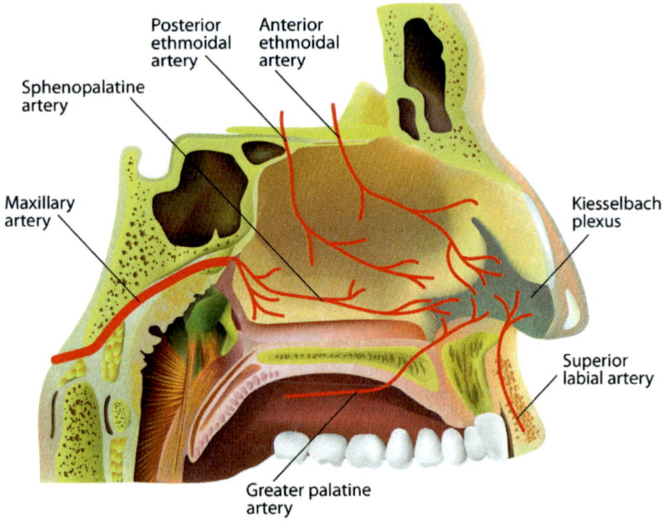

FIGURE 10.6.5 - Kiesselbach Plexus

IV. Posterior Epistaxis
   A. Bleeding from the posterior segment of nostril
   B. Life-threatening: bleeding can cause aspiration
   C. Often occurs in older patients
   D. Source of bleeding
      1. Sphenopalatine artery (most common)
      2. Other branches of maxillary artery

V. Etiology
   A. Trauma
   B. Hypertension
   C. Allergic rhinitis
   D. Nasal angiofibromas
   E. Bleeding disorders

VI. Treatment
   A. Nasal packing (e.g. nasal tampons, gauze)
   B. Ligation
   C. Local anesthetics/vasoconstrictors
   D. Blood pressure control in hypertensive patients
   E. Surgical resection

REVIEW QUESTIONS ?

1. A 23-year-old male presents to the emergency department with a nosebleed. His symptoms began after he got into a bar fight. He denies dizziness, shortness of breath, double vision, hemoptysis, or hematemesis. Family history is unremarkable. His heart rate is 85 beats/minute, blood pressure is 120/75 mm Hg, and temperature is 37 °C (98.6 °F). On physical examination, there is small volume bleeding of the nose. Rupture of which of the following blood vessels is the likely source of bleeding?

   A. Middle meningeal artery
   B. Internal carotid artery
   C. Superior labial artery
   D. Ophthalmic artery

- **The correct answer is C.**
- The Kiesselbach plexus is an anastomosis of several arteries that supply the nasal septum, including the superior labial artery, anterior and posterior ethmoidal arteries, greater palatine artery, and sphenopalatine artery.
- A is incorrect because the rupture of the middle meningeal artery causes epidural hematoma and is often secondary to skull fracture.
- B is incorrect because although the internal carotid artery is near the head and neck, rupture of this artery is very unlikely to cause a nosebleed.
- D is incorrect because although the ophthalmic artery is in the head, damage to the ophthalmic artery would cause vision problems.

Section III - Head and Neck Cancer

Cancer	Affected Tissue	Associations	Clinical Presentation
Nasopharyngeal carcinoma	- Nasopharyngeal epithelium	- EBV infection (infectious mononucleosis) - Chinese adults - African children	- Nasal obstruction - Epistaxis - Early metastasis to cervical lymph nodes
Oropharyngeal carcinoma	- Oropharyngeal epithelium	- HPV-16 - Younger individuals	- Non-healing ulcer - Sore throat
Laryngeal carcinoma	- Epithelial lining of vocal cords	- Males - Heavy smokers - Alcoholics	- Persistent hoarseness - Dysphonia - Dysphagia

TABLE 10.6.2 - Types of Head and Neck Cancer

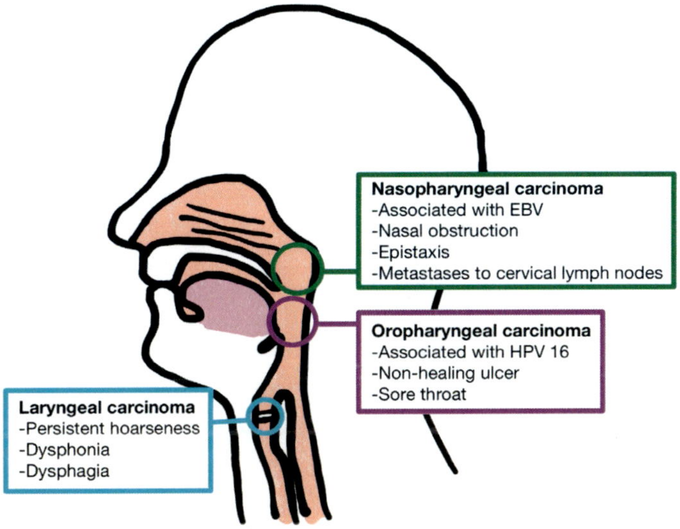

FIGURE 10.6.6 - Anatomical Locations of Head and Neck Cancers

I. Field Cancerization
   A. Chronically affected mucosal area is prone to multiple primary tumors and/or local recurrence
   B. Due to prolonged exposure of the area to carcinogens
   C. Cancers may not share same genetic alteration
   D. May occur in other regions but predilection for head and neck

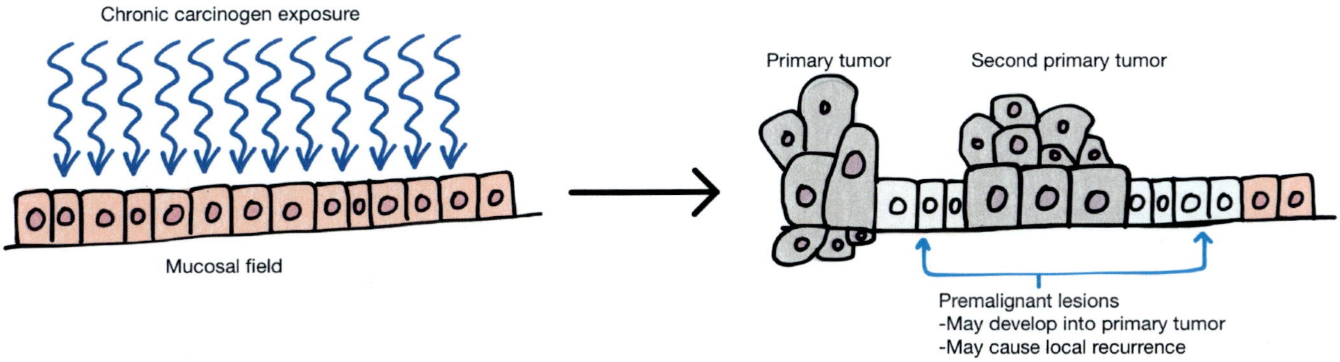

FIGURE 10.6.7 - Field Cancerization

II. Major Risk Factors for HNSCC
  A. Smoking
  B. Alcohol
  C. EBV (especially nasopharyngeal cancer)
  D. HPV-16 (especially oropharyngeal cancer)

III. Diagnosis of HNSCC
  A. Biopsy: keratin-positive syncytium-like clusters of epithelial cells ("keratin pearls")
  B. Keratin pearls are frequently seen in all types of squamous cell carcinomas

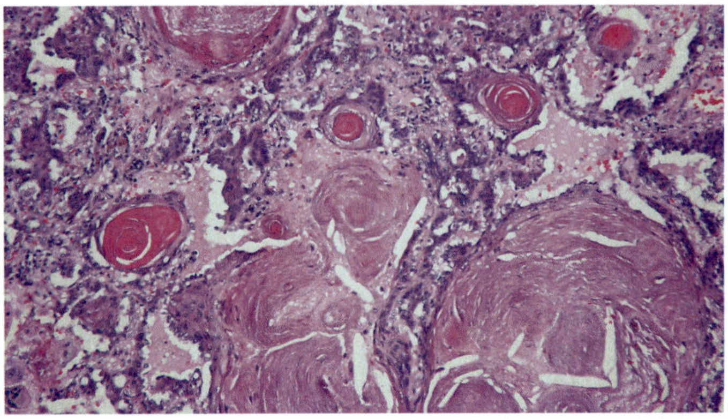

FIGURE 10.6.8 - Keratin Pearls in Squamous Cell Carcinoma

IV. Treatment
  A. Radiation therapy

REVIEW QUESTIONS ?

1. A 40-year-old Chinese male presents to his physician with complaints of fever and a sore throat. Physical examination shows cervical and axillary lymphadenopathy and splenomegaly. A complete blood count shows elevated white blood cells. Horse erythrocytes agglutinate when exposed to the patient's serum. The pathogen most likely responsible for the patient's condition is also associated with which of the following disorders?

   A. Anal carcinoma
   B. Glomerulonephritis
   C. Oropharyngeal carcinoma
   D. Nasopharyngeal carcinoma

- **The correct answer is D.**
- This question describes a Chinese male who presents with fever, sore throat, lymphadenopathy, and splenomegaly. Also, labs show elevated white blood cells and the agglutination of horse erythrocytes tells us that the monospot test is positive.
- This points towards infectious mononucleosis or EBV infection, which is frequently associated with nasopharyngeal carcinoma.
- As answer choices A-C don't have a known association with EBV infection, they are incorrect.

Section IV - Deep Vein Thrombosis (DVT)

I. Basic Principles
   A. Blood clot that forms in the deep veins
   B. Most common place: lower extremities
   C. Can embolize to the lungs, which may be life-threatening

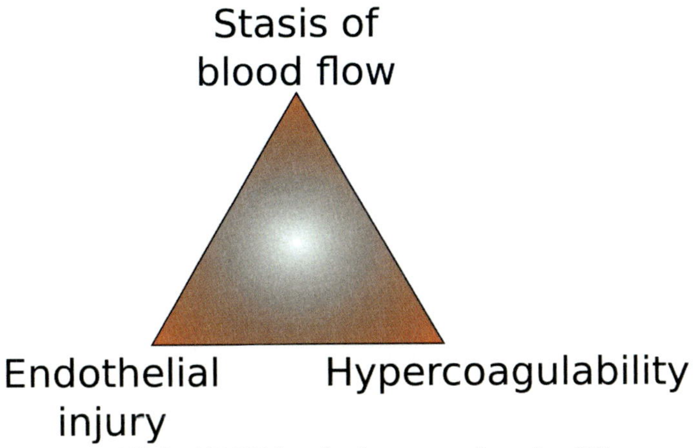

FIGURE 10.6.9 - Virchow's Triad

II. Virchow's Triad: Stasis
   A. Surgery
   B. Bed-bound patients
   C. Long hospitalization
   D. Long plane or car rides

III. Virchow's Triad: Endothelial Injury
   A. Damage to blood vessel
   B. Exposure of collagen and other chemicals
   C. Platelet activation and aggregation

IV. Virchow's Triad: Hypercoagulability
   A. Inherited: factor V Leiden, protein C or S deficiency, antithrombin III deficiency
   B. Not inherited: oral contraceptives, pregnancy, obesity, smoking
   C. Disease states: cancer, nephrotic syndrome

V. Physical Exam Findings
   A. Asymmetrical swelling of the leg
   B. Erythema
   C. Warmth
   D. Pain with dorsiflexion of the foot (Homan's sign)
   E. Asymmetric calf diameter

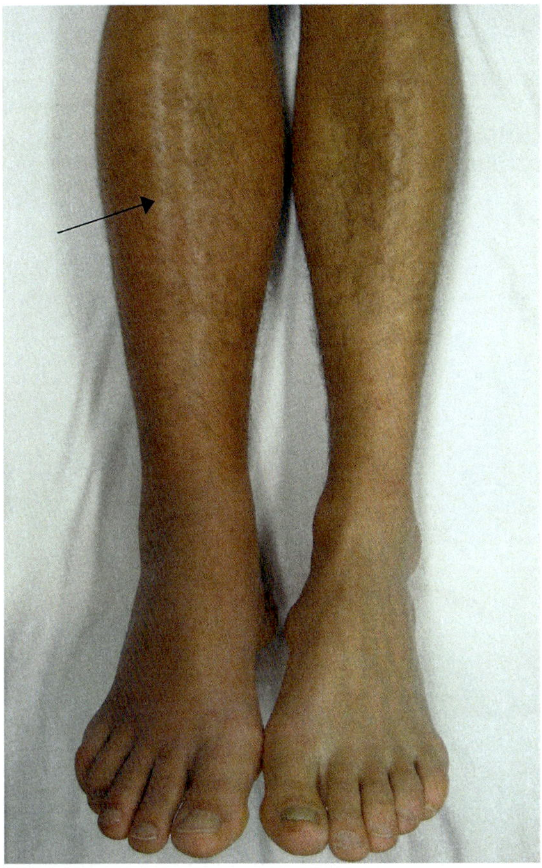

FIGURE 10.6.10 - DVT (Black Arrow) of Right Leg

VI. Diagnosis
   A. D-dimer
   B. Ultrasound with compression and doppler

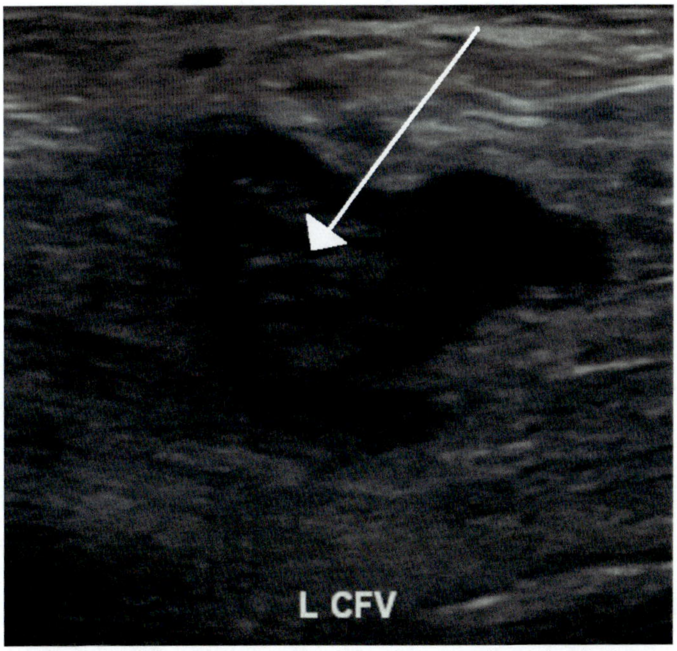

FIGURE 10.6.11 - Ultrasound of Blood Clot in Left Common Femoral Vein (White Arrow)

VII. Prophylaxis
   A. Sequential compression devices
   B. Ambulation
   C. Low molecular weight heparin (e.g. enoxaparin)
   D. Unfractionated heparin

VIII. Treatment
   A. Short term: unfractionated heparin or low molecular weight heparin
   B. Long term: oral anticoagulants, warfarin

REVIEW QUESTIONS ?

1. A 73-year-old male smoker presents to the emergency room because of pain in his left leg for the past 2 days. On exam, the left calf is edematous, erythematous, and warm to the touch. A CBC shows an elevated white blood cell count, hemoglobin of 14 g/dL (normal: 13.5-17.5 g/dL), and platelet count of 249,000/mm^3 (normal: 150,000 - 400,000/mm^3). An ultrasound with Doppler demonstrates a non-compressible left popliteal vein consistent with a clot. He reveals he had a total knee replacement 4 days ago and wasn't able to fill any of his postoperative prescriptions. Missing which of the following medications predisposed him to this pathology?

   A. Tylenol
   B. Oxycodone
   C. Enoxaparin
   D. Rifampin
   E. Cephalexin

- **The correct answer is C.**
- This is a 73-year-old male smoker who has acute onset left leg pain. Physical exam shows a swollen, red, warm left leg and a normal right leg. Ultrasound shows a noncompressible vein consistent with a clot. He recently had orthopedic surgery and wasn't taking any of his postoperative medicines. Enoxaparin is often given after surgery to prevent clots.
- A is incorrect because Tylenol is for pain, not to prevent blood clots.
- B is incorrect because oxycodone is a strong opioid pain medication and does not prevent blood clots.
- D and E are incorrect as both of these drugs are antibiotics and do not prevent blood clots.

Section V - Pulmonary Embolism

I. Basic Principles
   A. Blockage in one or more arteries of the lungs
   B. Multiple causes
   C. Travel from distant site to the lungs

II. Pathophysiology
   A. Area is ventilated, but not perfused
   B. Leads to V/Q mismatch
   C. V/Q approaches ∞
   D. Hypoxemia → tachypnea → low CO_2
      1. Causes respiratory alkalosis
      2. Hypoxemia will improve with 100% O_2

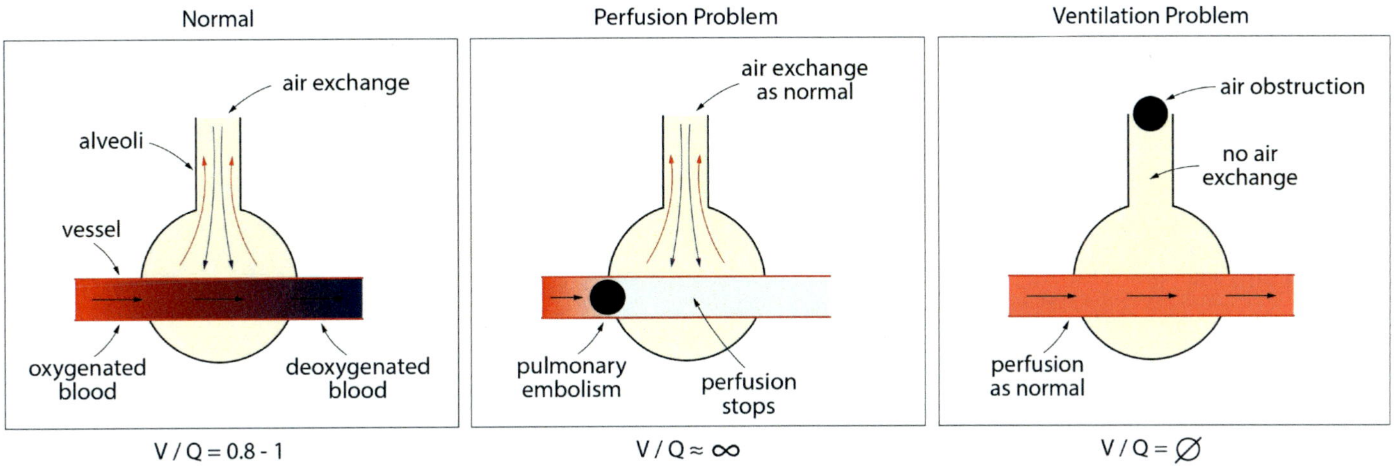

FIGURE 10.6.12 - Normal Ventilation (Left), Perfusion Problem (Middle), and Ventilation Problem (Right)

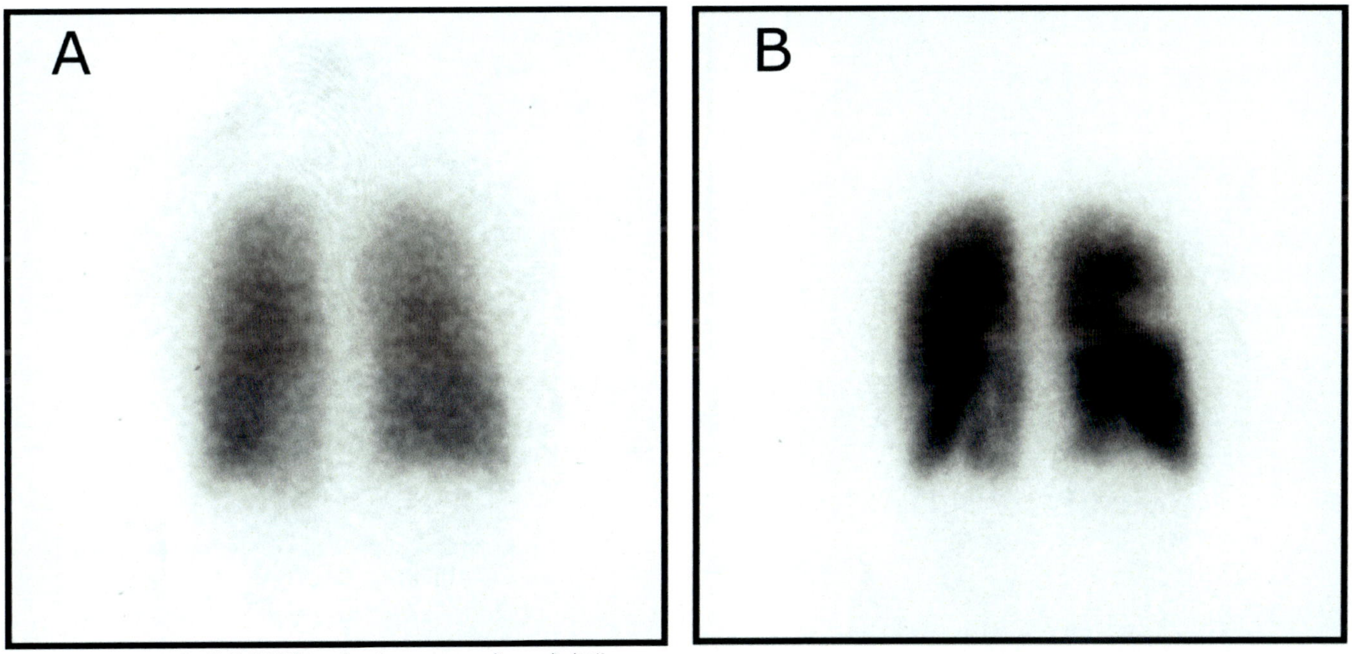

FIGURE 10.6.13 - V/Q Scan of Patient with PE Before (Left) and After (Right) IV Injection of a Radiolabeled Molecule

III. Types
   A. Bacterial
   B. Air
   C. Fat
   D. Amniotic fluid
   E. Blood clot (thrombus)

IV. Bacterial Embolism
   A. Also called septic pulmonary embolism
   B. Infectious nidus
   C. Some bacterial debris separates from nidus and travels to lungs
   D. Associated with bacterial endocarditis

V. Air Embolism
   A. Divers: decompression sickness
      1. Nitrogen precipitates in organs during descent and creates bubbles in bloodstream during rapid ascent
      2. Treat with hyperbaric oxygen
   B. Iatrogenic: central lines

VI. Fat Embolism
   A. Long bone fractures
   B. Liposuction
   C. Classic triad: hypoxemia, petechial rash, and neurologic changes

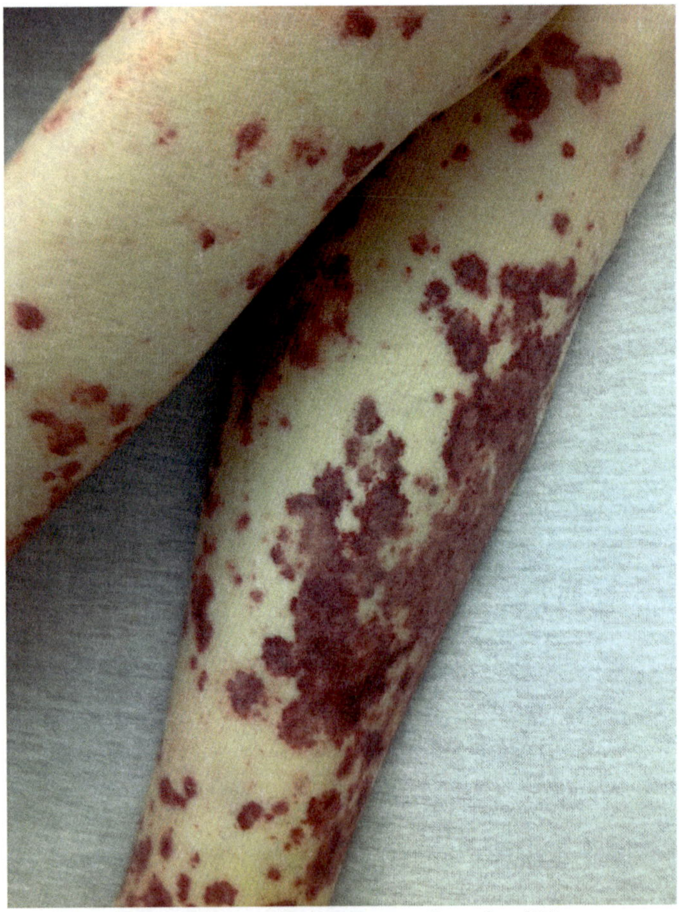

FIGURE 10.6.14 - Petechial Rash

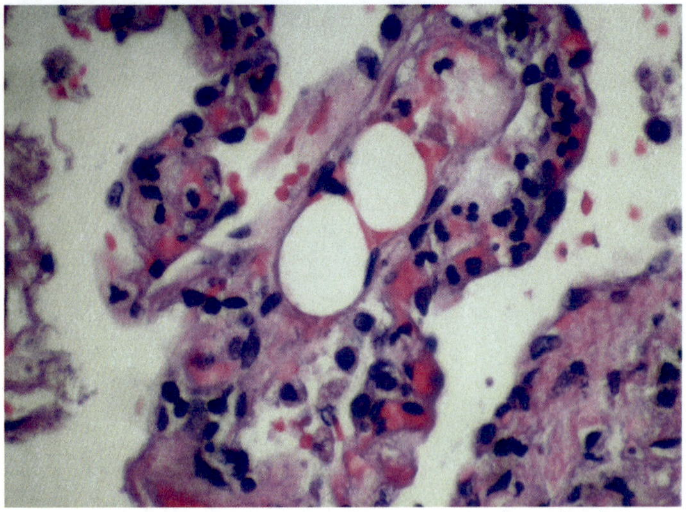

FIGURE 10.6.15 - Fat Embolism

VII. Amniotic Fluid Embolism
   A. Most common during or after labor
   B. Amniotic fluid enters mother's bloodstream
   C. Very high mortality
   D. Can cause disseminated intravascular coagulation (DIC)

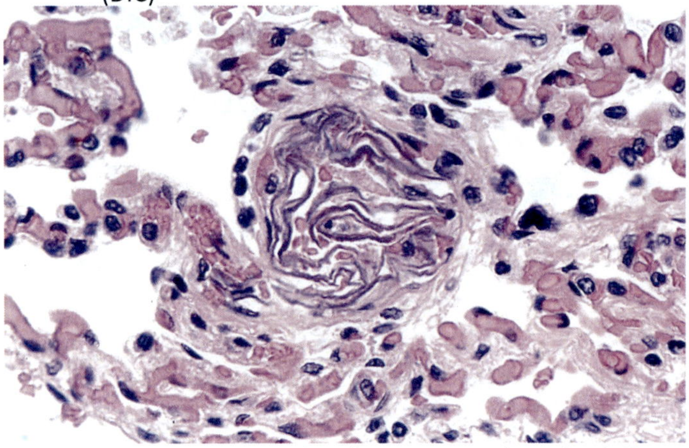

FIGURE 10.6.17 - Amniotic Fluid Embolism

VIII. Thrombus
   A. Most common cause of PE
   B. Arises from DVT in the lower extremities
   C. Travels from deep vein → inferior vena cava → right heart → lungs

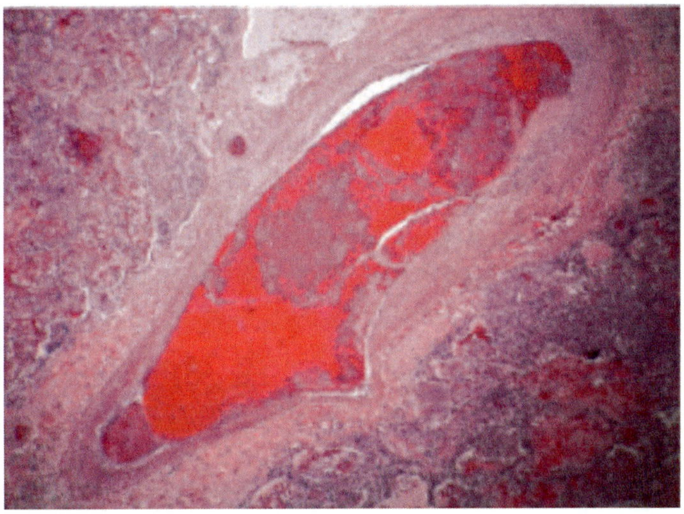

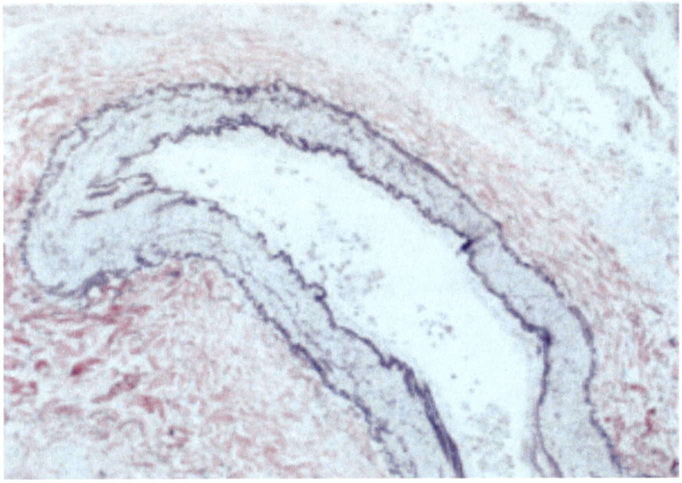

FIGURE 10.6.17 - Thrombus in Pulmonary Artery (Top) and Normal Pulmonary Artery (Bottom)

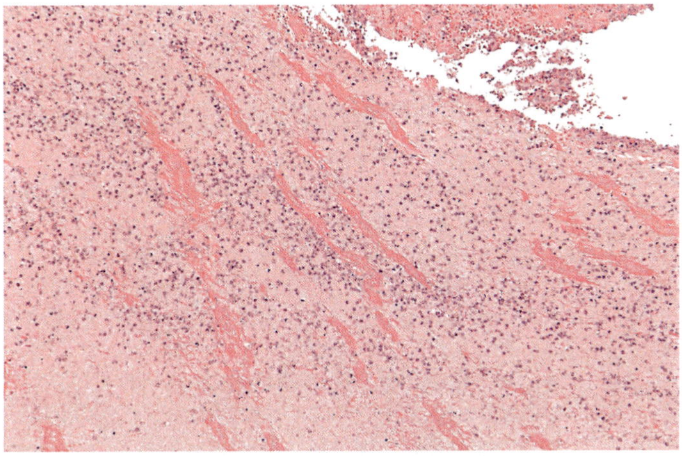

FIGURE 10.6.18 - Microscopic Image of Blood Clot

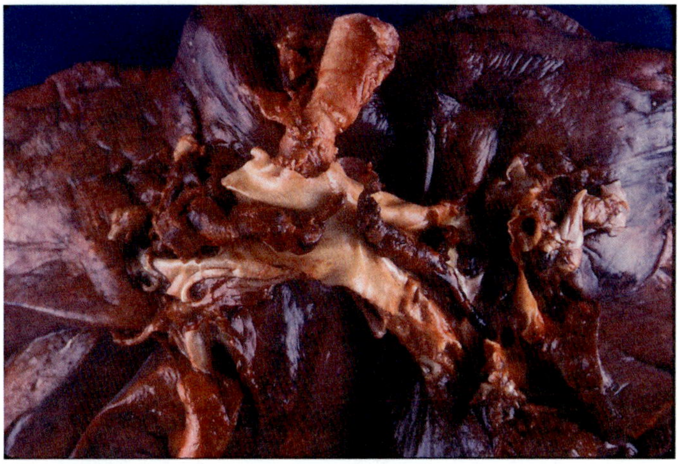

FIGURE 10.6.19 - Saddle Pulmonary Embolus

IX. Symptoms
   A. Pleuritic chest pain
   B. Dyspnea
   C. Cough
   D. Hemodynamic instability
   E. DVT symptoms
      1. Asymmetric legs, warmth, swelling, pain with dorsiflexion of the foot

X. EKG Findings
   A. S1Q3T3
   B. Pulseless electrical activity (PEA)

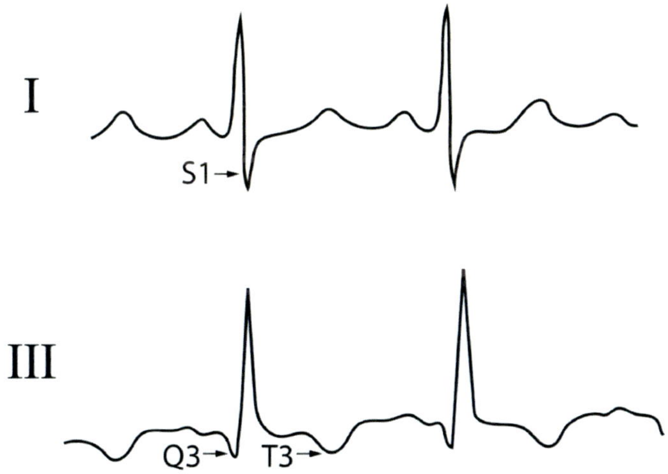

FIGURE 10.6.20 - S1Q3T3 Finding on EKG

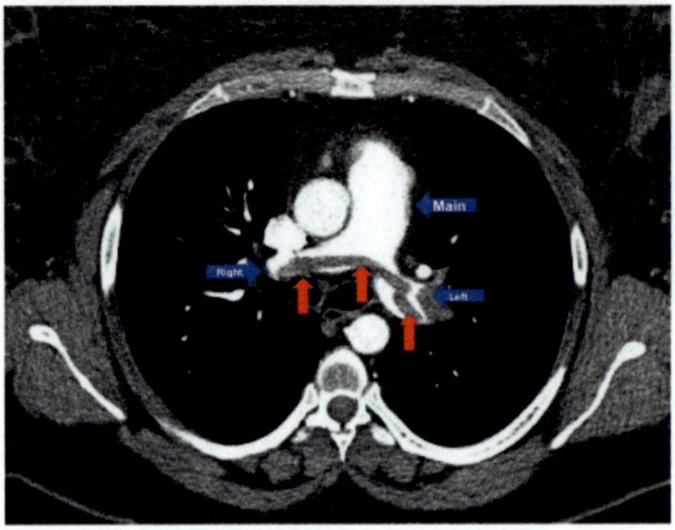

FIGURE 10.6.21 - CT Angiography of Saddle Pulmonary Embolus

XI. Prophylaxis
   A. Low molecular weight heparin (enoxaparin)
   B. Unfractionated heparin
   C. Sequential compression devices
   D. Ambulation

REVIEW QUESTIONS

1. A 75-year-old woman undergoes a left total hip replacement. She is discharged home on postoperative day 2. Her hospital course was uncomplicated. Three days later, a family member finds her unresponsive in bed. She is unable to be revived. During autopsy, a blood clot is found in the main pulmonary artery that extends into the left and right pulmonary arteries. Microscopy reveals the image below.

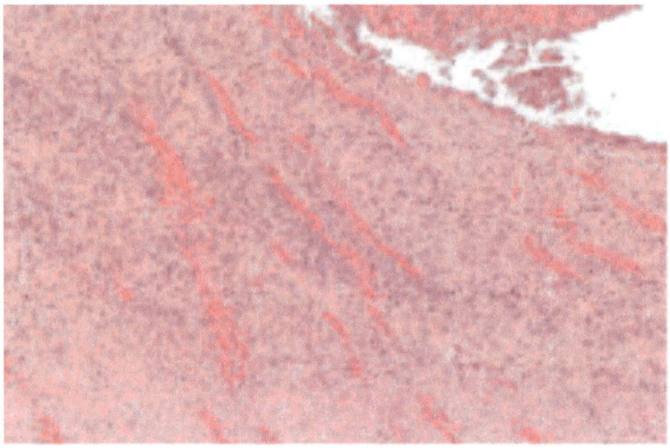

Which of the following should have been initiated for prophylaxis after surgery?

A. Aspirin
B. Atorvastatin
C. Warfarin
D. Enoxaparin
E. Acetaminophen

- **The correct answer is D.**
- The blood clot from her autopsy shows lines of Zahn, which are made of platelets, fibrin, and RBCs. They are seen only in blood clots that are formed when the patient is alive. The blood clot is in the main pulmonary artery and extends into the left and right pulmonary arteries. Thus, the diagnosis is a saddle pulmonary embolism. The medication that would have been appropriate for DVT and PE prophylaxis is a low molecular weight heparin, such as enoxaparin.
- A is incorrect because although aspirin is an antiplatelet agent, it alone would not be sufficient to prevent a DVT or PE.
- B is incorrect because statins are used to manage high cholesterol.
- C is incorrect because starting Warfarin immediately without a bridge would make the patient more likely to have a DVT or PE.
- E is incorrect because acetaminophen is not an anticoagulant. It is an analgesic and antipyretic.

Section VI - Mediastinal Pathology

I. Anatomy
   A. Heart, thymus, lymph nodes, esophagus, and aorta
   B. Superior mediastinum (above the T4 vertebra)
   C. Inferior mediastinum (below the T4 vertebra)
      1. Anterior mediastinum
      2. Middle mediastinum
      3. Posterior mediastinum

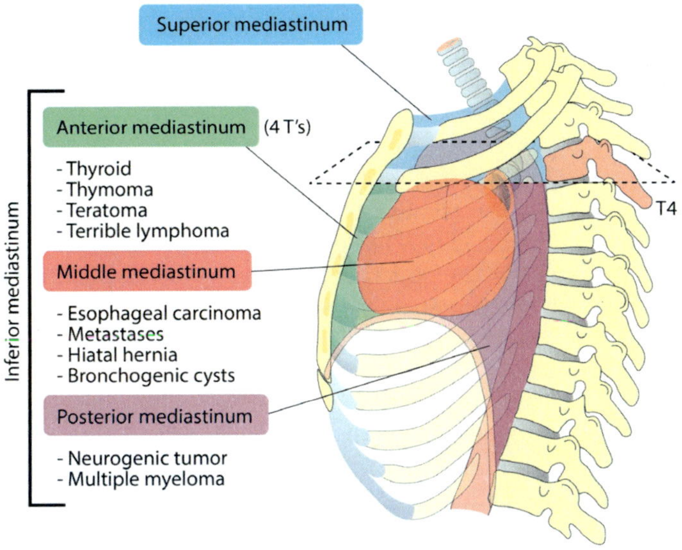

FIGURE 10.6.22 -Anatomy of Mediastinum

II. Mediastinitis
   A. Inflammation of mediastinal tissues
   B. Common causes
      1. Post-operative complications of cardiothoracic procedures (≤ 2 weeks)
      2. Esophageal perforation
      3. Contiguous spread of odontogenic/ retropharyngeal infection

III. Chronic Mediastinitis
   A. "Fibrosing mediastinitis"
   B. Increased proliferation of connective tissue in mediastinum
   C. *Histoplasma capsulatum* is the most common cause
   D. Idiopathic fibrosing mediastinitis is less common
      1. Associated with autoimmune diseases (especially granulomatosis with polyangiitis)
      2. Radiation therapy

IV. Clinical Features
   A. Fever
   B. Increased WBCs
   C. Pain in chest
   D. Tachycardia
   E. Sternal wound drainage

V. Pneumomediastinum
   A. Air within the mediastinum
   B. Causes
      1. Spontaneous: rupture of a central pulmonary bleb
      2. Secondary causes: trauma, iatrogenic, and Boerhaave syndrome

VI. Clinical Features
   A. Dyspnea
   B. Chest pain
   C. Positive Hamman sign (crunch sound that is heard during systole)
   D. Subcutaneous emphysema
   E. Cough
   F. Hoarseness

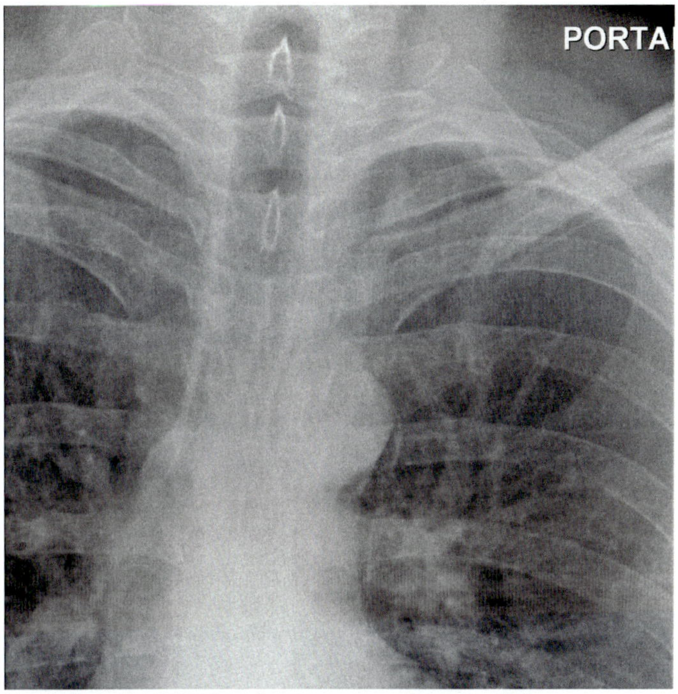

FIGURE 10.6.23 - X-ray of Mediastinum

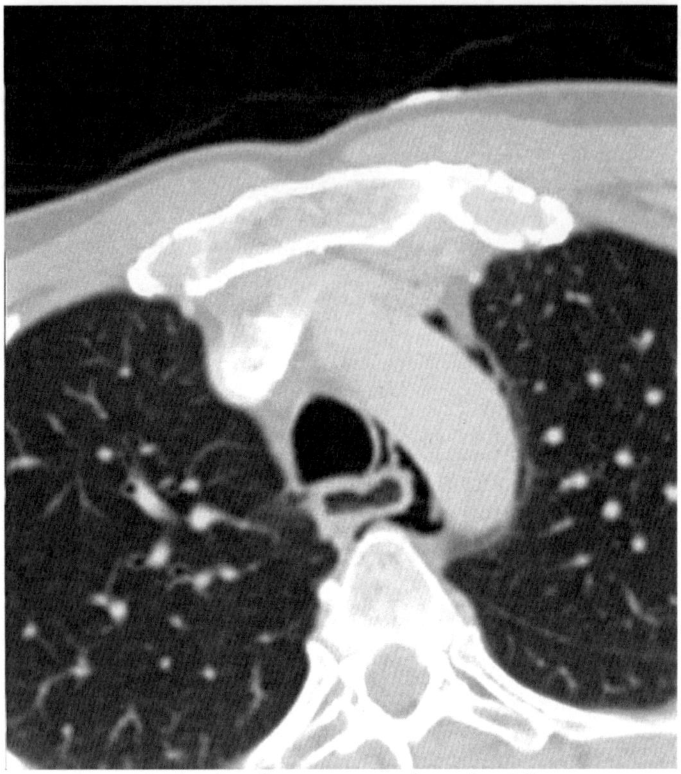

FIGURE 10.6.24 - CT Scan of Thorax

REVIEW QUESTIONS ?

1. A 24-year-old male presents with nausea, vomiting, and chest pain. On physical examination, a "rice-crispy-like" crackling under the skin around his neck is appreciated with palpation. The patient has a past medical history significant for alcohol abuse disorder and takes no medications. A chest X-ray reveals the presence of air in the mediastinum. What is the most likely diagnosis?

   A. Mallory-Weiss syndrome
   B. Myocardial infarction
   C. Boerhaave syndrome
   D. Gastroesophageal reflux disease

- **The correct answer is C.**
- The rice-crispy-like description of air under the skin of the neck raises suspicion that the patient has subcutaneous emphysema. This coupled with chest pain, chronic vomiting, and the imaging findings of air in the mediastinum make pneumomediastinum likely. These presentations along with pneumomediastinum make Boerhaave syndrome the most likely diagnosis.
- Choice A is incorrect because Mallory-Weiss syndrome does not involve transmural rupture of the esophagus. Only the mucosa is damaged, so there is no leakage of air into the mediastinum.
- Choices B and D are associated with chest pain, but since neither of them involves pneumomediastinum, both are incorrect.

Section VII - Obstructive Lung Disease

I. Basic Principles
   A. Group of lung diseases characterized by small airway inflammation and airway flow obstruction

II. Emphysema: Etiology
   A. Emphysema: tobacco smoke, pollution, alpha-1-antitrypsin deficiency

III. Emphysema: Pathophysiology
   A. Inflammatory response due to inhalational exposure to caustic substances
   B. Excess protease activity leads to lung tissue damage and mucus hypersecretion
   C. Loss of elastic lung recoil

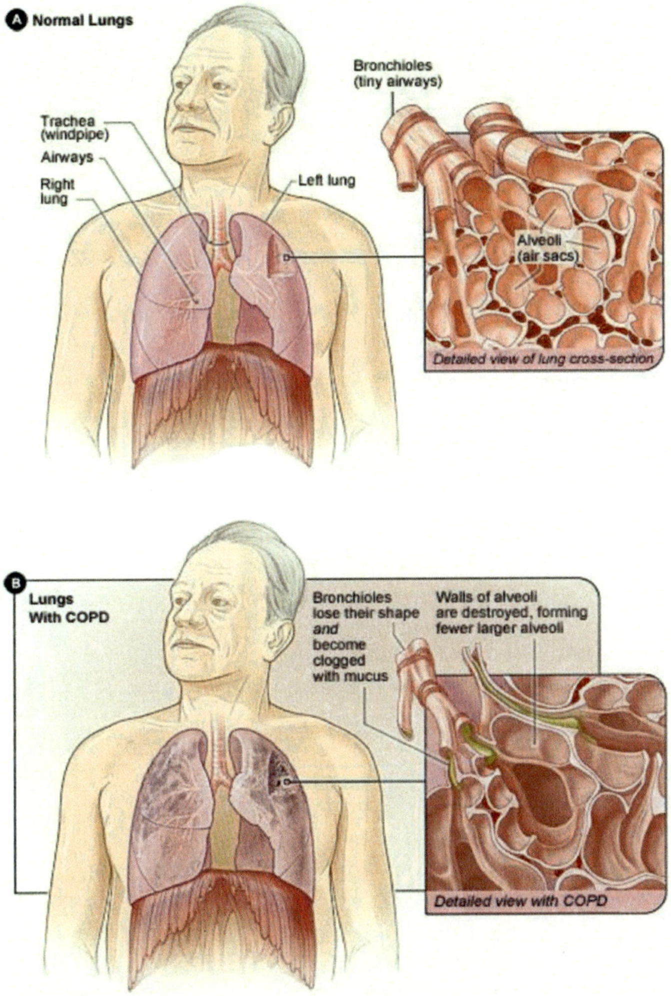

Photo Credit: National Heart Lung and Blood Institute [Public domain]

FIGURE 10.6.25 - Contrast between Normal Lungs and Emphysematous Lungs

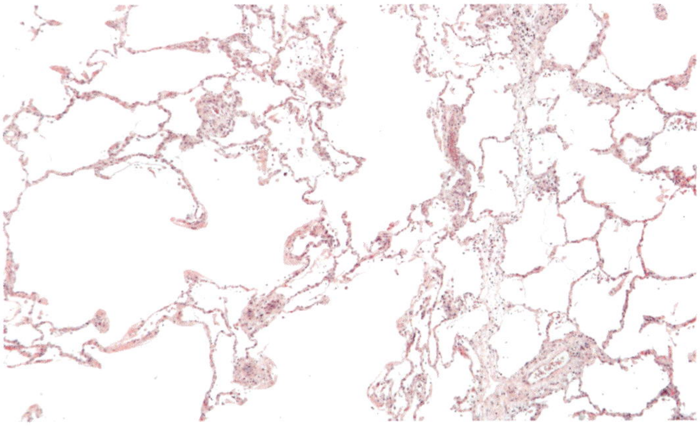

Photo Credit: Nephron [CC BY-SA (https://creativecommons.org/licenses/by-sa/3.0)]

FIGURE 10.6.26 - Alveolar Wall Destruction

   D. Protease activity is normally inhibited by anti-proteases such as alpha-1-antitrypsin (necessary for lung tissue homeostasis)
   E. Patients with an alpha-1-antitrypsin deficiency will have excess protease activity, which leads to chronic obstructive pulmonary disease

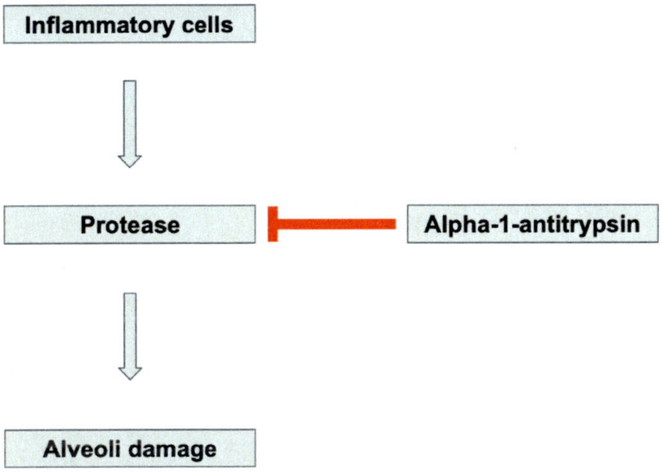

FIGURE 10.6.27 - Pathogenesis of Emphysema

   F. Centrilobular emphysema is seen in smokers and affects the upper lobes
   G. Panlobular emphysema is seen in alpha-1-antitrypsin deficiency and affects the lower lobes

IV. Emphysema: Clinical Features
   A. Symptoms: dyspnea, chronic productive cough, wheezing
   B. Physical exam: decreased lung sounds, pursed lip breathing, barrel chest, decreased tactile fremitus
   C. Diagnosis: clinical presentation and pulmonary function testing

V. Emphysema: Chest X-ray
   A. Increased anterior-posterior chest diameter
   B. Flattened diaphragms
   C. Hyperinflated lungs
   D. Elongated heart
   E. Reduced lung markings

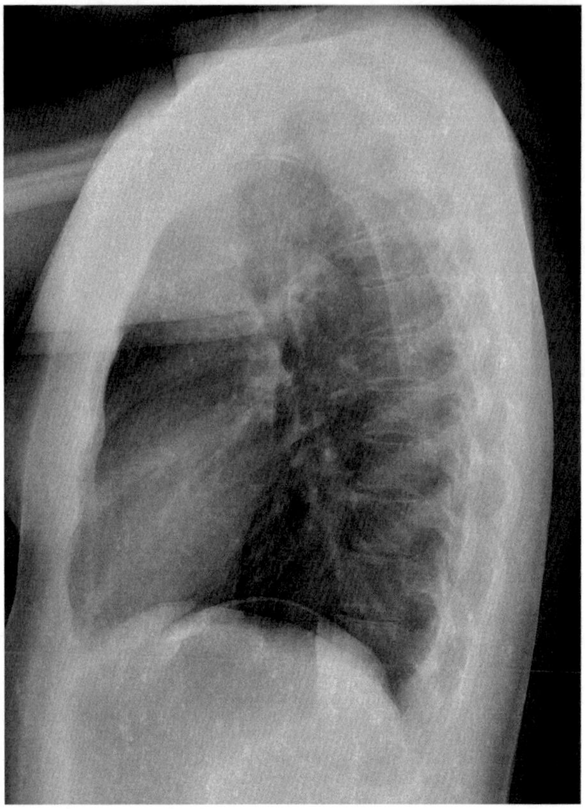

Photo Credit: Mikael Häggström [CC0]

FIGURE 10.6.28 - Normal Lateral Chest X-Ray

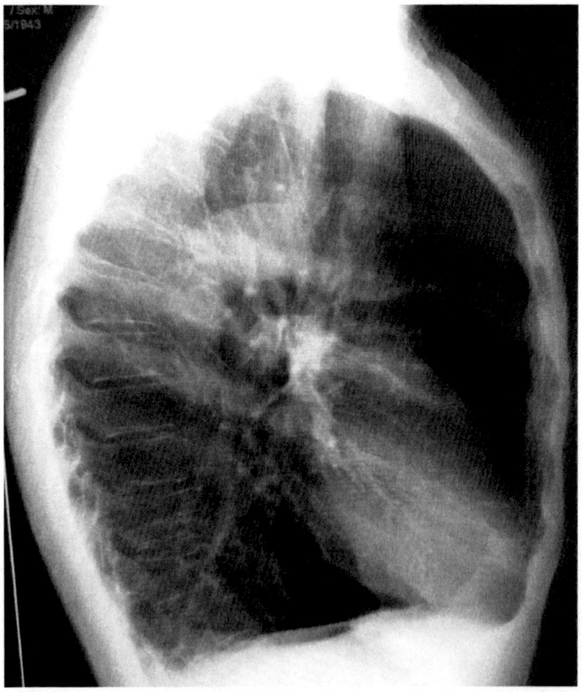

Photo Credit: James Heilman, MD [CC BY-SA (https://creativecommons.org/licenses/by-sa/3.0)]

FIGURE 10.6.29 - Lateral Chest X-Ray of Emphysema

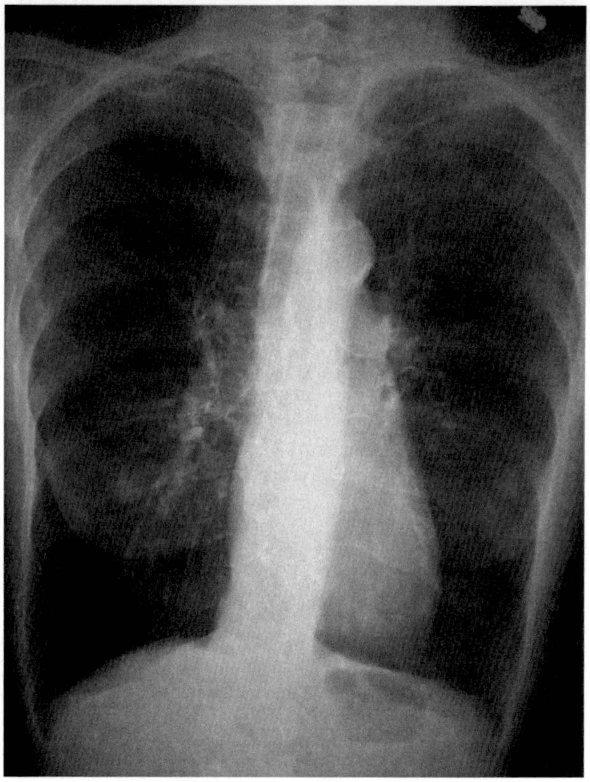

Photo Credit: James Heilman, MD [CC BY-SA (https://creativecommons.org/licenses/by-sa/3.0)]

FIGURE 10.6.30 - Posteroanterior Chest X-Ray of Emphysema

VI. Chronic Bronchitis: Etiology
   A. Most common cause: tobacco smoke

VII. Chronic Bronchitis: Pathophysiology
   A. Inflammatory response due to inhalational exposure to tobacco smoke
   B. Excess protease activity leads to hypertrophy of bronchial mucosal glands and mucus hypersecretion

VIII. Chronic Bronchitis: Histopathology
   A. Reid index used in assessment of chronic bronchitis
   B. Reid index > 0.5 is seen in patients with chronic bronchitis

IX. Chronic Bronchitis: Clinical Features
   A. Symptoms: dyspnea and chronic productive cough
   B. Physical exam findings: wheezing, inspiratory crackles, and cyanosis
   C. Diagnosis: productive cough for ≥ 3 months in a year for 2 consecutive years

X. Bronchiectasis: Etiology
   A. Chronic lung infection, Kartagener syndrome, cystic fibrosis

XI. Bronchiectasis: Pathophysiology
   A. Necrotizing inflammation
   B. Permanent bronchi and bronchiole dilatation

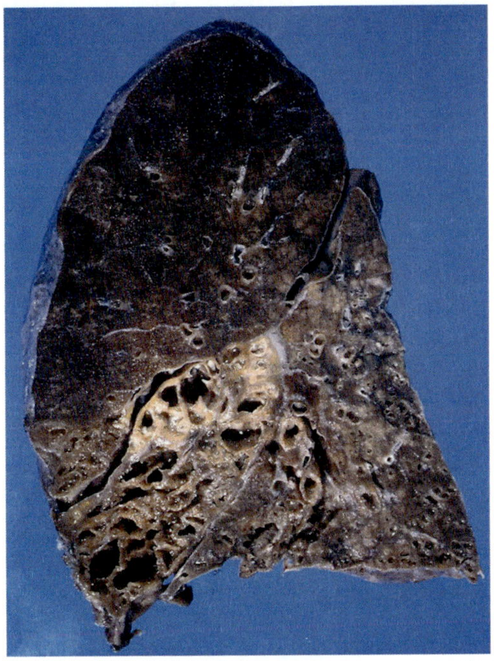

FIGURE 10.6.31 - Dilated Bronchioles in Bronchiectasis

XII. Bronchiectasis: Clinical Features
   A. Symptoms: dyspnea, hemoptysis, cough with foul-smelling sputum
   B. Physical exam findings: wheezing, digital clubbing, cyanosis
   C. Diagnosis: clinical presentation and pulmonary function testing

XIII. Asthma: Etiology
   A. Allergen-mediated, drug sensitivity, virus-induced

XIV. Asthma Pathophysiology
   A. Type 1 hypersensitivity reaction
   B. Bronchoconstriction and smooth muscle hypertrophy

XV. Asthma: Histopathology
   A. Charcot-Leyden crystals and Curschmann spirals

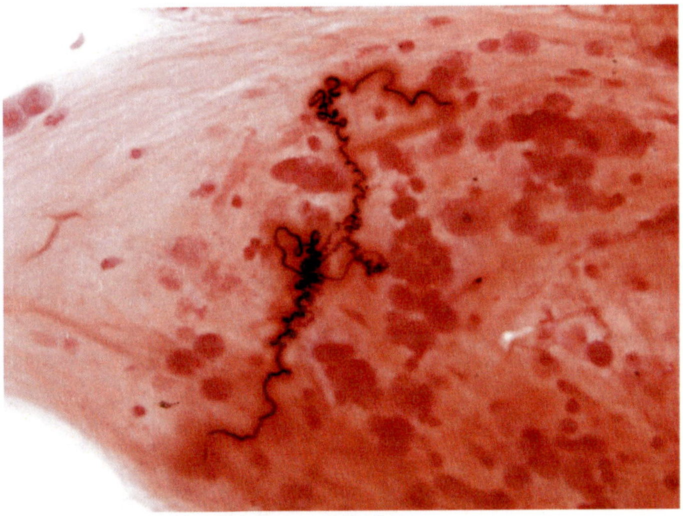

FIGURE 10.6.32 - Curschmann Spirals

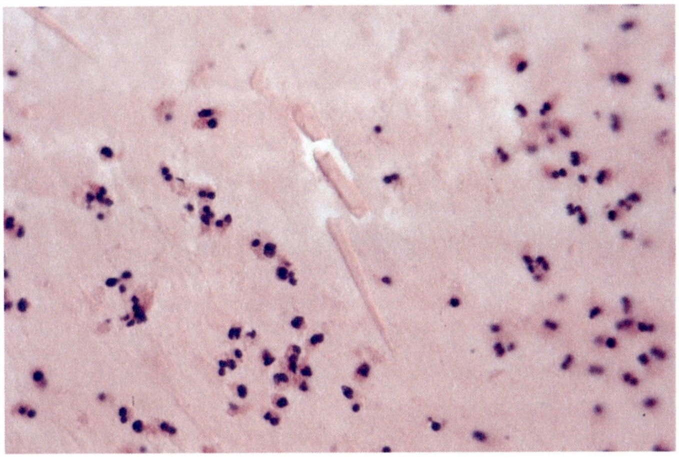

FIGURE 10.6.33 - Charcot-Leyden Crystals

XVI. Asthma: Clinical Features
   A. Symptoms: dyspnea and productive or nonproductive cough
   B. Physical exam findings: wheezing, hypoxemia, mucus plugs
   C. Diagnosis: pulmonary function testing and methacholine challenge test

XVII. Pulmonary Function Testing
   A. FEV1/FVC < 70%
   B. Increased residual volume, functional residual capacity, total lung capacity
   C. Decreased DLCO in emphysema
   D. Normal DLCO in chronic bronchitis, bronchiectasis and asthma

XVIII. Complications
   A. Cor pulmonale
   B. Respiratory infections

REVIEW QUESTIONS

1. A 62-year-old male with a past medical history of type 2 diabetes mellitus, hypertension, hyperlipidemia, and 35 pack-years of smoking presents to the physician with a chief complaint of a productive cough for the past 4 months. The patient's current temperature is 98.7 °F (37 °C), blood pressure is 134/88 mm Hg, heart rate is 72 beats/min, and the respiratory rate is 15 breaths/min. The patient states he has had mild exertional dyspnea but denies any hemoptysis, chest pain, fever, nausea, or diaphoresis. The patient has been experiencing this cough on and off for the past few years. Which of the following is associated with this patient's condition?

    A. Increased DLCO
    B. Reid index of 0.6
    C. Elevated serum ACE
    D. Decreased residual volume

- **The correct answer is B.**
- The important thing to recognize here is that this patient has 35 pack-years of smoking and meets the clinical criteria for chronic bronchitis, which is a form of COPD.
- Chronic bronchitis is a purely clinical diagnosis. Patients must have a productive cough for greater than or equal to 3 months in a year for 2 consecutive years.
- The Reid index is a histological measurement used in patients with chronic bronchitis. It is the ratio of thickness between mucus-secreting glands and epithelium and cartilage that covers the bronchi. Patients with chronic bronchitis will have a Reid index greater than 0.5.
- A is incorrect because the DLCO is either normal or decreased in COPD. DLCO is normal in chronic bronchitis and alpha-1-antitrypsin deficiency. Patients who have emphysema will have a decreased DLCO.
- C is incorrect because serum ACE levels are not affected in COPD. ACE levels may be increased in certain lung pathologies, such as sarcoidosis.
- D is incorrect because residual volume increases in patients with chronic bronchitis. Residual volume decreases in restrictive lung disease, like as pulmonary fibrosis.

Section VIII - Restrictive Lung Diseases

I. Restrictive Lung Diseases
   A. Group of diseases that restrict lung expansion, causing decreased lung volumes

II. Types
   A. Extrinsic (extrapulmonary)
   B. Intrinsic (intrapulmonary)

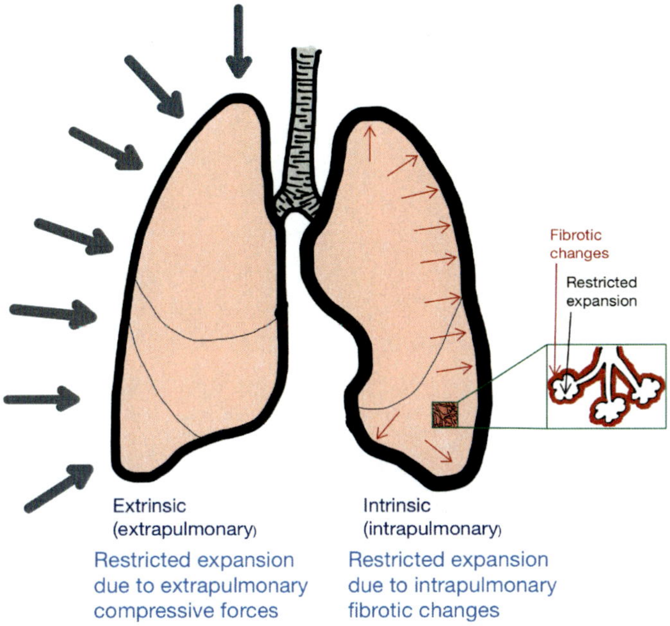

FIGURE 10.6.34 - Extrinsic (Right Lung) vs. Intrinsic (Left Lung) Restrictive Lung Diseases

III. Extrinsic: Etiology
   A. Poor breathing mechanics
      1. Structural (e.g. chest wall deformities such as scoliosis and morbid obesity)
      2. Neuromuscular (e.g. polio, myasthenia gravis, Guillain-Barre syndrome)

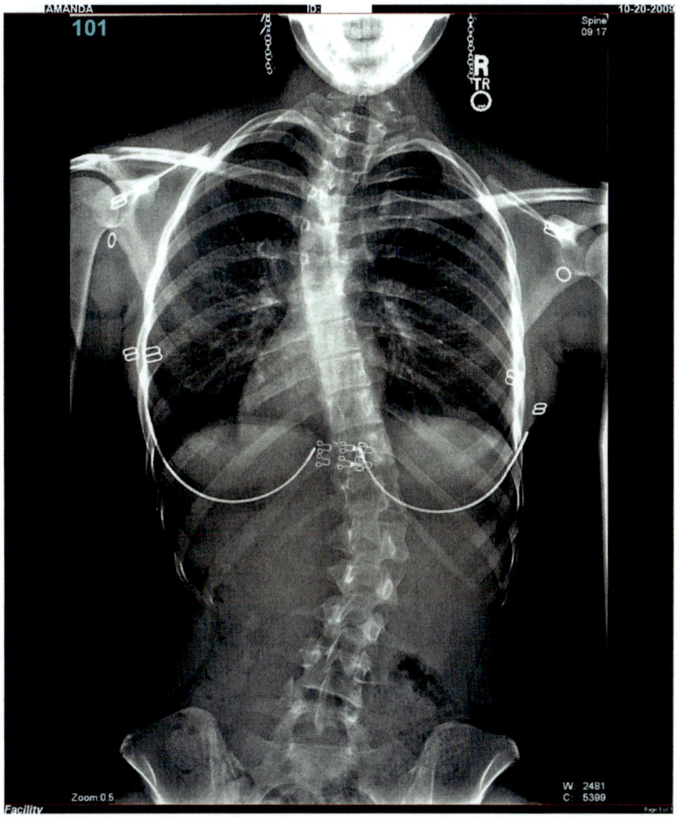

Photo Credit: University of Utah Hospital - Radiology Department [Public domain]

FIGURE 10.6.35 - X-Ray of Patient with Scoliosis

IV. Extrinsic: Pathophysiology
   A. Mechanical compression of the lung
   B. Normal DLCO
   C. Normal A-a gradient

V. Intrinsic: Etiology
   A. Interstitial lung diseases
      1. Pneumoconiosis (e.g. coal workers' pneumoconiosis, silicosis, asbestosis)
      2. Sarcoidosis
      3. Idiopathic pulmonary fibrosis
      4. Granulomatosis with polyangiitis (formerly known as Wegener's granulomatosis)
      5. Drug toxicity (e.g. bleomycin, busulfan, methotrexate, amiodarone)
      6. Hypersensitivity pneumonitis

VI. Intrinsic: Pathophysiology
   A. Decreased compliance
   B. Alveolar macrophages
   C. Repetitive injury → inflammation → disordered healing → focal loss of type 1 pneumocytes → hyperplasia of type 2 pneumocytes in basement membrane → eventual fibrosis → honeycomb lung
   D. Decreased DCLO
   E. Increased A-a gradient

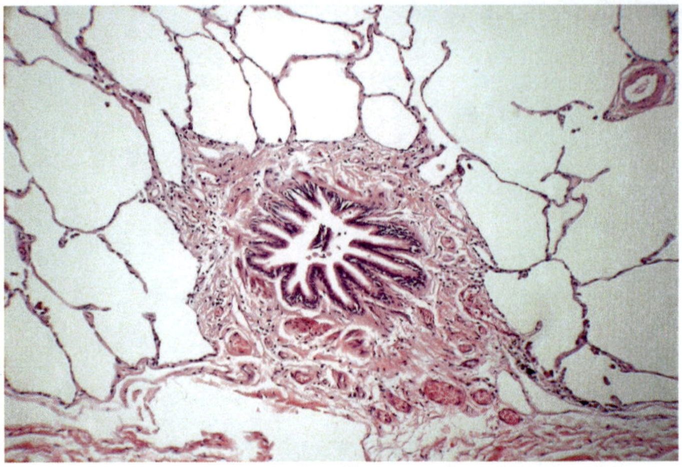

Photo Credit: Yale Rosen from USA [CC BY-SA (https://creativecommons.org/licenses/by-sa/2.0)]

FIGURE 10.6.36 - Histological slide of Normal Lung Parenchyma

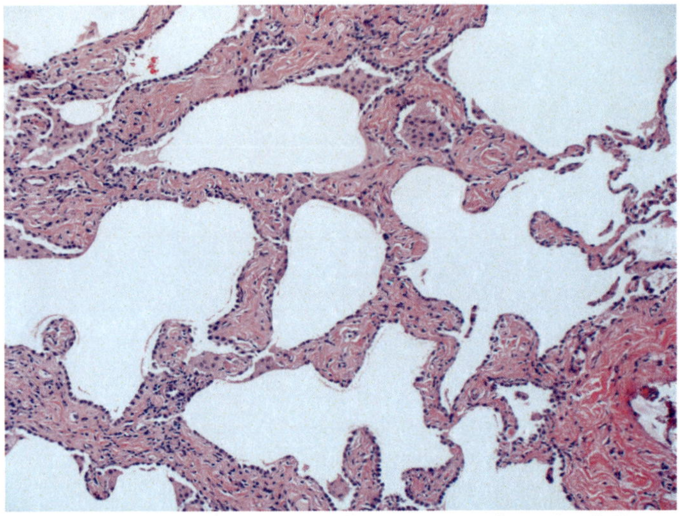

Photo Credit: Yale Rosen from USA [CC BY-SA (https://creativecommons.org/licenses/by-sa/2.0)]

FIGURE 10.6.37 - Histopathological Slide of Fibrotic Changes in Lung Tissue

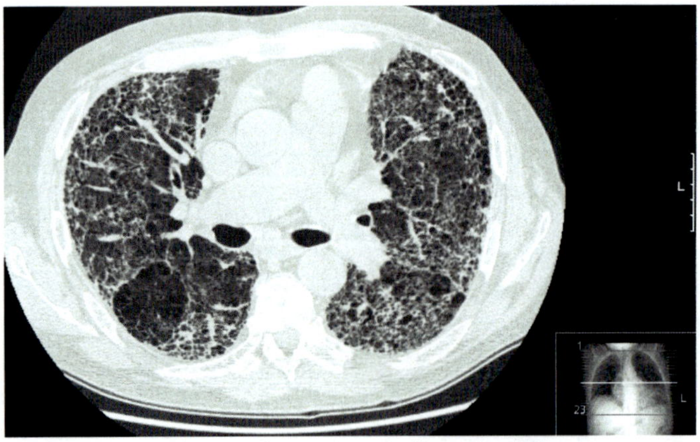

Photo Credit: Drriad [CC BY-SA (https://creativecommons.org/licenses/by-sa/3.0)]

FIGURE 10.6.38 - CT Scan of Advanced Interstitial Lung Disease and Fibrosis

VII. Hypersensitivity Pneumonitis
   A. Mixed type III/IV hypersensitivity reaction to environmental antigen
   B. Often seen in farmers and those exposed to birds or chemicals
   C. Causes dyspnea, cough, chest tightness, fever, headache
   D. Reversible in early stages if stimulus is avoided

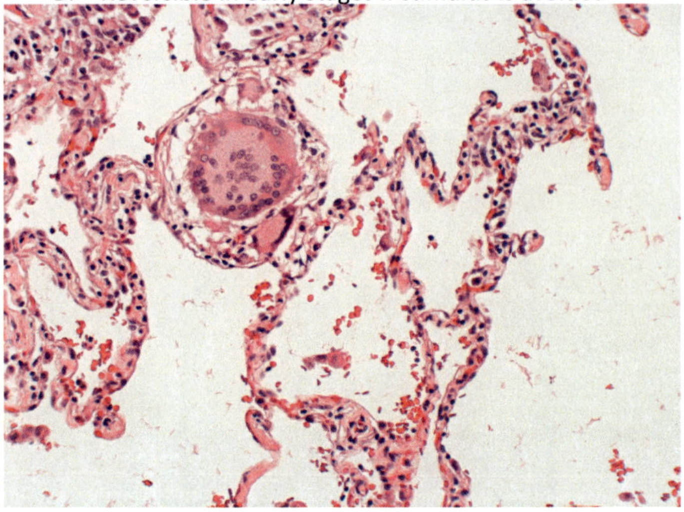

Photo Credit: By Yale Rosen from USA - Hypersensitivity pneumonitis Case 132, CC BY-SA 2.0, https://commons.wikimedia.org/w/index.php?curid=82806328

FIGURE 10.6.39 - Histological Slide of Lung with Hypersensitivity Pneumonitis

VIII. Pulmonary Function Test
   A. Decreased total lung capacity (TLC)
   B. Decreased FEV1 and FVC
   C. Normal or increased FEV1/FVC ratio
   D. Increased maximal expiratory rate due to radial traction
   E. Decreased FRC, RV, and VC

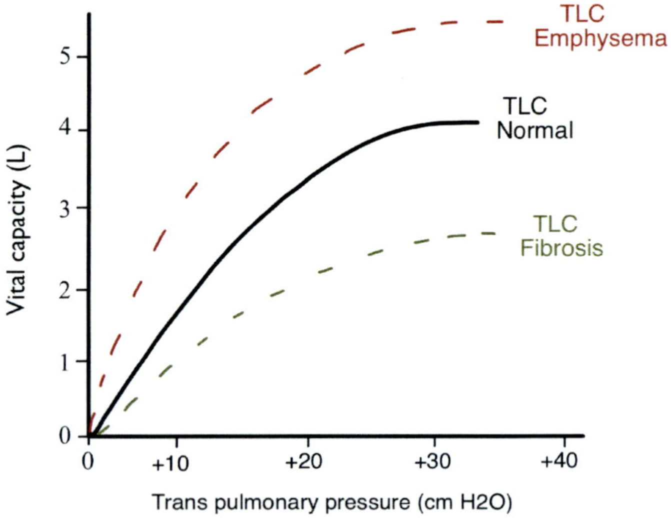

FIGURE 10.6.40 - Changes in Vital Capacity vs. Transpulmonary Pressure in Obstructive and Restrictive Lung Disease

IX. Diagnosis: Physical Findings
  A. Progressive dyspnea, short shallow breaths
  B. Inspiratory crackles
  C. Digital clubbing due to chronic hypoxia (hypertrophic osteoarthropathy)

X. Diagnosis: Imaging
  A. Chest X-ray
  B. CT/HRCT

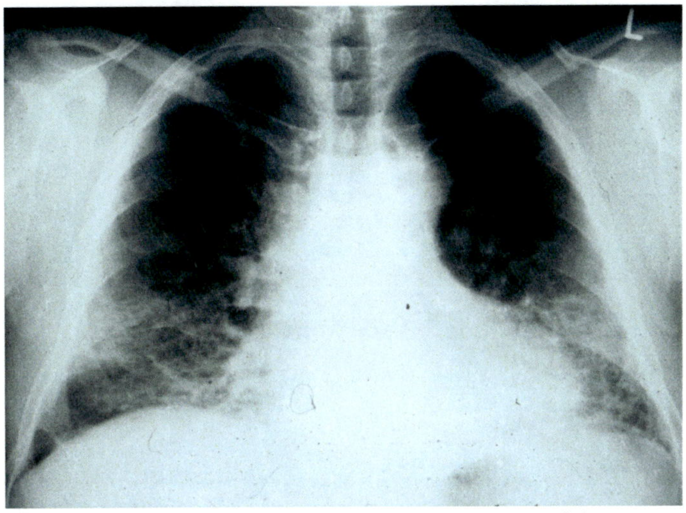

FIGURE 10.6.41 - X-Ray of Bilateral Diffuse Reticular Opacities

XI. Diagnosis: Microscopy
  A. Patchy interstitial fibrosis
  B. Fibroblastic foci
  C. Alveolar walls are thickened by collagenous fibrosis

XII. Treatment
  A. Underlying cause
  B. Extrinsic
    1. Weight loss for obesity
    2. Surgery/bracing for scoliosis
  C. Intrinsic
    1. Corticosteroids/immunosuppressive therapy
    2. Colchicine (antifibrotic)
    3. Lung transplantation (curative for end-stage disease)

REVIEW QUESTIONS

1. A 60-year-old man comes to the physician due to progressive dyspnea and cough. He says his symptoms have been getting worse. He is a lifelong smoker. On physical exam, inspiratory crackles are evident. He has rheumatoid arthritis and is compliant with his medications. His spirometry results indicate a decrease in total lung capacity and decreased residual volume. What additional findings would be expected in this patient?

    A. Decreased maximal expiratory rate
    B. Increased FEV1
    C. Increased functional residual capacity
    D. Increased FEV1/FVC ratio

- **The correct answer is D.**
- The patient has progressive dyspnea and cough. The inspiratory crackles and spirometry results, which indicate a decrease in total lung capacity and residual volume, point towards an interstitial lung disease that is causing a restrictive lung disease pattern. You would therefore expect to see an increased FEV1/FVC ratio.
- A is incorrect because restrictive lung diseases cause an increased maximal expiratory rate. In these diseases, the fibrotic lung collapses faster, allowing the air to be pushed out faster.
- B is incorrect because restrictive lung diseases cause a decreased FEV1. In these diseases, the stiffness of the lung limits the amount of air that can be inhaled, which also limits the amount of air that can be exhaled.
- C is incorrect because increased lung stiffness increases the tendency of the lung to collapse. This means that there is less air left in the lung after normal exhalation, which is the functional residual capacity.

Section IX - Sarcoidosis

I. Basic Principles
   A. Immune-mediated multisystem inflammatory disorder
   B. Most commonly involves the lungs
   C. Many other organs may be affected

II. Pathophysiology
   A. CD4+ T-cells responding to an antigen → macrophage activation → noncaseating granulomas at multiple different organ sites
   B. Noncaseating granulomas involve hilar and/or mediastinal lymph nodes → interstitial fibrosis → restrictive lung disease

III. Affected Organs
   A. Lungs: restrictive lung disease
   B. Heart: dilated & restrictive cardiomyopathy, myocarditis, heart block, and ventricular arrhythmias
   C. Kidney: acute interstitial nephritis
   D. Liver: hepatomegaly
   E. Eyes: uveitis
   F. Skin: erythema nodosum
   G. Glands: Sjogren-like syndrome
   H. Nervous system: Bell palsy

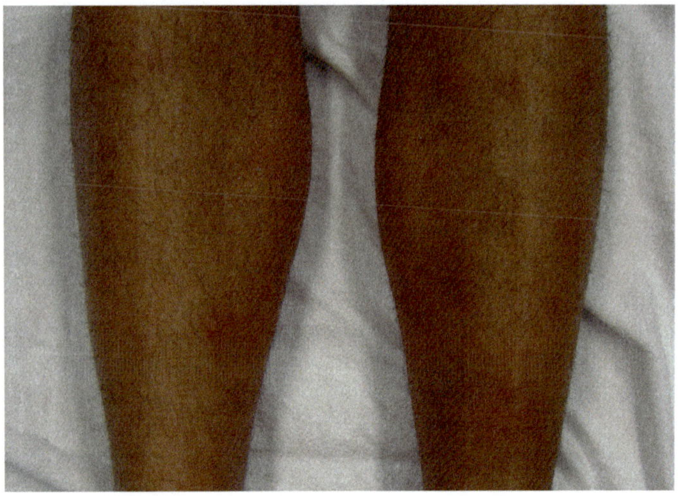

FIGURE 10.6.42 - Erythema Nodosum

IV. Histology
   A. Noncaseating granulomas of epithelioid cells
   B. Giant multinucleated cells
   C. Stellate "asteroid" inclusions inside giant cells

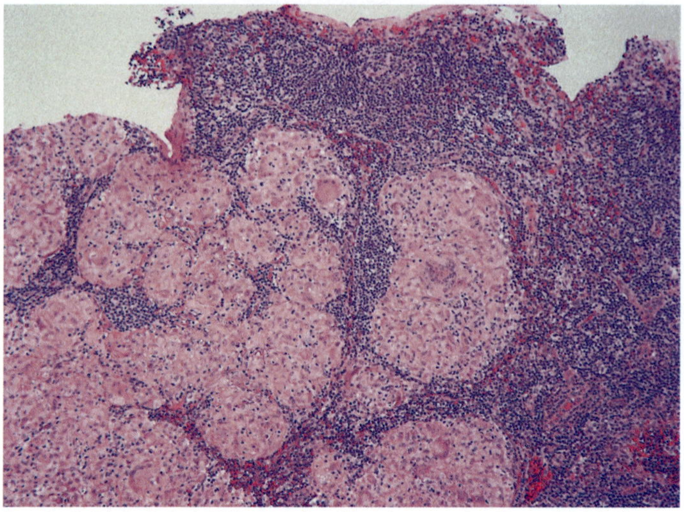

FIGURE 10.6.43 - Lymph Node with Non-Caseating Granulomas

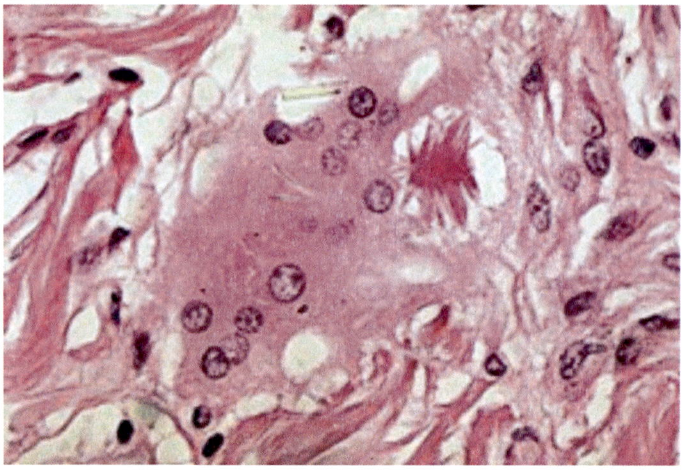

FIGURE 10.6.44 - Asteroid Body

V. Imaging
   A. Chest X-ray
      1. Bilateral hilar and mediastinal adenopathy
      2. Coarse opacities

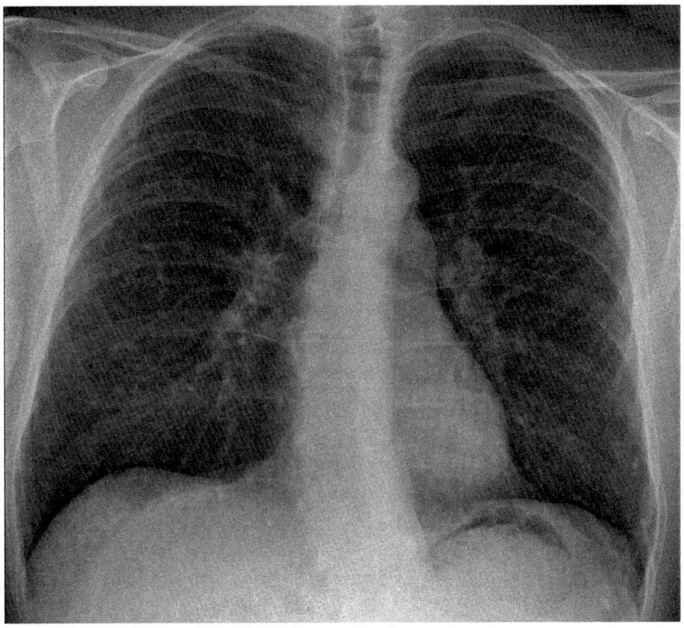

Photo Credit: Mikael Häggström [CC0]

FIGURE 10.6.45 - Bilateral Hilar Lymphadenopathy

VI. Clinical Presentation
   A. Classic presentation: African American female with shortness of breath and cough
   B. Hypercalcemia
   C. Elevated ACE
   D. Elevated CD4+/CD8+ ratio
   E. Enlarged bilateral hilar/mediastinal lymph nodes on X-ray

VII. Treatment
   A. Self-limiting
   B. Steroids

REVIEW QUESTIONS

1. A 34-year-old African American female comes to the office presenting with shortness of breath, cough, weight loss, and weakness of her facial muscles on the left side. She has also noticed that her mouth and eyes have been very dry recently. What substance will most likely be elevated in this patient?
   A. 25-hydroxyvitamin D
   B. 1,25-hydroxyvitamin D
   C. Parathyroid hormone
   D. Parathyroid hormone-related protein
   E. Calcitonin

- **The correct answer is B.**
- This African American female has shortness of breath, cough, weakness of her facial muscles, and dry eyes. Collectively, these clues should have helped you recognize that this patient has sarcoidosis.
- The two main lab values we will see are elevated ACE and calcium. None of these options relate to ACE, so this question must be referring to hypercalcemia. The question is essentially asking which of these substances will lead to hypercalcemia when elevated
- In sarcoidosis, activated macrophages will stimulate the activation of the enzyme 1-alpha-hydroxylase. This enzyme is responsible for the formation of 1,25-hydroxyvitamin D, which is the active form of vitamin D. This can lead to hypervitaminosis D.
- The other answer choices are incorrect because these substances will not necessarily be elevated in a patient with sarcoidosis.

Section X - Inhalation Injury

I. Inhalation Injury
   A. Nonspecific term for airway irritation
   B. Any part of the airway can be affected
   C. Can cause a systemic reaction

II. Pathophysiology
   A. Small particles (< 1μm), heat, or irritants damage the distal airway
   B. Insult to the airway → inflammation → tracheobronchitis and edema
   C. Pulmonary dysfunction and prolonged mechanical ventilation can lead to pneumonia and ARDS

III. Causes
   A. Heat
   B. Chemicals
   C. Smoke

IV. Chemicals
   A. Carbon monoxide (CO)
   B. Cyanide
   C. Arsenic
   D. Ammonia (NH_3)
   E. Mustard gas (agents of war)

V. Smoke
   A. Most often from household or building fires
   B. Can be fatal
   C. Physical exam findings
      1. Burns, singed nasal hairs, soot in pharynx, mucosal ulcerations, airway edema

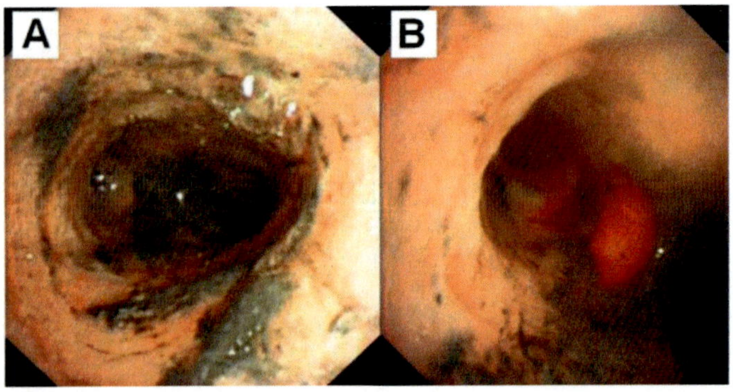

Photo Credit: Bai C, et al. 2013. Diagnostic Pathology. doi: 10.1186/1746-1596-8-174

FIGURE 10.6.46 - Bronchoscopy Showing Soot Deposition

VI. Treatment
   A. Smoke and heat: supportive care
      1. IV fluids, supplemental O_2, intubation
   B. Chemicals: chemical-specific medication

REVIEW QUESTIONS ?

1. A 25-year-old man is brought to the emergency room by ambulance after being rescued from a burning home. He is fatigued and is having difficulty talking in full sentences. He has singed nasal hair and burns on approximately 57% of his total body surface area. IV fluids are started. Shortly after arriving at the hospital he is gasping for air. A physical exam is repeated. What physical exam finding would suggegst that the medical team should prepare for intubation?

   A. Singed nasal hairs
   B. Skin burns
   C. Pharyngeal edema
   D. Cherry red skin
   E. Petechiae

- **The correct answer is C.**
- This is a 25-year-old man at high risk for inhalation injury because he was rescued from a burning building.
- He has singed nasal hairs and significant burns and is having difficulty speaking in full sentences, indicating shortness of breath.
- This is concerning for smoke inhalation injury.
- After his IV fluids are started, he becomes increasingly short of breath. This is likely secondary to pharyngeal edema from the fluid resuscitation.
- A is incorrect. Singed nasal hairs alone do not require intubation. However, they should prompt you to look in the patient's mouth at his pharynx.
- B is incorrect. Skin burns alone do not require intubation.
- D is incorrect. However, this might be seen in carbon monoxide or cyanide poisoning.
- E is incorrect. Petechiae are associated with platelet disorders.

Section XI - Pneumoconioses

I. Pneumoconioses
  A. Types
    1. Asbestosis
    2. Berylliosis
    3. Coal workers' pneumoconiosis
    4. Silicosis
  B. Restrictive lung disease
  C. Dyspnea on exertion and dry cough

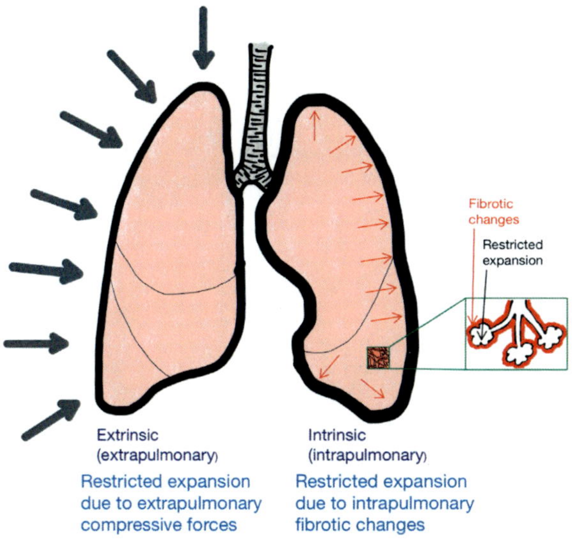

FIGURE 10.6.47 - Extrinsic vs. Intrinsic Restrictive Lung Diseases

Type	Occupation	Pathology	Risks	Histology	Imaging
Asbestos	- Shipbuilding - Roofing - Plumbing - Insulation manufacturing	- Asbestos exposure → macrophage activation → fibrosis of lung and pleura	- Bronchogenic lung cancer → mesothelioma - Pleural effusion	- Long, golden-brown, barbell-shaped fibers with associated iron	- Calcified bilateral lower lobe lesions on CXR - Pleural opacities ("pleural plaques") on CT
Berylliosis	- Aerospace - Nuclear weapons manufacturing	- Beryllium exposure → macrophage activation → granuloma formation	- Lung cancer - Cor pulmonale	- Noncaseating granulomas	- Upper lobe lesions on CXR
Coal workers' pneumoconiosis	- Coal mining	- Prolonged exposure to coal → carbon-laden macrophages → inflammation/fibrosis → black lung - Exposure to sooty air in urban areas → anthracosis (asymptomatic) → black lung	- No risk of lung cancer - Caplan syndrome	- Accumulation of black, carbon-laden macrophages	- Micronodular opacities of upper lobes on CXR
Silicosis	- Sandblasting - Silica mining - Foundry work (metal casting)	- Silica exposure → macrophage activation → release of fibrogenic factors → fibrosis - Silica → phagolysosome disruption → impaired macrophages → TB	- TB - Lung cancer - Cor pulmonale - Caplan syndrome	- Birefringent silica particles inside whorled collagen nodules surrounded by dust-laden macrophages	- Egg-shell calcifications of upper lobe hilar lymph nodes on CXR

TABLE 10.6.3 - Types of Pneumoconioses

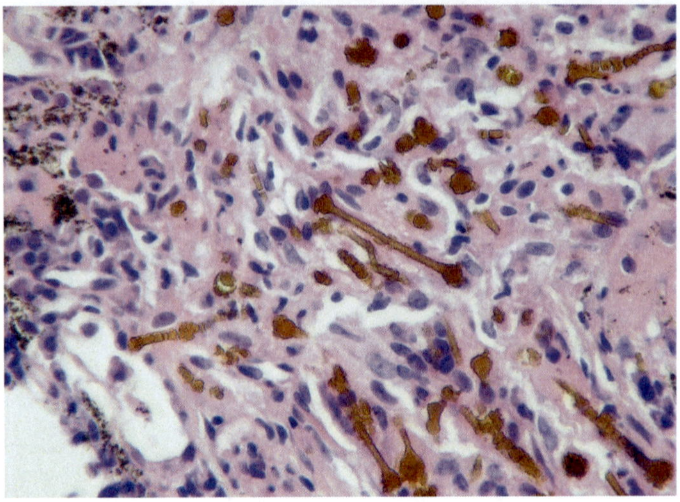

Photo Credit: Yale Rosen from USA [CC BY-SA (https://creativecommons.org/licenses/by-sa/2.0)]

FIGURE 10.6.48 - Barbell-Shaped Asbestos Bodies in Asbestosis

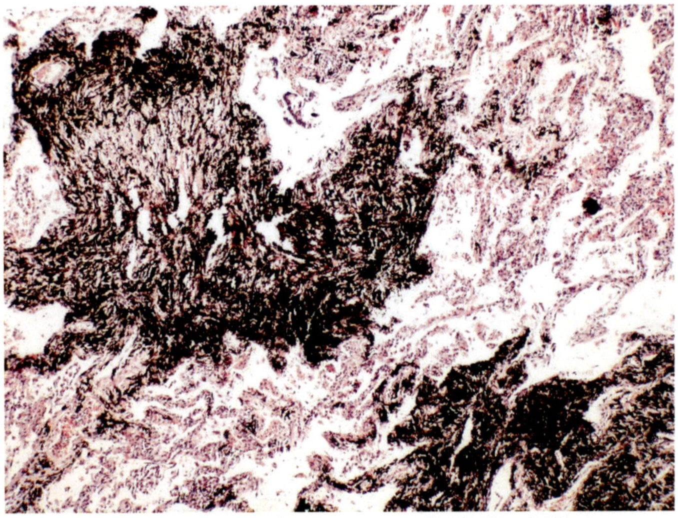

Photo Credit: Yale Rosen [CC BY-SA (https://creativecommons.org/licenses/by-sa/2.0)]

FIGURE 10.6.49 - Carbon-Laden Macrophages in Coal Workers' Pneumoconiosis

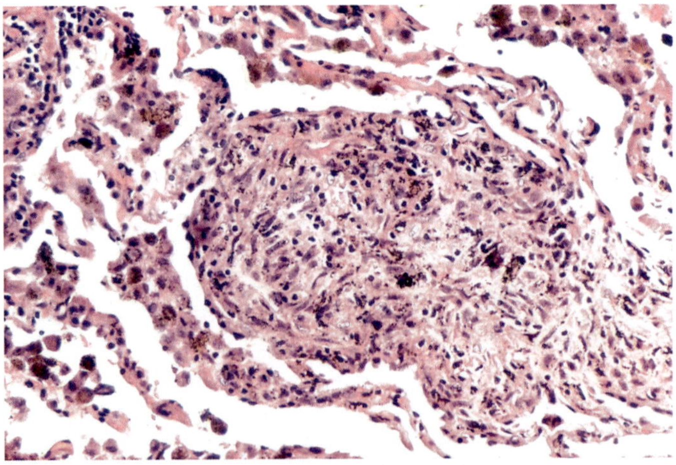

Photo Credit: Yale Rosen from USA [CC BY-SA (https://creativecommons.org/licenses/by-sa/2.0)]

FIGURE 10.6.50 - Whorled Collagen Nodules in Silicosis

REVIEW QUESTIONS

1. A 45-year-old man presents with progressive dyspnea on exertion and a dry cough. He has owned his own roofing business for years and has been unable to work due to the new onset of symptoms. There are crackles on lung auscultation and a chest X-ray reveals lower lobe lesions. CT imaging shows small, hyalinized lesions. A biopsy of this patient's lung will most likely reveal which of the following?

   A. Whorled collagen nodules
   B. Carbon-laden macrophages
   C. Barbell fibers with associated iron
   D. Noncaseating granulomas
   E. Small, round, oval cells with a high nuclear-to-cytoplasmic ratio

- **The correct answer is C.**
- This patient has asbestosis. Recall that asbestosis is the only pneumoconiosis where you'll see lower lobe lesions. He's in the roofing business, which is an occupation with a higher risk for asbestosis. The stem is also describing pleural plaques, which is specific to asbestosis.
- On histology, patients with asbestos will have barbell-shaped fibers with associated iron.
- A is describing silica exposure.
- B is describing coal workers' pneumoconiosis or anthracosis
- D is describing berylliosis.
- E is describing small cell lung cancer.

Section XII - Mesothelioma

I. Basic Principles
   A. Malignant neoplasm of mesothelial cells
   B. Visceral and parietal pleurae are both lined by mesothelial cells
   C. Mesothelial cells lubricate the pleural space → facilitate movement

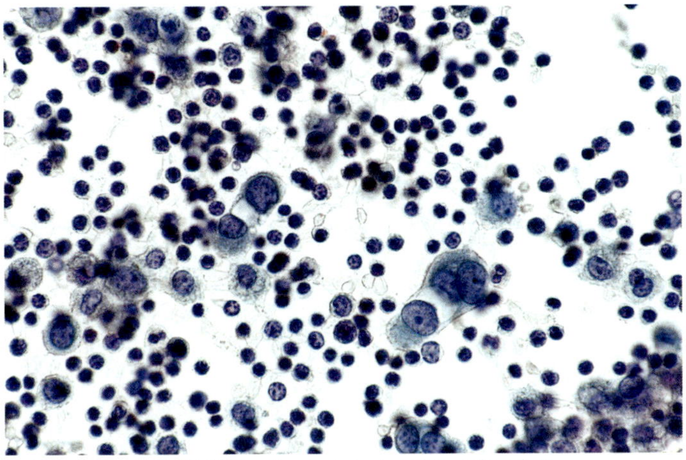

Photo Credit: Nephron [CC BY-SA (https://creativecommons.org/licenses/by-sa/3.0)]

FIGURE 10.6.51 - Mesothelial Cells

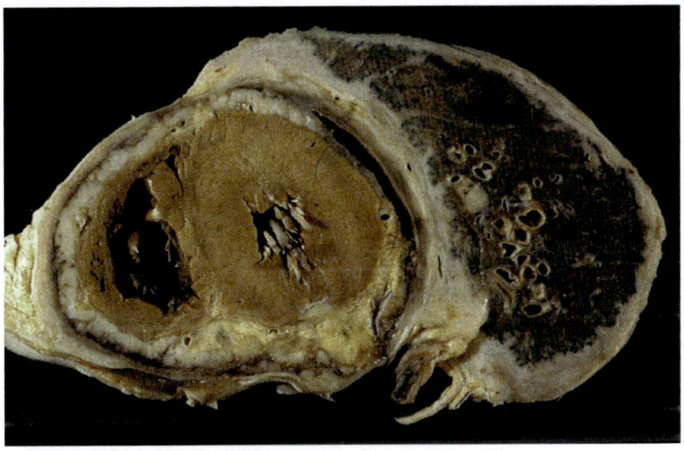

Photo Credit: The Armed Forces Institute of Pathology (AFIP) [Public domain]

FIGURE 10.6.52 - Mesothelioma

II. Risk Factors
   A. Asbestos is the only known risk factor
      1. Asbestos mining, insulation, shipbuilding
   B. Smoking is NOT a risk factor

III. Symptoms
   A. Dyspnea
   B. Cough
   C. Chest pain

IV. Findings
   A. Hemorrhagic pleural effusion
   B. Nodular or smooth unilateral pleural thickening
   C. Histology: psammoma bodies

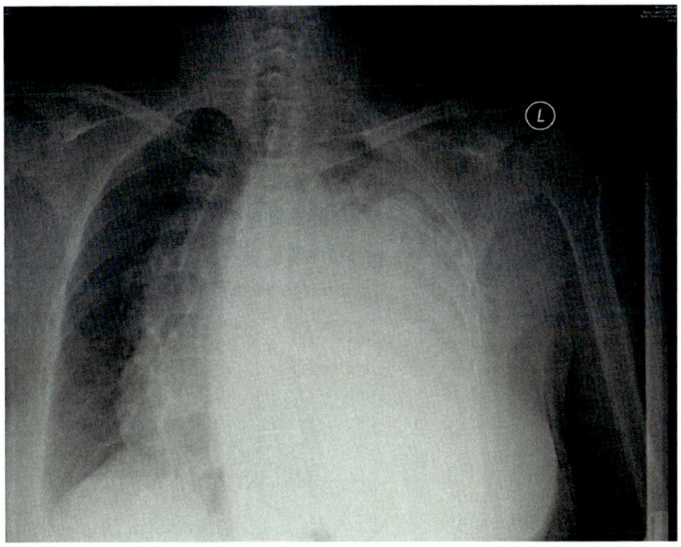

Photo Credit: Yale Rosen from USA [CC BY-SA (https://creativecommons.org/licenses/by-sa/2.0)]

FIGURE 10.6.53 - Chest X-Ray of Pleural Effusion

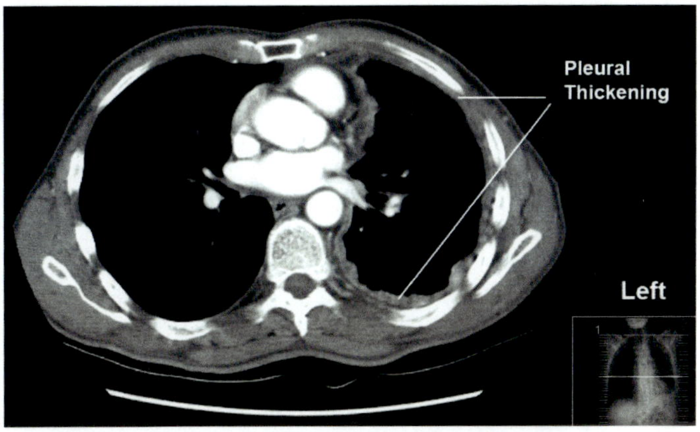

Photo Credit: I, Drriad [CC BY-SA (http://creativecommons.org/licenses/by-sa/3.0/)]

FIGURE 10.6.54 - Pleural Thickening

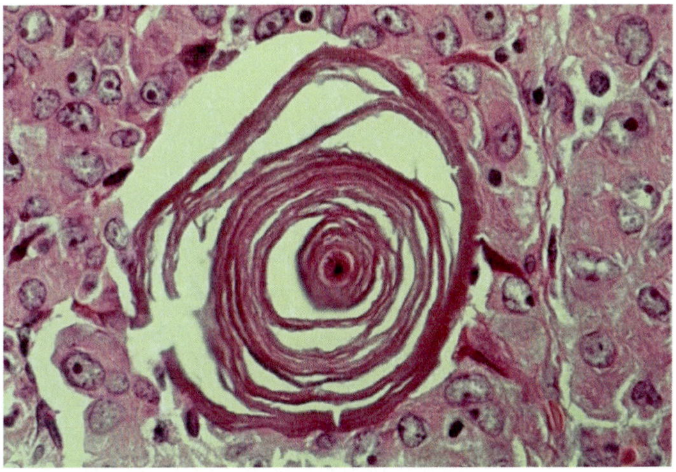

Photo Credit: The Armed Forces Institute of Pathology [Public domain]

FIGURE 10.6.55 - Psammoma Bodies

V. Immunohistochemical Markers
   A. Calretinin
   B. Cytokeratin 5
   C. Cytokeratin 6

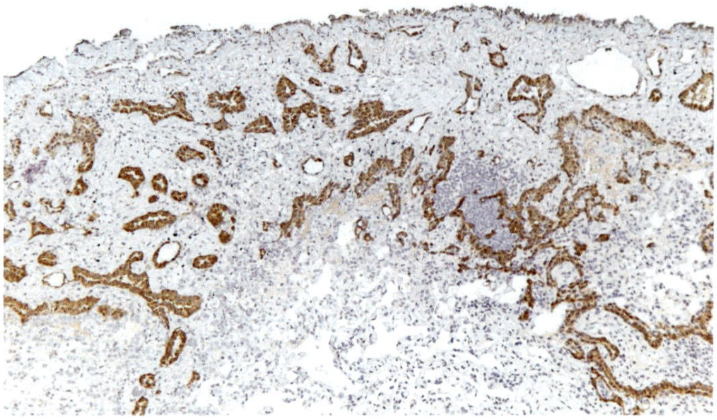

Photo Credit: Nephron [CC BY-SA (https://creativecommons.org/licenses/by-sa/3.0)]

FIGURE 10.6.56 - Mesothelioma

REVIEW QUESTIONS

1. A 59-year-old male presents to the clinic with worsening cough and chest pain. He smoked 3 packs of cigarettes daily for 32 years, but quit 2 years ago. He is a construction worker who spent 25 years working in a shipyard. Upon examination, there are decreased breath sounds and percussive dullness in the region of the right middle lobe. A chest CT shows pleural thickening. Which of the following histologic features would likely be found in a pleural biopsy from this patient?

    A. Onion-skinned and calcified deposition
    B. Clear, empty-appearing nuclei and nuclear grooves
    C. Perivascular pseudorosettes
    D. Small, round blue cells

- **The correct answer is A.**
- This is a 59-year-old male who was previously a chronic smoker presenting with worsening cough and chest pain. He was also a shipyard worker, which should make you suspicious of exposure to asbestos. His chest CT scan shows pleural thickening. This should all lead you to think this patient has mesothelioma. The biopsy would show psammoma bodies, which are laminated concentric spherules with dystrophic calcification and are described as "onion-skinned and calcified" in appearance.
- B is incorrect because this is the "Orphan Annie eye" appearance seen in papillary carcinoma of thyroid.
- C is incorrect because perivascular pseudorosettes are seen in ependymoma, a malignant tumor of ependymal cells.
- D is incorrect because small round blue cells are characteristically seen in neuroblastoma, rhabdomyosarcoma, non-Hodgkin's lymphoma, and Ewing sarcoma.

Section XIII - ARDS

I. Definition
   A. Form of respiratory failure
   B. Seen in critically ill or severely injured patients
   C. Acute onset
   D. Diffuse injury to the lungs
   E. High mortality rate

II. Berlin Definition of ARDS
   A. Acute onset within the last 7 days
   B. Bilateral opacities with pulmonary edema on chest x-ray or CT
   C. Impaired oxygenation causing hypoxemia, with severity defined by PaO_2/FiO_2 ratio
      1. Mild: 200-300
      2. Moderate: 100-200
      3. Severe: <100

III. Pathophysiology
   A. Lung insult → inflammatory mediators (cytokines) → neutrophils recruited and activated → ROS and protease release
      1. Capillary leakage → pulmonary edema, hyaline membrane formation (diffuse alveolar damage)
      2. Death of type I and II pneumocytes
      3. End result: diffuse alveolar damage

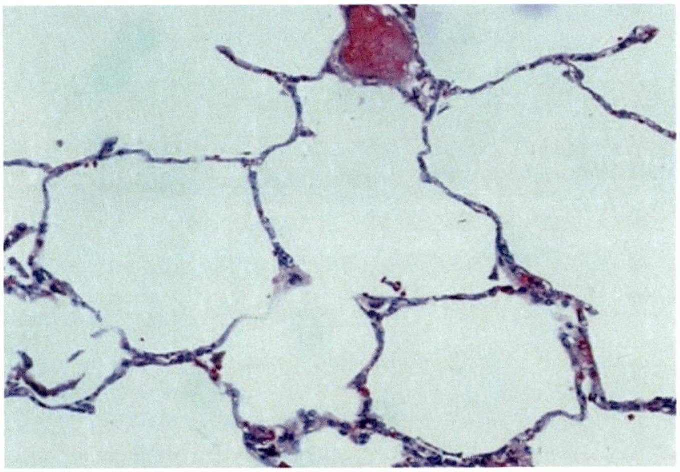

Photo Credit: https://www.flickr.com/photos/pulmonary_pathology/3678762542

FIGURE 10.6.57 - Normal Alveoli

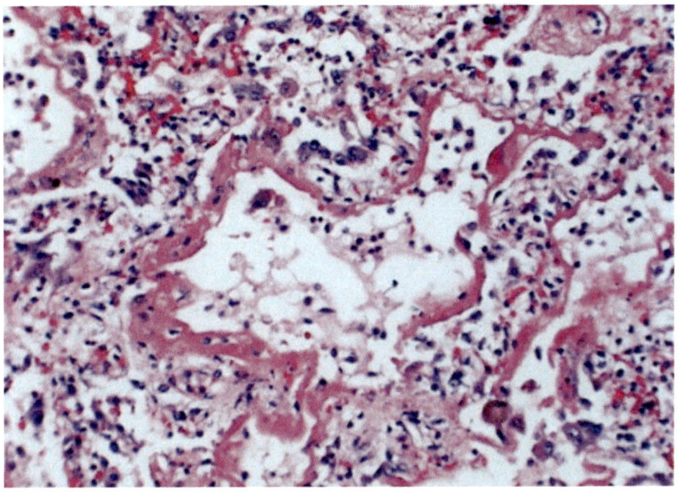

Photo Credit: https://www.flickr.com/photos/pulmonary_pathology/4564039878

FIGURE 10.6.58 - Diffuse Alveolar Damage

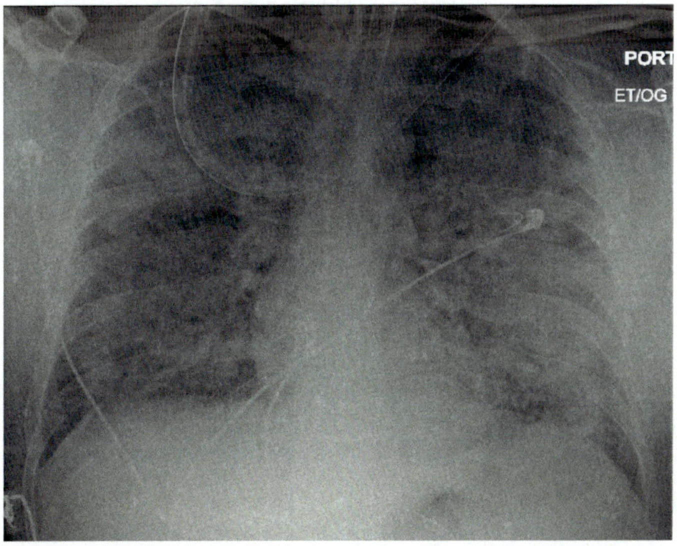

Photo Credit: James Heilman, MD / CC BY-SA (https://creativecommons.org/licenses/by-sa/4.0)

FIGURE 10.6.59 - Chest X-Ray of a Patient with ARDS

IV. Causes
  A. Sepsis
  B. Pneumonia (viral, bacterial, fungal)
  C. Aspiration or inhalation
  D. Pancreatitis
  E. Trauma
  F. Iatrogenic (chemotherapy, radiation)

V. Treatment
  A. Primary goal: treat underlying cause
  B. Respiratory support: mechanical ventilation
    1. PEEP: positive end-expiratory pressure
    2. Low tidal volume

REVIEW QUESTIONS

1. A 55-year-old man is admitted to the hospital for bacterial pneumonia. A chest X-ray at admission shows consolidation of the right lower lobe of the lung. He is started on antibiotics. Two days after admission, he becomes increasingly hypoxic. His O_2 saturation is currently 70% with maximum supplemental O_2 delivered by nasal cannula. A repeat chest X-ray is obtained and is shown below.

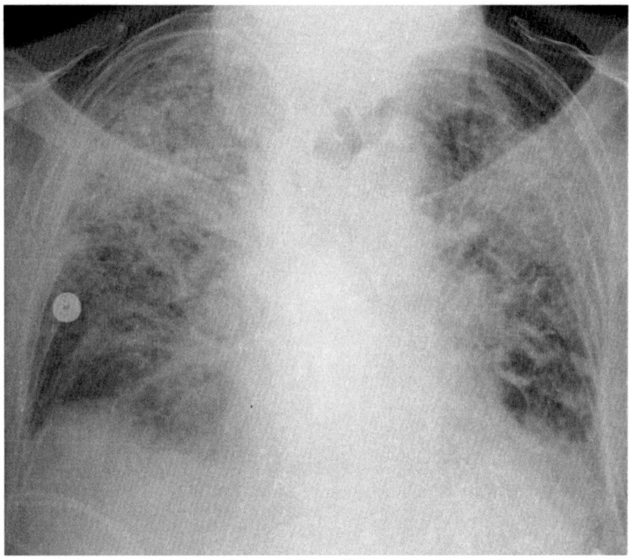

Photo Credit: James Heilman, MD / CC BY-SA (https://creativecommons.org/licenses/by-sa/3.0)

He is transferred to the ICU for escalation of care. Which of the following is an appropriate next step in treatment?
   A. Discontinue antibiotics
   B. Intubate and start PEEP with low tidal volumes
   C. Intubate and start PEEP with high tidal volumes
   D. Emergent surgery
   E. Administer supplemental surfactant

- **The correct answer is B.**
- This is a 55-year-old male who was recently admitted for pneumonia. At admission, his chest X-ray showed a simple pneumonia and he was started on antibiotics. However, two days later he is hypoxic despite supplemental oxygen. Repeat chest X-ray shows bilateral opacities consistent with ARDS. He needs to be intubated and started on PEEP with low tidal volumes.
- A is incorrect because part of treating ARDS is treating the underlying cause, which in this case is bacterial pneumonia.
- C is incorrect because high tidal volumes would not be appropriate.
- D is incorrect because ARDS is not a surgical problem.
- E is incorrect. Although patients with ARDS have decreased levels of surfactant, supplemental surfactant has not been shown to be beneficial.

Section XIV - Sleep Apnea

I. Basic Principles
   A. Pausing of breathing during sleep, lasting > 10 seconds
   B. Disrupted sleep and daytime somnolence

II. Central Sleep Apnea
   A. CNS injury → decreased respiratory drive
   B. Associated with an underlying chronic condition
   C. No breathing effort
   D. Cheyne-Stokes respirations
   E. Treat with continuous positive airway pressure (CPAP)

III. Obstructive Sleep Apnea
   A. Interaction between anatomic upper airway susceptibility and sleep-related changes
   B. Bulky tongue/crowded oropharynx and weak upper airway dilator muscles → airway narrowing → airway collapse → hypoxia
   C. Loud snoring and gasping respirations
   D. Classic presentation: Obese, non-smoker presenting with daytime somnolence, morning headaches, loud snoring, and unrefreshing sleep
   E. Will have breathing effort
   F. Normal arterial blood gas values
   G. Treat with CPAP, weight loss, or hypoglossal nerve stimulation

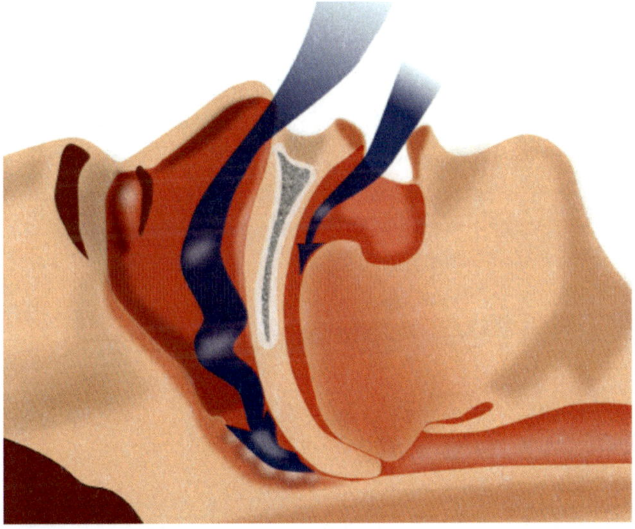

Photo Credit: Dyolf77 [Public domain]

FIGURE 10.6.60 - Blocked Airway from Crowded Oropharynx

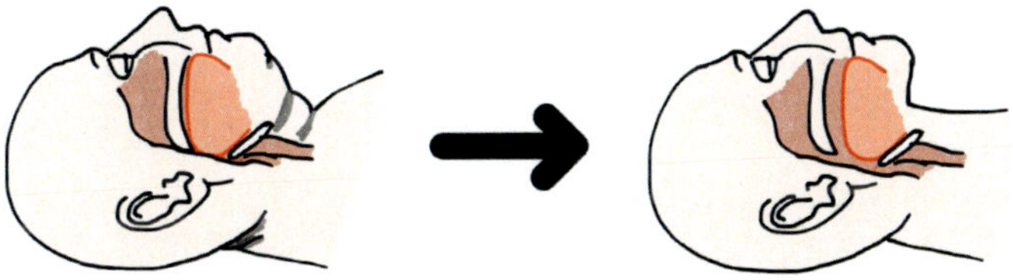

FIGURE 10.6.61 - Before (Right) and After (Left) Weight Loss to Improve Symptoms of Obstructive Sleep Apnea

IV. Obesity Hypoventilation Syndrome
   A. Presentation often confused with obstructive sleep apnea
   B. Severe obesity → restricted chest expansion → hypoventilation
   C. Elevated PCO_2 and decreased PO_2
   D. Normal A-a gradient
   E. Fatigue, dyspnea, difficulty concentrating, obesity
   F. Treat with weight loss

V. Complications of Apnea
   A. Systemic hypertension
   B. Pulmonary hypertension
   C. Right heart failure
   D. 2° polycythemia
   E. Increased risk for cardiac events

REVIEW QUESTIONS

1. A 38-year-old man presents to the clinic due to lack of feeling refreshed after sleeping. A few days ago, he fell asleep while having a conversation with his boss. He finds himself abruptly gasping for breath in the middle of the night and his wife has been sleeping in the guest room due to his loud snoring. His BMI is 32. Blood gases are normal. What could be a potential consequence of his underlying disorder?
   A. Atelectasis
   B. Pneumothorax
   C. Cor pulmonale
   D. Cardiac tamponade
   E. Left heart failure

- **The correct answer is C.**
- This person has obstructive sleep apnea, which is typically seen in obese patients. This patient is also presenting with a history of snoring, gasping, unrefreshing sleep, and falling asleep at random times during the day. Systemic hypertension, pulmonary hypertension, right heart failure, secondary polycythemia, and increased risk for cardiac events are all complications that can be seen with apnea.
- A, B, D, and E are incorrect because they do not characterize the consequences of sleep apnea.

Section XV - Pulmonary Hypertension

I. Definition
   A. Mean pulmonary artery pressure ≥ 25 mmHg at rest
      1. Normal: 10-15 mmHg
   B. Right heart catheterization is the gold standard for measurement

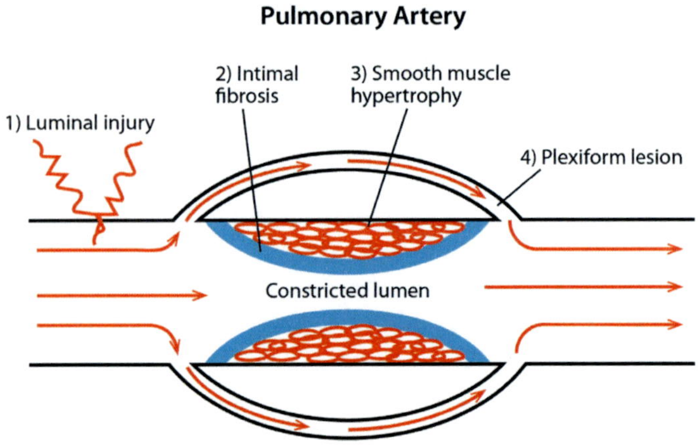

FIGURE 10.6.62 - Morphological Changes due to Pulmonary Hypertension

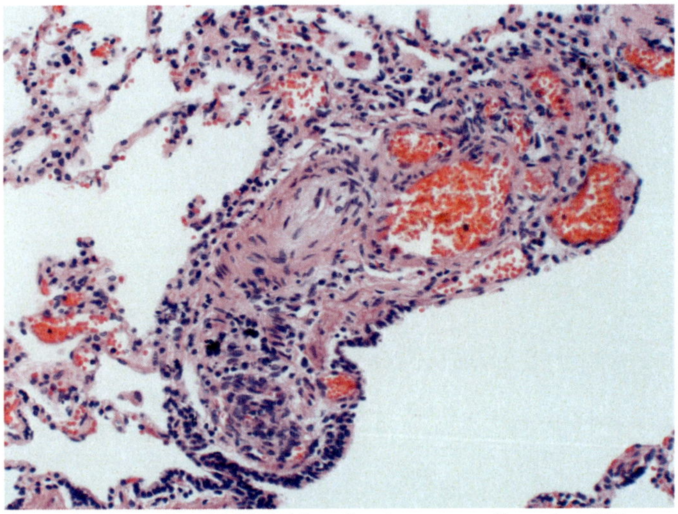

FIGURE 10.6.63 - Plexiform Lesions in Pulmonary Hypertension

II. Pathophysiology
   A. Increased pulmonary pressure
      1. Luminal injury to the pulmonary artery
      2. Intimal fibrosis
      3. Smooth muscle cell hypertrophy
      4. Formation of plexiform lesions
      5. Atherosclerosis of the pulmonary trunk

III. Findings
   A. Exertional dyspnea
   B. Right ventricular hypertrophy
   C. Cor pulmonale (right-sided heart failure)
      1. Jugular venous distention
      2. Peripheral edema
      3. Loud pulmonic S2 component (pathological splitting)
      4. Prominent "a wave" on jugular venous pressure waveform

IV. Primary Pulmonary Hypertension
   A. Idiopathic or hereditary
   B. Young adult females
   C. Inactivating mutation of *BMPR2* gene
   D. Excess smooth muscle proliferation of the pulmonary artery
   E. ↑ vasoconstrictors (e.g. endothelin)
   F. ↓ vasodilators (e.g. nitric oxide, prostacyclin synthase)

V. Secondary Pulmonary Hypertension
   A. Occurs secondary to an underlying pathology
      1. Hypoxemia (e.g. COPD, interstitial lung disease)
      2. ↑ blood volume in pulmonary circulation (Eisenmenger syndrome)
      3. Recurrent pulmonary embolisms
      4. Autoimmune (e.g. systemic sclerosis, SLE, RA)

VI. Treatment
   A. No cure
   B. Supplemental oxygen and diuretics for symptoms of heart failure
   C. Prostacyclin analogues (epoprostenol, iloprost)
   D. Endothelin-1 receptor antagonist (bosentan)
   E. Phosphodiesterase-5 (PDE-5) inhibitors (sildenafil)

REVIEW QUESTIONS

1. A healthy 40-year-old woman comes to the clinic with a 4-month history of shortness of breath on exertion. Lungs are clear on auscultation. Cardiac examination reveals a loud pulmonic component of S2 and a prominent "a wave" on the JVP waveform. Expression of what molecule is most likely upregulated in the pulmonary vasculature of this patient?

    - **The correct answer is endothelin.**
    - Note that this woman has a history of progressive shortness of breath on exertion, a loud pulmonic component of S2, and a prominent "a wave" on the JVP tracing, which are all key findings of pulmonary hypertension.
    - Since she does not have a significant past medical history, we can conclude that she has primary pulmonary hypertension.
    - Recall that in primary pulmonary hypertension, there is an overall increased expression of vasoconstrictive molecules within the pulmonary vasculature and a decreased expression of vasodilative molecules, in addition to excessive smooth muscle proliferation of the pulmonary artery.
    - The most potent vasoconstrictor of the pulmonary vasculature involved in pulmonary hypertension is endothelin, which is the correct answer here.
    - On the other hand, substances like nitric oxide and prostacyclin synthase are responsible for vasodilation and would be downregulated in this setting.
    - In fact, the activation and inhibition of these mediators is the basis of treatment of pulmonary hypertension.

2. A 40-year-old woman comes to her physician complaining about exertional dyspnea and fatigue. She experiences discoloration of her fingers when exposed to the cold and tightening of the skin on her hands. She has a 3-year history of difficulty swallowing and joint stiffness. Cardiac examination reveals a loud S2 over the upper left sternal border. The abdomen is soft with mild hepatomegaly and there is bilateral lower extremity pitting edema. Lung function tests are normal. Which of the following is the cause of the patient's dyspnea?

    A. Hypoxia-induced vasoconstriction
    B. Intimal thickening of pulmonary arterioles
    C. Pulmonary interstitial fibrosis
    D. Right-sided valvular heart disease

    - **The correct answer is B.**
    - Hopefully from the question stem you realize that this patient with progressive exertional dyspnea with a history of difficulty swallowing and joint stiffness has the diffuse type of systemic sclerosis.
    - This can be further confirmed by the fact that she is experiencing Raynaud phenomenon and sclerodactyly, or tightening of the skin.
    - She also shows symptoms of right-sided heart failure like hepatomegaly and bilateral lower extremity pitting edema.
    - Systemic sclerosis plus right-sided heart failure leads us to believe that her dyspnea is due to pulmonary hypertension.
    - Remember that the increased pulmonary artery pressure in pulmonary hypertension leads to intimal thickening, making choice B the correct answer.
    - Answer choices A and C are incorrect because although they could cause pulmonary hypertension, the lung function tests would be abnormal.
    - Answer choice D is wrong because the patient's history and cardiac examination do not indicate any valvular anomalies.

Section XVI - Atelectasis

I. Atelectasis
   A. Loss of lung volume due to collapse of lung tissue
   B. Can affect part of or an entire lung
   C. Results in impaired exchange of O_2 and CO_2

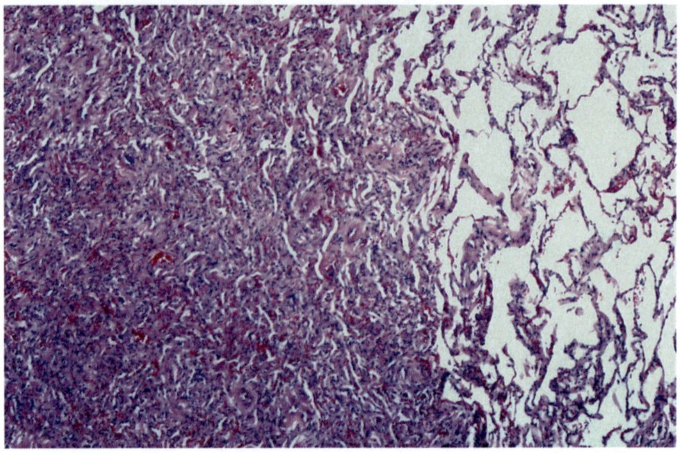

FIGURE 10.6.64 - Atelectasis

II. Obstructive Atelectasis: Etiology
   A. Lung collapse caused by an obstruction of the airway, preventing ventilation
   B. Examples: tumor, foreign body, mucus plug

III. Obstructive Atelectasis: Pathophysiology
   A. Obstruction of the airways
   B. Lung is not ventilated
   C. The air that is trapped in the lung distal to the obstruction gets absorbed into the pulmonary capillary system
   D. Loss of lung volume

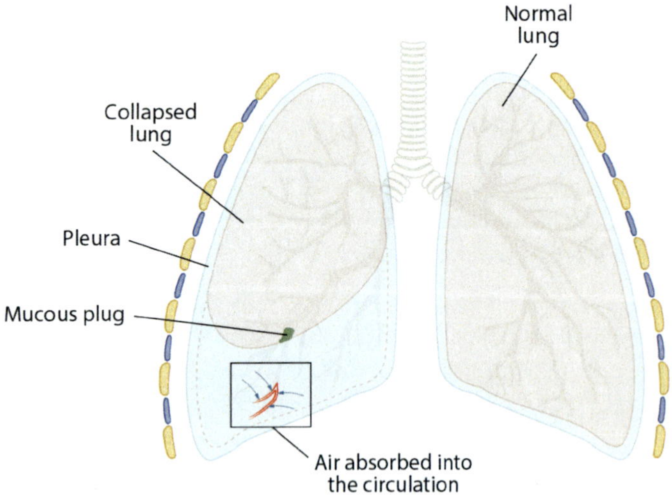

FIGURE 10.6.65 - Pathophysiology of Obstructive Atelectasis

IV. Compressive Atelectasis: Etiology
   A. Caused by external compression of the lung by a space-occupying lesion
   B. Examples: loculated pleural effusions, elevated hemidiaphragm, solid mass

V. Compressive Atelectasis: Pathophysiology
   A. External pressure on the lung by a space-occupying lesion
   B. Pressure on the lung causes loss of lung volume
   C. Decrease in functional residual capacity compared to normal

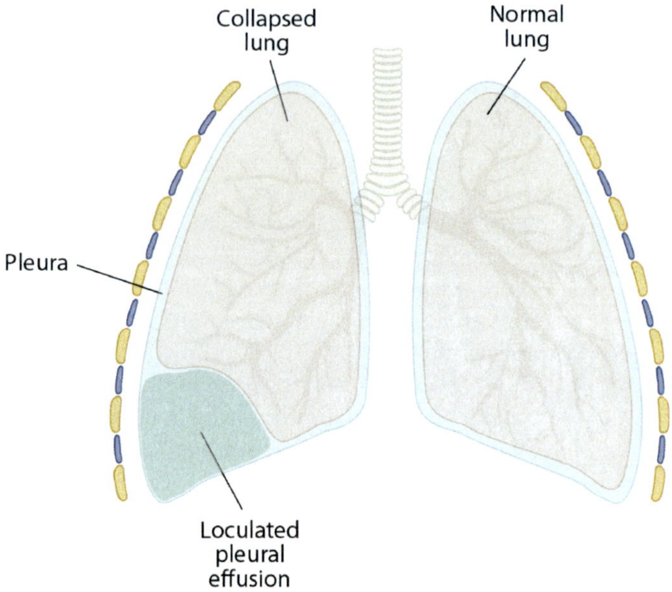

FIGURE 10.6.66 - Pathophysiology of Compressive Atelectasis

VI. Passive Atelectasis: Etiology
   A. Due to loss of contact between the visceral and parietal pleurae
   B. Examples: pleural effusion, pneumothorax, hemothorax, emphysema

VII. Passive Atelectasis: Pathophysiology
   A. Loss of negative intrapleural pressure
   B. Loss of contact between the two layers of the pleurae
   C. Lung is not expanded but "relaxed"
   D. Unopposed elastic recoil of the lung causes it to collapse
   E. Similar to compressive atelectasis but the compressive subtype is more focal or localized

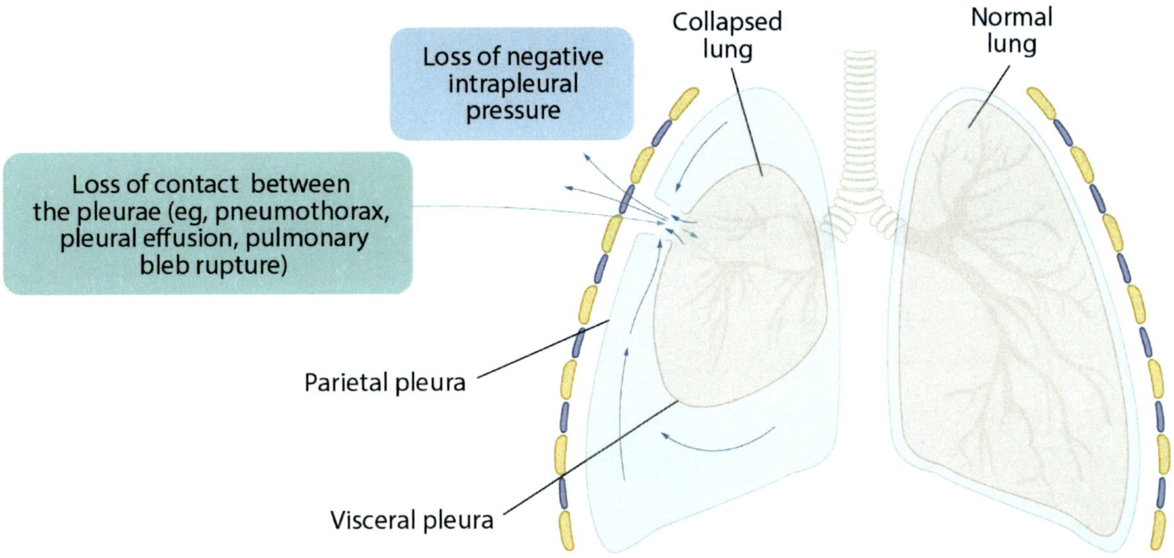

FIGURE 10.6.67 - Pathophysiology of Passive Atelectasis

VIII. Contraction Atelectasis: Etiology
  A. Lung collapse due to scarring
  B. Examples: granulomatous disease (classically TB), sarcoidosis, radiation fibrosis

IX. Contraction Atelectasis: Pathophysiology
  A. Scarring and fibrosis of the lung parenchyma
  B. Decreases lung ability to expand

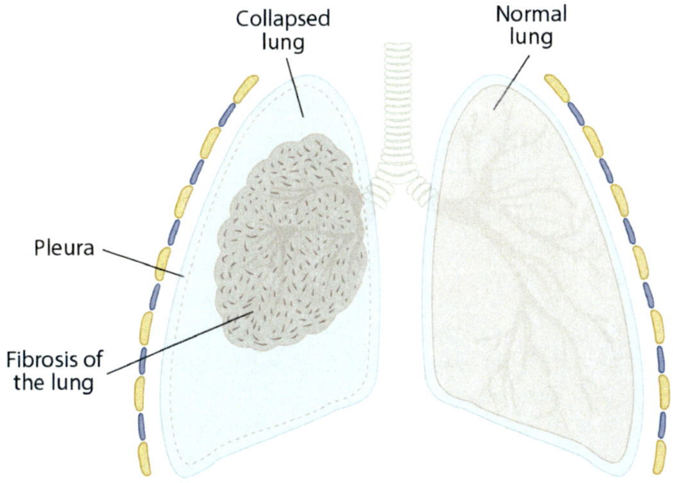

FIGURE 10.6.68 - Pathophysiology of Contraction Atelectasis

X. Adhesive Atelectasis: Etiology
  A. Due to lack of surfactant from lamellar bodies of type II pneumocytes
  B. Examples: NRDS and ARDS

XI. Adhesive Atelectasis: Pathophysiology
  A. Surfactant normally reduces surface tension and keeps alveoli open
  B. Loss of surfactant due to decreased production or inactivation
  C. Alveolar instability and collapse

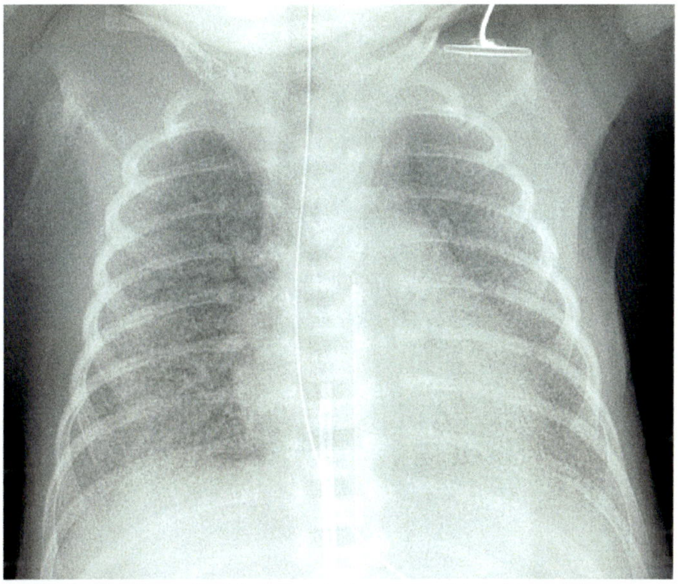

Photo Credit: Mikael Häggström, M.D. - Author info - Reusing images Written informed consent was obtained from a parent of the individual, including for online publication. [CC0]

FIGURE 10.6.69 - Chest X-Ray of Adhesive Atelectasis due to NRDS

XII. Absorption Atelectasis: Etiology
  A. Replacement of nitrogen with 100% oxygen, causing oxygen to be absorbed into the blood
  B. Examples: delivery of 100% oxygen and PEEP

XIII. Absorption Atelectasis: Pathophysiology
  A. 100% oxygen delivery
  B. Nitrogen in the alveoli is washed out and replaced with oxygen
  C. The higher solubility of oxygen causes it to diffuse into the blood more quickly
  D. This occurs quickly so there is not enough gas in the alveoli left to maintain their patency causing the alveoli to collapse

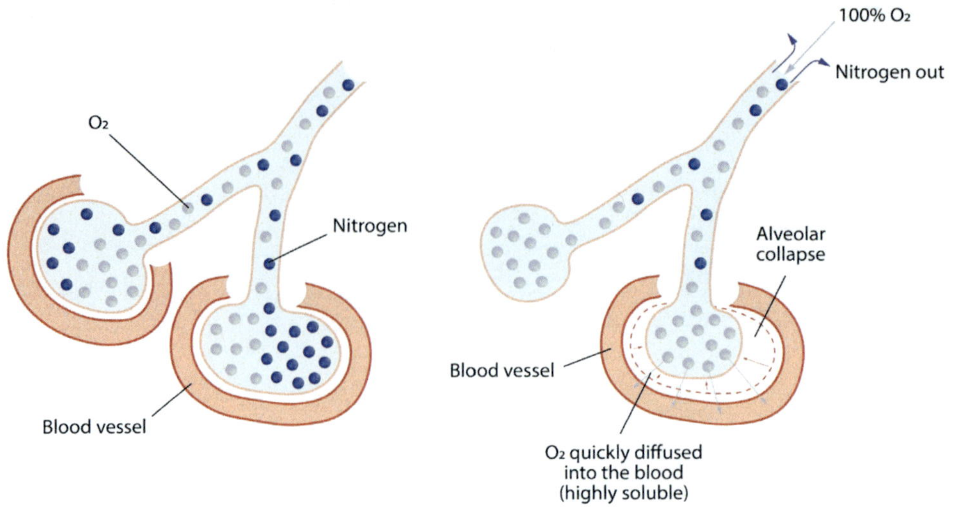

FIGURE 10.6..70 - Pathophysiology of Absorption Atelectasis

XIV. Diagnosis: Physical Findings
   A. Could be asymptomatic
   B. Decreased breath sounds
   C. Dullness to percussion
   D. Decreased tactile fremitus

XV. Diagnosis: Imaging
   A. Depends on the size of the area affected
   B. Opacifications on chest X-ray
   C. Mediastinal shift towards the side of the lesion could be evident

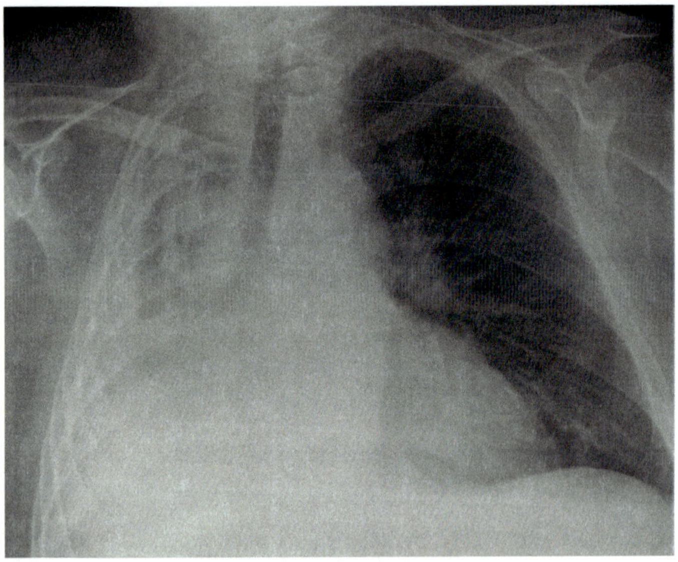

FIGURE 10.6.71 - Chest X-Ray of Absorption Atelectasis

XVI. Diagnosis: Labs
   A. Could be normal because of compensatory mechanism
   B. Decreased PaO_2 (hypoxemia) if a large area is involved
   C. $PaCO_2$ could be normal/decreased due to compensatory increased minute ventilation
   D. Check WBCs to rule out pneumonia

REVIEW QUESTIONS

1. A 48-year-old woman comes to the physician due to difficulty breathing. She says her breathing has become shallow recently. She has no fever and no other symptoms. Her history is significant for breast carcinoma, for which she has undergone bilateral mastectomy and radiation therapy. What is the pathophysiological mechanism of this patient's disease?

   A. Obstruction
   B. Loss of negative intrapleural pressure
   C. Increased fibrous deposition
   D. Inflammation of the lung

- **The correct answer is C.**
- This patient has a history of breast cancer that was treated with radiation, which can cause fibrosis of the lungs as a complication. Therefore, this patient has contraction atelectasis.
- A is incorrect because obstruction due to a foreign object or a tumor is highly unlikely, since she has no other symptoms.
- B is incorrect, because it refers to pneumothorax, but there was no history of trauma or anything else that can cause you to suspect pneumothorax
- D is incorrect because it refers to pneumonia, which is unlikely in this case because she has no fever and no other symptoms of pneumonia.

Section XVII - Pleural Effusions

I. Basic Principles
   A. Excess accumulation of fluid between pleural layers
   B. Restricted lung expansion during inspiration

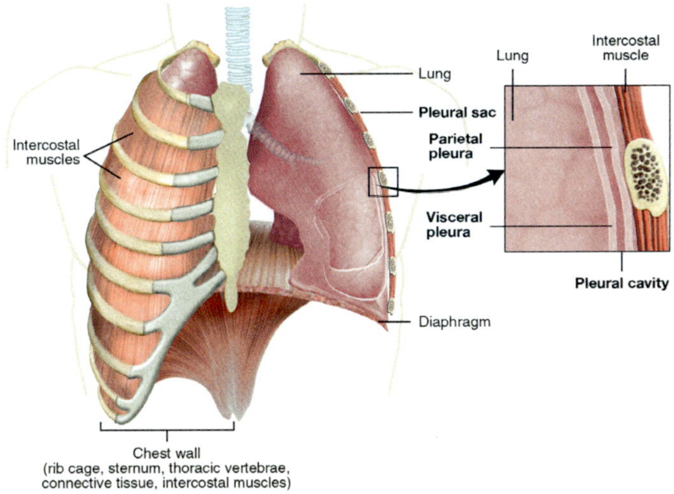

Photo Credit: OpenStax College [CC BY (https://creativecommons.org/licenses/by/3.0)]

FIGURE 10.6.72 - Parietal and Visceral Pleura of Lung

II. Symptoms
   A. Dyspnea
   B. Orthopnea
   C. Dry, nonproductive cough
   D. Chest pain

III. Findings
   A. Decreased breath sounds
   B. Decreased fremitus
   C. Dullness to percussion
   D. Blunting of costophrenic angle
   E. Tracheal deviation away from side of lesion (if large)

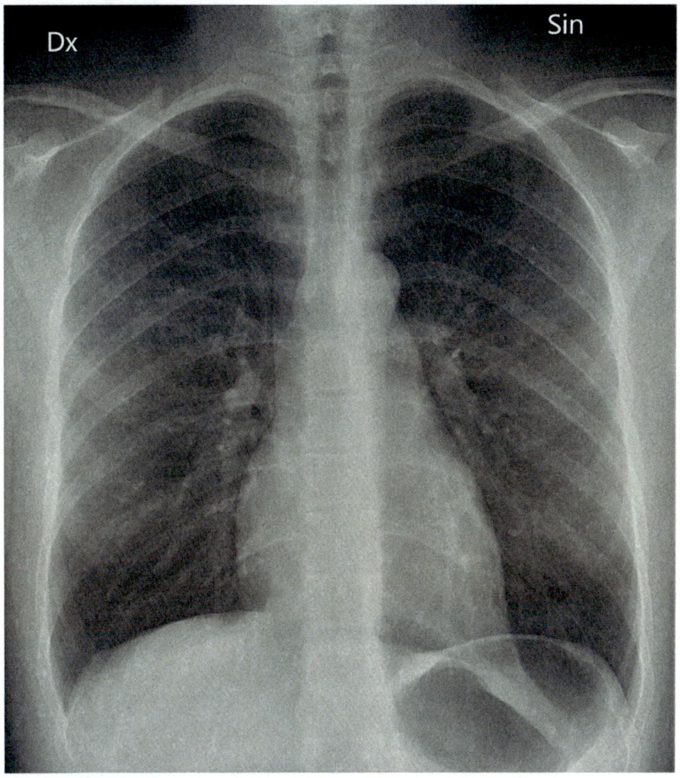

Photo Credit: Mikael Häggström [CC0]

FIGURE 10.6.73 - Normal Chest X-Ray

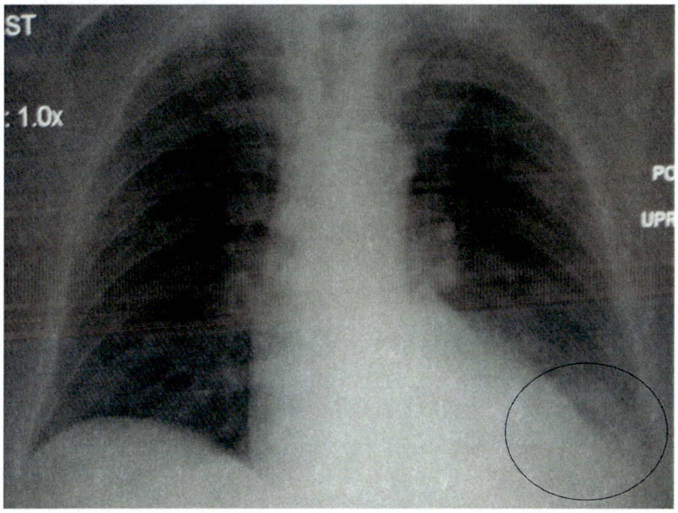

Photo Credit: James Heilman, MD [CC BY-SA (https://creativecommons.org/licenses/by-sa/3.0)]

FIGURE 10.6.74 - Blunting of the Left Costophrenic Angle in Pleural Effusion

IV. Complications
   A. Compressive atelectasis
   B. Infection

Effusion type	Fluid findings	Etiology	Treatment
Transudate	- ↓ Protein content - Watery	- Increased capillary hydrostatic pressure (e.g. heart failure) - Decreased oncotic pressure (e.g. nephrotic syndrome, cirrhosis)	- Treat underlying condition
Exudate	- ↑ Protein content - Cloudy	- Malignancy - Pneumonia - Collagen vascular disease - Trauma	- Thoracentesis
Lymphatic	- ↑ Protein content - Milky-appearing fluid	- Thoracic duct injury from trauma - Malignancy	- Treat underlying causes - Thoracentesis

TABLE 10.6.4 - Types of Pleural Effusions

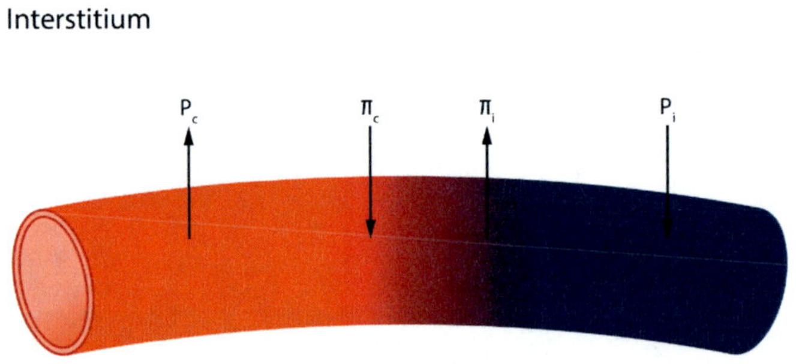

Net fluid flow = $K_f\,[\,(P_c - P_i) - \sigma(\pi_c - \pi_i)\,]$

K_f = capillary permeability to fluid
P_c = capillary pressure
P_i = interstitial pressure
σ = capillary permeability to protein
π_c = plasma oncotic pressure
π_i = interstial oncotic pressure

FIGURE 10.6.75 - Pathophysiology of Pleural Effusion

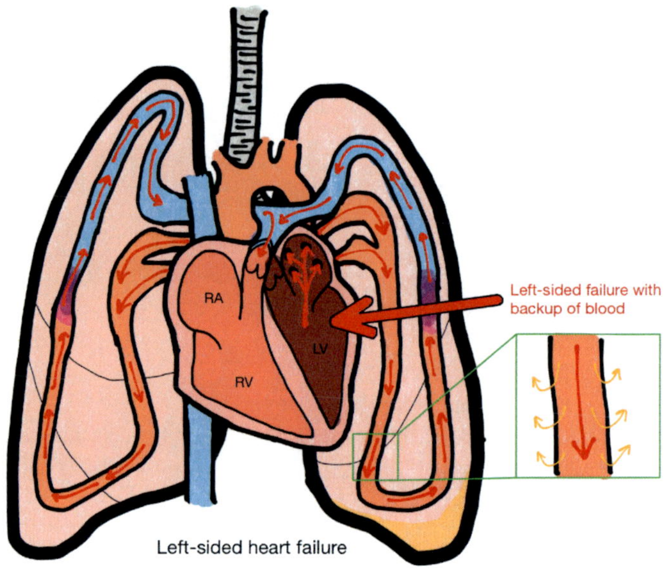

FIGURE 10.6.76 - Balance of Hydrostatic and Oncotic Pressures

V. Transudate: Pathophysiology
   A. CHF → congestion of blood in the lungs → increased capillary hydrostatic pressure in lungs → increased fluid in pleural space
   B. Nephrotic syndrome and cirrhosis → decreased plasma proteins → decreased plasma oncotic pressure → increased fluid in pleural space

VI. Exudate: Pathophysiology
   A. Inflammation → pleural damage → vascular damage → increased protein permeability of capillaries (σ) → increased escape of proteins into pleural space

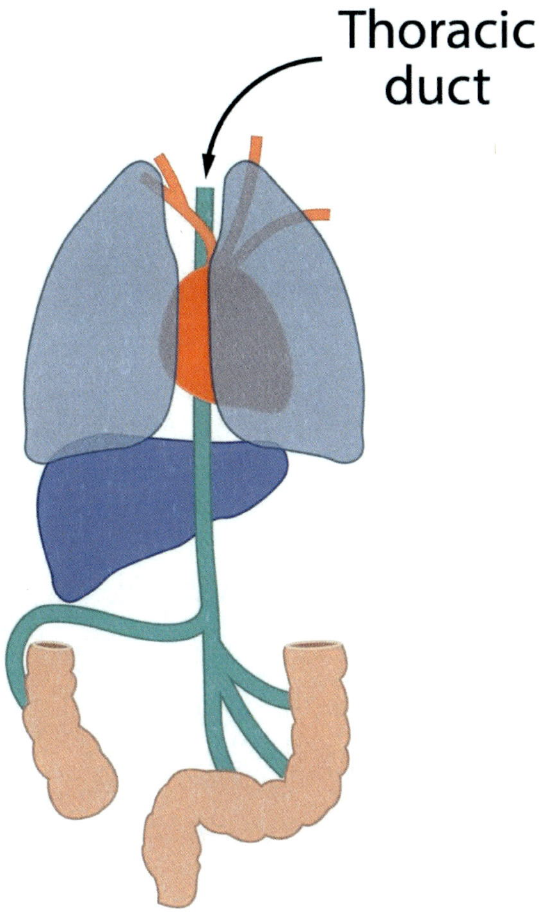

FIGURE 10.6.77 - Location of Thoracic Duct Relative to Lungs

VII. Lymphatic Effusion: Pathophysiology

A. Lymphatic blockage → lymphatic leakage → increased triglyceride levels in pleural space

REVIEW QUESTIONS

1. If the capillary hydrostatic pressure is elevated above normal and the interstitial fluid pressure remains the same, will the amount of fluid in the interstitium increase, decrease, or remain the same?
    - **The amount of fluid will increase.**
    - Remember, the capillary hydrostatic pressure and the interstitial fluid colloid osmotic (or oncotic) pressure push fluid out of the capillaries.

REVIEW QUESTIONS

2. A 23-year-old African American woman with a history of arthritis presents with progressive dyspnea, a nonproductive cough, and orthopnea for 3 weeks. Physical examination reveals a red rash on her cheeks, decreased breath sounds on auscultation, dullness on percussion, and decreased fremitus. A chest X-ray reveals a midline trachea. A fluid sample from the pleural space reveals high protein levels. How should this patient's condition be treated?

    A. Thoracentesis
    B. Immediate needle decompression and chest tube placement
    C. Gentamicin
    D. Treat the underlying cause

    - **The correct answer is A.**
    - Notice that the patient has an exudative pleural effusion due to systemic lupus.
    - She is an African American woman, she has a maculopapular rash (red rash), and she has a history of arthritis.
    - She also has signs of a pleural effusion.
    - She has progressive dyspnea, a nonproductive cough, and orthopnea.
    - She also presents with decreased breath sounds, dullness on percussion, and decreased fremitus.
    - Other evidence of pleural effusion in the question is the high protein level.
    - From these clues, we can determine that the correct answer is thoracentesis.
    - Exudative pleural effusion presents with an increased protein content, is caused by collagen vascular disease (such as SLE), and is treated with thoracentesis.
    - B is wrong because this is the treatment option for a tension pneumothorax.
    - Tension pneumothorax presents with decreased breath sounds and decreased fremitus, like pleural effusion, but with hyperresonance on percussion.
    - C is wrong because this is treatment for lobar pneumonia.
    - Gentamicin is a fluoroquinolone antibiotic used to treat lobar pneumonia caused by *Legionalla*.
    - Lobar pneumonia presents with dullness on percussion, bronchial breath sounds, and increased fremitus.
    - D is wrong because this is treatment for transudative pleural effusion.
    - Transudative pleural effusion does not present with high protein levels.

Section XVIII - Pneumothorax

I. Pneumothorax
   A. Presence of air in pleural cavity between visceral and parietal pleura

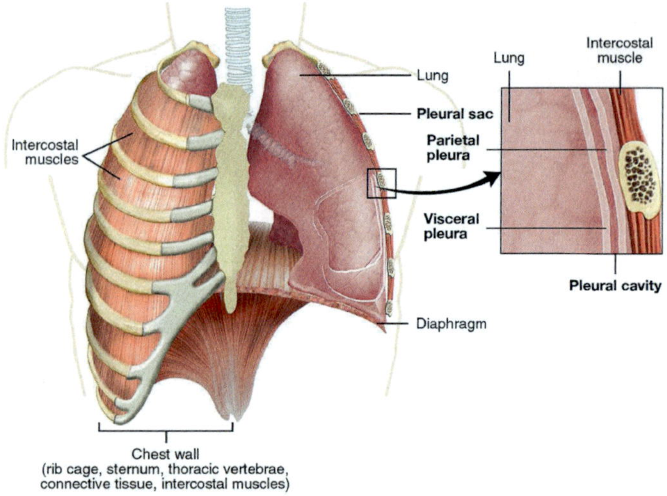

Photo Credit: https://commons.wikimedia.org/wiki/File:2313_The_Lung_Pleurea.jpg

FIGURE 10.6.72 - Anatomy of Pleural Space

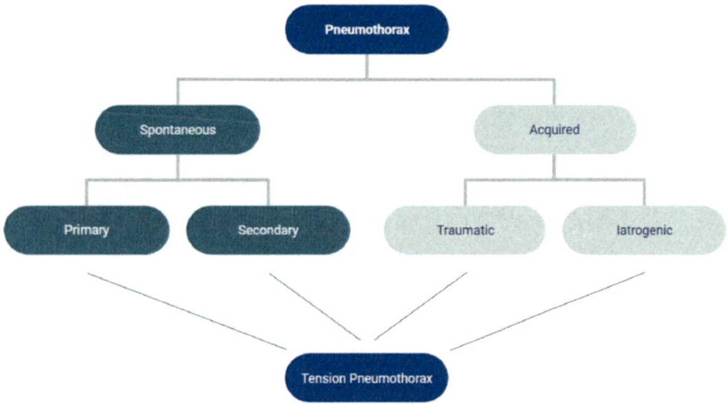

FIGURE 10.6.78 - Types of Pneumothorax

II. Primary Spontaneous Pneumothorax (PSP)
   A. Occurs without a pre-existing lung disease
   B. Classic presentation: Tall, thin young male
   C. More common in smokers

III. Secondary Spontaneous Pneumothorax (SSP)
   A. Occurs due to a pre-existing lung disease
   B. Obstructive airway disease (COPD, emphysema)
   C. Connective tissue disease (Marfan, Ehlers-Danlos)
   D. Mechanical ventilation (PEEP)
   E. Infection (abscess)
   F. Interstitial lung disease (sarcoidosis)
   G. Scuba diving
   H. Thoracic endometriosis (catamenial pneumothorax)
   I. Malignancy

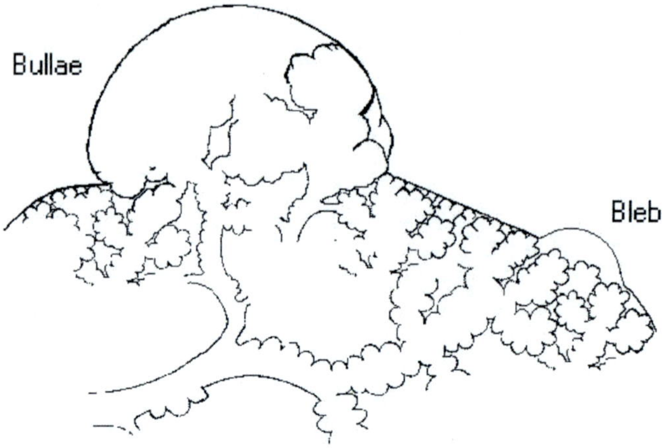

Photo Credit: https://commons.wikimedia.org/wiki/File:Pneumot_rax_bullae.JPG

FIGURE 10.6.79 - Diagram of Bulla and Bleb

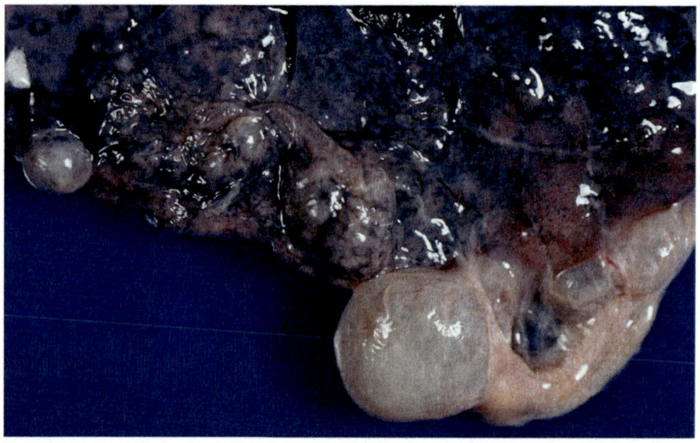

Photo Credit: https://commons.wikimedia.org/wiki/File:Emphysema,_bullous,_subpleural_(4563271452).jpg

FIGURE 10.6.80 - Gross Pathology of a Subpleural Bulla

IV. Spontaneous Pneumothorax: Pathophysiology
   A. Spontaneous rupture of apical subpleural bleb, cyst, bullae
   B. Air from lungs leaks into the pleural space changing negative pressure into positive
   C. Loss of lung volume and increase in pleural space pressure cause a portion or all of lung to collapse
   D. Trachea may deviate to same side of collapsed lung (spontaneous = same side)

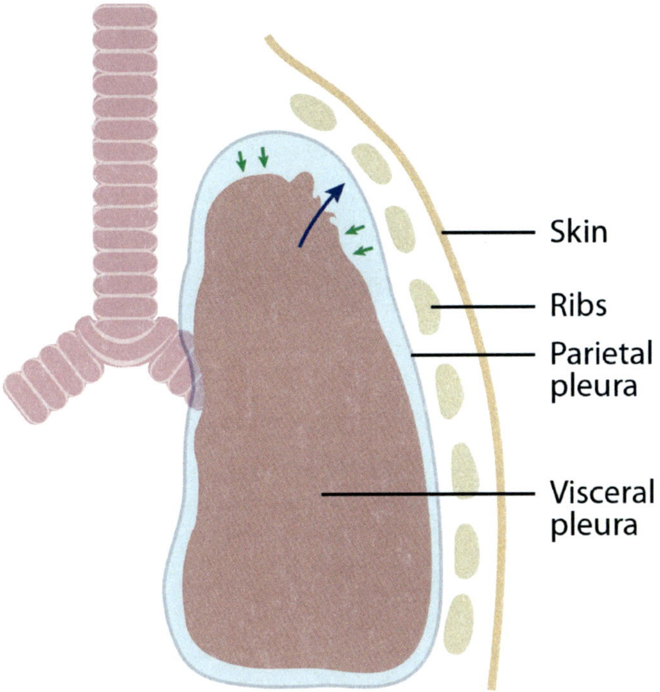

FIGURE 10.6.81 - Pathophysiology of a Apontaneous Pneumothorax

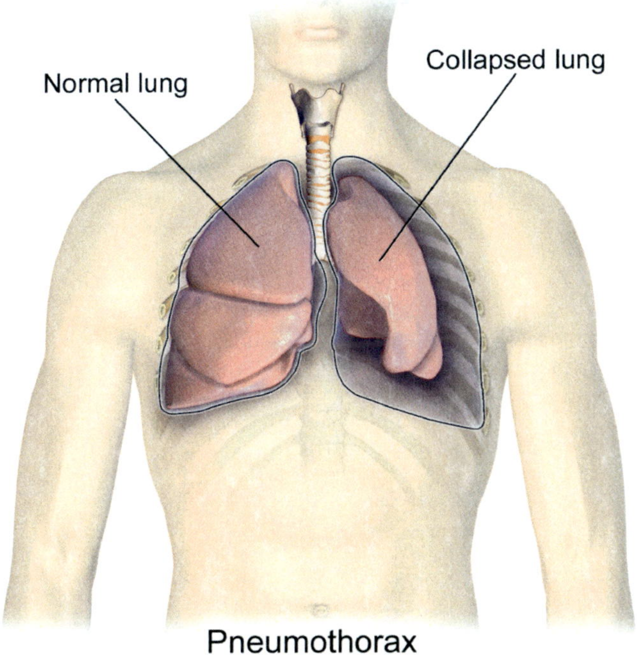

Photo Credit: https://commons.wikimedia.org/wiki/File:Blausen_0742_Pneumothorax.png

FIGURE 10.6.82 Normal Lung (Right) vs. Atelectasis (Left)

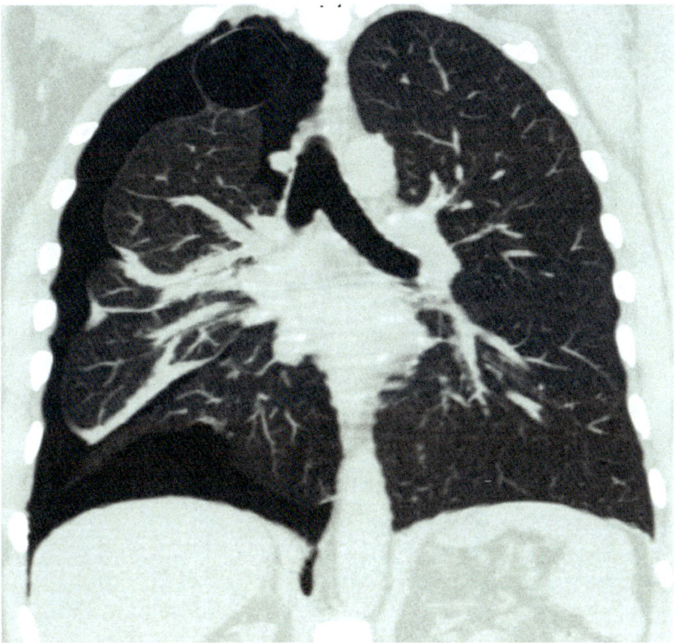

Photo Credit: https://commons.wikimedia.org/wiki/File:Pneumot%C3%B3rax_espont%C3%A2neo.png

FIGURE 10.6.83 - T Scan of Apical Bulla (Right) Resulting in Atelectasis

V. Traumatic Pneumothorax
   A. Pneumothorax due to trauma
   B. Blunt or closed: intact skin
   C. Penetrating or open: open skin

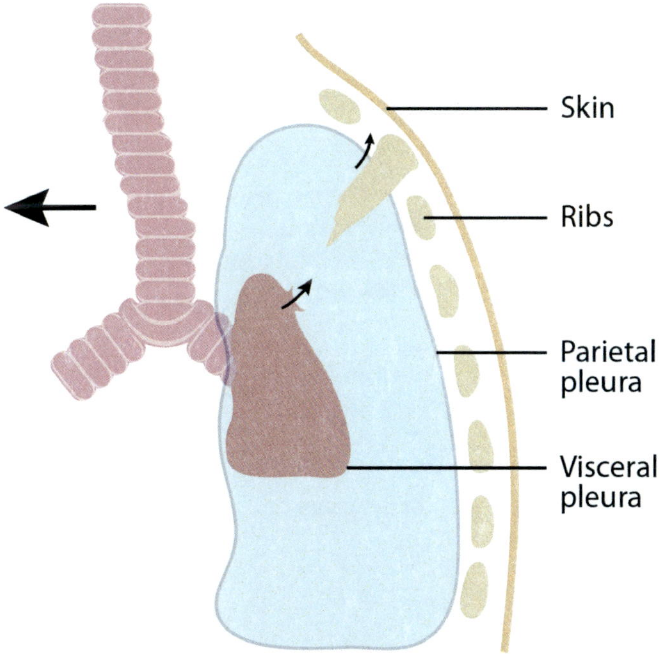

FIGURE 10.6.84 - Pathophysiology of Closed Traumatic Pneumothorax

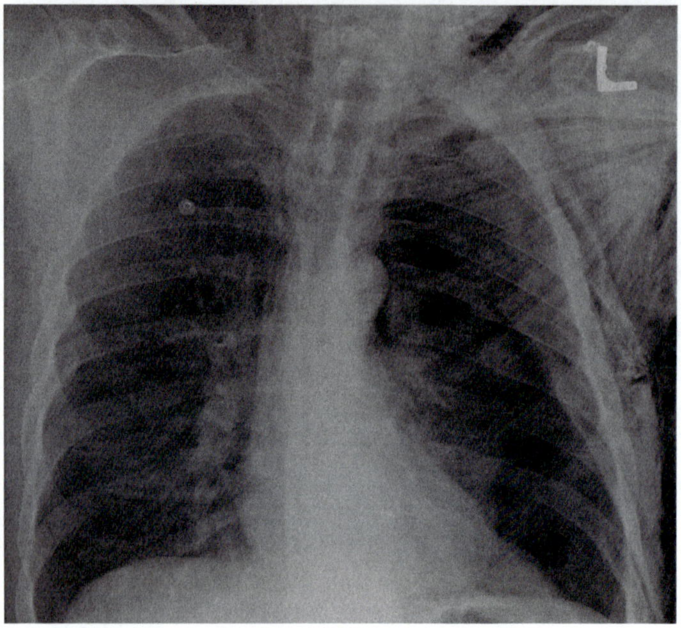

Photo Credit: https://commons.wikimedia.org/wiki/File:Tpneumopneumomed.png

FIGURE 10.6.85 - Rib Fractures Causing Pneumothorax

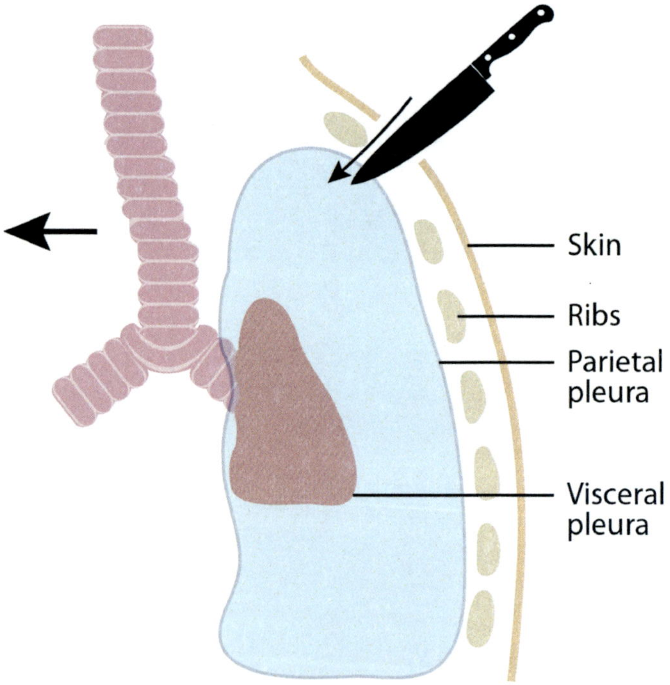

FIGURE 10.6.86 - Pathophysiology of Open Traumatic Pneumothorax

VI. Iatrogenic Pneumothorax
   A. Pneumothorax due to invasive diagnostic or therapeutic interventions
   B. Needle-related (central venous catheter placement, transthoracic needle aspiration, thoracocentesis, lung biopsy)
   C. Tube-related (tracheostomy, bronchoscopy, NG tube, mechanical ventilation)

VII. Tension Pneumothorax
   A. Pneumothorax that causes physical disruption of visceral and parietal pleura and tracheobronchial tree

VIII. Tension Pneumothorax: Etiology
   A. Spontaneous pneumothorax
   B. Traumatic pneumothorax
   C. Acquired pneumothorax

IX. Tension Pneumothorax: Pathophysiology
   A. One-way valve
   B. Air enters the pleural space on inspiration but cannot leave on expiration
   C. IIncrease in intrapleural pressure collapses the lung (compression atelectasis), leading to reduced vital capacity (VC) of lung
   D. Collapsed lung coupled with mass effect shifts trachea away (keep tension away)
   E. If mediastinum shifts to the right, it bends the IVC, which reduces venous return and cardiac output, causing obstructive shock
   F. Hypotension and respiratory and cardiac arrest ensues, which can be fatal

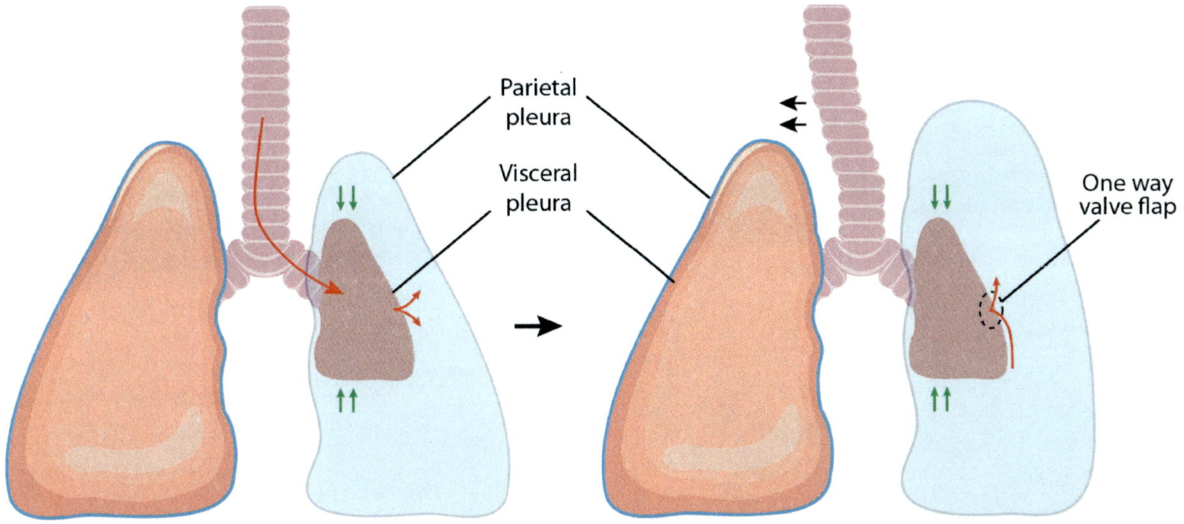

FIGURE 10.6.87 - Pathophysiology of Tension Pneumothorax

X. Pneumothorax: Findings
   A. Sudden pleuritic chest pain
   B. Dyspnea
   C. Flail chest (uneven rise/fall with respiration)
   D. Hyperresonant to percussion
   E. Diminished breath sounds on auscultation
   F. Tactile fremitus decreased
   G. Hemodynamic instability: pulsus paradoxus, tachycardia, Beck's triad (distended neck veins, distant heart sounds, hypotension)
   H. Cyanosis

XI. Pneumothorax: Diagnosis
   A. Upright chest X-ray
   B. CT scan if needed

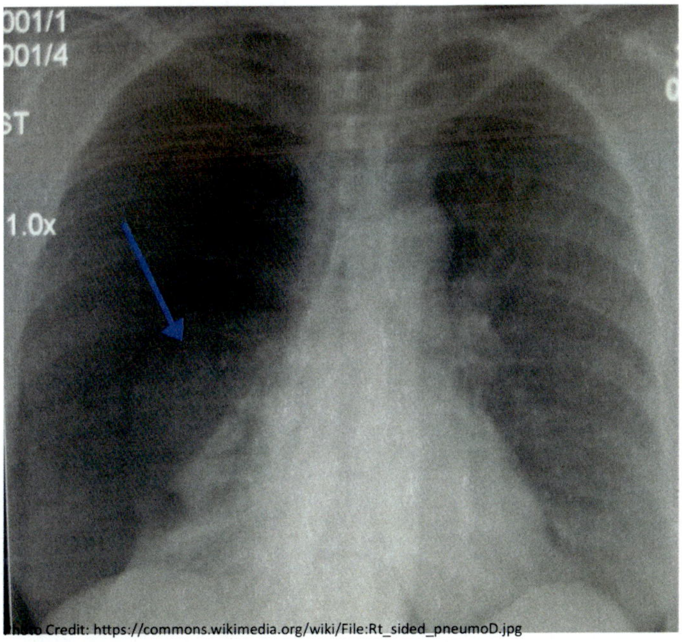

Photo Credit: https://commons.wikimedia.org/wiki/File:Rt_sided_pneumoD.jpg

FIGURE 10.6.88 - X-ray Showing Pneumothorax (Blue Arrow)

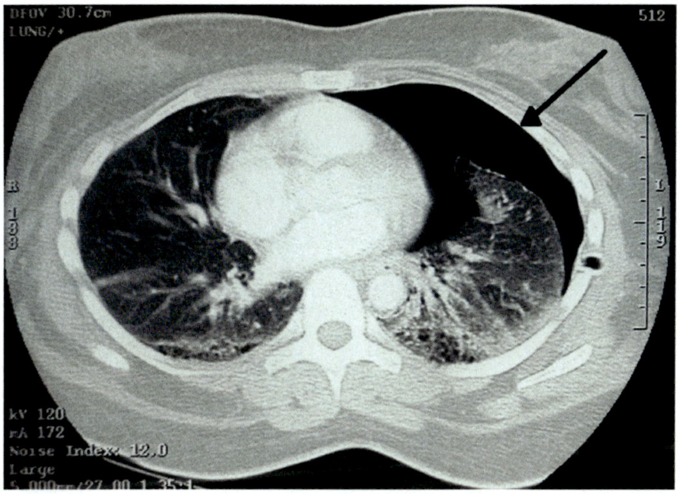

Photo Credit: https://commons.wikimedia.org/wiki/File:Pneumothorax_CT.jpg

FIGURE 10.6.89 - CT of Left-Sided Pneumothorax

XII. Pneumothorax: Treatment
   A. If small (<2 cm), observe, monitor with CXR
   B. If large, perform needle decompression followed by tube thoracostomy (chest tube placement)

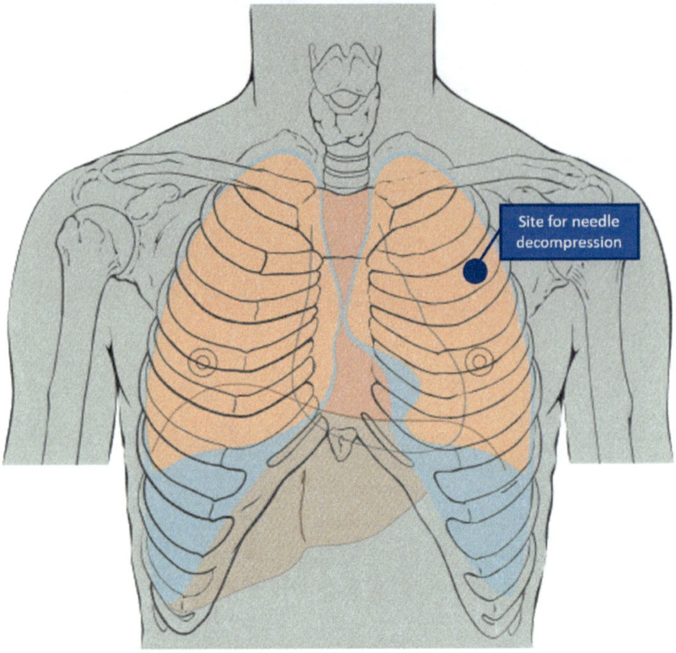

Photo Credit: https://commons.wikimedia.org/wiki/File:Thoracic_landmarks_anterior_view.svg

FIGURE 10.6.90 - Site of Needle Decompression

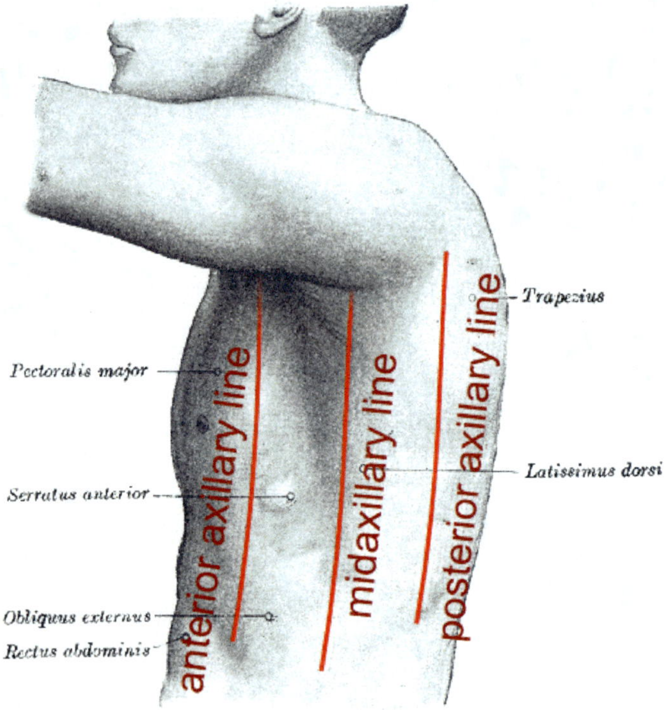

Photo Credit: https://commons.wikimedia.org/wiki/File:Axillary_lines.png

FIGURE 10.6.91 - Site of Chest Tube Placement

REVIEW QUESTIONS

1. A 25-year-old soldier is shot in the chest in a battlefield. The medic notices that the bullet narrowly missed the heart on the left side. The soldier is having difficulty breathing. The rise and fall of the left side of the chest is not matching with the right side of the chest. Jugular venous distension is noted and pulses are getting weaker. There are no breath sounds on the left side of the chest. What is the diagnosis?

   A. Spontaneous pneumothorax
   B. Cardiac tamponade
   C. Right-sided heart failure
   D. Tension pneumothorax

- **The correct answer is D.**
- The patient took a bullet that penetrated the thoracic cavity and disrupted the pleural space. The patient has dyspnea, a flail chest, and jugular venous distention. The JVD is indicative of impaired venous return, possibly due to obstruction of inferior vena cava. Pulses are getting weaker and there are no breath sounds on the left side of the chest. Together, this presentation indicates a pneumothorax.
- In a tension pneumothorax, air entering the lung escapes to the pleural cavity and is unable to get back in the lung parenchyma. The hole acts as one-way valve that causes a buildup of intrapleural pressure that compresses and collapses the lung. This results in the trachea deviating away from the collapsed lung.
- A is incorrect because the pneumothorax did not occur spontaneously but due to the trauma of a gunshot wound.
- B is incorrect because in cardiac tamponade, breath sounds are normal bilaterally even though a patient may have jugular venous distention and hypotension.
- C is incorrect because right-sided heart failure is a chronic process that arises primarily due to left-sided heart failure or a pulmonary pathology, such as pulmonary hypertension.

Section XIX - Pneumonia

I. Pathophysiology
   A. Infection of pulmonary parenchyma
      1. Lungs sterile below first major bronchial division
   B. Pulmonary defense mechanisms
      1. Turbulence and abrupt changes of airflow in nasal passages
      2. Mucociliary escalator
      3. Resident alveolar macrophages
   C. Disruption of pulmonary defense mechanisms → pneumonia
   D. Factors that compromise pulmonary defense mechanisms
      1. Loss or suppression of cough reflex (comatose, anesthetized)
      2. Mucociliary escalator injury (viral infection, smoking, genetic)
      3. Accumulation of secretions (bronchial obstruction, cystic fibrosis)
      4. Acute injury to the lung (trauma)

II. Clinical Features
   A. Fever and chills (IL-1 and TNF)
   B. Peripheral leukocytosis and ↑ total leukocyte count
   C. Productive cough and hemoptysis
   D. Hypoxemia → tachypnea, pleuritic chest pain, and dyspnea
   E. Auscultation: decreased breath sounds and crackles
   F. Dullness to percussion
   G. CXR: radiographic infiltrate

III. Diagnosis
   A. CBC: neutrophilic leukocytosis
   B. Sputum gram stain and culture
   C. Blood culture
   D. CXR (gold standard): lobar opacification or patchy infiltrates

IV. Classification
   A. Lobar pneumonia
   B. Bronchopneumonia
   C. Interstitial (atypical) pneumonia

Types	Features	Etiology
Lobar pneumonia	- Diffuse inflammation → consolidation of an entire lobe - CXR: lobar consolidation	- *Streptococcus pneumoniae* - *Klebsiella pneumoniae* (red currant jelly sputum) - Memory aid: -pneumo
Bronchopneumonia	- Infection of terminal bronchioles → widespread focal/patchy consolidation of many lobules - CXR: patchy consolidations scattered throughout lung	- *Pseudomonas aeruginosa* - *Haemophilus influenzae* - *Legionella pneumophila* - *Moraxella catarrhalis* - *Staphylococcus aureus* - Memory aid: PHLegMS
Interstitial (atypical, walking) pneumonia	- Infection of interstitial lung tissue - Causative organisms not usually gram stainable or culturable - Minimal alveolar exudate	- *Mycoplasma pneumoniae* (most common) - *Influenza pneumoniae* (elderly, immunosuppressed) - *Chlamydia pneumoniae* (2nd most common) - *Cytomegalovirus* (post-transplant) - *Coxiella burnetii* (Q fever) - Respiratory syncytial virus (RSV) - Memory aid: MICRo

TABLE 10.6.5 - Anatomical Classification of Pneumonia

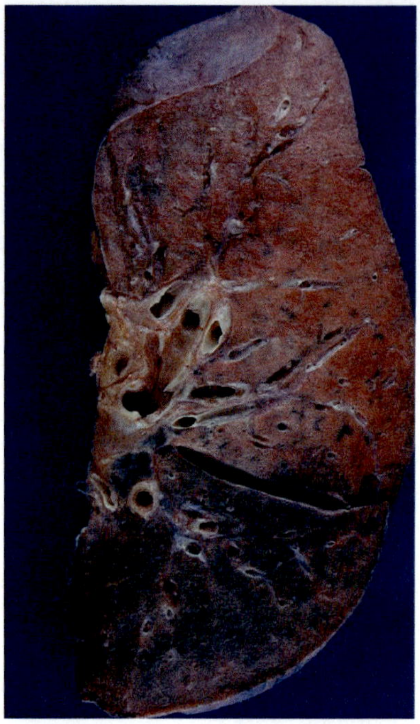

Photo Credit: Yale Rosen [CC BY-SA (https://creativecommons.org/licenses/by-sa/2.0)]

FIGURE 10.6.92 - Lobar Pneumonia

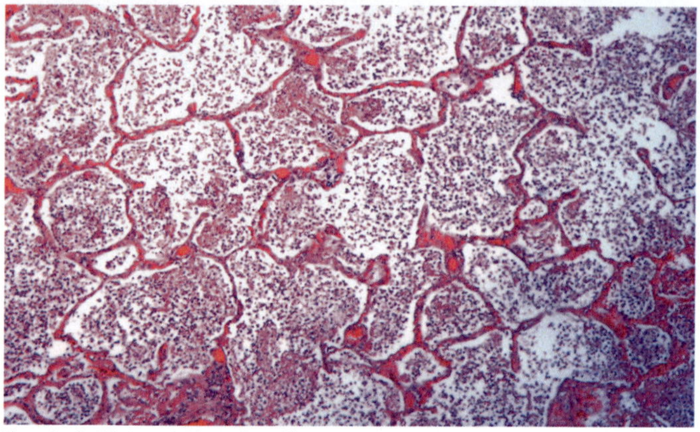

Photo Credit: Yale Rosen [CC BY-SA (https://creativecommons.org/licenses/by-sa/2.0)]

FIGURE 10.6.95 - Congestion Phase of Lobar Pneumonia

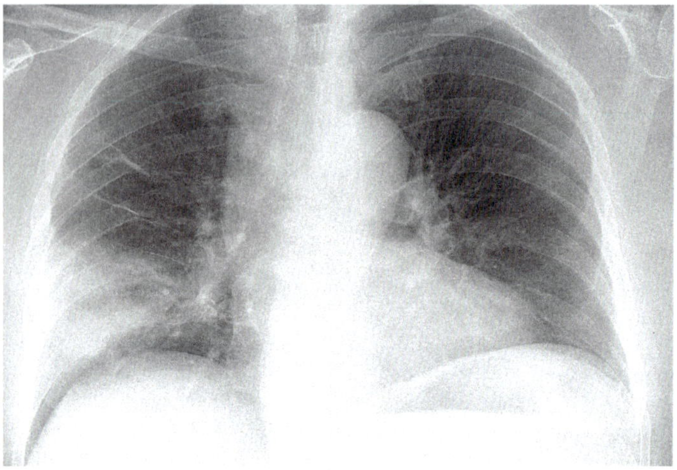

Photo Credit: Mikael Häggström, M.D. - Author info - Reusing images Written informed consent was obtained from the individual, including online publication. [CC0]

FIGURE 10.6.93 - Chest X-Ray of Lobar Pneumonia

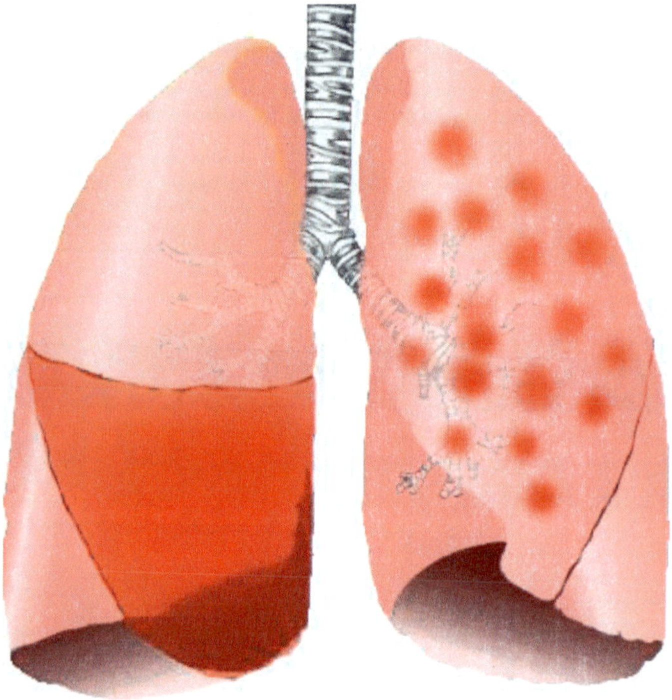

Photo Credit: Suraj at Malayalam Wikipedia [Public domain]

FIGURE 10.6.96 - Lobar Pneumonia (Right Lung) and Bronchopneumonia (Left Lung)

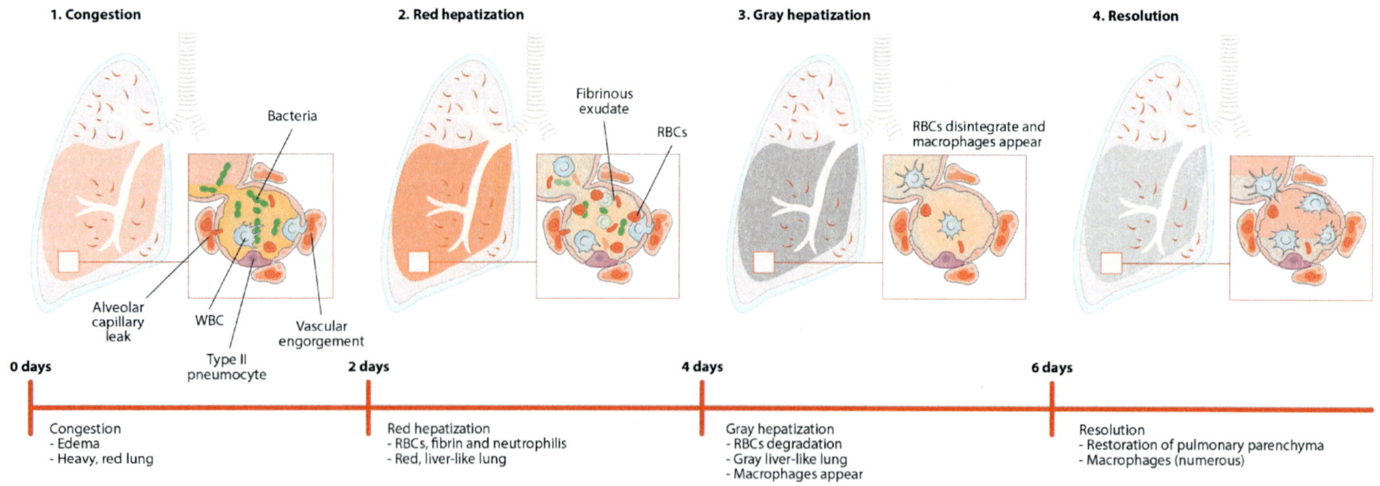

FIGURE 10.6.94 - 4 Classic Inflammatory Phases of Lobar Pneumonia

V. Cryptogenic Organizing Pneumonia
   A. Formerly known as bronchiolitis obliterans organizing pneumonia (BOOP)
   B. Rare, noninfectious pneumonia of unknown etiology
   C. Ages 50-60
   D. Cough and dyspnea
   E. Inflammation of bronchioles and small airways → plugging
   F. Alone or secondary to connective tissue disease, medication (e.g. amiodarone), or malignancy
   G. Treatment: corticosteroids

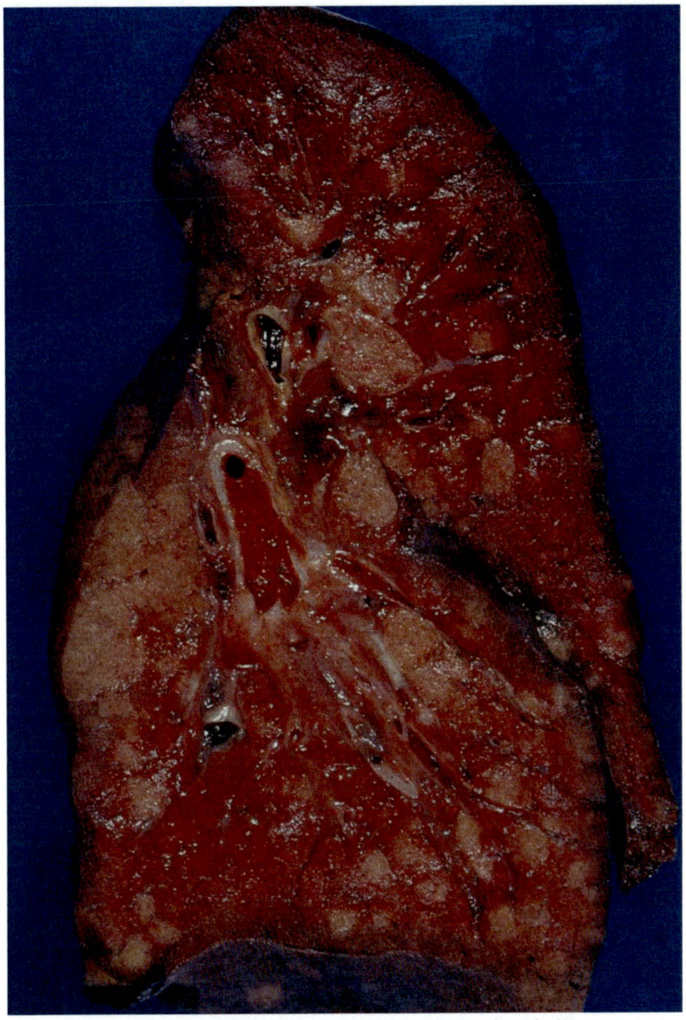

Photo Credit: Yale Rosen [CC BY-SA (https://creativecommons.org/licenses/by-sa/2.0)]

FIGURE 10.6.97 - Bronchopneumonia

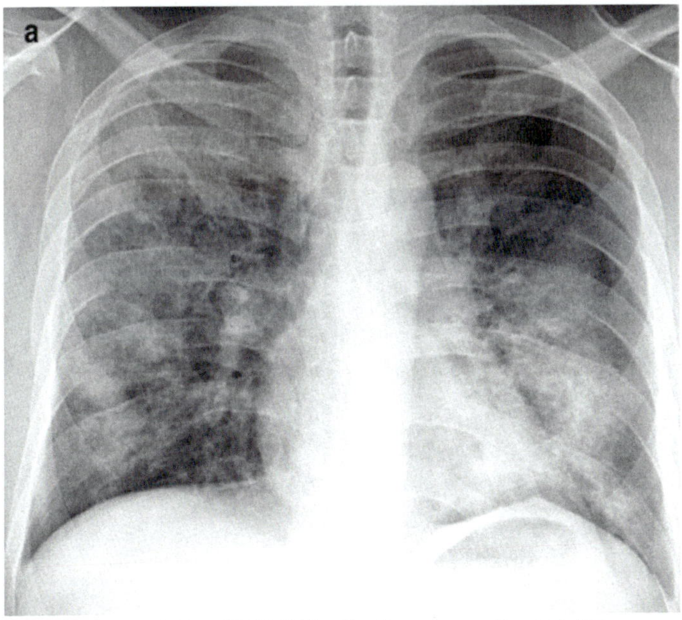

Photo Credit: Franquet T., Chung J.H. / CC BY (https://creativecommons.org/licenses/by/4.0)

FIGURE 10.6.98 - Chest X-Ray of Bronchopneumonia

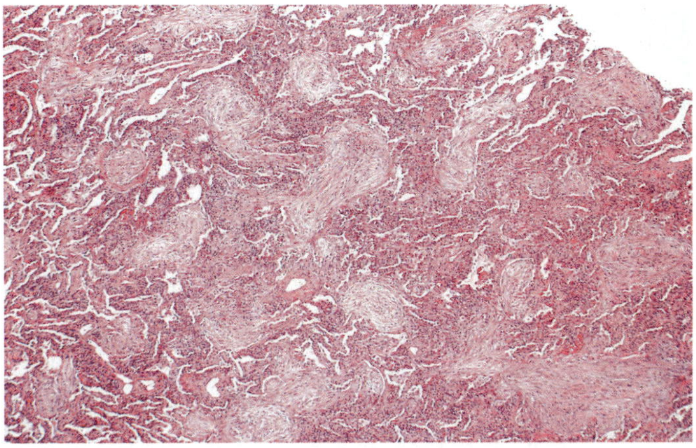

Photo Credit: Yale Rosen [CC BY-SA (https://creativecommons.org/licenses/by-sa/2.0)]

FIGURE 10.6.99 - Cryptogenic Organizing Pneumonia

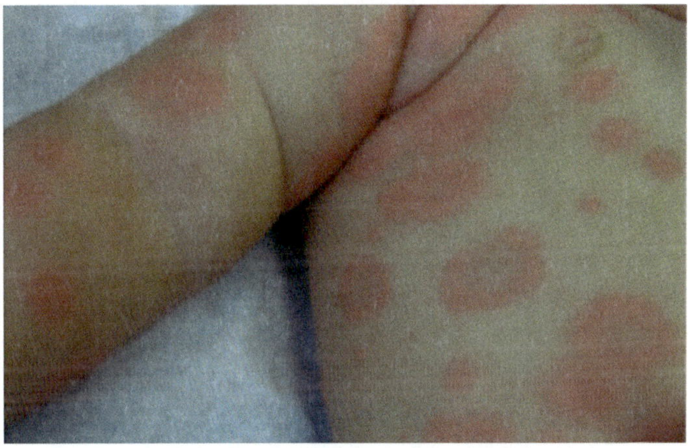

Photo Credit: Grook Da Oger / CC BY-SA (https://creativecommons.org/licenses/by-sa/3.0)

FIGURE 10.6.100 - Erythema Multiforme

Association	Characteristics	Organisms
Secondary pneumonia	- Primary viral infection → secondary bacterial infection	- *Streptococcus pneumoniae* - *Staphylococcus aureus*
Aspiration pneumonia	- Aspiration of gastric contents - Due to unconsciousness or vomiting - Common in alcoholics, comatose patients, and patients with difficulty swallowing - Necrotizing and fulminant	- Anaerobes: *Bacteroides, Fusobacterium, Peptococcus*
Cystic fibrosis	- Autosomal recessive mutation of CFTR gene - Mucus plugs → pneumonia	- *Pseudomonas aeruginosa*
Erythema multiforme	- Targetoid skin lesion - Others: HSV-1, medications	- *Mycoplasma pneumoniae*

TABLE 10.6.6 - Important Associations for Pneumonia

REVIEW QUESTIONS

1. A 65-year-old male presents to the office with shortness of breath and a fever. A chest X-ray reveals consolidation in the right middle lobe. Despite aggressive measures, the patient suddenly dies. An autopsy is performed and microscopy of the alveoli reveals an abundance of red blood cells, fibrin, and neutrophils, but no macrophages. Leading up to the time of death, how many days had it most likely been since the patient developed pneumonia?

- **The answer is 4 days.**
- An abundance of RBCs, fibrin, and neutrophils occurs as part of red hepatization around 4 days following infection.
- The absence of macrophages means we haven't yet reached day 6 or beyond.

2. A 24-year-old man presents with complaints of a headache, myalgias, a nonproductive cough, and a rash. Respiratory examination reveals dullness to percussion and inspiratory crackles on auscultation. A maculopapular rash of targetoid appearance is noted on the extremities and torso. The patient denies the use of any medications. Which of the following microbes is the most likely cause of his symptoms?

   A. *Pseudomonas aeruginosa*
   B. *Staphylococcus aureus*
   C. *Fusobacterium necrophorum*
   D. *Mycoplasma pneumoniae*

- **The correct answer is D.**
- This patient has classic findings of pneumonia, like cough, dullness to percussion, and inspiratory crackles. A maculopapular rash of targetoid appearance refers to erythema multiforme, which is associated with *Mycoplasma pneumoniae*.
- There are other causes of erythema multiforme, like herpes simplex virus (HSV) and medications.
- A is incorrect because *Pseudomonas aeruginosa* is a common cause of pneumonia in cystic fibrosis patients but does not cause erythema multiforme.
- B is incorrect because *Staphylococcus aureus* is a common cause of secondary pneumonia but does not explain the targetoid rash.
- C is incorrect because *Fusobacterium* is an anaerobe and is commonly implicated in aspiration pneumonia.

Section XX - Lung Cancer

I. Epidemiology
   A. Lung cancer is the leading cause of cancer death

II. Risk Factors
   A. Smoking/secondhand smoke
   B. Radon
   C. Asbestos
   D. Family history

III. Clinical Findings
   A. Cough
   B. Hemoptysis
   C. Wheezing
   D. Primary: pneumonic "coin" lesion on CXR or noncalcified nodule on CT
   E. Metastasis: multiple lung lesions

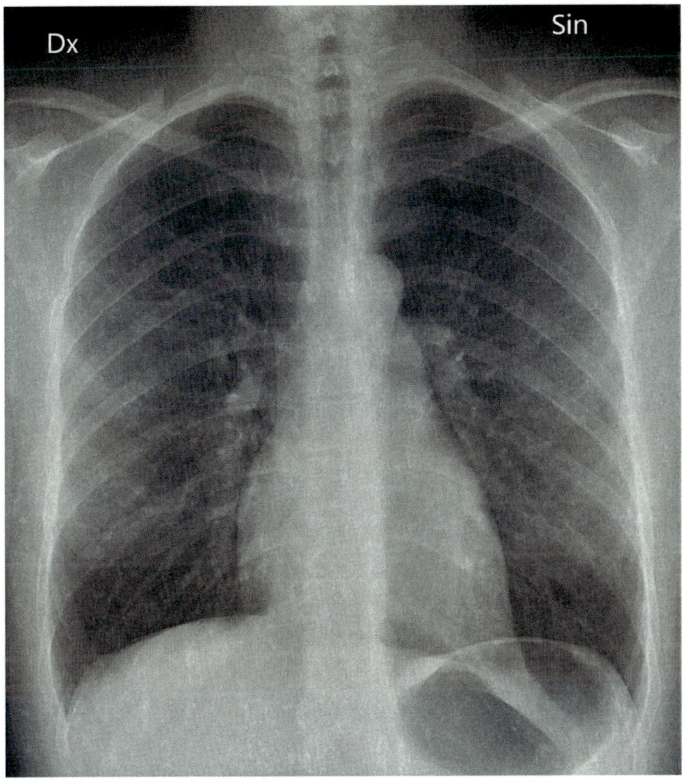

Photo Credit: Mikael Häggström [CC0]

FIGURE 10.6.73 - Normal Chest X-ray

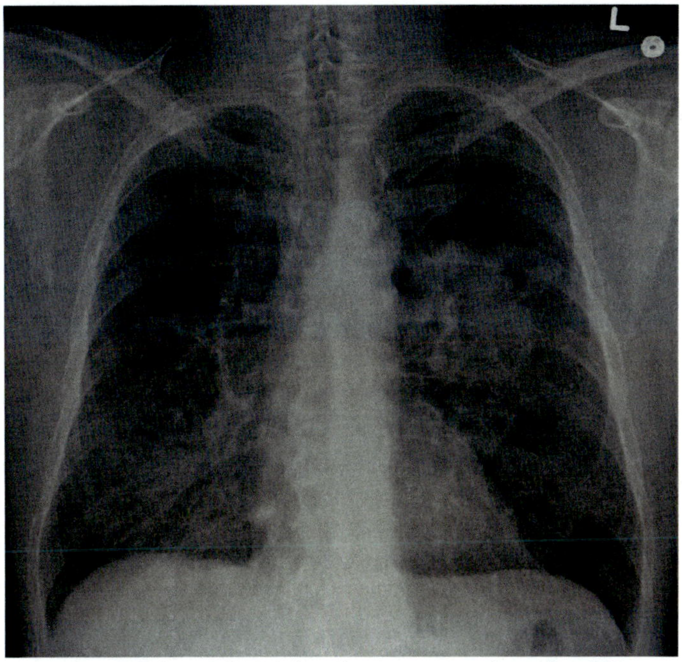

Photo Credit: James Heilman, MD [CC BY-SA (https://creativecommons.org/licenses/by-sa/4.0)]

FIGURE 10.6.101 - Chest X-Ray Showing Coin-Sized Lesion in the Left Lung

IV. Complications
   A. Compression of local structures (e.g. superior vena cava, recurrent laryngeal nerve, stellate ganglion, brachial plexus)

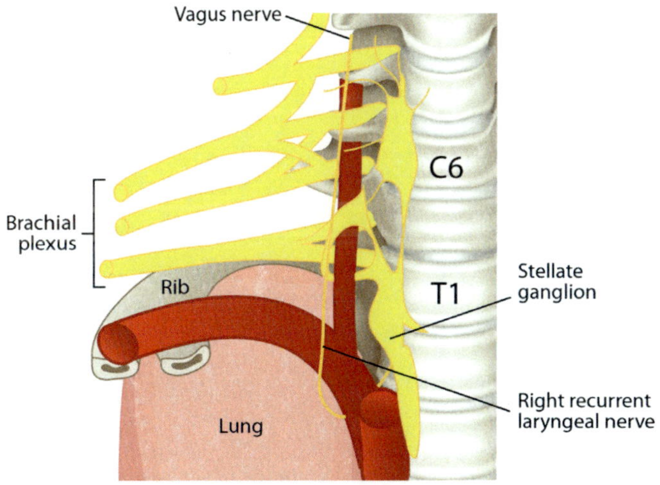

FIGURE 10.6.102 - Anatomy Surrounding the Apex of the Lungs

V. Sites of Metastases
  A. Metastases to lung from breast, colon, pancreas, and bladder
  B. Metastases from lung
    1. Liver → jaundice and hepatomegaly
    2. Bone → pathological fractures
    3. Brain → headaches or seizures
    4. Pleura of lung and pericardium → pericardial or pleural effusion
    5. Adrenal glands

Type	Location	Characteristics	Clinical Associations	Treatment
Small cell carcinoma	Central	- Smokers - Males > females - Undifferentiated - IHC: chromogranin A, neuron-specific enolase, synaptophysin	- Cushing syndrome - Lambert-Eaton myasthenic syndrome (LEMS) - Syndrome of inappropriate antidiuretic hormone (SIADH)	- Chemotherapy Radiation
Adenocarcinoma	Peripheral	- Nonsmokers - Females > males - IHC: mucin	- Hypertrophic osteoarthropathy (digital clubbing)	- Surgery
Squamous cell carcinoma	Central	- Smokers - Hilar mass arising from-bronchus - Cavitation	- Hypercalcemia	- Surgery
Large cell carcinoma	Peripheral	- Smokers - Undifferentiated - Poor prognosis		- Surgery
Bronchial carcinoid tumor	Central or peripheral	- Metastasis rare - Excellent prognosis	- Carcinoid syndrome	- Surgery - Chemotherapy

TABLE 10.6.7 - Main Types of Lung Cancer

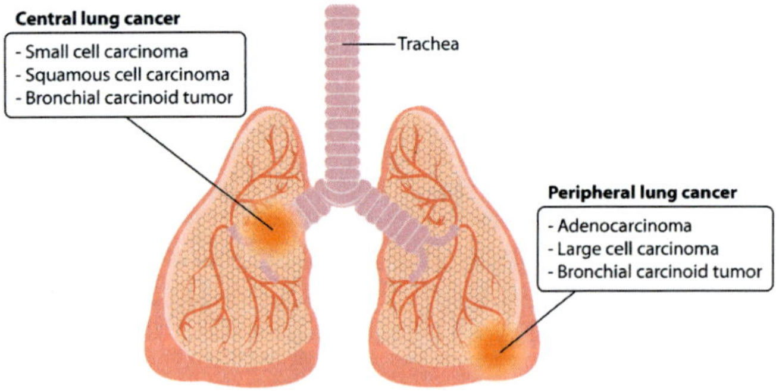

FIGURE 10.6.103 - Location of Various Lung Cancers

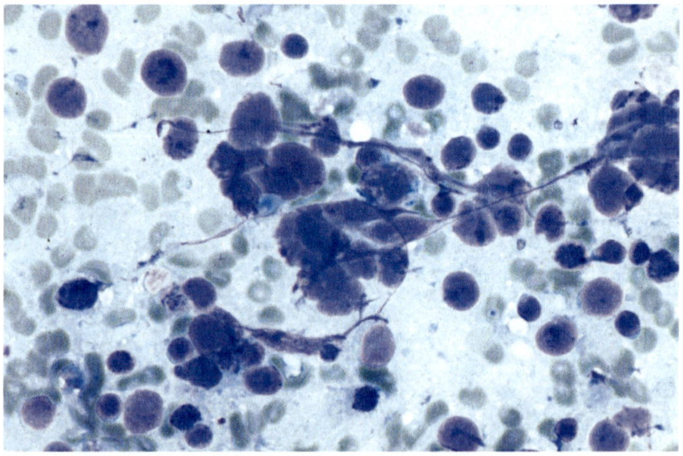

Photo Credit: Nephron [CC BY-SA (https://creativecommons.org/licenses/by-sa/3.0)]

FIGURE 10.6.104 - Kulchitsky Cells

VI. Cushing Syndrome
   A. Excess cortisol
   B. Muscle weakness
   C. Moon facies, buffalo hump, and truncal obesity with thin extremities
   D. Abdominal striae
   E. Hypertension with hypokalemia and metabolic alkalosis
   F. Elevated ACTH not suppressed by administration of dexamethasone

VII. Lambert-Eaton Myasthenic Syndrome (LEMS)
   A. Autoantibodies against presynaptic Ca^{2+} channels
   B. Impaired acetylcholine release
   C. Proximal muscle weakness that improves with use
   D. Resolves with resection of cancer

VIII. Syndrome of Inappropriate ADH (SIADH)
   A. Excess ADH secretion
   B. Hyponatremia and low serum osmolality
   C. Mental status changes and seizures

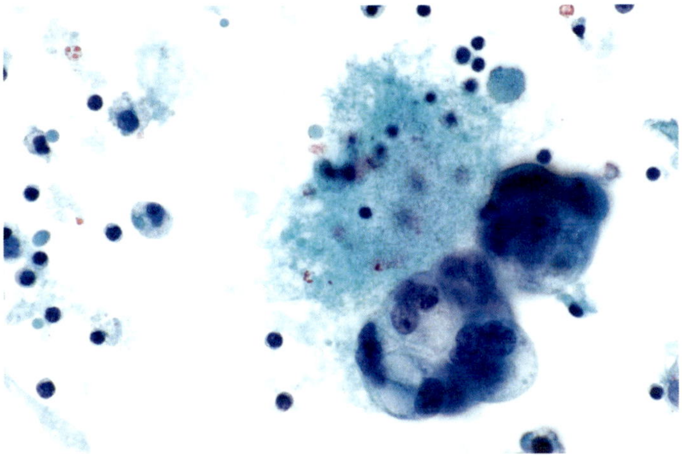

FIGURE 10.6.105 - Micrograph of Adenocarcinoma

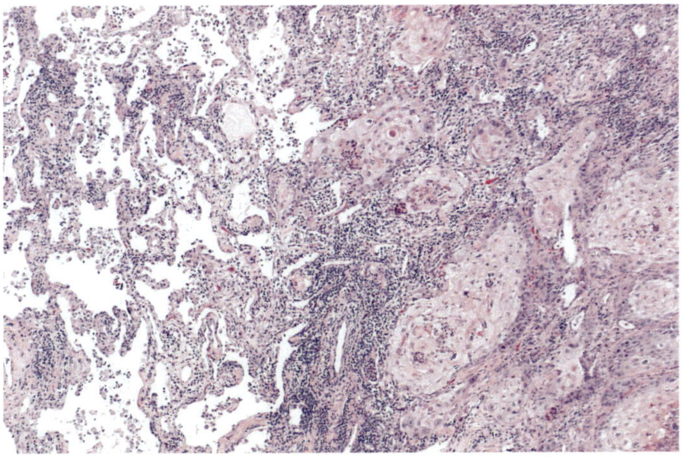

FIGURE 10.6.106 - Small Cell Carcinoma

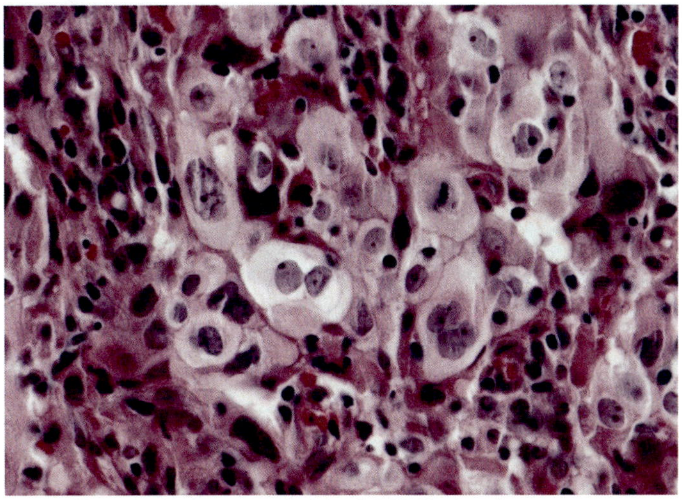

FIGURE 10.6.107 - Large Cell Carcinoma with Pleomorphic Giant Cells

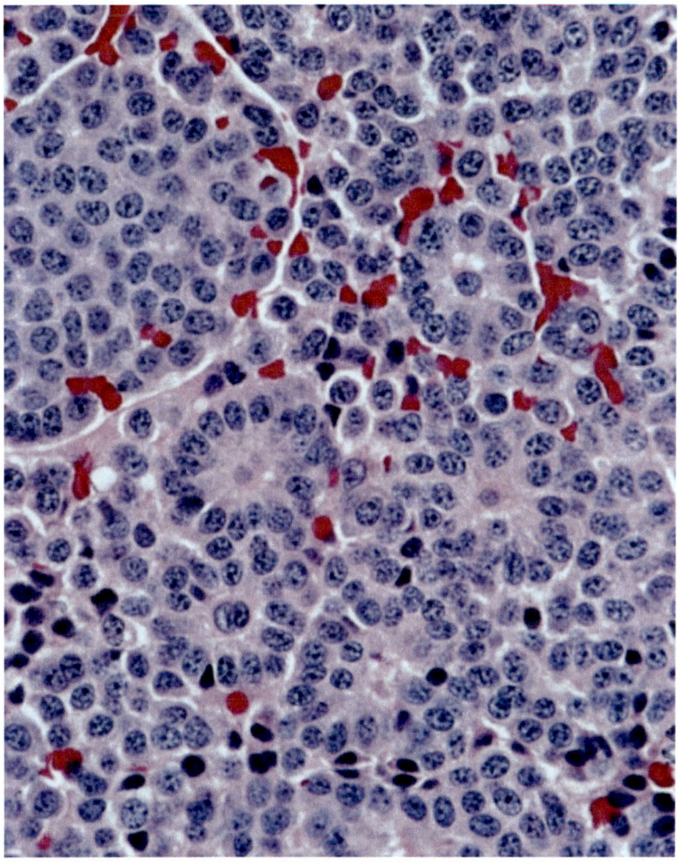

FIGURE 10.6.108 - Carcinoid Tumor

REVIEW QUESTIONS

1. A 50-year-old man with a 30 pack-year smoking history presents with progressive dyspnea, decreased proximal strength, and scattered ecchymoses. Physical examination reveals darkening of the skin, a round face, hyperglycemia, and decreased breath sounds on auscultation. A chest X-ray reveals a lung mass in the right lower lobe. Serum cortisol level is elevated and is not suppressed following the administration of dexamethasone. ACTH is also elevated. What is the most likely cause of the elevated ACTH?

    A. Exogenous steroids
    B. Large cell carcinoma
    C. Small cell carcinoma
    D. Pituitary adenoma

- **The correct answer is C.**
- This patient has decreased proximal strength, scattered ecchymoses, darkening of the skin, a round face, hyperglycemia, and elevated cortisol levels. These symptoms are indicative of Cushing syndrome. The patient also has progressive dyspnea, decreased breath sounds on auscultation, and a right lower lung mass, which all points to lung cancer. The ACTH is elevated and not suppressed following administration of dexamethasone, which means the ACTH is being secreted by an ectopic source. The only lung cancer that secretes ACTH is small cell carcinoma, which is associated with SIADH and Cushing syndrome.
- A is incorrect because if our patient were overusing steroids, ACTH would be low and not elevated.
- B is incorrect because large cell lung carcinoma is not associated with Cushing syndrome.
- D is incorrect because if the patient had a pituitary adenoma, ACTH levels would be suppressed by a dexamethasone test.

Section XXII - Lung Abscess

I. Definition
   A. Liquefactive necrosis of lung parenchyma due to microbial infection
   B. Collection of pus within the lung

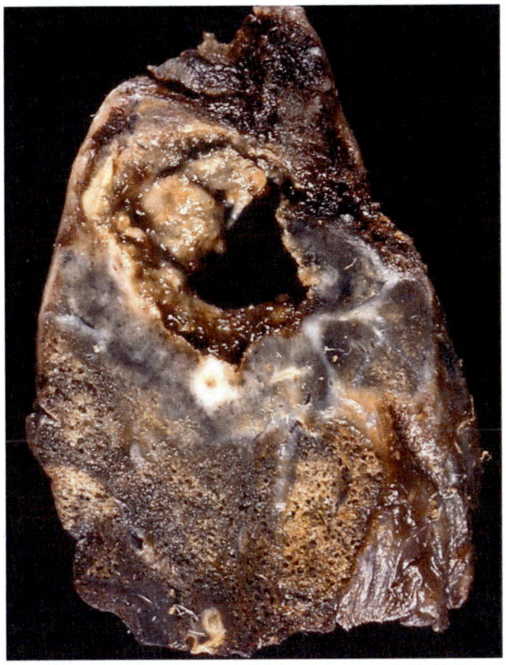

Photo Credit: https://commons.wikimedia.org/wiki/File:Lung_abscess_(7468374664).jpg

FIGURE 10.6.109 - Lung Abscess

II. Presentation and Findings
   A. Productive cough with foul-smelling sputum
   B. Fever
   C. Night sweats
   D. Weight loss
   E. Crackles on auscultation
   F. CXR: cavitary lesion with air-fluid level

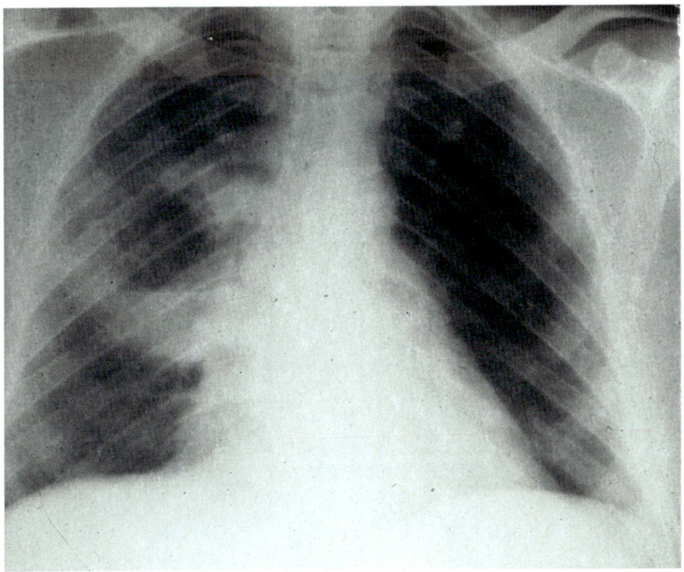

Photo Credit: https://www.flickr.com/photos/pulmonary_pathology/7468374820

FIGURE 10.6.110 - Chest X-Ray Showing Lung Abscess

III. Causes
   A. Aspiration
   B. Bacterial pneumonia
   C. Bacteremia or infective endocarditis
   D. Other (e.g. bronchial obstruction, tuberculosis)

IV. Causes: Aspiration
   A. Most common cause of lung abscess
   B. Caused by a combination of normal anaerobic flora of the mouth (*Peptostreptococcus*, *Fusobacterium*, *Bacteroides*) and aerobic organisms (*Streptococcus*)
   C. Increased risk with loss ofconsciousness (alcoholism, epilepsy) or impaired swallowing (neurologic disease, diverticula)
   D. Most often found in the right lung

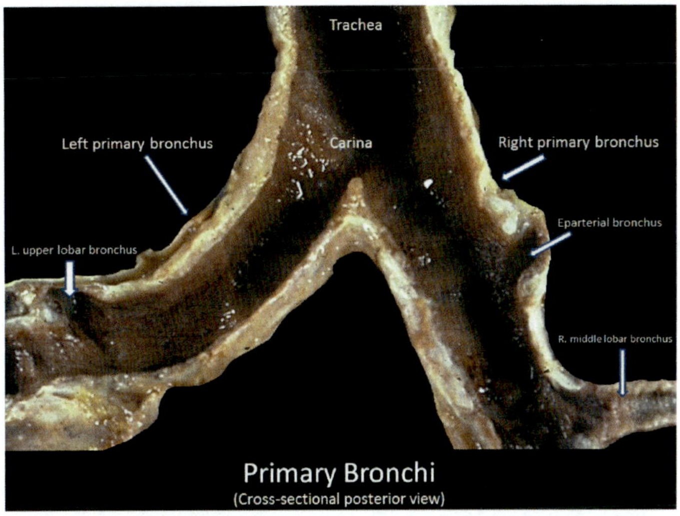

Photo Credit: https://commons.wikimedia.org/wiki/File:Primary_bronchi_cross-sectional_posterior_view.PNG

FIGURE 10.6.111 - Primary Bronchi

   E. If patient is upright, abscess will be in the right lower lobe
   F. If patient is lying down in supine position, abscess will be in the right upper or middle lobes

V. Causes: Bacterial Pneumonia
   A. Commonly caused by *S. aureus*, *E. coli*, *Klebsiella pneumoniae*, or *Pseudomonas aeruginosa*
   B. Occurs in immunosuppressed or elderly patients with underlying lung disease
   C. Often arises in hospitals

VI. Causes: Bacteremia or Infective Endocarditis
   A. Hematogenous spread
   B. Multiple monomicrobial abscesses
   C. Commonly *Staphylococcus* or *Streptococcus*

VII. Causes: Other
   A. Bronchial obstruction: cancers
      1. Post-obstructive pneumonia leads to lung abscess

B. Tuberculosis
   1. Primary: enlarged hilar lymph nodes, Ghon focus in middle/lower lobes (Ghon complex)
   2. Reactivation/secondary: cavitary lesion in apex of lung

Primary Tuberculosis

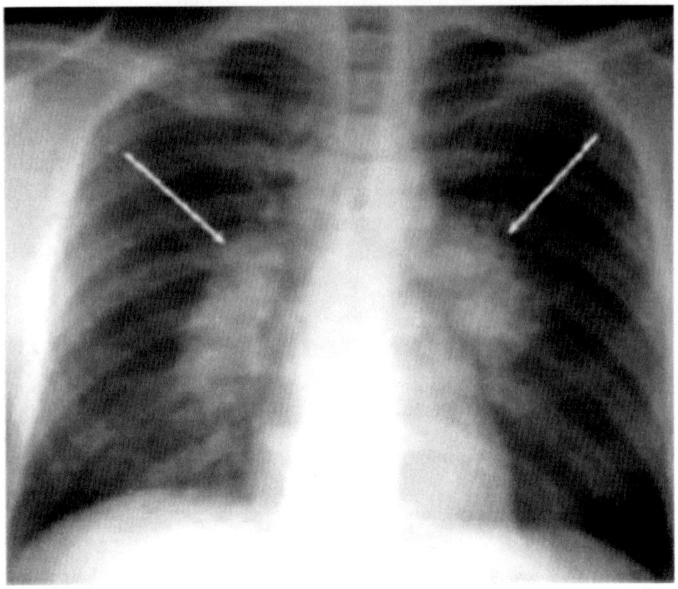

Reactivation Tuberculosis

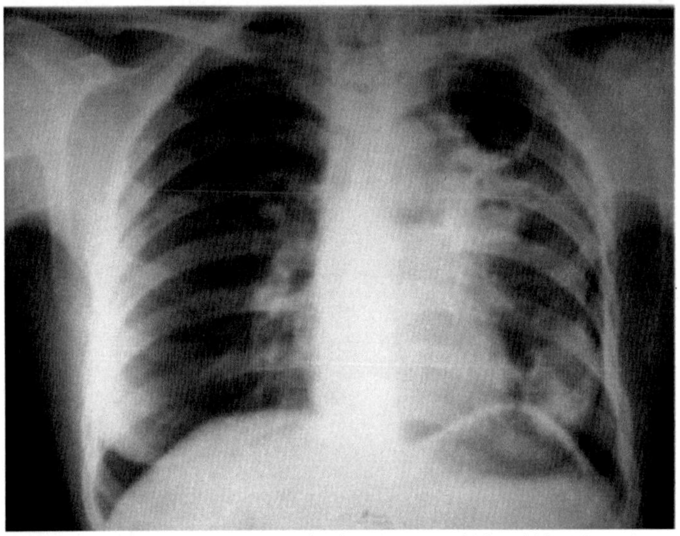

Photo Credit: https://commons.wikimedia.org/wiki/File:Chest_x-ray_of_bilateral_hilar_adenopathy_of_primary_pulmonary_tuberculosis.jpg
https://commons.wikimedia.org/wiki/File:Chest_plain_film._Fibrotic_cavitary_Tuberculosis.jpg

FIGURE 10.6.112 - Chest X-Rays Showing Primary and Reactivation Tuberculosis

VIII. Treatment
   A. IV antibiotics: clindamycin – watch for *C.difficile*
   B. Drainage and surgery if the patient does not respond to antibiotics

REVIEW QUESTIONS

1. A 65-year-old man with a history of dysphagia due to Parkinson's disease presents with a productive cough with thick, foul-smelling sputum for the past 2 weeks. He also complains of night sweats. Physical examination reveals crackles in the right lower lobe of his lung. A chest X-ray reveals a cavitary lesion with an air-liquid interface. Aspiration and culture of the lesion's contents would reveal which of the following bacterial causes?
   A. *Klebsiella pneumoniae*
   B. *Peptostreptococcus* spp.
   C. *Staphylococcus aureus*
   D. *Pseudomonas aeruginosa*
   E. *Mycobacterium tuberculosis*

- **The correct answer is B.**
- This patient has a history of trouble swallowing and has a productive cough with foul-smelling sputum.
- He also has night sweats and crackles on auscultation.
- The chest X-ray shows a cavitary lesion with an air-liquid interface.
- All of these clues should make you think he has a lung abscess.
- His history of trouble swallowing should clue you into aspiration as the probable cause.
- Lung abscesses due to aspiration are usually caused by anaerobes of the normal mouth flora.
- The answer is B, *Peptostreptococcus spp.*, as this is the only anaerobe listed.
- A, C, D, and E are incorrect because these bacteria are not anaerobes that are part of the normal mouth flora.
- *Klebsiella, Staphylococcus aureus,* and *Pseudomonas* are associated with a lung abscess due to bacterial pneumonia.
- *Mycobacterium tuberculosis* is the causative agent of tuberculosis.
- This patient does not have a history or chest X-ray consistent with tuberculosis.

Section XXII - Pancoast Tumor

I. Pancoast Tumor
   A. Carcinoma that occurs in the apex of the lung
   B. Involves the superior sulcus
   C. Complications due to mass effect

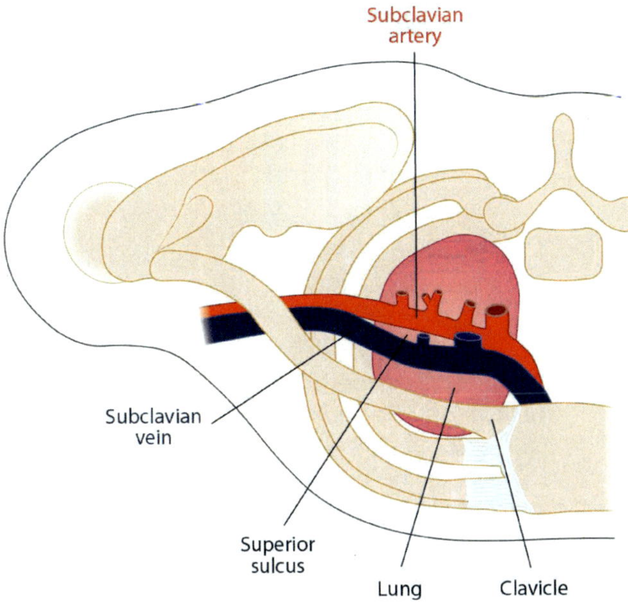

FIGURE 10.6.113 - Transverse Section of Superior Sulcus of Right Lung

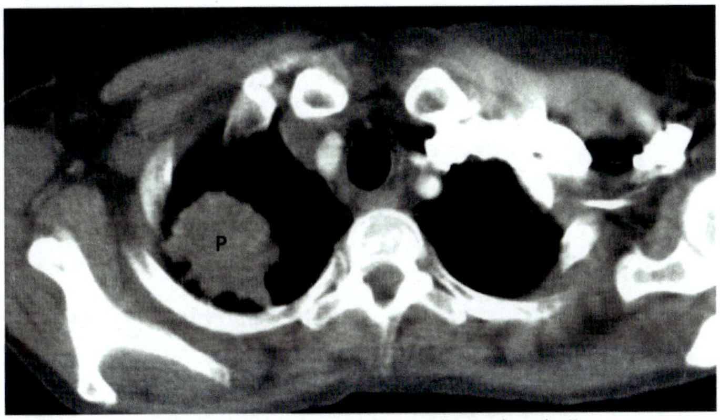

FIGURE 10.6.114 - CT Scan Showing a Pancoast Tumor

II. Complications: Structures Involved
   A. Stellate ganglion
   B. Recurrent laryngeal nerve
   C. Superior vena cava
   D. Brachiocephalic vein
   E. Brachial plexus
   F. Phrenic nerve

III. Complications: Clinical Features

Stellate ganglion → Horner syndrome

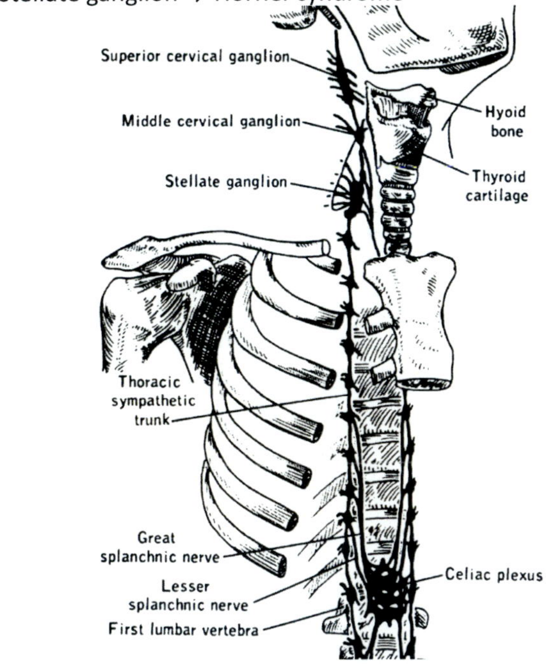

FIGURE 10.6.115 - Stellate Ganglion in Anatomical Context

   A. Recurrent laryngeal nerve → hoarseness

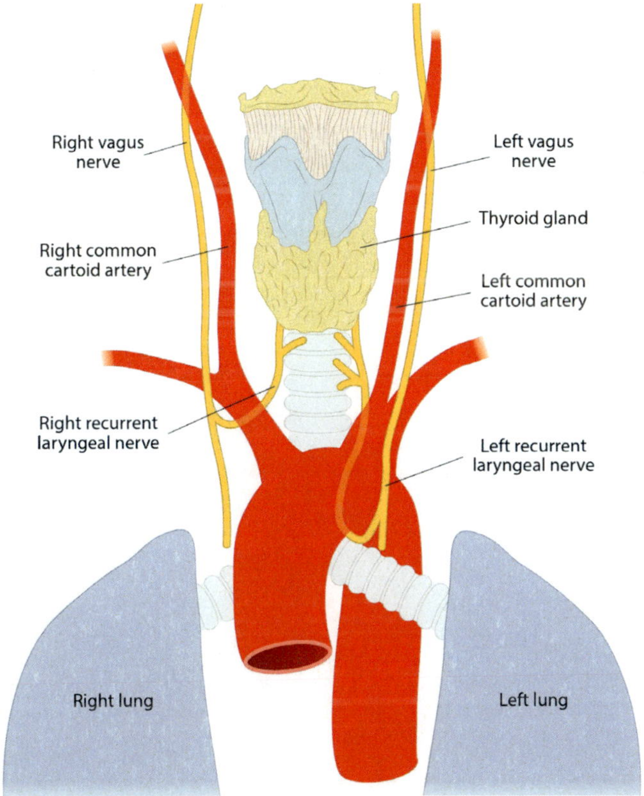

FIGURE 10.6.116 - Recurrent Laryngeal Nerve in Anatomical Contex

   B. Superior vena cava → SVC syndrome
   C. Brachiocephalic vein → brachiocephalic syndrome

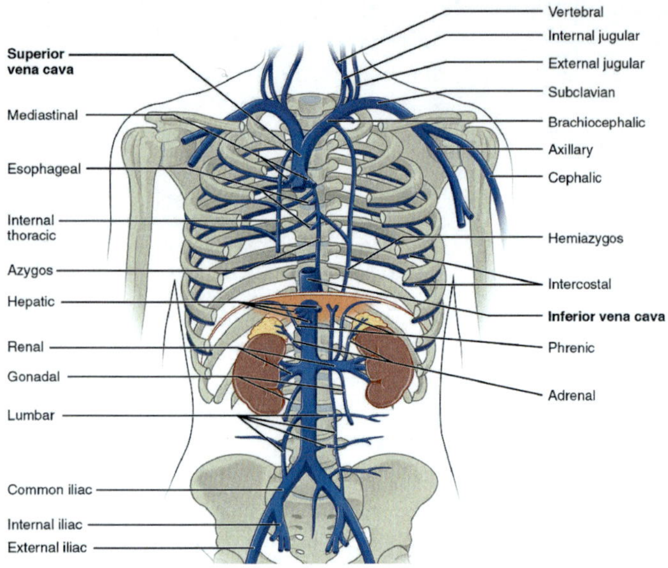

FIGURE 10.6.117 - Venous Drainage of the Upper Body

D. Brachial plexus → sensorimotor deficits

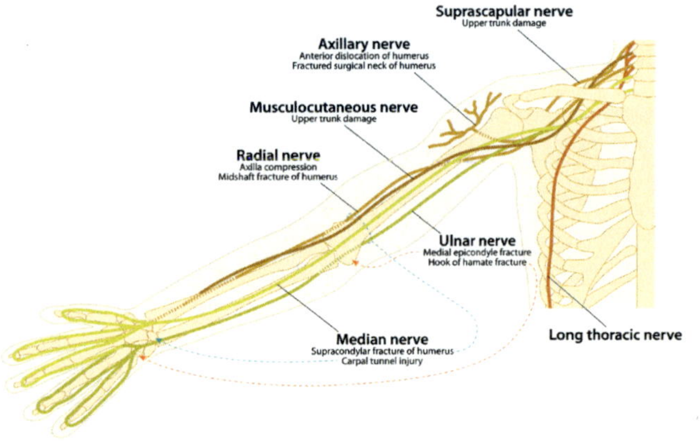

FIGURE 10.6.118 - Branches of Brachial Plexus

E. Phrenic nerve → hemidiaphragm paralysis

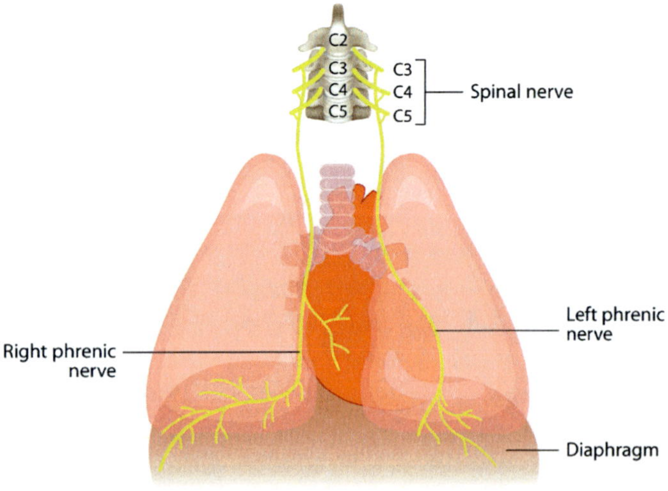

FIGURE 10.6.119 - Phrenic Nerves

REVIEW QUESTIONS ?

1. A 48-year-old woman presents to the clinic with shortness of breath and muscle weakness, especially in the arms. She also explains that when she is reading a book, she has double vision. Her heart rate is 85 beats/minute, blood pressure is 140/75 mmHg, and temperature is 37 °C (98.6 ° F). Upon physical examination, her upper eyelids are drooping. A tensilon test is performed and the patient immediately notices an improvement in muscle strength in her arms. Which of the following is the most likely cause of this patient's symptoms?

   A. Small cell carcinoma
   B. Trochlear nerve lesion
   C. Pancoast tumor
   D. Myasthenia gravis

- **The correct answer is D.**
- The patient's muscle weakness improved upon the tensilon test. Tensilon, or edrophonium, is an anticholinesterase that prevents a breakdown of acetylcholine at the neuromuscular junction. Myasthenia gravis is an autoimmune phenomenon that causes weakness in the skeletal muscles, including the muscles of the respiratory system. This is due to anti-acetylcholine receptor antibodies, which destroy acetylcholine receptors. Administering an anticholinesterase such as tensilon prolongs the presence of acetylcholine, thereby improving the symptoms of muscle weakness.
- A is incorrect because small cell carcinoma is associated with paraneoplastic syndromes, such as SIADH, Cushing syndrome, or Lambert-Eaton syndrome. None of these symptoms are seen in the vignette.
- B is incorrect because although diplopia can be observed with trochlear nerve lesion, no other symptoms seen in the vignette indicate this type of pathology.
- C is incorrect because although someone with a Pancoast tumor would have weakness of the arms, ptosis, and shortness of breath, this patient doesn't have any symptoms that would indicate lung cancer, such as prolonged smoking history or worsening cough.

Section XXIII - Superior Vena Cava Syndrome

I. Basic principles
  A. Compression of superior vena cava (SVC) → impaired venous return from upper body
  B. Medical emergency

II. Etiology
  A. Caused by mediastinal mass
    1. Lung cancer (most common)
    2. Non-Hodgkin lymphoma
    3. Thrombosis from indwelling catheter

III. Anatomy
  A. SVC provides venous drainage for upper body
    1. Formed from joining of right and left brachiocephalic veins
    2. Drains directly into right atrium
  B. Thin-walled, so easily compressed
    1. Compression impairs venous drainage, causing venous congestion in head, neck, and upper extremities

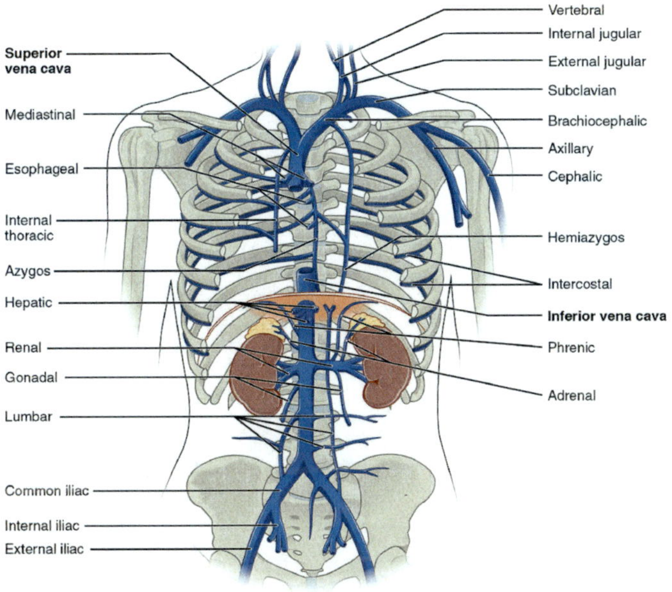

FIGURE 10.6.117 - Venous Drainage of the Upper Body

IV. Symptoms
  A. Dyspnea
  B. Cough
  C. Swelling of face, neck, upper extremities
  D. Jugular venous distension
  E. Headache, dizziness, confusion
    1. Can cause rupture of intracranial arteries

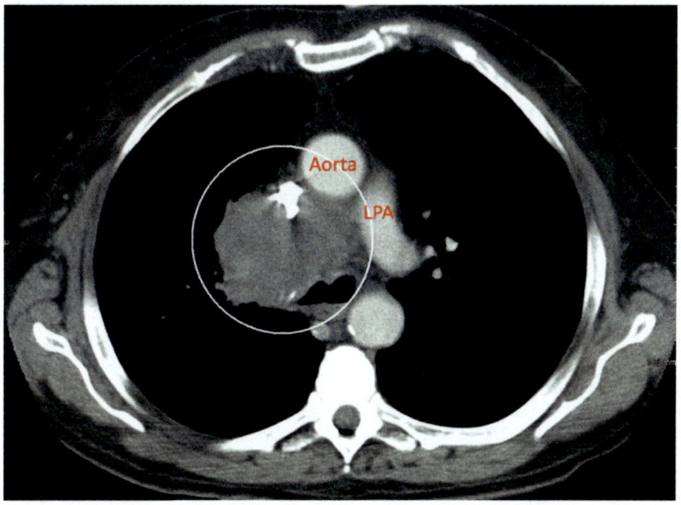

FIGURE 10.6.120 - Axial Chest CT of Mediastinal Mass Causing Uerior Vena Cava Syndrome

V. Treatment
  A. Remove obstruction

REVIEW QUESTIONS

1. A 67-year-old man with a history of smoking presents to his primary care physician complaining of trouble breathing and a chronic cough for the past few months. He also notes frequent headaches and dizziness. On physical exam, there is swelling of the face and neck with jugular venous distension. He has normal heart sounds. Which of the following is the likely cause of these symptoms?

    A. Pneumonia
    B. Mitral valve stenosis
    C. Mediastinal mass
    D. Pulmonary hypertension

- **The correct answer is C.**
- We have a 67-year-old smoker with dyspnea and a cough. He also has headaches and dizziness, with facial swelling and jugular venous distension. He also has normal heart sounds.
- The neurological symptoms combined with swelling and JVD should make you think about SVC syndrome. SVC syndrome is caused by compression of the SVC by a mediastinal mass.
- A is incorrect because pneumonia usually presents with an acute cough and dyspnea, and this patient is presenting with a chronic cough.
- B is incorrect because mitral valve stenosis presents with abnormal heart sounds, namely a diastolic decrescendo murmur with an opening snap.
- D is incorrect because pulmonary hypertension presents with abnormal heart sounds, usually a murmur on the right side of the heart.

ENDOCRINE PATHOLOGY

Section I - Pituitary

I. Hypopituitarism
   A. Undersecretion of pituitary hormones
   B. Initial symptoms are subtle but gradually get worse over time
   C. Etiologies
      1. Pituitary apoplexy
      2. Sheehan syndrome
      3. Empty sella syndrome

II. Hypopituitarism: Clinical Features
   A. Fatigue
   B. Dizziness
   C. Difficulty concentrating
   D. Lethargy
   E. Decreased libido
   F. Female: failure to lactate, galactorrhea, and menstrual irregularities

III. Hypopituitarism: Pituitary Apoplexy
   A. Sudden hemorrhage of pituitary gland
   B. Preexisting pituitary adenoma
   C. Presentation
      1. Sudden-onset severe headache
      2. Visual impairment (e.g. bitemporal hemianopsia, diplopia)
      3. Features of hypopituitarism

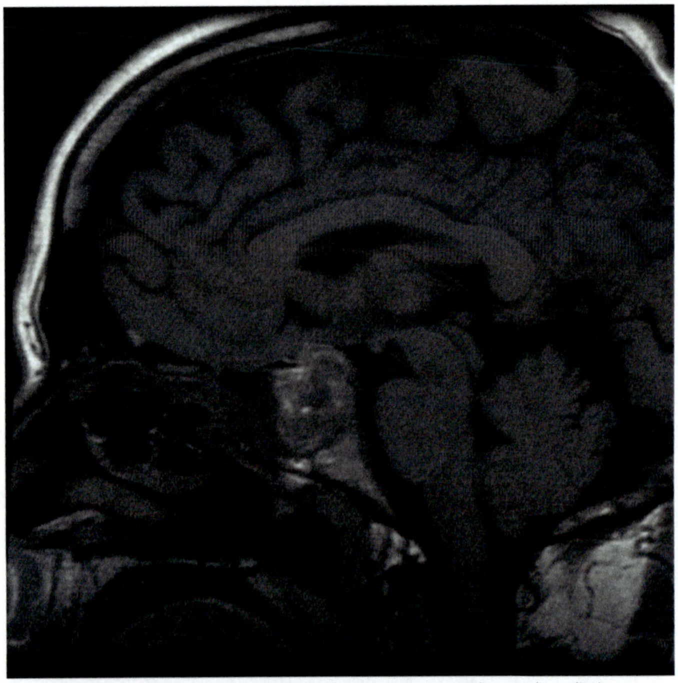

FIGURE 10.7.1 - Sagittal Brain MRI of Pituitary Apoplexy

IV. Hypopituitarism: Sheehan Syndrome
   A. Infarction of the pituitary gland following postpartum bleeding
      1. Pituitary grows bigger, but blood supply does not increase
      2. Excess blood loss during labor worsens infarction
   B. Presentation
      1. Inability tobreastfeed
      2. Loss of pubic and underarm hair
      3. Weight gain and intolerance to cold

V. Hypopituitarism: Empty Sella Syndrome
   A. Atrophy or compression of the pituitary in the sella turcica
   B. Obese women
   C. CSF buildup in sella turcica → compression and destruction of the pituitary gland
   D. Imaging: pituitary gland is absent (empty sella)

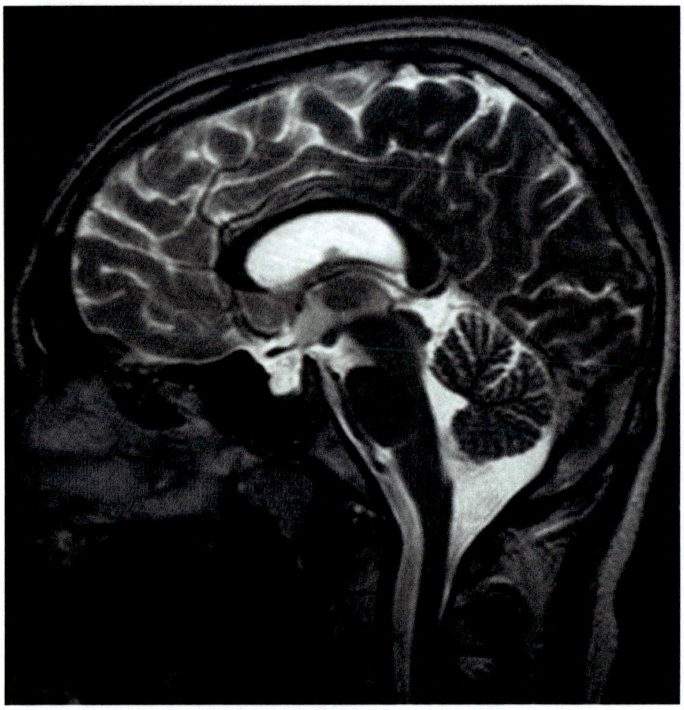

FIGURE 10.7.2 - Sagittal Brain MRI of Empty Sella Syndrome

VI. Pituitary Adenoma
   A. Benign tumor of the pituitary gland
   B. Functioning tumors: hormone-producing
      1. Presentation depends on type of hormone produced
   C. Nonfunctioning tumors: hormonally silent
      1. Mass effect: headache, bitemporal hemianopsia

VII. Functional Pituitary Adenoma: Types
   A. Rare: TSH, LH, or FSH-producing adenomas
   B. Cushing syndrome: ACTH-producing adenoma
   C. Prolactinoma
   D. Gigantism
   E. Acromegaly

VIII. Functional Pituitary Adenoma: Prolactinoma
   A. Prolactin-secreting
   B. Most common type of pituitary adenoma
   C. ↑ prolactin → ↓ GnRH → ↓ LH and FSH
   D. Females present with galactorrhea and amenorrhea
   E. Males present with decreased libido and infertility
   F. Treatment: dopamine agonists (bromocriptine, cabergoline), surgery

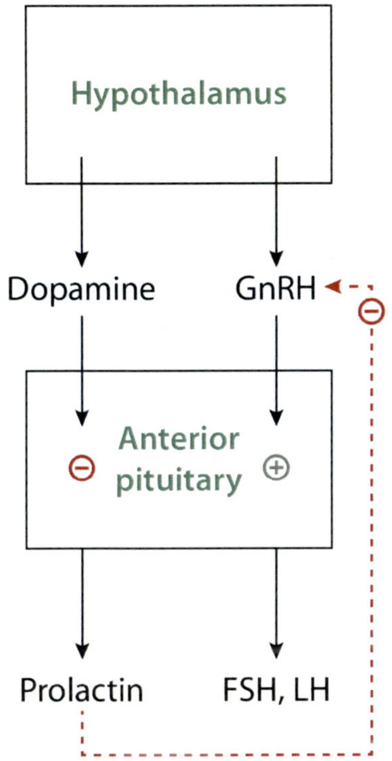

FIGURE 10.7.3 - Hypothalamic-Pituitary Axis in Prolactinoma

IX. Functional Pituitary Adenoma: Gigantism
   A. Growth hormone cell adenoma in children
   B. Increased linear bone growth prior to closure of epiphyseal plates
   C. Diagnosis
      1. Elevated GH and IGF-1
      2. Lack of GH suppression by oral glucose

X. Functional Pituitary Adenoma: Acromegaly
   A. Growth hormone cell adenoma in adults
   B. Enlarged bones of hands and feet, coarsening of facial features, enlarged tongue, growth of visceral organs
   C. Secondary diabetes mellitus often present
   D. Diagnosis
      1. Elevated GH and IGF-1
      2. Lack of GH suppression by oral glucose

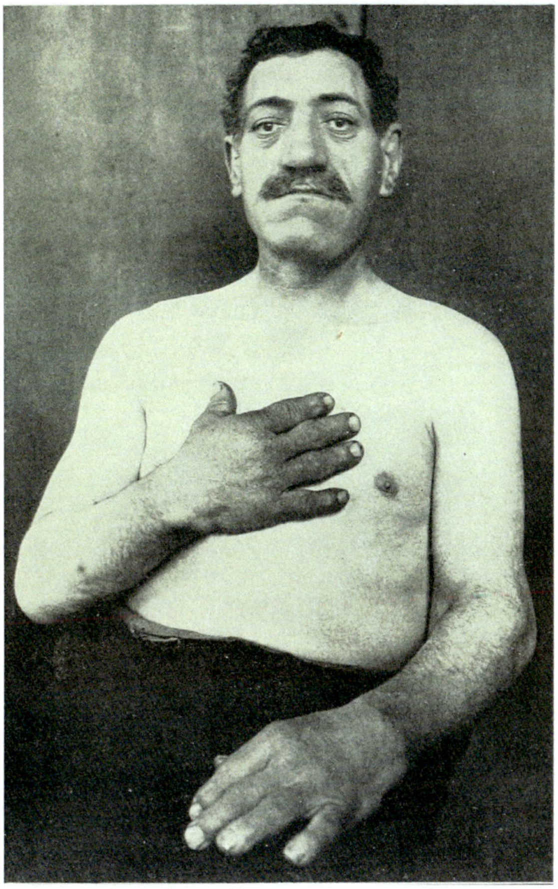

Photo Credit: Internet Archive Book Images / No restrictions

FIGURE 10.7.4 - Acromegaly

REVIEW QUESTIONS

1. A 23-year-old woman presents to the clinic with complaints of undesirable weight gain and an inability to lactate following the recent delivery of a healthy baby boy. She has been feeding him only with formula. Past medical history confirms that she had a spontaneous vaginal delivery complicated by severe postpartum hemorrhage. What is the most likely cause of her symptoms?

- **The correct answer is pregnancy-related infarction of the pituitary gland, or Sheehan syndrome.**
- This is a 23-year-old woman presenting with undesirable weight gain and failure to lactate. History is notable for spontaneous vaginal delivery complicated by postpartum hemorrhage.
- She has a pregnancy-related infarction of the pituitary gland, also known as Sheehan syndrome.Pituitary infarction often occurs during pregnancy and blood loss during parturition precipitates the infarction.

2. A 31-year-old woman presents with a complaint of milky nipple discharge for the past 2 weeks. She does not recall any instance of trauma to the area. On physical examination, she is found to have a severe visual defect with impaired peripheral vision bilaterally. Which of the following sets of laboratory results would be expected from this patient's serum?

   A. Increased prolactin, decreased LH, decreased FSH
   B. Increased prolactin, increased LH, increased FSH
   C. Decreased prolactin, decreased LH, decreased FSH
   D. Decreased prolactin, increased LH, increased FSH

- **The correct answer is A.**
- This is a 31-year-old woman presenting with milky nipple discharge for the past 2 weeks. She also has bitemporal hemianopsia. A woman with galactorrhea and bitemporal hemianopsia is a classic presentation of prolactinoma. In someone with prolactinoma, elevated levels of prolactin are present, along with decreased levels of FSH and LH due to negative feedback.
- An elevated level of prolactin in someone with prolactinoma suppresses GnRH, which decreases FSH and LH, which then decreases the production of estrogen and testosterone.
- B is incorrect because increased levels of prolactin would suppress the production of GnRH, which would result in decreased levels of LH and FSH.
- C and D are incorrect because prolactin levels are elevated in a prolactinoma.

Section II - Hyperthyroidism

I. Basic Principles
  A. Increased production of thyroid hormone
    1. Increased synthesis of Na^+/K^+ ATPase → increased basal metabolic rate (BMR)
    2. Increased expression of beta-adrenergic receptors → increased sympathetic nervous system activity

II. Clinical Features
  A. Weight loss despite increased appetite
  B. Heat intolerance
  C. Tachycardia
  D. Arrhythmia
  E. Tremor, anxiety, insomnia, and heightened emotions
  F. Diarrhea
  G. Bone resorption with hypercalcemia
  H. Decreased muscle mass with weakness
  I. Hypocholesterolemia
  J. Hyperglycemia

III. Graves Disease
  A. Autoantibody (IgG) stimulates TSH receptor → overproduction of thyroid hormone
  B. Most common cause of hyperthyroidism
  C. Women under age 40
  D. Histology: irregular follicles with scalloped colloid

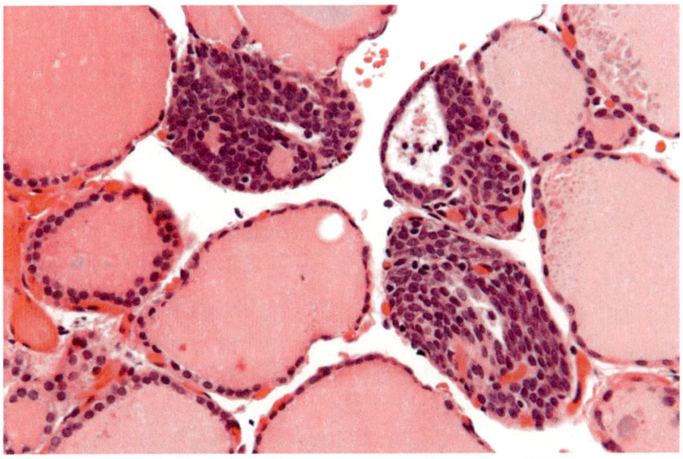

FIGURE 10.7.5 - Normal Histological Image of Thyroid

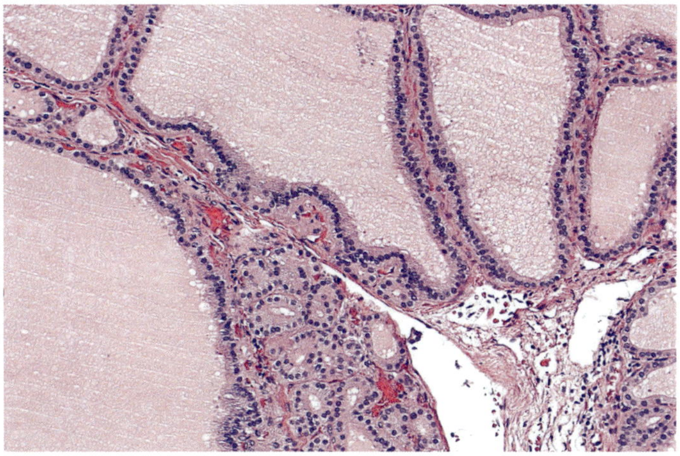

FIGURE 10.7.6 - Histopathology of Graves disease

IV. Graves Disease: Findings
  A. Hyperthyroidism
  B. Diffuse goiter
  C. Exophthalmos and pretibial myxedema
  D. Lab findings
    1. ↑ total T4, ↑ free T4, ↓ TSH
    2. Hypocholesterolemia
    3. Hyperglycemia

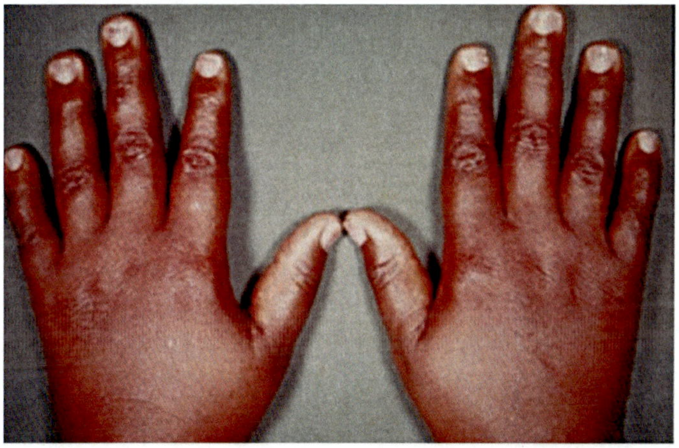

FIGURE 10.7.7 - Hands of a Patient with Graves Disease

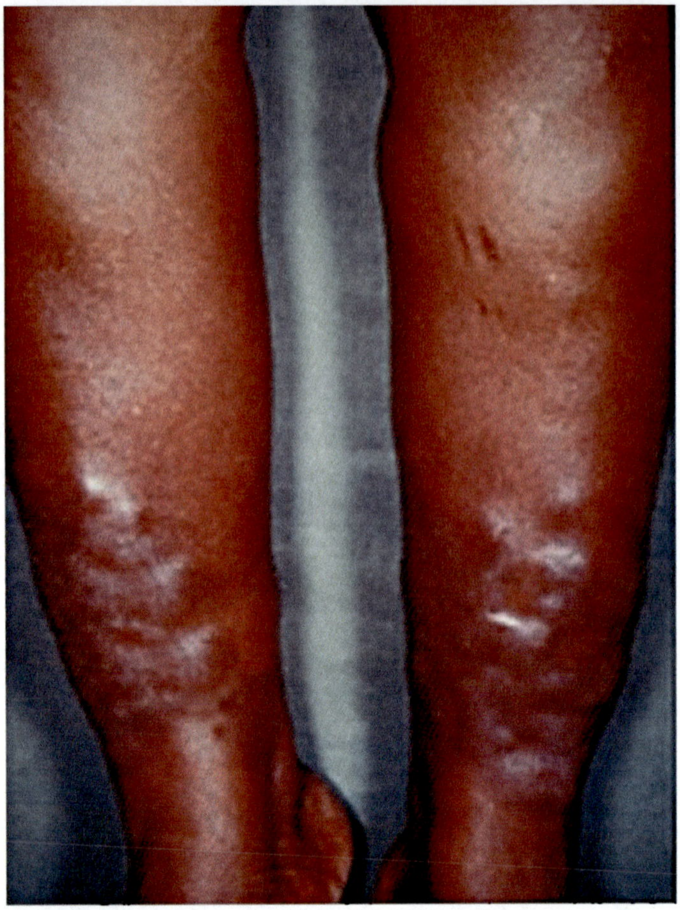

Photo Credit: Herbert L. Fred, MD and Hendrik A. van Dijk / CC BY (https://creativecommons.org/licenses/by/2.0)

FIGURE 10.7.8 - Legs of a Patient with Graves Disease

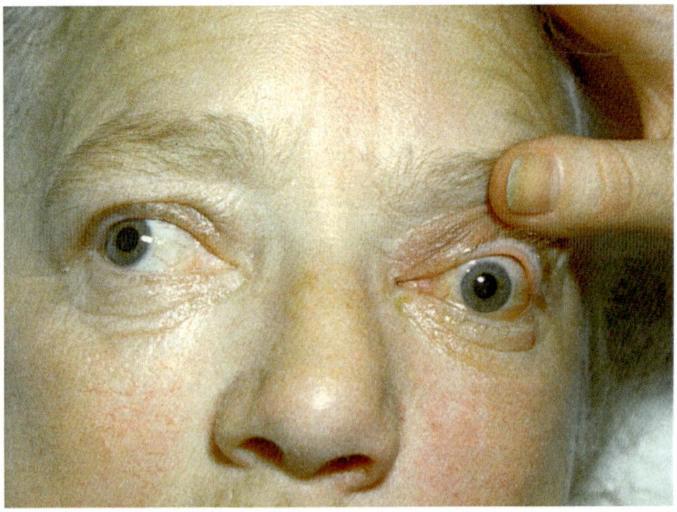

Photo Credit: CDC/Dr. Sellers/Emory University / Public domain

FIGURE 10.7.9 - Exophthalmos

V. Graves Disease: Treatment
   A. Beta blockers
   B. Thioamide (PTU and methimazole)
   C. Radioiodine ablation

VI. Graves Disease: Thyroid Storm
   A. Life-threatening complication of Graves disease
   B. Massive surge of catecholamines in response to stress (e.g. infection, trauma, surgery)
   C. Tachyarrhythmia, hyperthermia, persistent sweating, coma
   D. Treatment: PTU, beta blockers, steroids

VII. Multinodular Goiter
   A. Enlarged thyroid gland with multiple nodules
   B. Etiology:
      1. Relative iodine deficiency
      2. Goitrogens in food (e.g. cabbage, Brussel sprouts, cauliflower)
   C. Usually euthyroid
   D. Rarely, can be toxic multinodular goiter or non-toxic

REVIEW QUESTIONS

1. A 26-year-old woman presents to the clinic with complaints of diarrhea and muscle weakness. She mentions that she has lost 8 pounds over the past month despite an increased appetite. She is a vegetarian. On physical exam, the patient seems very anxious and has bilateral exophthalmos. Lab studies show high total and free T4 levels and low TSH levels. Which of the following is the most likely cause of her symptoms?

   A. Goitrogens in food
   B. Relative iodine deficiency
   C. IgM autoantibody
   D. IgG autoantibody

- **The correct answer is D.**
- A 26-year-old woman is presenting with diarrhea, muscle weakness, and unintentional weight loss. On physical exam, she seems very anxious and has bilateral exophthalmos. Lab work shows that total and free T4 levels are higher than normal and her TSH level is low. All these findings are characteristic of Graves disease. Graves disease is characterized by IgG autoantibodies that stimulate the TSH receptor, which results in increased synthesis and release of thyroid hormone.
- A is incorrect because goitrogens in food, such as cabbage, brussel sprouts, and cauliflower, would cause multinodular goiter, not Graves disease.
- B is incorrect because relative iodine deficiency would also cause multinodular goiter.
- C is incorrect because it is not an IgM autoantibody, but an IgG autoantibody, that stimulates TSH receptors.

Section III - Hypothyroidism

I. Cretinism
   A. Severe deficiency of thyroid hormone in newborns
   B. Thyroid hormone essential for proper brain and skeletal development
      1. Intellectual disability
      2. Growth abnormalities/developmental delays
      3. Coarse facial features
      4. Enlarged tongue
      5. Umbilical hernia

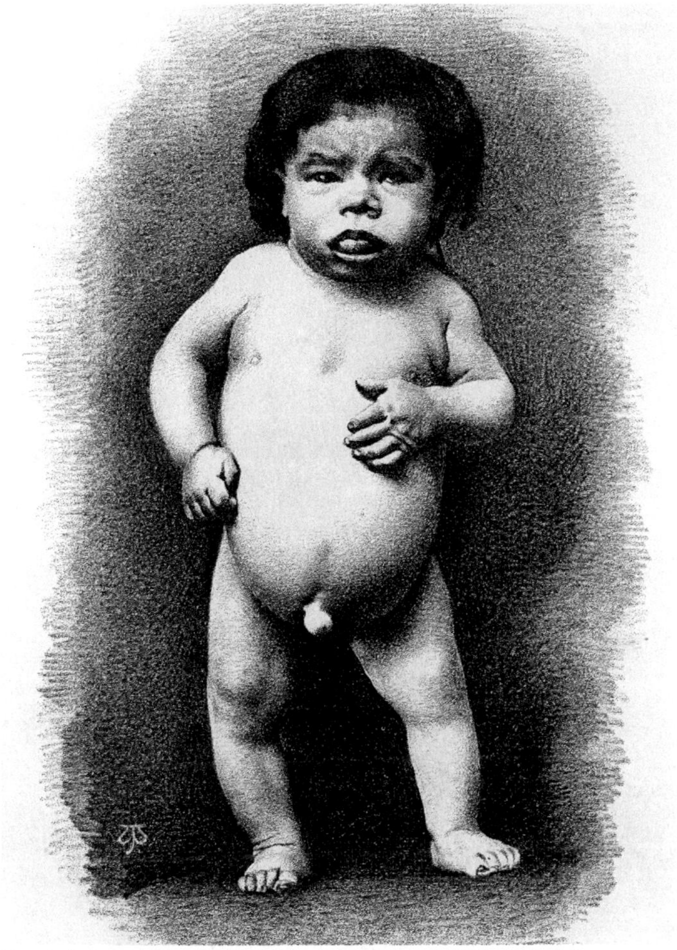

FIGURE 10.7.10 - Patient With Cretinism

II. Cretinism: Etiology
   A. Maternal hypothyroidism during early pregnancy
   B. Iodine deficiency
   C. Thyroid agenesis
   D. Dyshormonogenetic goiter
      1. Congenital defect in thyroid hormone production
      2. Most commonly involves thyroid peroxidase

III. Myxedema
   A. Severe hypothyroidism in older children and adults
   B. Etiology
      1. Iodine deficiency (common)
      2. Hashimoto thyroiditis (common)
      3. Drugs (e.g. lithium)
      4. Thyroidectomy

IV. Myxedema: Clinical Features
   A. Deepening of voice, large tongue
   B. Constipation
   C. Weight gain
   D. Muscle weakness/pain
   E. Decreased sweating
   F. Bradycardia with decreased cardiac output → shortness of breath, fatigue
   G. Oligomenorrhea
   H. Hypercholesterolemia
   I. Sensitivity to cold

REVIEW QUESTIONS

1. A 6-week-old neonate presents with hypotonia and an umbilical hernia. His parents mention that he was healthy at birth. On physical examination, he has coarse facial features and his height is less than the 3rd percentile. What is the most likely cause of his symptoms?
   A. Hashimoto thyroiditis
   B. Maternal hyperthyroidism
   C. Dyshormonogenetic goiter
   D. Thyroid hyperplasia

- **The correct answer is C.**
- This is a 6-week-old neonate with hypotonia and umbilical hernia. He was otherwise healthy at birth. On exam, he is found to have coarse facial features and his height is less than the 3rd percentile. Based on the age and the presentation, this neonate has cretinism.
- There are many causes of cretinism, including maternal hypothyroidism, thyroid agenesis, dyshormonogenetic goiter, and iodine.
- A is wrong because Hashimoto thyroiditis is a common cause of myxedema, which refers to hypothyroidism in older children and adults.
- B is wrong because maternal hyperthyroidism would not cause cretinism; rather, it is maternal hypothyroidism that results in cretinism.
- D is wrong because thyroid hyperplasia would cause symptoms of hyperthyroidism.

Section IV - Thyroid Neoplasia

I. Basic Principles
   A. Tumor of the thyroid gland
   B. Presents as a solitary nodule
   C. ^{131}I radioactive uptake studies useful to characterize nodules
      1. Increased uptake ("hot" nodules) → Graves disease
      2. Decreased uptake ("cold" nodules) → adenoma and carcinoma
   D. Diagnosed by fine-needle aspiration (FNA)

II. Follicular Adenoma
   A. Benign tumor of thyroid gland surrounded by fibrous capsule
   B. Growth completely contained by thin fibrous capsule
   C. Does not cause dysregulation of thyroid hormone, but may rarely secrete thyroid hormone

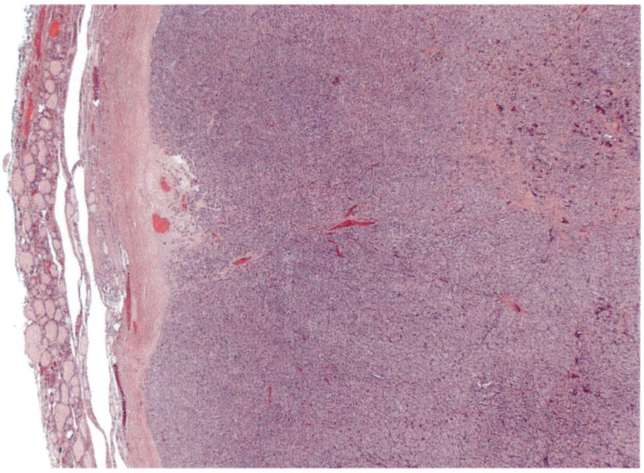

FIGURE 10.7.11 - Follicular Adenoma

III. Follicular Carcinoma
   A. Invasive growth of follicles surrounded by fibrous capsule
      1. Invasion through fibrous capsule
   B. Diagnosis of follicular carcinoma cannot be made by fine-needle aspiration
      1. FNA can examine only the follicles, not the capsule
   C. Diagnosed by complete removal of the thyroid mass
   D. Metastasis occurs hematogenously

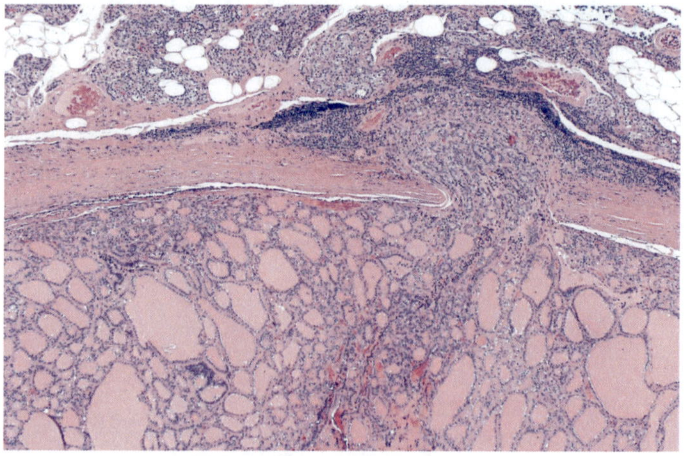

FIGURE 10.7.12 - Follicular Carcinoma

IV. Papillary Carcinoma
   A. Most common type of thyroid carcinoma
   B. Exposure to ionizing radiation in childhood
   C. Histology
      1. Papillae lined by cells with clear "Orphan Annie eye" nuclei
      2. Nuclear grooves
      3. Psammoma bodies
   D. Often spreads to cervical lymph nodes

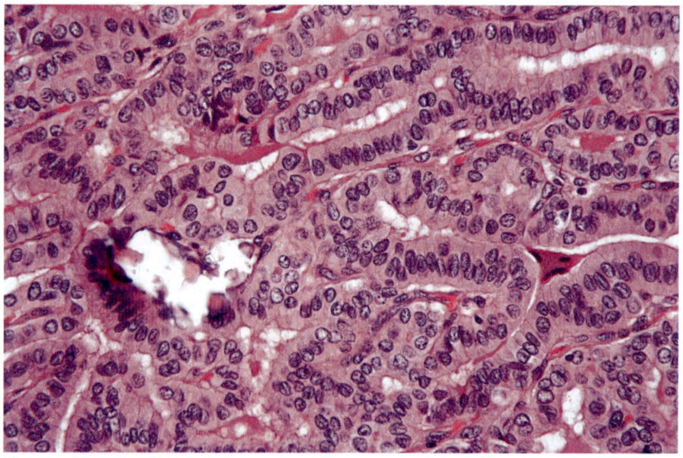

FIGURE 10.7.13 - "Orphan Annie Eye" Nuclei and Nuclear Grooves in Papillary Carcinoma

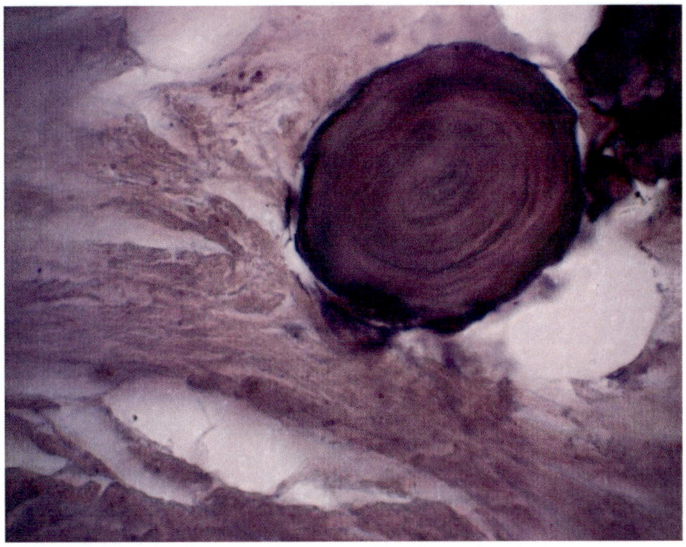

Photo Credit: Eriugen / CC BY-SA (https://creativecommons.org/licenses/by-sa/4.0)

FIGURE 10.7.14 - Psammoma Bodies in Papillary Carcinoma

V. Medullary Carcinoma
   A. Thyroid carcinoma that originates from parafollicular C cells
      1. C cells: neuroendocrine cells that produce calcitonin
   B. Calcitonin reduces calcium levels by decreasing the resorption of calcium in the kidneys
      1. Excess calcitonin produced by tumor → hypocalcemia
      2. Calcitonin may deposit as amyloid in the tumor

VI. Medullary Carcinoma: Findings
   A. Biopsy: sheets of polygonal cells in an amyloid stroma (Congo red stain)
   B. Familial cases due to MEN 2A and 2B syndromes
      1. Gain-of-function germline mutations in the *RET* gene
      2. Detection of RET mutation → prophylactic thyroidectomy

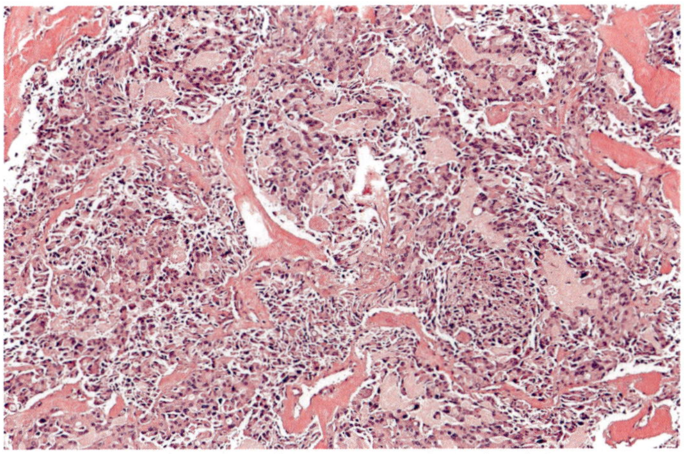

Photo Credit: Nephron / CC BY-SA (https://creativecommons.org/licenses/by-sa/3.0)

FIGURE 10.7.15 - Medullary Carcinoma

VII. Anaplastic Carcinoma
   A. Aggressive form of thyroid tumor
   B. Undifferentiated malignant cells on microscopy
   C. More common in elderly patients.
   D. Spreads quickly to other adjacent organs
   E. Compresses and invades local structures
      1. Esophagus → dysphagia
      2. Trachea → respiratory compromise

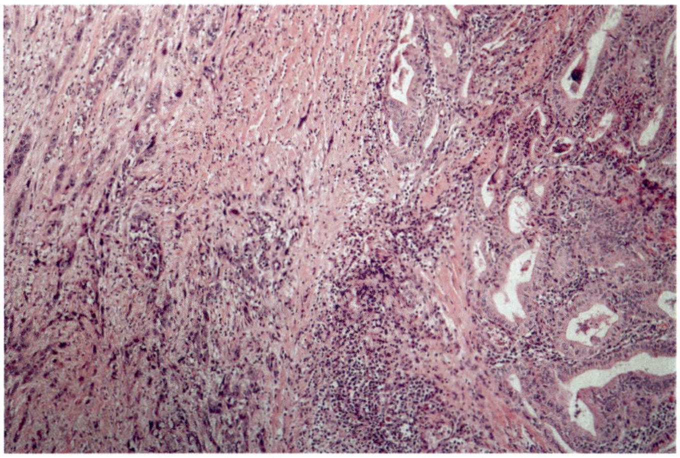

Photo Credit: Nephron / CC BY-SA (https://creativecommons.org/licenses/by-sa/3.0)

FIGURE 10.7.16 - Anaplastic Carcinoma

VIII. Treatment
   A. Thyroidectomy
   B. Complications
      1. Removal of parathyroid glands → hypocalcemia
      2. Transection of recurrent laryngeal nerve during ligation of inferior thyroid artery → dysphagia and hoarseness

REVIEW QUESTIONS

1. A 42-year-old woman comes to the clinic with a sense of fullness in her neck. She is asymptomatic with no complaint of hoarseness or dysphagia. On physical examination, there is a thyroid mass that was not present previously. Fine-needle aspiration reveals cells with empty-appearing nuclei and nuclear grooves. What would a radioactive iodine uptake study (thyroid scintigraphy) most likely reveal?

   - **The correct answer is decreased iodine uptake of the nodule, or cold nodule.**
   - This is a 42-year-old woman with a sense of fullness in her neck. On physical exam, there is a thyroid mass, in which the fine-needle aspiration biopsy reveals cells with empty-appearing nuclei and nuclear grooves. The above findings indicate a diagnosis of papillary carcinoma of the thyroid.
   - ^{131}I radioactive uptake studies are useful to further characterize nodules. An adenoma or a carcinoma would have a decreased iodine uptake, also known as "cold" nodules, on thyroid scintigraphy.
   - In this case, the patient has thyroid carcinoma so there will be decreased uptake, resulting in a 'cold' nodule.

2. A 33-year-old woman comes to the clinic with a complaint of a choking sensation around her neck. On physical exam, there is a thyroid mass. Her heart rate is 72 beats/minute, blood pressure is 120/75 mmHg, and temperature is 37 °C (98.6 °F). Lab studies are notable for hypocalcemia. Biopsy of the thyroid reveals sheets of polygonal cells with an amyloid stroma when stained with Congo red. Which of the following most likely describes the malignancy?

   A. Comprised of cells with empty-appearing nuclei and nuclear grooves
   B. Malignant proliferation of follicles invading the fibrous capsule
   C. Malignant proliferation of parafollicular C cells
   D. Undifferentiated malignant tumor of the thyroid

   - **The correct answer is C.**
   - This is a 33-year-old female presenting with a thyroid mass. Her lab is notable for hypocalcemia. Biopsy of the thyroid reveals sheets of polygonal, or irregularly-shaped, cells in an amyloid stroma when stained with Congo red. All of these findings are consistent with medullary carcinoma of the thyroid.
   - High levels of calcitonin due to the proliferation of parafollicular C cells lead to hypocalcemia and excess calcitonin deposited within the tumor as amyloid. Therefore, the correct answer is malignant proliferation of parafollicular C cells. Medullary carcinoma is a thyroid carcinoma that originates from parafollicular C cells, is associated with hypocalcemia, and results in amyloid deposition.
   - A is incorrect because a malignancy comprised of cells with empty-appearing nuclei and nuclear grooves best describes papillary carcinoma.
   - B is incorrect because a malignant proliferation of follicles invading the fibrous capsule best describes follicular carcinoma.
   - D is incorrect because an undifferentiated malignant tumor of the thyroid best describes anaplastic carcinoma.

Section V - Thyroiditis

I. Hashimoto Thyroiditis
  A. Chronic lymphocytic thyroiditis
  B. Autoimmune destruction of the thyroid gland (HLA-DR5)
  C. Most common cause of hypothyroidism
  D. Histology: lymphoplasmacytic infiltrate with germinal centers, follicular destruction, Hürthle cells (thyroid tissue that has enlarged eosinophilic cells)

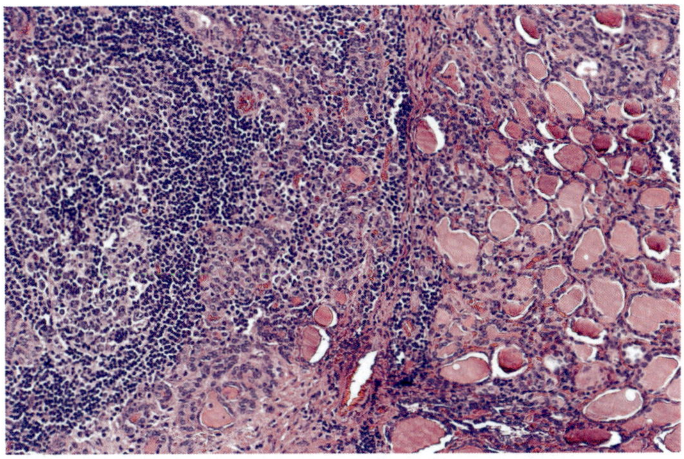

FIGURE 10.7.17 - Germinal Centers and Hürthle Cells in Hashimoto Thyroiditis

II. Hashimoto Thyroiditis: Clinical Features
  A. Hyperthyroidism (initially): destruction of thyroid follicles → leakage of thyroid hormones
  B. Hypothyroidism (later)
  C. Lab results: antithyroglobulin and antithyroid peroxidase antibodies
  D. Increased risk for B-cell (marginal zone) lymphoma

III. Subacute Granulomatous (De Quervain) Thyroiditis
  A. Granulomatous thyroiditis after a viral infection
  B. Most common cause of a painful thyroid gland
  C. Transient hyperthyroidism (initially) → may progress to hypothyroidism (15% of cases)
  D. "A young woman with a tender thyroid"
  E. Self-limited

IV. Riedel Fibrosing Thyroiditis
  A. Chronic inflammation of the thyroid gland characterized by a fibrous tissue that replaces normal thyroid parenchyma
  B. Hypothyroidism with a painless thyroid
  C. Classic presentation: A young woman with a non-tender, hard-as-wood thyroid

V. Riedel Fibrosing Thyroiditis: Complications
  A. Fibrosis invades surrounding structures (e.g. trachea, esophagus)
  B. Signs of dysphagia or respiratory compromise
  C. Mimics anaplastic carcinoma, but often occurs in middle-aged women and malignant cells are absent when biopsied

REVIEW QUESTIONS

1. A 41-year-old woman presents with complaints of progressively worsening fatigue and constipation over the past few months. She also mentions that she has been experiencing shortness of breath. Physical exam reveals diffuse enlargement of the thyroid gland that was not present previously. A biopsy of this patient's thyroid gland would most likely reveal what prominent pathological features?

   - **The correct answer is lymphoplasmacytic infiltrate with germinal centers, follicular destruction, and Hürthle cells (thyroid tissue that has enlarged eosinophilic cells).**
   - This is a 41-year-old woman with progressively worsening fatigue, constipation, and shortness of breath. The physical exam reveals a diffuse enlargement of the thyroid gland that was not present previously. These findings characterize someone with Hashimoto thyroiditis.
   - The biopsy of someone with Hashimoto thyroiditis would show lymphoplasmacytic infiltrate with germinal centers, follicular destruction, and Hürthle cells.

2. A 30-year-old female presents to the clinic complaining of increased weight despite a normal appetite along with muscle weakness and cold intolerance. On physical exam, the thyroid gland is very tender on palpation. Her heart rate is 47 beats/minute, blood pressure is 125/95 mmHg, and temperature is 37 °C (98.6 °F). A biopsy of the thyroid gland reveals granulomatous inflammation. Which of the following most likely precipitated the patient's condition?

   A. Autoimmune destruction of the thyroid
   B. IgG autoantibody stimulating the TSH receptor
   C. Viral infection
   D. Goitrogens

   - **The correct answer is C.**
   - This is a 30-year-old female presenting with increased weight despite normal appetite, muscle weakness, and cold intolerance. These symptoms are all consistent with hypothyroidism. On physical exam, her thyroid is very tender on palpation and she is bradycardic. Biopsy of her thyroid reveals granulomatous inflammation.
   - A young woman with tender thyroid that reveals granulomatous inflammation on biopsy along with signs of hypothyroidism is a classic case of subacute granulomatous (De Quervain) thyroiditis. Subacute granulomatous (De Quervain) thyroiditis is characterized by granulomatous thyroiditis after a viral infection.
   - A is incorrect because autoimmune destruction of the thyroid gland characterizes Hashimoto thyroiditis, which does not present with granulomatous inflammation of the thyroid.
   - B is incorrect because IgG autoantibody that stimulates the TSH receptor would cause Graves disease, which presents with symptoms of hyperthyroidism.
   - D is wrong because goitrogens in food, such as cabbage, Brussel sprouts, cauliflower, would cause multinodular goiter, which can present with symptoms of hyperthyroidism.

Section VI - Endocrine Pancreas

I. Basic Principles
   A. Islets of Langerhans
   B. Single islet composed of multiple cell types, each producing a single hormone
   C. Insulin secreted by beta cells
   D. Glucagon secreted by alpha cells

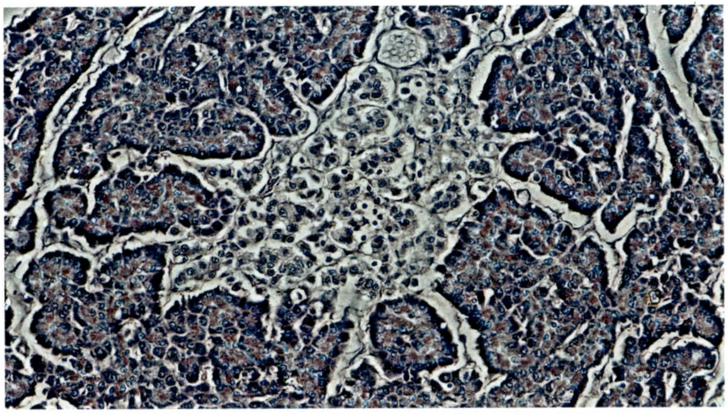

FIGURE 10.7.18 - Islet of Langerhans

II. Long-Term Consequences of Diabetes: Introduction
   A. Causes
      1. Nonenzymatic glycosylation of vascular basement membranes
      2. Osmotic damage
   B. Peripheral neuropathy

III. Long-term Consequences of Diabetes: Non-Enzymatic Glycosylation
   A. Large and medium-sized vessels: atherosclerosis
      1. Cardiovascular disease: leading cause of death (40%)
      2. Peripheral artery disease: amputation
   B. Small vessels: hyaline arteriolosclerosis
      1. Renal, retinal, endoneurial arterioles
      2. Kimmelstiel-Wilson nodules
   C. Hemoglobin A1c (HbA1c)

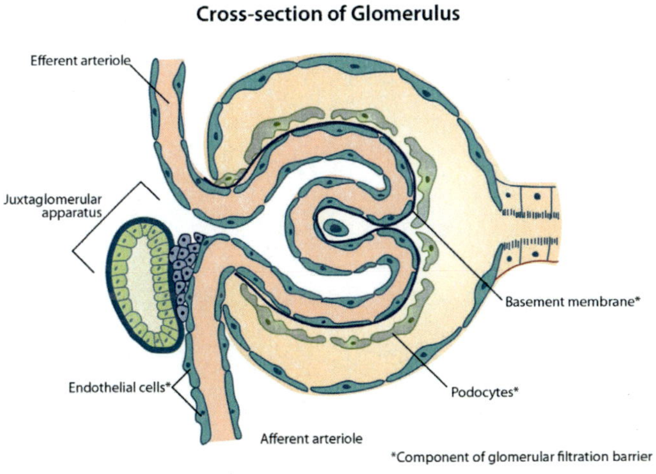

FIGURE 10.2.4 - Cross-Section of Glomerulus

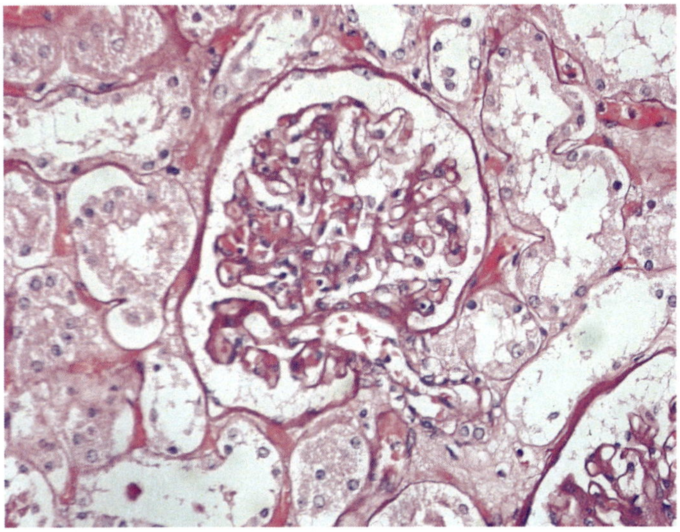

FIGURE 10.7.19 - Normal Glomerulus

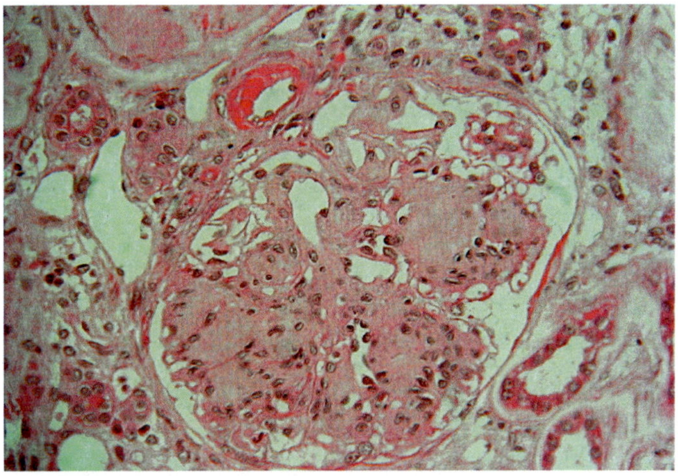

FIGURE 10.7.20 - Glomerulus in a Diabetic Patient

IV. Long-Term Consequences of Diabetes: Osmotic Damage
   A. Glucose enters Schwann cells, pericytes of retinal blood vessels, and the lens
   B. Aldose reductase converts glucose to sorbitol, which cannot cross cell membranes
   C. Intracellular osmotic shift
   D. Peripheral neuropathy, gastroparesis, impotence, blindness, and cataracts

V. Long-Term Consequences of Diabetes: Peripheral Neuropathy
   A. Caused by both non-enzymatic glycosylation and osmotic damage
   B. Length-dependent axonopathy
      1. Foot ulcers
      2. Charcot foot, hammer toes
   C. Small-fiber damage: positive symptoms (pins and needles, pain)
   D. Large-fiber damage: negative symptoms (numbness, proprioception)

VI. Pancreatic Endocrine Neoplasms
   A. Tumors of islet cells account for < 5% pancreatic neoplasms
   B. Can be part of MEN1 along with parathyroid hyperplasia and pituitary adenomas

VII. Insulinoma
   A. Tumor derived from beta cells
   B. Episodic hypoglycemia with mental status changes relieved by administration of glucose
   C. Lab findings
      1. Decreased serum glucose (< 50 mg/dL)
      2. Increased insulin
      3. Increased c-peptide

VIII. Gastrinoma
   A. Tumor of G cells in duodenum, pancreas, or stomach
   B. Treatment-resistant peptic ulcers (Zollinger-Ellison syndrome)
   C. Ulcers are extensive and can extend into jejunum
   D. Secretin stimulation test
      1. Increases gastrin secretion

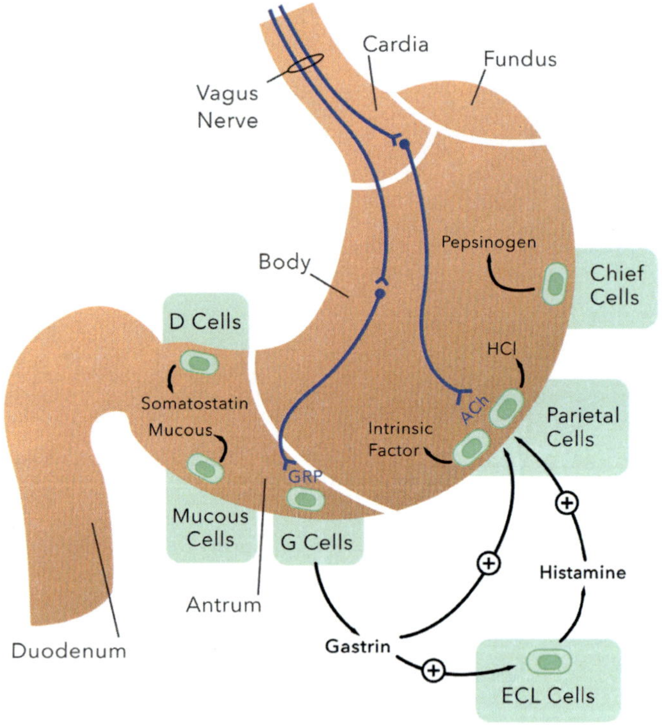

FIGURE 10.7.21 - Enzymes Released by the Stomach

IX. Somatostatinoma
   A. Tumor of delta cells in the pancreas
   B. Mild diabetes (inhibition of insulin)
   C. Achlorhydria (inhibition of gastrin)
   D. Cholelithiasis with steatorrhea (inhibition of cholecystokinin)
   E. Elevated serum somatostatin

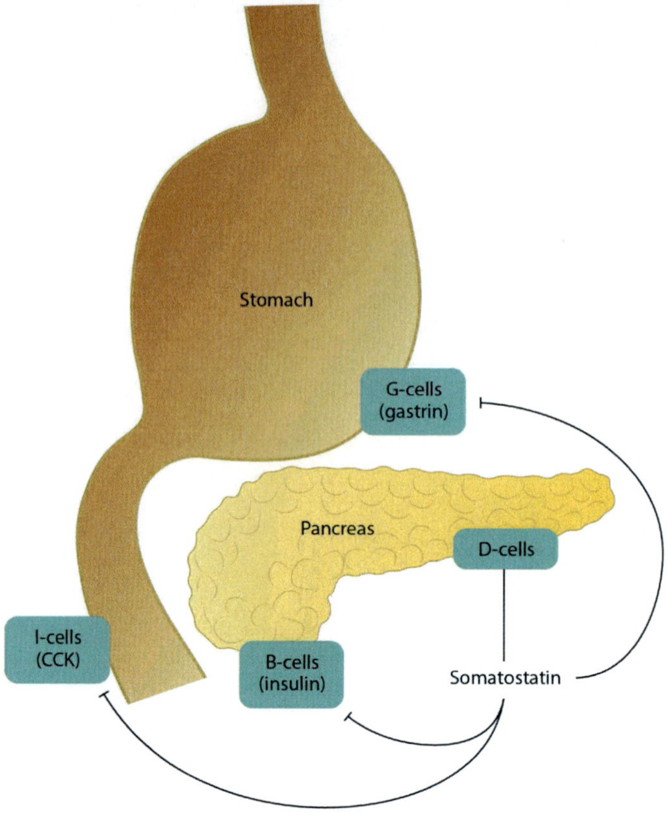

FIGURE 10.7.22 - Action of Somatostatin

X. VIPoma
   A. Tumor of vasoactive intestinal peptide-secreting non-beta pancreatic endocrine cells
   B. WDHA syndrome
      1. Watery diarrhea
      2. Hypokalemia
      3. Achlorhydria

REVIEW QUESTIONS

1. A 72-year-old woman with a history of type 2 diabetes presents to the clinic complaining of a burning pain in both feet. She states that she has had issues with balance for the past few years and that she has noticed increasing numbness and discomfort in both feet. Physical examination reveals a non-infected 1 cm ulcer at the base of the right first metatarsal and decreased sensation in both feet up to the ankles. The patient also has a positive Romberg sign. What condition associated with this patient's diabetes carries the highest risk of mortality?

- **The correct answer is cardiovascular disease.**
- In this question, we are presented with a patient with type 2 diabetes who has significant peripheral neuropathy with a foot ulcer on her right foot.
- She also has decreased proprioception as indicated by her history and a positive Romberg sign.
- We are then asked what the highest risk of mortality is for this patient.
- Although this patient is certainly at a higher risk of developing peripheral vascular disease and may need an amputation in the future secondary to her foot ulcers, remember that the overall leading cause of mortality in patients with diabetes is cardiovascular disease, or myocardial infarction.
- Thus, most of the information in this vignette serves as a distraction from the answer, which is cardiovascular disease.

2. A 48-year-old woman who recently immigrated from Sudan presents to the clinic complaining of stomach pain. She has had issues with "dyspepsia" in the past and has tried multiple remedies with minimal relief. Esophagogastroduodenoscopy reveals twelve ulcers present in the GI tract extending into the jejunum. She is tested for *H. pylori*, but the results are negative. What is the most likely cause of this patient's symptoms?

   A. Parasitic infection
   B. Excessive ibuprofen use
   C. Pancreatic beta cell tumor
   D. Pancreatic G cell tumor
   E. Pancreatic delta cell tumor

- **The correct answer is D.**
- In this vignette we are presented with a patient who has significant peptic ulcer disease, extending past the duodenal bulb into the jejunum.
- Recall that the most common causes of peptic ulcer disease are *H. pylori* infection and NSAID use; however, this patient is negative for *H. pylori* and has no evidence of NSAID use.
- A patient presenting with extensive ulcers that extend into the jejunum should make you suspicious for Zollinger-Ellison syndrome, a syndrome characterized by extensive peptic ulcers caused by a proliferation of gastrin-secreting G cells, or gastrinoma.
- G cells are present in the duodenum, pancreas, and stomach, and a tumor can arise from any of these locations.
- A is incorrect because while this patient is from a developing country, Sudan, which may predispose her to parasitic infection, parasites are almost never associated with peptic ulcers, making this very unlikely.
- B is incorrect because there is no evidence that this patient is using ibuprofen in the vignette and the presence of extensive ulcers past the jejunum make Zollinger-Ellison syndrome more likely.
- C is incorrect because a pancreatic beta cell tumor describes an insulinoma, which would present with hypoglycemia, not peptic ulcers.
- E is incorrect because a pancreatic delta cell tumor describes a somatostatinoma, which would present with mild diabetes, achlorhydria, and cholelithiasis with steatorrhea, not peptic ulcers.

Section VII - Hyperaldosteronism

I. Adrenal Cortex Physiology
   A. Outer portion of adrenal gland
   B. Three hormone-secreting layers
      1. Zona glomerulosa → mineralocorticoids (aldosterone)
      2. Zona fasciculata → glucocorticoids (cortisol)
      3. Zona reticularis → weak androgens (DHEA)

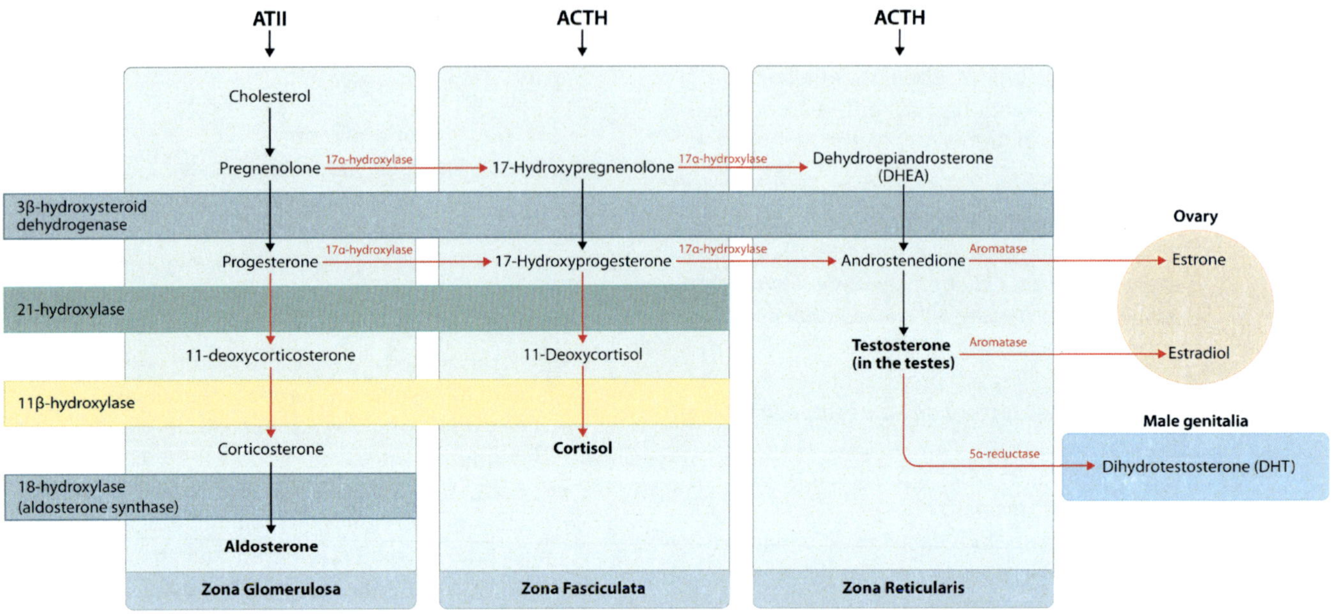

FIGURE 10.7.23 - Hormonal Production of the Layers of the Adrenal Medulla

II. Definition
   A. Excess aldosterone
      1. Increases Na^+ absorption, K^+ and H^+ secretion in renal distal tubule and collecting duct
   B. Presentation
      1. Hypertension
      2. Hypokalemia
      3. Metabolic alkalosis

III. Primary Hyperaldosteronism
   A. Intrinsic adrenal pathology
   B. Most common: bilateral adrenal hyperplasia
      1. Treatment: mineralocorticoid receptor antagonist (spironolactone, eplerenone)
   C. Other causes: adrenal adenoma (Conn syndrome) and adrenal carcinoma (rare)
      1. Treatment: surgical resection

IV. Secondary Hyperaldosteronism
   A. Due to activation of renin-angiotensin-aldosterone system (RAAS)
      1. Renovascular hypertension
      2. Congestive heart failure

V. Primary vs. Secondary Hyperaldosteronism
   A. Distinguished based on plasma renin level and presence of edema
      1. Primary: low renin without edema (aldosterone escape)
      2. Secondary: high renin with edema

VI. Glucocorticoid-Remediable Aldosteronism (GRA)
   A. Genetic mutation resulting in abnormal expression of aldosterone synthase in zona fasciculata
      1. Autosomal dominant
      2. Familial hyperaldosteronism
   B. Child with hypertension and hypokalemia
      1. High aldosterone and low renin
   C. Responds to administration of dexamethasone

Subtype	Cause	Presentation	Lab Findings	Diagnosis	Treatment
Liddle syndrome	- Genetic mutation resulting in decreased degradation of Na^+ channels in renal collecting tubules - Autosomal dominant	- HTN - Hypokalemia - Metabolic alkalosis	- Low aldosterone - Low renin	- Genetic testing	- K^+ -sparing diuretics (amiloride, triamterene)
Syndrome of apparent mineralocorticoid excess (SAME)	- 11β-HSD2 deficiency - Autosomal recessive - Licorice intake	- HTN - Hypokalemia - Metabolic alkalosis	- Low aldosterone - Low renin - Low urinary free cortisone	- Urinary free cortisone - Genetic testing	- Spironolactone

TABLE 10.7.1 - Types of Hyperaldosteronism Mimics

REVIEW QUESTIONS

1. A previously healthy 8-year-old boy is brought in by his mother due to recurring headaches and blurry vision for the past month. His past medical history is unremarkable. His blood pressure is 160/90 mmHg, heart rate is 90 beats per minute, and respiratory rate is 14 breaths per minute. Physical exam shows no gross abnormalities. Lab results indicate normal serum sodium, low serum potassium levels, and a metabolic alkalosis. What other lab tests should be run in order to properly diagnose this patient?

   - **The correct answer is serum aldosterone and renin levels.**
   - Here we have a boy with headaches and blurry vision with hypertension. His labs indicate he also has hypokalemia and metabolic alkalosis. These are all signs of hyperaldosteronism. However, to properly diagnose him with the correct subtype of hyperaldosteronism, more lab tests are needed and this is exactly what the question is asking for.
   - To diagnose the correct subtype of hyperaldosteronism, you would need to know:
     - his serum aldosterone level, to distinguish between true hyperaldosteronism and its mimics
     - his serum renin level, to distinguish between primary and secondary hyperaldosteronism.

2. A 14-year-old male presents with headaches and excessive fatigue. His past medical history is significant for treatment-resistant hypertension. Past lab tests indicate hypokalemia with metabolic alkalosis. His mother notes that she has experienced similar symptoms in the past. New lab tests show increased serum aldosterone with low renin. Serum aldosterone levels decrease following the administration of dexamethasone. Which of the following is the most likely cause of this patient's symptoms?

   A. Decreased degradation of renal sodium channels
   B. Bilateral adrenal hyperplasia
   C. 11β-hydroxysteroid dehydrogenase 2 deficiency
   D. Aberrant enzyme expression in the zona fasciculata

   - **The correct answer is D.**
   - Here we have a teenage boy with treatment-resistant hypertension, hypokalemia, and metabolic alkalosis. These are all signs of hyperaldosteronism. His mom has also had similar symptoms, likely indicating a genetic disorder as the cause. Further lab tests show high aldosterone with low renin. Importantly, his aldosterone levels are suppressed following administration of dexamethasone. This is the clinical picture for glucocorticoid remediable aldosteronism (GRA).
   - Recall that GRA is caused by a genetic mutation resulting in aberrant expression of aldosterone synthase in the zona fasciculata. This mutation is inherited in an autosomal dominant fashion and can lead to familial hyperaldosteronism, as indicated in the question since his mom experiences similar symptoms.
   - Lab results usually show high levels of aldosterone with low levels of renin. Importantly, GRA responds to dexamethasone administration since the zona fasciculata is controlled by ACTH levels.
   - A is incorrect, as this is describing the cause of Liddle syndrome. Liddle syndrome is a hyperaldosteronism mimic and presents with low serum aldosterone levels.
   - B is incorrect, as this is describing a cause of primary hyperaldosteronism. Primary hyperaldosteronism does not correct upon administration of dexamethasone.
   - C is incorrect, as this is describing syndrome of apparent mineralocorticoid excess (SAME). SAME is another hyperaldosteronism mimic, and presents with low serum aldosterone levels.

Section VIII - Hypercortisolism

I. Definition
   A. Excess cortisol secretion
   B. Cushing syndrome

II. Presentation
   A. Muscle weakness
   B. Thin extremities

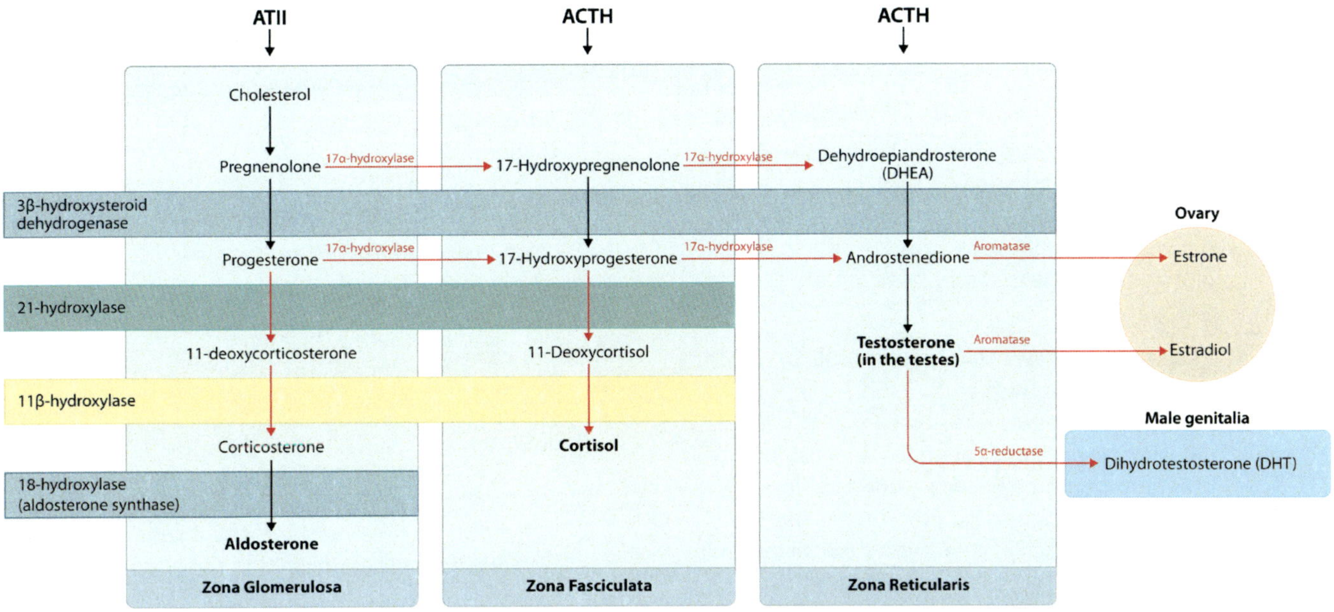

FIGURE 10.7.23 - Hormonal Production of the Layers of the Adrenal Medulla

   C. Buffalo hump, moon facies, and rotund abdomen
   D. Abdominal striae
   E. Hypertension, hypokalemia, and metabolic acidosis
   F. Osteoporosis
   G. Immunosuppression: recurrent infections

III. Lab Findings
   A. Increased 24-hour urine cortisol level
   B. Increased late night salivary cortisol level
   C. Failure to suppress cortisol levels with low-dose dexamethasone

IV. Subtypes
   A. Plasma ACTH level used to determine if the cause is ACTH-independent or ACTH-dependent
      1. ACTH-independent: low ACTH → adrenal imaging
      2. ACTH-dependent: high ACTH → high-dose dexamethasone test

V. Cushing Disease: Nelson Syndrome
   A. Bilateral adrenalectomy causes growth of the pituitary (adenoma)
      1. Hyperpigmentation
      2. Headache
      3. Bitemporal hemianopsia

Plasma ACTH	Cause	High Dose Dexamethasone	Imaging Findings	Treatment
Low (ACTH - independent)	- Exogenous glucocorticoid use	- N/A	- N/A	- Taper glucocorticoids
	- Primary adrenal pathology (hyperplasia, adenoma, carcinoma)	- N/A	- Unilateral adrenal mass, contralateral atrophy - Bilateral hyperplasia	- Resection of affected adrenal gland - Hormone replacement if bilateral
High (ACTH - dependent)	- ACTH-secreting pituitary adenoma (Cushing disease)	- Suppression	- Pituitary mass	- Removal of adenoma via transsphenoidal resection
	- Ectopic ACTH secretion	- No change	- Lung mass (small cell lung carcinoma, carcinoid tumor)	- Resection of lung mass

TABLE 10.7.2 - Subtypes of Hypercortisolism

REVIEW QUESTIONS

1. A 35-year-old woman presents with visual disturbances and a chronic cough. She has been suffering from mild fatigue and a nonproductive cough for the past 3 months, despite completing 2 full courses of antibiotics. Her blood pressure is 170/90 mmHg. Her temperature is 38.4 °C (101.2 °F). Physical exam reveals a bump on the back of her neck and scattered dark patches of skin. Rhonchi are heard on lung auscultation. Lab results show an elevated serum and urine cortisol, not suppressed following the administration of dexamethasone. What is the likely physiologic cause behind the prolonged upper respiratory infection she is experiencing?

    - **The correct answer is hypercortisolism resulting in immunosuppression.**
    - The patient has visual disturbances and an illness resulting in a cough for the past 2 months that has persisted despite using antibiotics. She also has high blood pressure, a "buffalo hump," and ecchymoses, with rhonchi on lung auscultation. Labs are consistent with hypercortisolism. High levels of cortisol can result in immunosuppression, which presents as recurrent infections. Therefore, the answer is hypercortisolism resulting in immunosuppression prolonging her URI.

2. A 65-year-old man presents with headaches and generalized muscle weakness. He has a 45 pack-year smoking history. His blood pressure is 165/95 mmHg. Physical exam reveals a swollen face, rotund abdomen, thin and weak extremities, and scattered ecchymoses. Lung auscultation reveals decreased breath sounds over the base of the left lung. Imaging confirms a mass in this area. Lab tests show hyperglycemia and elevated urinary free cortisol. Which of the following changes in cortisol levels is expected following the administration of a low and high dose of dexamethasone, respectively?

    A. No change, no change
    B. No change, decrease
    C. No change, increase
    D. Decrease, no change

    - **The correct answer is A.**
    - The patient has a significant smoking history and moon face. Lab results show high urinary cortisol. Taken together, these findings should suggest hypercortisolism. There is also a mass in his left lung, which should make you suspicious of lung cancer such as small cell carcinoma that can secrete ACTH and cause Cushing syndrome.
    - Since the source is ectopic, these patients usually do not respond to low-dose or high-dose dexamethasone administration. In all listed causes of hypercortisolism, cortisol levels are not suppressed following administration of low-dose dexamethasone.The ectopic ACTH secretion is considered to be an ACTH-dependent cause of hypercortisolism, which is usually followed up with a high-dose dexamethasone test. In the event of ectopic ACTH secretion, like in lung cancer, cortisol levels are not changed by high-dose dexamethasone because the ACTH is secreted by a tumor, not the pituitary gland.
    - B is incorrect, because suppression of cortisol levels following high dose dexamethasone administration better describes a pituitary adenoma or Cushing disease.
    - C is incorrect, because cortisol levels will not increase following dexamethasone administration.
    - D is incorrect, because cortisol levels do not decrease following low-dose dexamethasone administration in hypercortisolism.

Section IX - Adrenal Insufficiency

I. Definition
   A. Adrenal hormone deficiency
   B. Subtypes
      1. Acute
      2. Chronic (Addison disease)

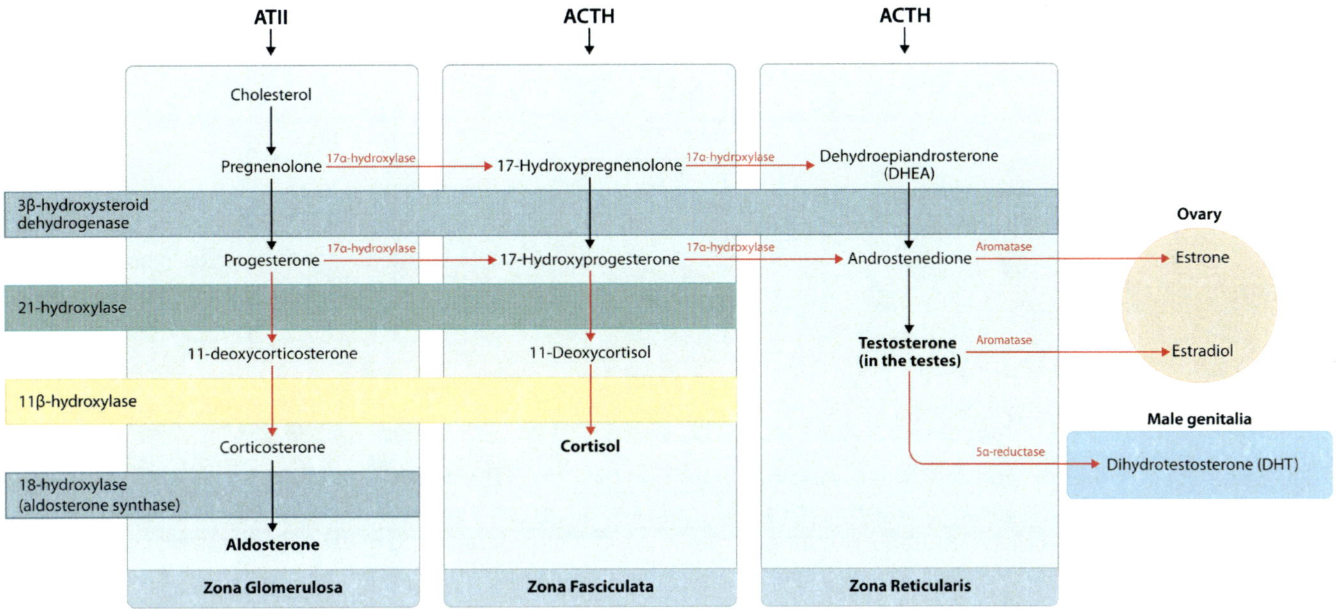

FIGURE 10.7.23 - Hormonal Production of the Layers of the Adrenal Medulla

II. Acute Adrenal Insufficiency
   A. Presentation: weakness and shock
   B. Causes
      1. Sudden glucocorticoid withdrawal
      2. Cushing syndrome treatment
      3. Waterhouse-Friderichsen syndrome

III. Waterhouse-Friderichsen Syndrome
   A. Bilateral hemorrhagic adrenal gland necrosis
      1. Children with *N. meningitidis* infection
   B. Presentation
      1. DIC due to sepsis → low platelet count, petechial rash, abnormal bleeding
      2. Cortisol deficiency → hypoglycemia
      3. Aldosterone deficiency → hyponatremia, hyperkalemia

IV. Chronic Adrenal Insufficiency (Addison Disease)
   A. Progressive damage to adrenal glands
      1. Developed countries: autoimmune destruction
         a) Associated with autoimmune polyendocrine syndromes
      2. Developing countries: tuberculosis
      3. Metastatic lung carcinoma

V. Chronic Adrenal Insufficiency (Addison Disease): Presentation
   A. Vague, progressive symptoms
      1. Hypotension
      2. Weakness
      3. Fatigue
      4. Nausea and vomiting
      5. Weight loss

VI. Chronic Adrenal Insufficiency (Addison Disease): Subtypes
   A. Primary: adrenal gland
   B. Secondary: pituitary gland
   C. Tertiary: hypothalamus

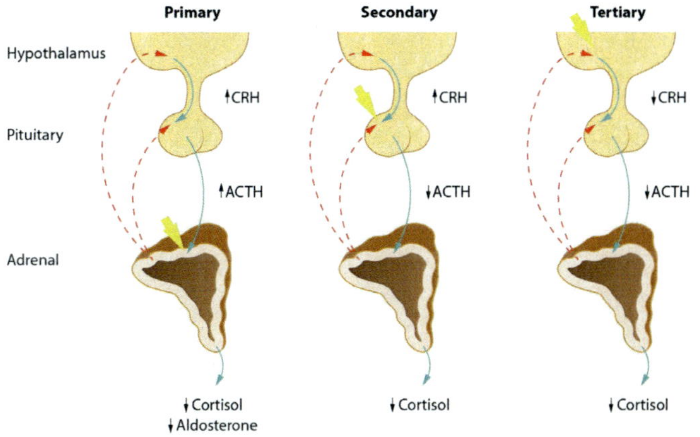

FIGURE 10.7.24 - Hypothalamic-Pituitary-Adrenal Axis in Adrenal Insufficiency

Subtype	Location of Problem	Cortisol	Aldosterone	ACTH	CRH	Clinical Findings
Primary adrenal insufficiency	- Adrenal gland	- Low	- Low	- High	- High	- Hyperpigmentation - Hyperkalemia
Secondary adrenal insufficiency	- Pituitary gland	- Low	- Normal	- Low	- High	- No hyperpigmentation - No hyperkalemia
Tertiary adrenal insufficiency	- Hypothalamus	- Low	- Normal	- Low	- Low	- No hyperpigmentation - No hyperkalemia

TABLE 10.7.3 - Types of Adrenal Insufficiency

REVIEW QUESTIONS

1. A 45-year-old woman presents with complaints of progressive fatigue and dizziness over the past 6 months. She has also had multiple vomiting episodes per week for the past 3 weeks. She has unintentionally lost weight during this time period, but believes this is due to constant nausea, which has suppressed her appetite. On physical exam, she has uniformly dark, bronze-colored skin throughout. Her blood pressure is 100/60 mmHg. Initial lab results indicate hyperkalemia. Which of the following additional lab results are expected in this patient?

	Cortisol	ACTH	CRH
A.	Low	Low	Low
B.	Low	Low	High
C.	Low	High	High
D.	High	Low	Low

- **The correct answer is C.**
- Here we have a woman with progressive fatigue, dizziness, vomiting, and weight loss. Her physical exam reveals hyperpigmentation and hypotension. Her lab results reveal hyperkalemia. These findings should make you suspicious for adrenal insufficiency. Specifically, since she has hyperpigmentation and hyperkalemia, you should be suspicious of primary adrenal insufficiency.
- Primary adrenal insufficiency is a problem with the adrenal gland, resulting in low cortisol and low aldosterone with high ACTH and high CRH. Clinically, this means you will see hyperpigmentation and hyperkalemia.
- A is incorrect because ACTH and CRH will both be low in tertiary adrenal insufficiency, which is a problem in the hypothalamus and does not present with hyperpigmentation or hyperkalemia.
- B is incorrect because ACTH will be low with high CRH in secondary adrenal insufficiency, which is a problem in the pituitary gland and does not present with hyperpigmentation or hyperkalemia.
- D is incorrect because adrenal insufficiency presents with low cortisol levels. High cortisol levels better describe Cushing syndrome, or hypercortisolism.

Section X - Adrenal Medulla

I. Basic Principles
   A. Composed of chromaffin cells (derived from neural crest)
   B. Main source of circulating catecholamines (epinephrine and norepinephrine)

II. Pheochromocytoma
   A. Tumor of chromaffin cells
      1. Zellballen pattern on biopsy
   B. Symptoms due to episodic release of catecholamines
      1. Episodic hypertension, headache, sweating, tachycardia, tremor, and shortness of breath
   C. Diagnosis: increased catecholamines, metanephrines, and vanillylmandelic acid (VMA) in serum and urine

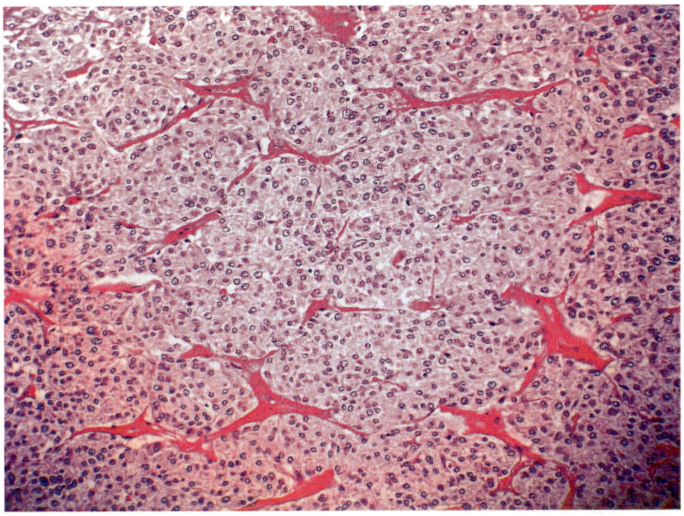

FIGURE 10.7.25 - Zellballen Pattern in Pheochromocytoma

III. Pheochromocytoma: Treatment
   A. Adrenalectomy
      1. Possibility of catecholamines leaking into circulation on handling of the tumor
      2. Phenoxybenzamine (irreversible alpha blocker) followed by beta blocker is administered preoperatively to prevent hypertensive crisis

IV. Pheochromocytoma: Rule of 10s
   A. 10% bilateral
   B. 10% familial, however, research is showing that many more pheochromocytomas may be genetic than was previously thought
   C. 10% malignant
   D. 10% located outside of adrenal medulla (e.g. bladder wall)

V. Pheochromocytoma: Associations
   A. MEN 2A and 2B (*RET* mutation)
   B. Von Hippel-Lindau disease
      1. Formation of tumors and cysts in multiple parts of body
   C. Neurofibromatosis type 1
      1. Changes in skin color and growth of benign tumors

REVIEW QUESTIONS ?

1. A 47-year-old male presents to the clinic with excessive sweating and palpitations. On physical exam, his blood pressure is 155/121 mmHg. On urinalysis, there is a 10-fold increase in the levels of metanephrines and catecholamines. Lab results also show elevated plasma vanillylmandelic acid. An adrenal mass is found on an abdominal CT scan. A pathological process involving which of the following cells is responsible for this patient's symptoms?

   A. C cells
   B. Chromaffin cells
   C. CD4+ T-cells
   D. Islet cells

- **The correct answer is B.**
- This is a 47-year-old hypertensive male presenting with excessive sweating and palpitations. On urinalysis, his metanephrine and catecholamine levels are significantly increased, as as are the plasma vanillylmandelic acid levels. On abdominal CT scan, there is an adrenal mass.
- This patient's findings are consistent with pheochromocytoma. Pheochromocytoma is a tumor of chromaffin cells.
- A is wrong because a tumor of C cells would cause medullary carcinoma of thyroid.
- C is wrong because a tumor of CD4+ T-cells would cause T-cell leukemias or lymphomas, or mycosis fungoides
- D is wrong because a tumor of the islet cells would cause insulinoma or glucagonoma.

Section XI - Multiple Endocrine Neoplasias

I. Definition
   A. Group of disorders that affects multiple endocrine organs
   B. Autosomal dominant inheritance

Subtype	Gene Mutation	Key Features
MEN 1	*MEN1* - Tumor suppressor - Chromosome 11	3Ps: - Pituitary tumors: secrete prolactin, GH; cause headache, visual defects - Primary hyperparathyroidism: hypercalcemia, hypophosphatemia, recurrent nephrolithiasis - Pancreatic endocrine tumors: gastrinoma, insulinoma, VIPoma, glucagonoma - Associated with angiofibroma, collagenoma, meningioma
MEN 2A	*RET* - Oncogene - Receptor tyrosine kinase - Mutation in cells derived from neural crest	2Ps + 1M: - Primary hyperparathyroidism - Pheochromocytoma: catecholamine-secreting tumor of chromaffin cells in adrenal medulla; HTN, headache, sweating, tachycardia - Medullary thyroid carcinoma: calcitonin-secreting neoplasm of parafollicular (C) cells; requires prophylactic thyroidectomy
MEN 2B		1P + 3Ms: - Pheochromocytoma - Medullary thyroid carcinoma - Mucosal neuromas: oral or intestinal painless flesh-colored papules - Marfanoid habitus: tall, slender build with disproportionately long arms, legs, and fingers

TABLE 10.7.4 - Types of MEN Syndromes

II. MEN 1: Pancreatic Endocrine Tumors
   A. Gastrinoma: gastrin-secreting tumor
      1. Causes Zollinger-Ellison syndrome
      2. Recurrent peptic ulcers, diarrhea, iron deficiency anemia
   B. Insulinoma: insulin-secreting tumor of pancreatic beta cells
      1. Hypoglycemia
   C. VIPoma: VIP-secreting neuroendocrine tumor
      1. Secretory diarrhea
   D. Glucagonoma: glucagon-secreting tumor of pancreatic alpha cells
      1. Rare
      2. Five Ds: dermatitis, diabetes, DVT, declining weight, depression

REVIEW QUESTIONS

1. A 35-year-old woman presents with a chief complaint of trouble seeing. Her past medical history is significant for recurrent nephrolithiasis and recent development of peptic ulcer disease. Physical exam reveals mild abdominal tenderness and milky white nipple discharge. An eye exam reveals bitemporal hemianopsia. Based on this patient's past medical history and current symptoms, what gene mutation does she likely carry and how was it inherited?

- **The correct answer is a mutation in the *MEN1* tumor suppressor with autosomal dominant inheritance.**
- This woman is having trouble seeing. Physical exam shows a milky white nipple discharge, and eye exam reveals bitemporal hemianopsia. These findings are consistent with a prolactinoma, or a prolactin-secreting pituitary adenoma, pressing on the optic chiasm.
- Her past medical history of recurrent nephrolithiasis and peptic ulcer disease also indicate she may have hyperparathyroidism and a gastrinoma, respectively. This constellation of symptoms should make you think of *MEN1* as a potential cause. *MEN1* is caused by a mutation in the *MEN1* tumor suppressor, and this disorder follows an autosomal dominant inheritance pattern.

2. A 27-year-old male presents to the physician due to abdominal pain and bloody urine. He says he has felt this pain on and off for a year, but this time it is more intense. Past medical history is significant for an adrenalectomy due to pheochromocytoma as a teenager. Physical exam shows severe abdominal tenderness. Urinalysis shows gross hematuria and hypercalciuria. Ultrasound confirms the presence of many small stones in the ureters. Which of the following steps should be taken to ensure long-term survival of this patient?

   A. Parathyroid resection
   B. Imaging for suspected mucosal neuromas
   C. Prophylactic removal of the thyroid gland
   D. Lab analysis of pancreatic secretions

- **The correct answer is C.**
- This patient has recurrent abdominal pain with hypercalciuria and hematuria, and an ultrasound shows stones in the ureters. This should make you suspicious for recurrent nephrolithiasis due to primary hyperparathyroidism. His past medical history is also significant for a pheochromocytoma.
- Patients with both primary hyperparathyroidism and pheochromocytoma likely have *MEN 2A*. *MEN 2A* is also characterized by medullary thyroid carcinoma, and these patients should receive a prophylactic thyroidectomy to prevent this.
- A is incorrect because although primary hyperparathyroidism is likely responsible for this patient's recurrent nephrolithiasis, resection of the parathyroids is not how this is treated.
- B is incorrect because mucosal neuromas are characteristic of *MEN 2B*, not *MEN 2A*.
- D is incorrect because pancreatic neuroendocrine tumors are characteristic of *MEN 1*, not *MEN 2A*.

Section I - Oral Cavity

I. Aphthous Ulcer
   A. Shallow, painful lesions of the oral mucosa
   B. Resolves spontaneously within days to weeks, but recurrent
   C. Clear base with erythematous surroundings

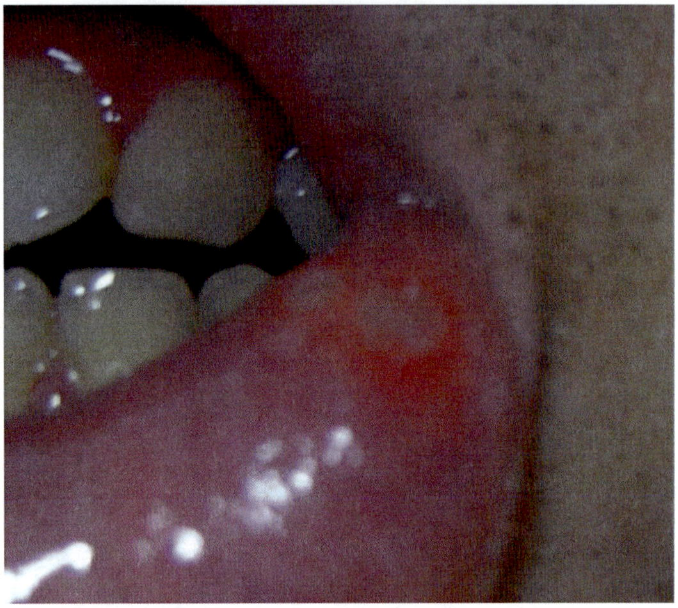

FIGURE 10.8.1 - Aphthous Ulcer

II. Behçet Syndrome
   A. Autoimmune disorder causing vasculitis throughout the body
   B. Findings: aphthous ulcers, genital ulcers, uveitis, skin rash
   C. Unknown etiology, but seen following viral infection

III. Oral Herpes
   A. Shallow, painful lesions of the oral mucosa that rupture
   B. Caused by HSV-1
   C. Primary episode of herpes infection occurs in childhood
   D. Virus lies dormant in the ganglia of the trigeminal nerve
   E. Viral infection, stress, exposure to sunlight → reactivation of virus → oral lesions

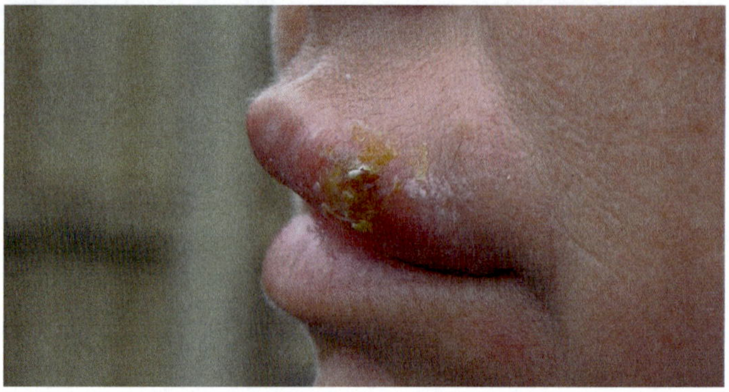

FIGURE 10.8.2 - Cold Sore

IV. 5. Squamous Cell Carcinoma
   A. Malignant proliferation of squamous cells lining lips and inside of mouth
   B. Risk factors: tobacco, heavy alcohol use, excessive sun exposure to lips
   C. Oral leukoplakia and erythroplakia are premalignant conditions
   D. Often biopsied to rule out squamous cell carcinoma

V. 6. Squamous Cell Carcinoma: Oral Leukoplakia
   A. Thickened, white patches that cannot be scraped off
   B. Different from oral candidiasis (thrush) and hairy leukoplakia
      1. Oral candidiasis: white patch on tongue, easily scraped off
      2. Hairy leukoplakia: white, rough (hairy) patch on lateral tongue

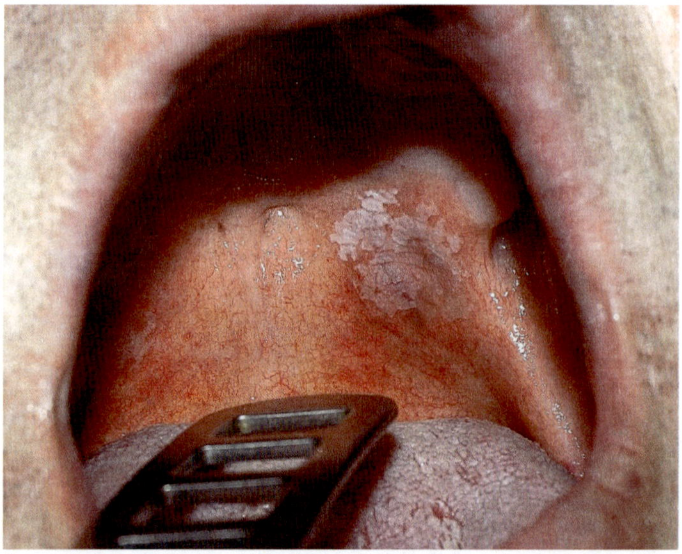

FIGURE 10.8.3 - Oral Leukoplakia

VI. Squamous Cell Carcinoma: Erythroplakia
  A. Erythematous plaque on oral mucous membrane
  B. Can develop into squamous cell carcinoma

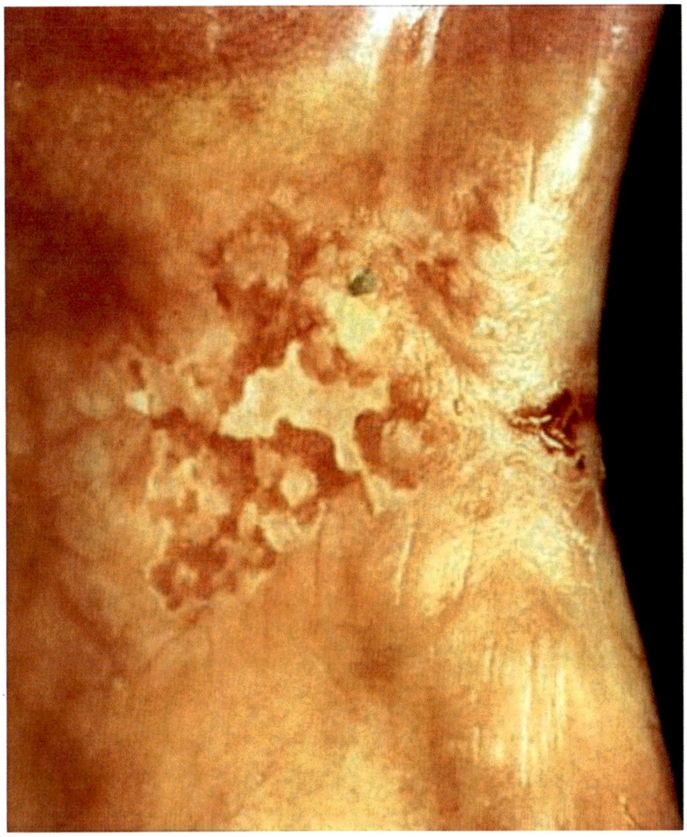

FIGURE 10.8.4 - Erythroplakia

REVIEW QUESTIONS

1. A 29-year-old female comes to the clinic for painful ulcers on her lips. She is afebrile. She is a law student and explains that she has been staying up late frequently for her final exams. On physical examination, a grayish base surrounded by erythema is observed on the upper lip. What most likely initiated this patient's condition?

- **The correct answer is stress.**
- A 29-year-old female law student who comes to
- Since she is afebrile, there are no painful vesicles found in her lips, oral herpes is unlikely.
- Rather, a grayish base surrounded by erythema is found on her lips, which characterizes aphthous ulcers.
- These ulcers are most likely triggered by stress since the patient has been staying up late for her law exams.

REVIEW QUESTIONS

2. A 58-year-old man presents with discomfort in his mouth. He denies any trauma to his oral mucosa. He has smoked cigarettes daily for the past 38 years. He drinks 2 cans of beer daily. His heart rate is 94 beats/minute, blood pressure is 142/74 mmHg, and the is 37° C (98.6 °F). On physical examination, the physician notices a plaque in the oral mucosa. Which of the following findings would most likely indicate the plaque is a premalignant lesion?

   A. A white deposit on the tongue that can be easily scraped off
   B. A white, rough patch on the lateral tongue
   C. A white plaque that cannot be scraped off
   D. A clear base surrounded by erythema

- **The correct answer is C.**
- This is a 58-year-old chronic smoker who presents to the clinic with discomfort in his mouth. He also drinks heavily.
- On examination, the physician notices a plaque in the oral mucosa.
- Oral leukoplakia and erythroplakia are premalignant conditions.
- A white plaque that cannot be scraped off describes oral leukoplakia.
- A is wrong because a white deposit on the tongue that can be easily scraped away refers to oral candidiasis or oral thrush.
- B is wrong because a white, rough patch on the lateral tongue refers to hairy leukoplakia.
- D is wrong because a grayish base surrounded by erythema of the oral mucosa describes aphthous ulcers.

Section II - Salivary Glands

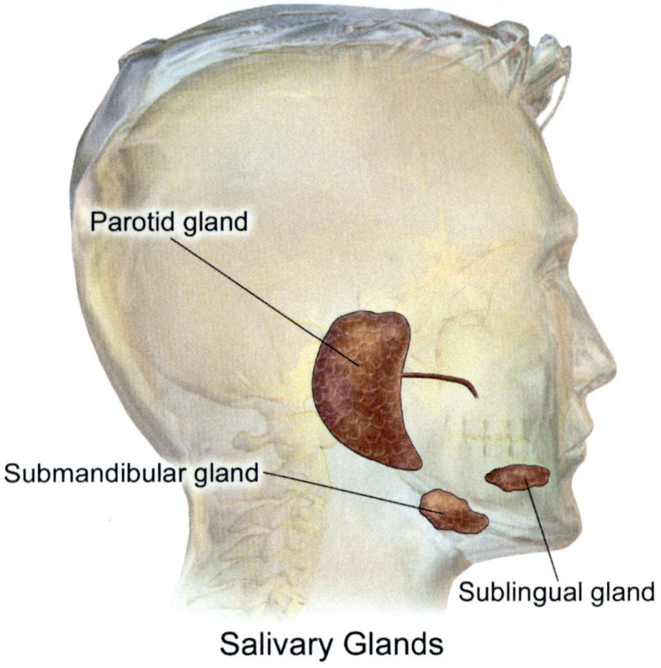

Photo Credit: Blausen.com staff (2014). "Medical gallery of Blausen Medical 2014". WikiJournal of Medicine 1 (2). DOI:10.15347/wjm/2014.010. ISSN 2002-4436. / CC BY (https://creativecommons.org/licenses/by/3.0)

FIGURE 10.8.5 - Anatomy of the Salivary Glands

I. Mumps
   A. Infection with mumps virus → bilateral inflammation of parotid glands and salivary glands
   B. Orchitis, pancreatitis, and aseptic meningitis can coexist with mumps

II. Mumps: Risk Factors
   A. Lack of MMR vaccination (measles, mumps, and rubella)
   B. Crowded living environment (e.g. college dorms)

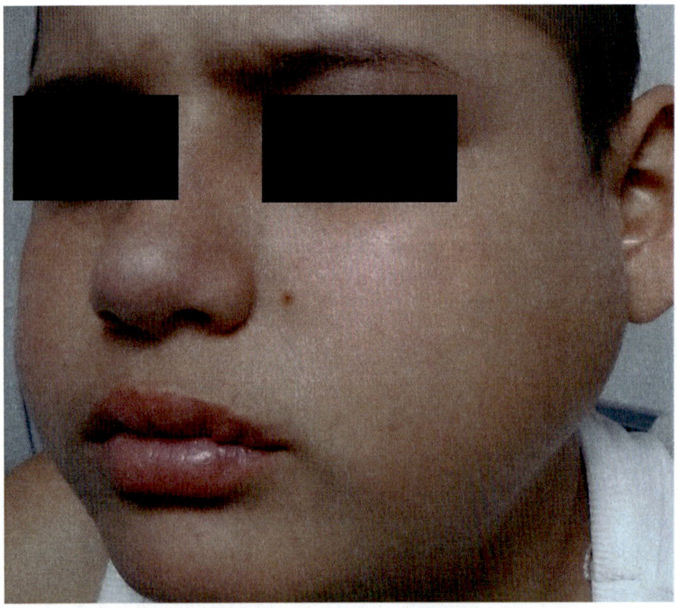

Photo Credit: Afrodriguezg / CC BY-SA (https://creativecommons.org/licenses/by-sa/3.0)

FIGURE 10.8.6 - Parotitis

III. Sialadenitis
   A. Inflammation of a salivary gland (usually unilateral)
   B. Often due to an obstructing salivary gland stone (sialolithiasis) leading to *S. aureus* infection

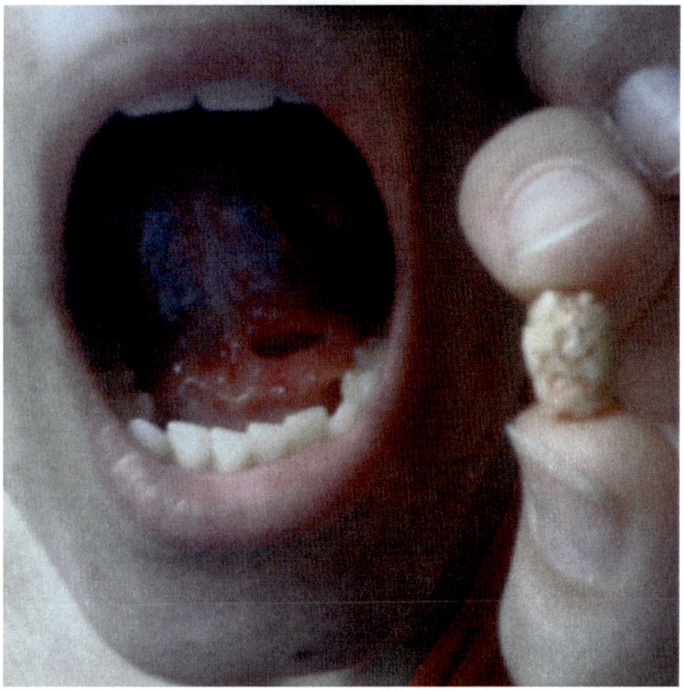

Photo Credit: Peternickson / CC0

FIGURE 10.8.7 - Sialadenitis Due to Sialolithiasis

IV. Pleomorphic Adenoma
   A. Common benign salivary gland neoplasm characterized by stromal and myoepithelial cells
   B. Often develops in parotid gland
   C. Slow-growing, painless, firm mass near the jaw
   D. High rate of recurrence
   E. Has potential to become malignant
      1. Signs of facial nerve damage

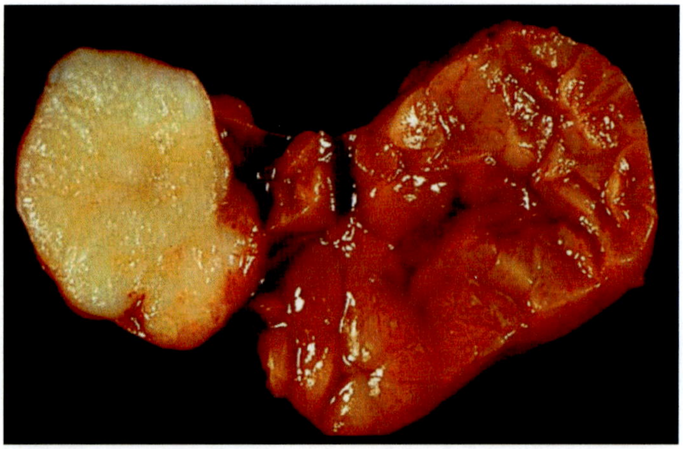

Photo Credit: Ed Uthman / Public domain

FIGURE 10.8.8 - Pleomorphic Adenoma

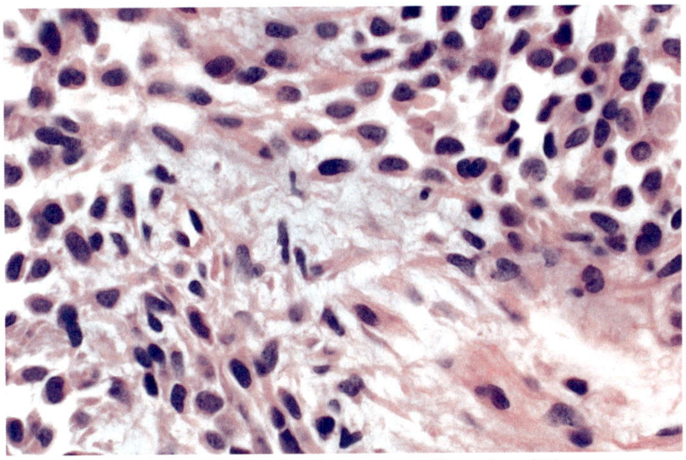

FIGURE 10.8.9 - Stromal and Myoepithelial Components of Pleomorphic Adenoma

V. Warthin Tumor
   A. Papillary cystadenoma lymphomatosum
   B. Benign cyst tumor with abundant lymphocytes and germinal centers
   C. Often develops in the parotid gland
   D. Typically found in smokers

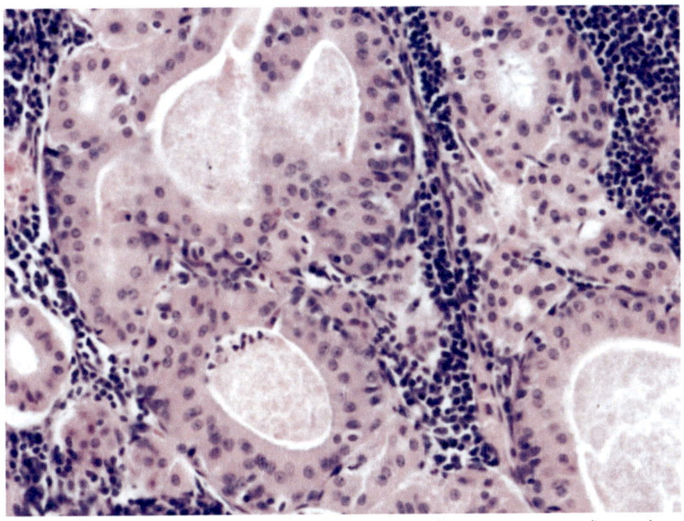

FIGURE 10.8.10 - Warthin Tumor

VI. Mucoepidermoid Carcinoma
   A. Mixed malignant salivary gland tumor characterized by the presence of squamous cells and mucin-secreting goblet cells
   B. Most common malignant tumor of the salivary glands
   C. Often develops in the parotid gland
   D. Signs of facial nerve damage

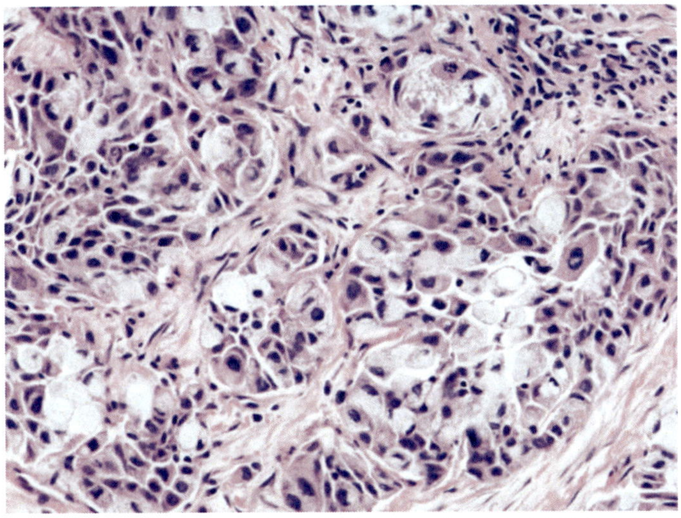

FIGURE 10.8.11 - Mucoepidermoid Carcinoma

REVIEW QUESTIONS

1. A 17-year-old boy presents to the emergency room with a swollen jaw and testicular pain. The patient immigrated from Haiti when he was 3 and does not recall if he has ever been vaccinated. On physical exam, he has a low-grade fever, and his parotid glands and testes are bilaterally swollen and tender on palpation. What other complications may be present in this patient?

    - **The correct answer is pancreatitis and aseptic meningitis.**
    - This is a potentially unvaccinated 17-year-old boy presenting with a swollen jaw and pain in the testes. He also has a low-grade fever as well as bilateral swollen and tender parotid glands and testes.
    - This is a classic presentation of a patient with mumps, which is characterized by bilateral parotitis as well as orchitis. In someone with mumps, pancreatitis and aseptic meningitis may also be present.

2. A 42-year-old male presents to the clinic with a lump in his jaw. He has smoked 2 packs of cigarettes daily for the past 33 years. His heart rate is 87 beats/minute, blood pressure is 132/72 mmHg, and temperature is 37° C (98.6 °F). He does not have any signs of facial nerve damage. Which of the following histopathological findings is most likely in this patient?

    A. Malignant tumor composed of mucinous and squamous cells
    B. Benign tumor composed of stromal and epithelial tissue
    C. Benign cystic tumor with abundant lymphocytes and germinal centers
    D. Malignant tumor composed of signet ring cells

    - **The correct answer is C.**
    - This is a 42-year-old male chronic smoker presenting with a lump in his jaw. Since he does not have any signs of facial nerve damage, malignancy is very unlikely. This is a classic finding of someone with Warthin tumor, which is typically found in smokers.
    - Warthin tumor is a benign cystic tumor with abundant lymphocytes and germinal centers.
    - A is incorrect because a malignant tumor composed of mucinous and squamous cells refers to mucoepidermoid carcinoma. Since this patient does not have any signs of facial nerve damage, a malignancy can be ruled out.
    - B is incorrect because a benign tumor composed of stromal and epithelial tissue refers to pleomorphic adenoma. Pleomorphic adenoma is not typically found in smokers.
    - D is incorrect because a malignant tumor composed of signet ring cells represents the diffuse type of gastric carcinoma.

Section III - Esophagus

I. Esophageal Web
   A. Protrusion of thin mucosal membrane in upper esophagus
   B. Dysphagia for solids
   C. Can lead to esophageal squamous cell carcinoma
   D. Plummer-Vinson syndrome: severe iron deficiency anemia, esophageal web, and glossitis

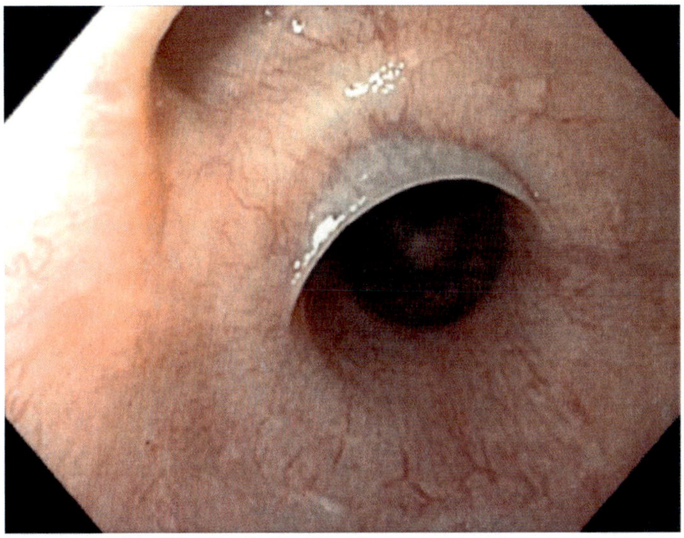

FIGURE 10.8.12 - Esophageal Web

II. Zenker Diverticulum
   A. Acquired herniation of pharyngeal mucosa
   B. False diverticulum
   C. Arises above upper esophageal sphincter at pharyngoesophageal junction
   D. Presents with dysphagia, cough, regurgitation, and halitosis

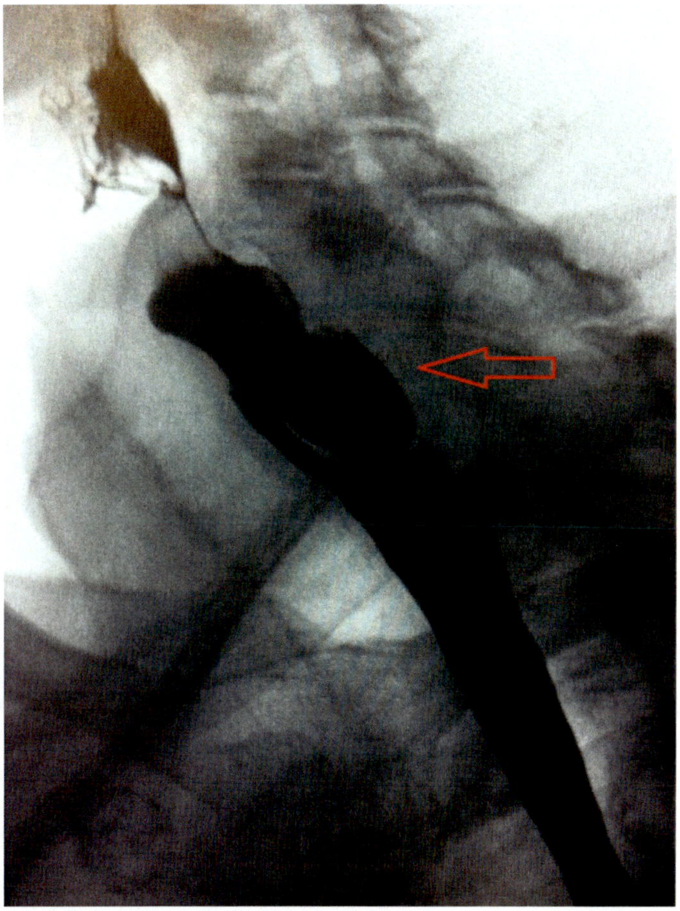

FIGURE 10.8.13 - Zenker Diverticulum

III. Mallory-Weiss Syndrome
   A. Superficial, longitudinal laceration of mucosa at the gastroesophageal junction
   B. Classicially caused by severe vomiting (due to alcoholism or bulimia)
   C. Often presents with painful hematemesis
   D. Risk of Boerhaave syndrome
      1. Esophageal rupture, leading to pneumomediastinum and subcutaneous emphysema

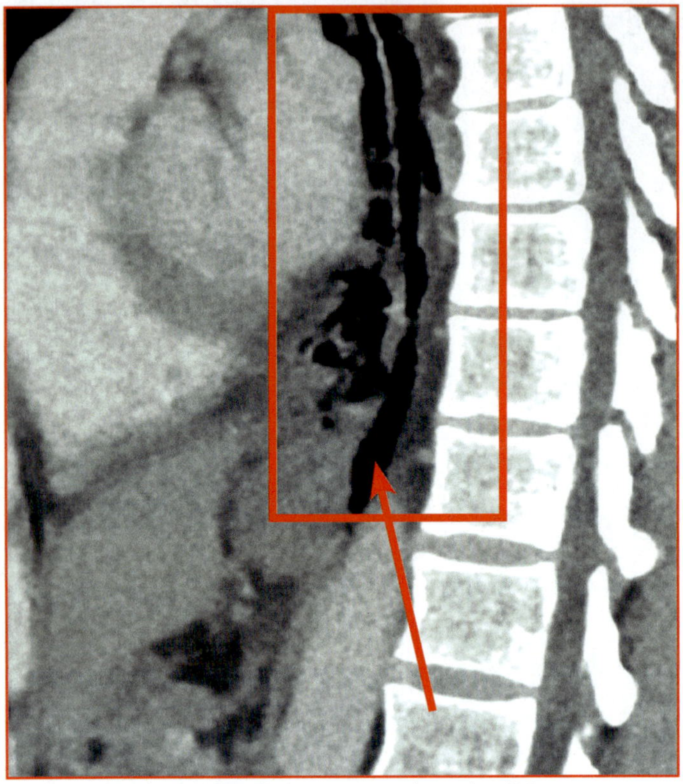

FIGURE 10.8.14 - Sagittal CT of Mallory-Weiss Syndrome

IV. Achalasia
   A. Failure of lower esophageal sphincter to relax
   B. Etiology: degeneration of inhibitory neurons in the myenteric (Auerbach's) plexus
      1. Secondary achalasia may arise from *Trypanosoma cruzi* infection in Chagas disease or extraesophageal malignancies
   C. Associated with increased risk of esophageal squamous cell carcinoma

V. Achalasia: Findings
   A. Progressive dysphagia to solid food and liquids
   B. Halitosis
   C. High lower esophageal sphincter pressure on esophageal manometry
   D. Dilated esophagus with an area of distal stenosis ("bird-beak" sign) on barium swallow study

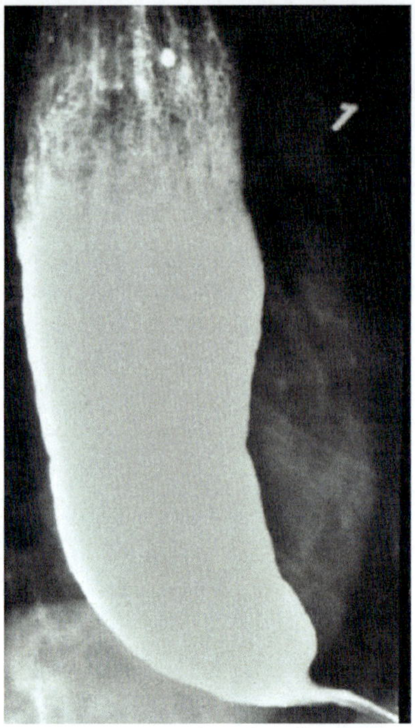

FIGURE 10.8.15 - "Bird-Beak" Sign of Achalasia

VI. Gastroesophageal Reflux Disease (GERD)
   A. Reflux of stomach acid due to transient decreases in lower esophageal sphincter tone
   B. Risk factors: alcohol, tobacco, obesity, fat-rich diet, caffeine, hiatal hernia
   C. Presentation: heartburn, regurgitation, chronic cough, hoarseness, damage to tooth enamel, adult-onset asthma
   D. Late complications: ulceration with stricture, Barrett esophagus

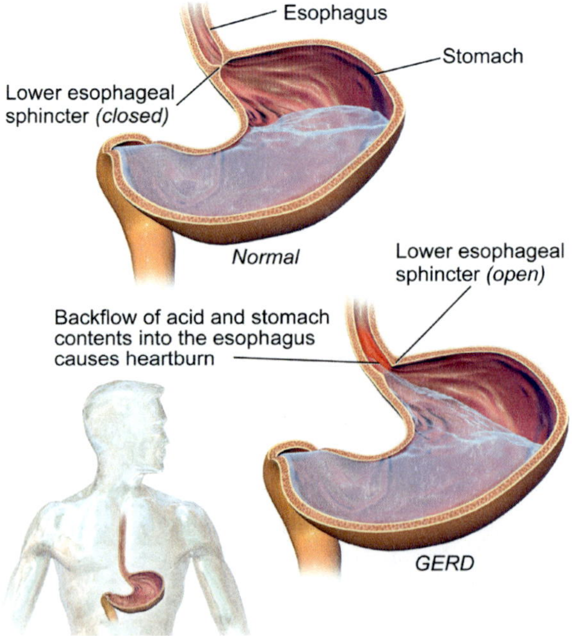

FIGURE 10.8.16 - Gastroesophageal Reflux Disease (GERD)

VII. Barrett Esophagus
   A. Specialized intestinal metaplasia
      1. Stratified squamous epithelium to nonciliated columnar epithelium with goblet cells
   B. Due to chronic GERD
      1. Response of lower esophageal mucosal cells to acidic stress
   C. Associated with increased risk of esophageal dysplasia and adenocarcinoma

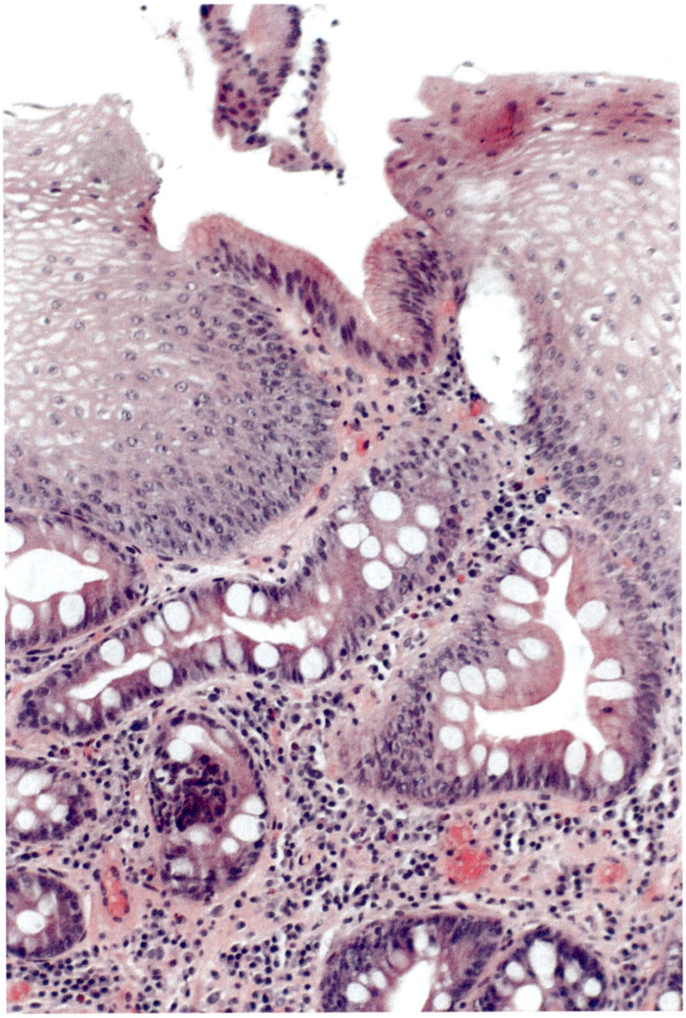

FIGURE 10.8.17 - Barrett Esophagus

VIII. Esophageal Carcinoma
   A. Two types
      1. Adenocarcinoma
      2. Squamous cell carcinoma

IX. Esophageal Carcinoma: Adenocarcinoma
   A. Malignant proliferation of glands in the esophagus
   B. More common in America
   C. Risk factors: preexisting Barrett esophagus, chronic GERD, obesity, smoking, achalasia
   D. Often involves lower one-third of esophagus

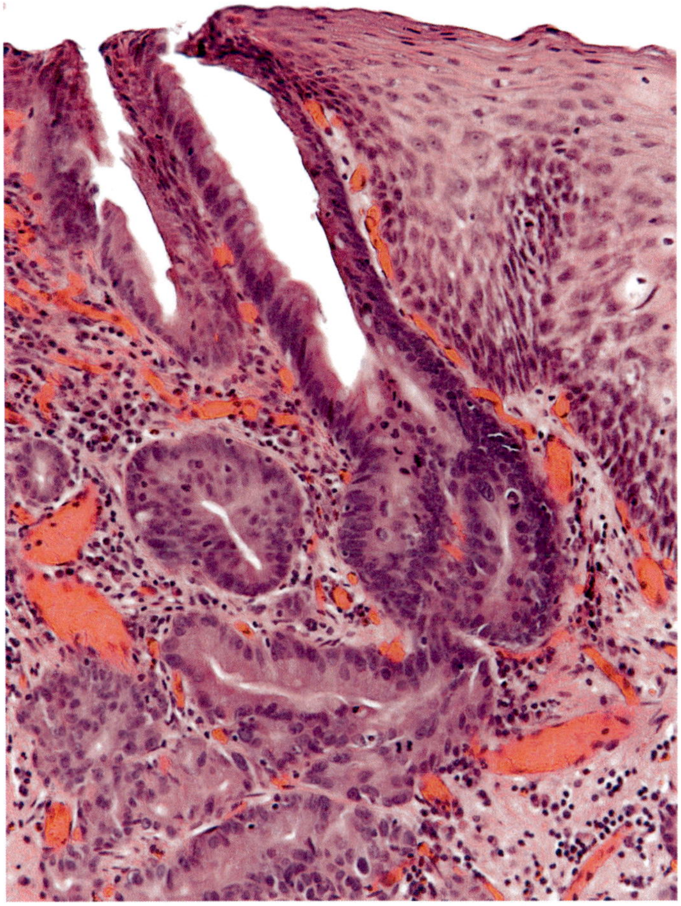

FIGURE 10.8.18 - Adenocarcinoma of the Esophagus

X. Esophageal Carcinoma: Squamous Cell Carcinoma
   A. Malignant proliferation of squamous cells in the esophagus
   B. More common worldwide
   C. Risk factors: alcohol and tobacco (most common), hot liquids, esophageal web (e.g. Plummer-Vinson syndrome), smoking, achalasia
   D. Often involves upper two-thirds of the esophagus

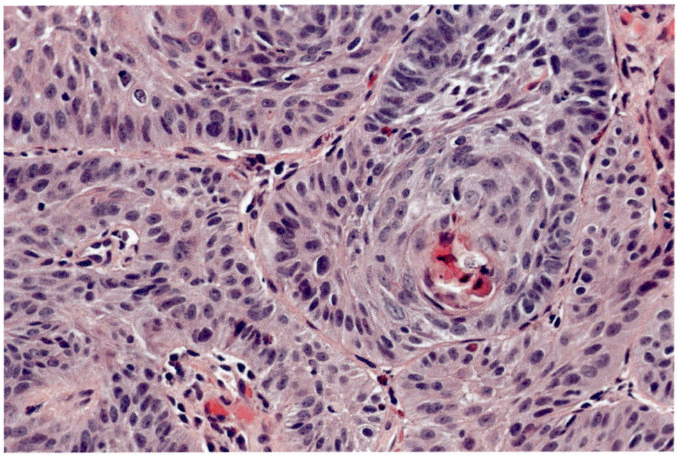

FIGURE 10.8.19 - Squamous Cell Carcinoma of the Esophagus

XI. Esophageal Carcinoma: Findings
- A. Progressive dysphagia (solids to liquids)
- B. Weight loss
- C. Hematemesis
- D. Hoarseness (recurrent laryngeal nerve)
- E. Cough (trachea)

XII. Esophageal Carcinoma: Lymph Node Involvement
- A. Location of lymph node spread depends on depth of involved esophagus
- B. Upper ⅓ - cervical nodes
- C. Middle ⅓ - mediastinal or tracheobronchial nodes
- D. Lower ⅓ - celiac and gastric nodes

REVIEW QUESTIONS

1. A 67-year-old man presents to the clinic with difficulty swallowing solid foods. His past medical history includes diabetes and iron deficiency anemia. On physical examination, he is pale, has spoon-shaped fingernails, and has a beefy-red tongue. Endoscopy reveals a thin protrusion of esophageal mucosa in the upper esophagus. If left untreated, what malignancy is this patient likely to develop?
   - **The correct answer is esophageal squamous cell carcinoma.**
   - All of these findings characterize Plummer-Vinson syndrome. If left untreated, this patient is likely to develop esophageal squamous cell carcinoma.

2. A 58-year-old chronic smoker presents to the clinic with chest pain. She mentions that her symptom worsens when she drinks coffee or energy drinks. When she takes a proton pump inhibitor, her symptom improves. On physical exam, there is significant damage to her tooth enamel. ECG shows a normal sinus rhythm with no significant abnormal findings. What is the cause of her chest pain?
   - **The correct answer is reflux of acid from the stomach.**
   - These findings characterize GERD. GERD is caused by a reflux of acid from the stomach due to reduced lower esophageal sphincter tone, which causes a transient lower esophageal sphincter relaxation. The reflux of acid from the stomach is what causes her chest pain.

3. A 52-year-old man presents to the clinic with weight loss and difficulty swallowing. He had difficulty swallowing solid food about 3 months ago, but it has since progressed to liquids. He has smoked 2 packs of cigarettes daily for the past 30 years. He also mentions that he drinks very hot tea every morning. An upper endoscopy demonstrates a malignancy in the upper one-third of the esophagus. The biopsy reveals nests of malignant squamous cells. Which of the following lymph nodes may be involved in the spread of this patient's condition?

   A. Celiac nodes
   B. Tracheobronchial nodes
   C. Gastric nodes
   D. Cervical nodes

   - **The correct answer is D.**
   - When there is a malignancy in the upper one-third of the esophagus, the cervical nodes are involved.
   - A is incorrect because the celiac nodes are involved when there is a malignancy in the lower one-third of the esophagus.
   - B is incorrect because the tracheobronchial nodes are involved when there is a malignancy in the middle one-third of the esophagus.
   - C is incorrect because the gastric nodes are involved when there is a malignancy in the lower one-third of the esophagus.

Section IV - Stomach

I. Acute Gastritis
   A. Injury to the gastric mucosa caused by stomach acid
   B. Loss of mucosal protective factors → stomach acid causes mucosal damage
   C. Complications include inflammation, erosion, or ulceration of the mucosa

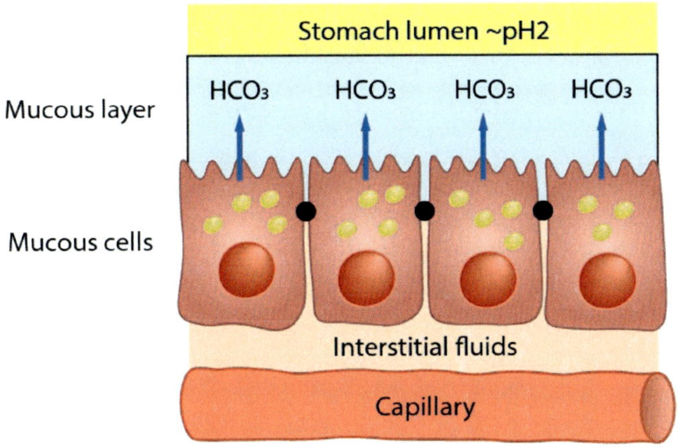

FIGURE 10.8.20 - Protective Factors of the Stomach

II. Acute Gastritis: Etiology
   A. NSAIDs (decrease PGE2, which is involved in mucus production)
   B. Alcohol abuse
   C. Hypovolemic shock → ischemia → multiple stress ulcers
   D. Severe burn injury → hypovolemia → Curling ulcers
   E. ↑ intracranial pressure → vagal stimulation → Cushing ulcer
   F. Chemotherapy

III. Chronic Gastritis
   A. Chronic inflammation of gastric mucosa → atrophy
   B. Two types
      1. Autoimmune gastritis
      2. *Helicobacter pylori* gastritis

IV. Autoimmune Gastritis: Pathophysiology
   A. T-cell mediated (type IV hypersensitivity) → atrophy of mucosa
   B. Antibodies against parietal cells and/or intrinsic factor located in body and fundus of stomach
   C. Impaired vitamin B12 absorption → pernicious anemia
   D. Intestinal metaplasia
   E. Achlorhydria → ↑ gastrin and antral G cell hyperplasia (loss of negative feedback from acid)
   F. ↑ risk for intestinal type gastric adenocarcinoma

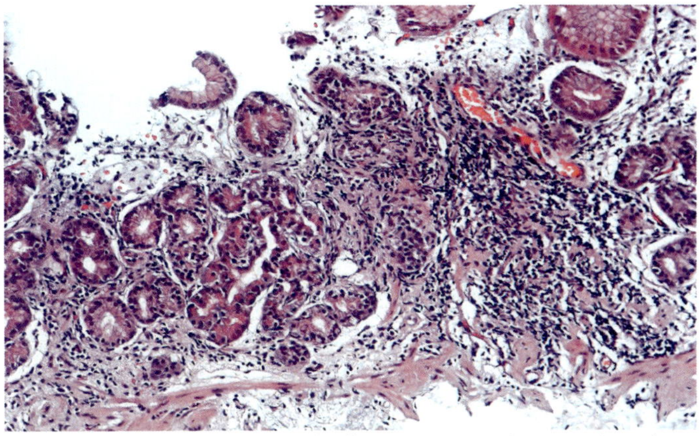

Photo Credit: https://commons.wikimedia.org/wiki/File:Autoimmune_atrophic_gastritis_(H%26E),_high_mag.jpg

FIGURE 10.8.21 - Atrophy of Oxyntic Mucosa in Autoimmune Atrophic Gastritis

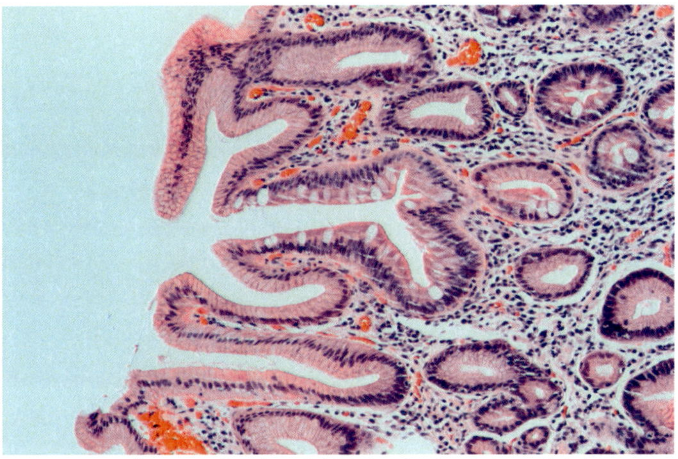

Photo Credit: https://commons.wikimedia.org/wiki/File:Complete_intestinal_metaplasia_in_a_case_of_chronic_gastritis,_HE_1.jpg

FIGURE 10.8.22 - Intestinal Metaplasia with Goblet Cells Due to Chronic Gastritis

V. *Helicobacter pylori* Gastritis
   A. Chronic gastritis caused by *H. pylori*
   B. Most common form
   C. Most common site: antrum
   D. Epigastric pain

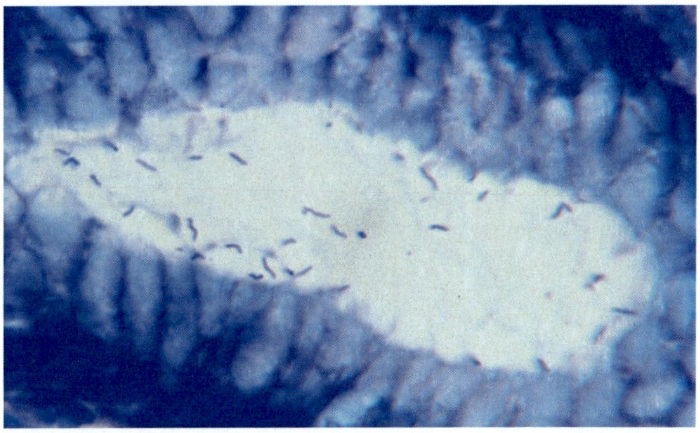

Photo Credit: https://commons.wikimedia.org/wiki/File:Helicobacter_pylori_in_a_case_of_gastritis.jpg

FIGURE 10.8.23 - *H. pylori* in Crypt of Foveolar Mucous Cells

VI. *Helicobacter pylori* Gastritis: Pathophysiology
   A. *H. pylori* enzymes (urease and protease) → inflammation of mucosa → ↓ mucosal protective factors
   B. Acute infection
      1. Decreased somatostatin → increased gastrin → duodenal ulcers
   C. Chronic infection
      1. Atrophy of mucosa in multiple locations + intestinal metaplasia
      2. Decreased acid secretion and hypochlorhydria
      3. ↑ risk of gastric ulcers, adenocarcinoma, and MALToma

VII. *Helicobacter pylori* Gastritis: Treatment
   A. Triple therapy (amoxicillin, clarithromycin, and a PPI)
   B. Urea breath test and stool antigen determines elimination of H. pylori

VIII. Peptic Ulcer Disease (PUD)
   A. Solitary ulcer of gastric or intestinal mucosa
      1. Proximal duodenum (90%)
      2. Distal stomach (10%)
   B. Types
      1. Duodenal *H. pylori* (> 95%); Zollinger-Ellison syndrome less common
      2. Gastric *H. pylori* (> 75%); NSAIDs and bile reflux less common

IX. Duodenal Ulcer: Pathophysiology
   A. *H. pylori* attaches to the mucosa of the gastric antrum (does not invade)
   B. *H. pylori* urease converts urea to ammonia, raising the gastric pH → injures mucosal epithelial cells → inflammation
   C. ↓ somatostatin → ↑ gastrin → ↑ acid secretion directly through CCK-B receptors and indirectly through histamine release of ECLs
   D. Cytotoxins impair production of duodenal bicarbonate → acidic chyme → ↑ duodenal ulcer formation

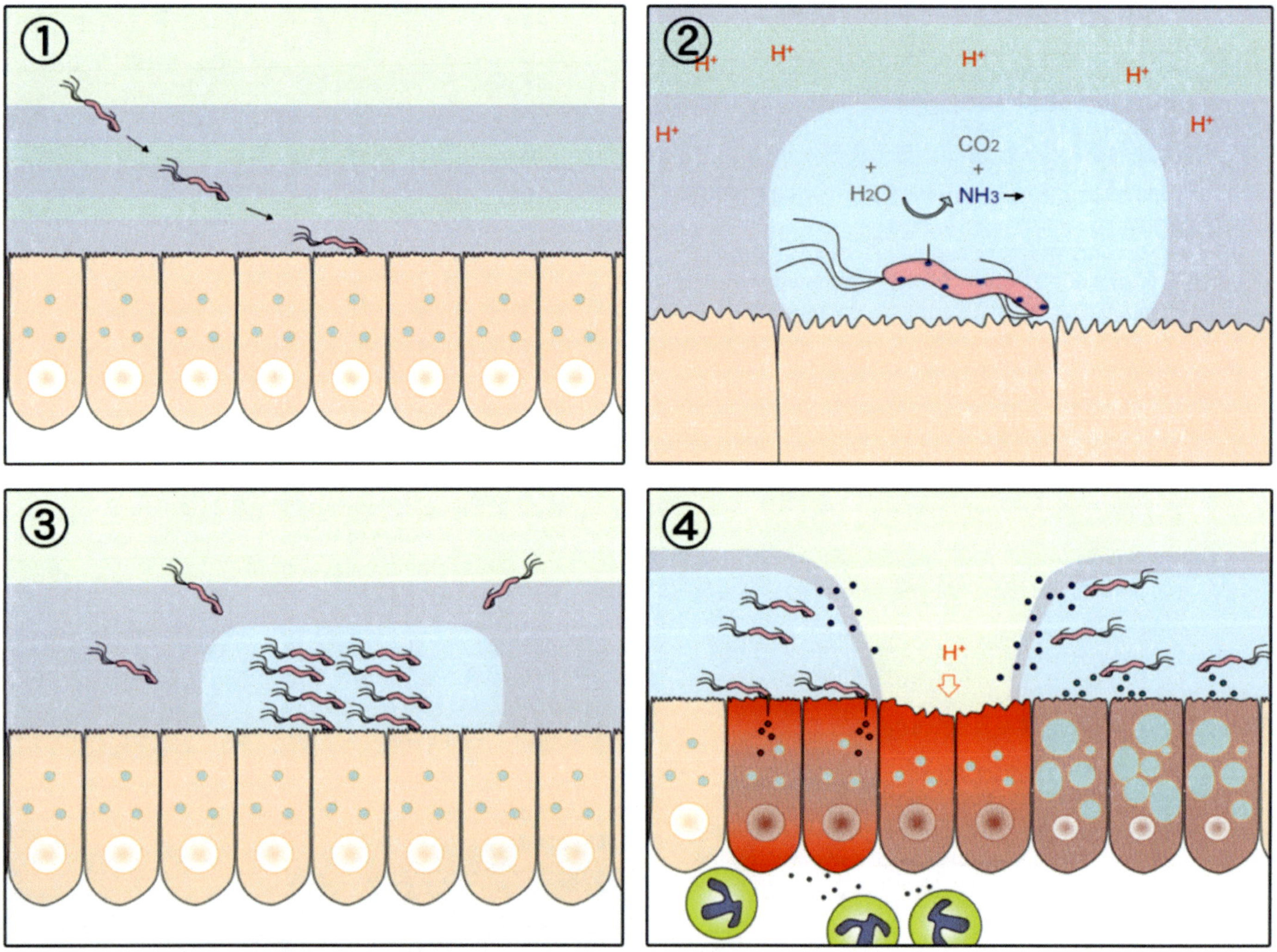

Photo Credit: https://commons.wikimedia.org/wiki/File:H_pylori_ulcer_diagram_en.png. This image may have been modified by cropping, labeling, and/or captions.

FIGURE 10.8.24 - Pathophysiology of *H. pylori*-Associated Peptic Ulcer Disease

X. Duodenal Ulcer: Findings
   A. Epigastric pain that is alleviated after eating
   B. Anterior duodenum affected
   C. Biopsy: Brunner gland hypertrophy
   D. If ulcer in posterior duodenum ruptures → erosion of gastroduodenal artery → internal hemorrhage
   E. Does not lead to malignancy

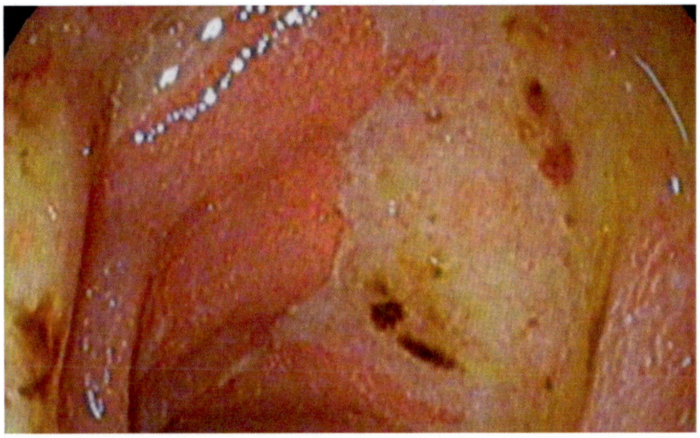

Photo Credit: https://commons.wikimedia.org/wiki/File:Duodenal_ulcer01.jpg

FIGURE 10.8.25 - Endoscopic image of a Duodenal Ulcer

XI. Gastric Ulcer: Pathology
   A. *H. pylori* colonizes body and lesser curvature of antrum of stomach → chronic inflammation → multifocal atrophic gastritis
   B. Delta cells in antrum that produce somatostatin are not affected → no major change in acid secretion
   C. Rupture of the ulcer may cause bleeding from left gastric artery
   D. Can cause gastric carcinoma (intestinal subtype)
   E. Biopsy to confirm diagnosis

XII. Gastric Ulcer: Findings
   A. Benign ulcers
      1. Small (< 3 cm)
      2. Punched out
      3. Surrounded by folds of symmetrically thickened mucosa
   B. Malignant ulcers
      1. Large and irregular
      2. Raised margins
   C. Epigastric pain that gets worse with meals

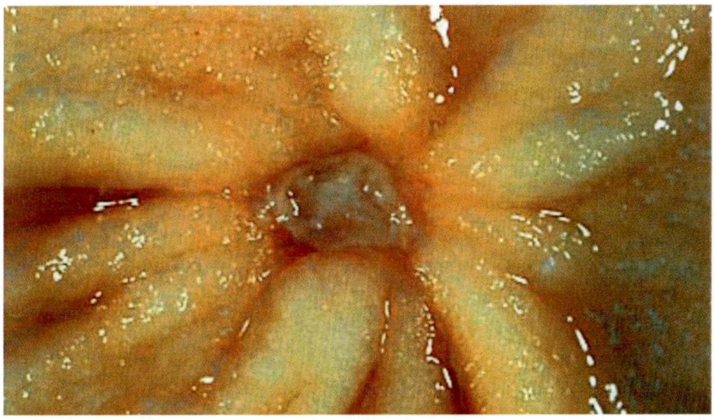

Photo Credit: https://commons.wikimedia.org/wiki/File:Benign_gastric_ulcer_1.jpg

FIGURE 10.8.26 - Small Benign Gastric Ulcer

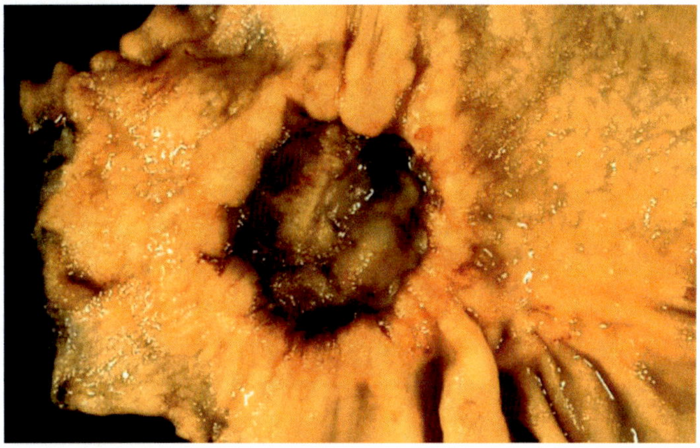

Photo Credit: https://commons.wikimedia.org/wiki/File:Adenocarcinoma_of_the_stomach.jpg

FIGURE 10.8.27 - Malignant Gastric Ulcer

XIII. Gastric Carcinoma
   A. Malignant proliferation of gastric epithelial cells → adenocarcinoma
   B. Types
      1. Intestinal
      2. Diffuse

XIV. Gastric Carcinoma Intestinal Type: Etiology
   A. Smoked foods high in nitrosamines (Japan)
   B. Intestinal metaplasia (due to gastritis)
   C. Tobacco smoking
   D. Achlorhydria
   E. Blood type A

XV. Gastric Carcinoma Intestinal Type: Pathology
   A. Defined glands that consist of columnar or cuboidal cells
   B. Presents as a nodular, polyp-like mass with a defined boundary that enlarges within the gastric lumen
   C. Large ulcer with irregular heaped-up margins on endoscopy
   D. Lesser curvature of antrum (most common)

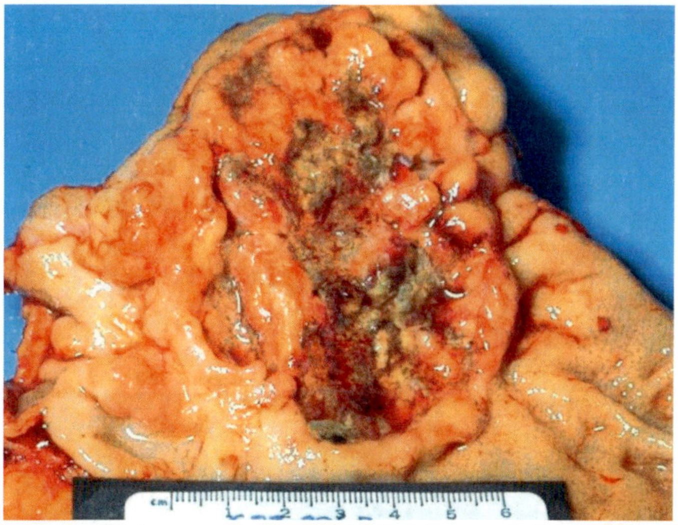

Photo Credit: https://commons.wikimedia.org/wiki/File:Adenocarcinoma,_stomach,_gross_pathology_IMG0037a_lores.jpg

FIGURE 10.8.28 - Gastric Adenocarcinoma

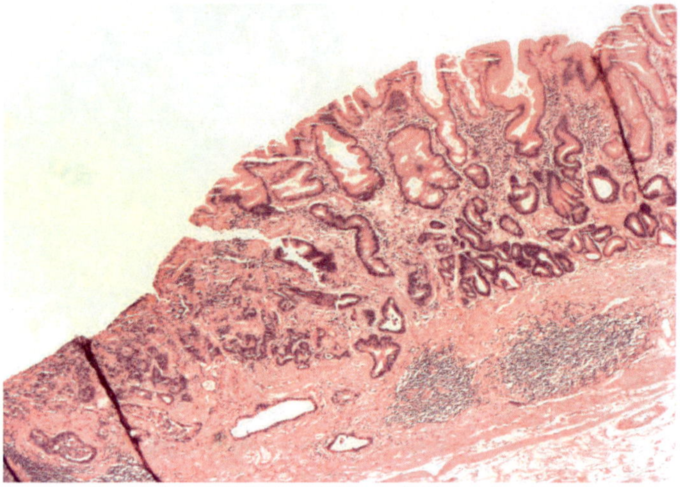

Photo Credit: https://commons.wikimedia.org/wiki/File:Gastric_adenocarcinoma.jpg

FIGURE 10.8.29 - Gastric Adenocarcinoma with Moderate to Poor Differentiation

XVI. Gastric Carcinoma Diffuse Type: Pathology

A. Diffuse infiltration of signet ring cells due to loss of E-cadherin
B. Plaque-like appearance and loss of rugae
C. Desmoplasia (fibrous and connective tissue growth) → diffuse thickening of stomach wall → "leather bottle stomach" (linitis plastica)
D. Prognosis depends on:
    1. Depth of invasion
    2. Metastasis to regional lymph node

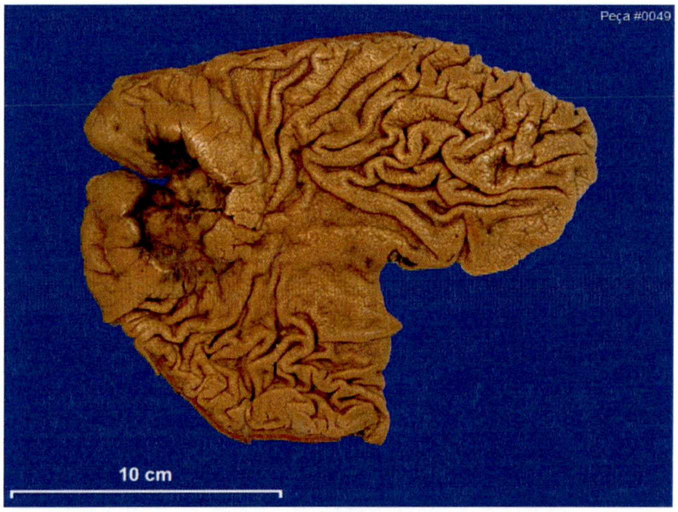

Photo Credit: https://commons.wikimedia.org/wiki/File:(UNESP-FMB_DEO_20180927-08)_Gastric_adenocarcinoma,_human.jpg

FIGURE 10.8.30 - Gastric Adenocarcinoma

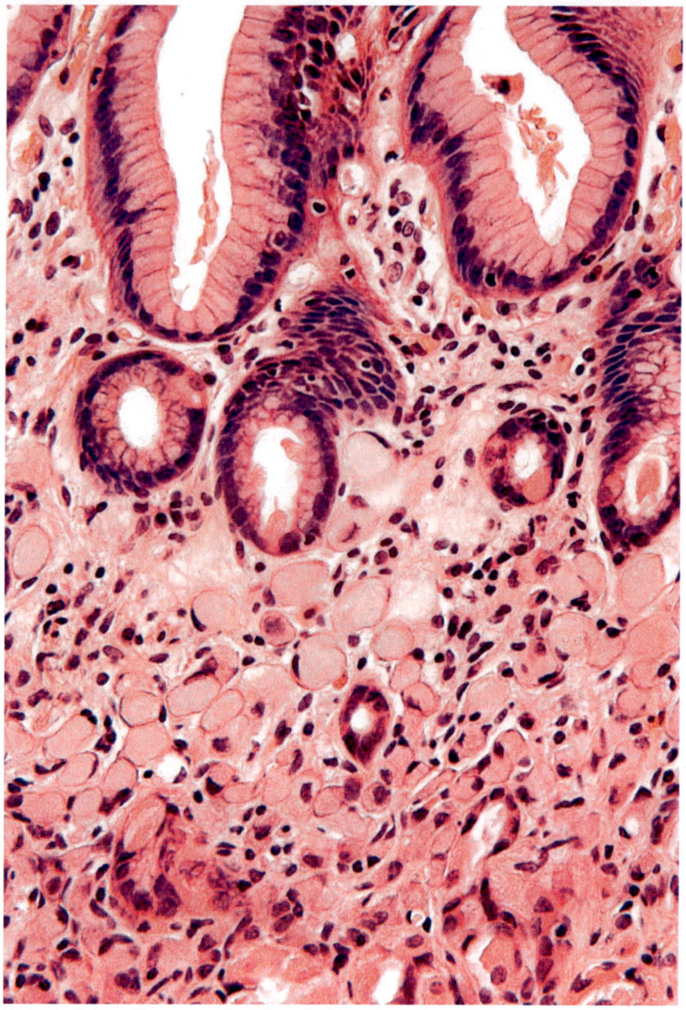

Photo Credit: https://commons.wikimedia.org/wiki/File:Signet_ring_cell_carcinoma_-_very_high_mag.jpg

FIGURE 10.8.31 - Gastric Adenocarcinoma with Diffuse Signet Cell Infiltration

XVII. Gastric Carcinoma: Findings

A. Abdominal Pain
B. Early feeling of fullness
C. Weight loss
D. Anemia
E. Acanthosis nigricans (hyperpigmented skin disorder)
F. Leser-Trélat sign: rapid onset of seborrheic keratosis is sign of internal malignancy (tumor cytokines or growth factors induced)

XVIII. Gastric Carcinoma: Metastasis

A. Liver
B. Left supraclavicular lymph node (Virchow node)
C. Periumbilical region (Sister Mary Joseph nodule): intestinal type
D. Bilateral ovaries (Krukenberg tumor): diffuse type
    1. Epigastric pain, early satiety, lower abdominal pressure
    2. US shows ovarian masses, CT shows stomach wall thickening

REVIEW QUESTIONS

1. A 62-year-old female presents with fatigue and shortness of breath. She complains of intermittent epigastric pain, lack of appetite, and nausea. Laboratory results show macrocytic anemia. Homocysteine and methylmalonic acid levels are elevated. Achlorhydria and elevated gastrin levels are also noted. What characteristic features from a biopsy of the body of the stomach will confirm the diagnosis?

   - **The correct answer is atrophy of the gastric mucosa along with intestinal metaplasia.**
   - This is an older female presenting with fatigue and shortness of breath along with epigastric pain, lack of appetite and nausea. She is also diagnosed with macrocytic anemia, which may be due to antibodies against intrinsic factor inhibiting the absorption of vitamin B12. Achlorhydria and elevated gastrin levels are also noted on lab results.
   - Considering her symptoms of epigastric pain, nausea and lack of appetite, and lab results of macrocytic anemia, achlorhydria and elevated gastrin levels, one can narrow down the diagnosis to autoimmune gastritis.
   - Endoscopic biopsy of the body of the stomach will show atrophy of gastric mucosa along with intestinal metaplasia.

2. A 39-year-old male presents with upper abdominal pain that improves with eating. He complains of waking up at night with epigastric pain that is burning in character. He also complains of belching, lack of appetite, and nausea. He has no vomiting, black or bloody stools, or weight loss. Endoscopy will show the ulcer in which area of the gastrointestinal system?

   - **The correct answer is the duodenum.**
   - This is a younger male presenting with upper abdominal pain that improves with eating along with epigastric pain that wakes him up at night, belching, lack of appetite, and nausea. He does not have vomiting, black or bloody stools or weight loss.
   - The fact that his epigastric pain improves with meals narrows the diagnosis to a duodenal ulcer. Hence, endoscopy will show an ulcer in the duodenum.

3. A 49-year-old male is being evaluated for fatigue and weight loss. He complains of epigastric pain after meals, lack of appetite, and nausea. He states that food is not appetizing to him anymore and that he gets full early after starting a meal. He states that his wife noticed black spots on his back, which began a few weeks ago. Physical exam reveals a rash on the upper back with pigmented macules with a greasy surface and well-demarcated borders. An endoscopy reveals a plaque-like ulcer and a thickened stomach wall. A biopsy of the lesion will show which of the following?

   A. Parietal cell hyperplasia
   B. Atrophy of the mucosa
   C. Finger-like projections with goblet cells
   D. Cells with a nucleus pushed to the periphery

   - **The correct answer is D.**
   - This is a middle-age male presenting with fatigue and weight loss along with epigastric pain, lack of appetite, nausea and early satiety. Physical exam also reveals a rash with pigmented macules with a greasy surface and well-demarcated borders. This rash is called seborrheic keratosis and is consistent with an underground malignancy.
   - EGD shows plaque-like ulcer with a thickened stomach wall, which shows that the entire stomach is affected. Collectively, these findings are consistent with a diagnosis of diffuse-type gastric carcinoma.
   - Endoscopic biopsy of a lesion will show diffuse infiltration of signet ring cells.
   - Option A is incorrect because parietal cell hyperplasia is a characteristic feature of gastronoma.
   - Option B is wrong because atrophy of the mucosa occurs in autoimmune and *H. pylori* gastritis and gastric ulcers.
   - Option C is wrong because the presents of finger like projections with goblet cells in the stomach mucosa is called intestinal metaplasia. This is a characteristic finding of autoimmune and *H. pylori* associated chonic gastritis and intestinal type gastric cancer, but not diffuse type cancer.

Section V - Small Bowel Pathology

I. Intussusception
   A. Telescoping of bowel
      1. Proximal segment into distal segment by peristalsis
   B. Associated with "leading edge"
      1. Children: lymphoid hyperplasia (rotavirus)
      2. Adults: tumor
   C. Intermittent abdominal pain, vomiting, "currant jelly" stools

II. Small Bowel Infarction
   A. Transmural infarction
      1. Thrombosis/embolism of SMA or thrombosis of mesenteric vein
   B. Mucosal infarction
      1. Hypotension
   C. Abdominal pain, bloody diarrhea, decreased bowel sounds

III. Small Bowel Infarction: Chronic Mesenteric Ischemia
   A. Atherosclerosis of the mesenteric arteries leading to diminished blood supply
   B. Most prominent after meals when more blood is needed
   C. Analogous to stable angina
   D. Epigastric pain after meals that doesn't respond to antacids
   E. Food aversion/weight loss

IV. Lactose Intolerance
   A. Decreased lactase function
      1. Brush border enzyme that breaks down lactose to galactose and glucose
   B. Abdominal distension and diarrhea after dairy consumption
   C. Can be congenital (autosomal recessive) or acquired
   D. Temporary deficiency seen after small bowel infarction

V. Celiac Disease: Cause
   A. Immune-mediated damage of small bowel villi due to gluten exposure
      1. Gluten present in wheat and grains (gliadin}
   B. Mechanism
      1. Gliadin deamidated by tissue transglutaminase (TTG)
      2. Deamidated gliadin is presented by antigen presenting cells via MHC class II
      3. Helper T cells mediate damage

VI. Celiac Disease: Laboratory Findings and Pathology
   A. Laboratory findings
      1. Associated with HLA-DQ2 and HLA-DQ8
      2. IgA and IgG antibodies against endomysium, tTG, or gliadin
   B. Histopathology (duodenal biopsy)
      1. Flattening of villi
      2. Hyperplasia of crypts
      3. Increased intraepithelial lymphocytes

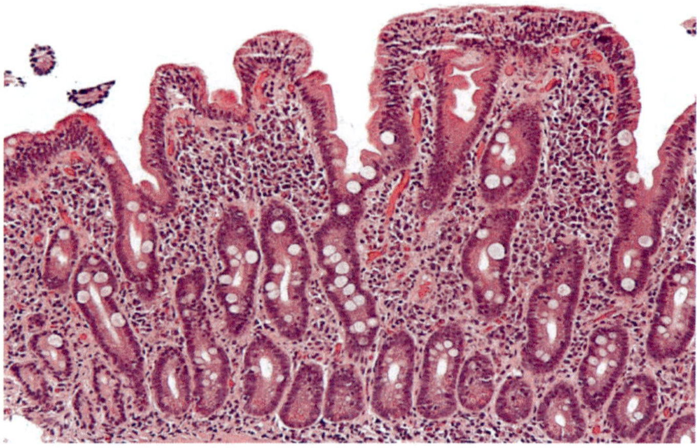

FIGURE 10.8.32 - Celiac Disease

VII. Celiac Disease: Clinical Presentation
   A. Children: abdominal distension, diarrhea, failure to thrive
   B. Adults: chronic diarrhea and bloating
   C. Dermatitis herpetiformis
      1. Blisters filled with watery fluid on extensor surfaces
      2. IgA deposition at the tips of dermal papillae
      3. Microabscesses at the dermal papillae tips containing fibrin and neutrophils

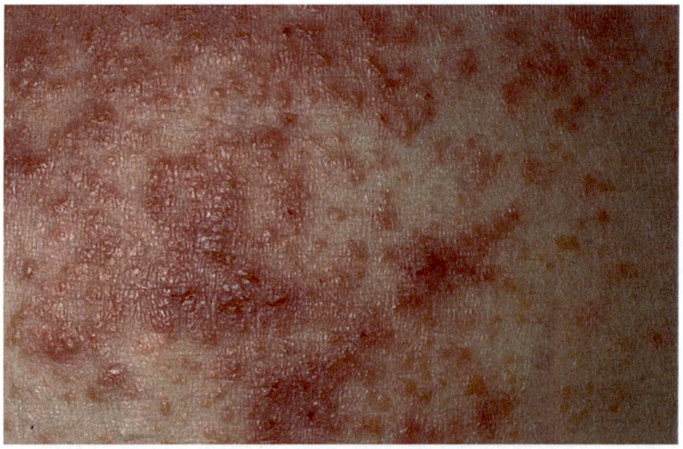

FIGURE 10.8.33 Dermatitis Herpetiformis

VIII. Celiac Disease: Treatment and Complications
A. Treatment
1. Gluten-free diet
B. Complications
1. Small bowel carcinoma
2. T cell lymphoma

IX. Tropical Sprue
A. Damage to small bowel villi due to unknown cause
B. Similar to celiac disease except
1. Occurs in tropical regions
2. Arises after infectious diarrhea and responds to antibiotics
3. Damage most prominent in jejunum and ileum (secondary B12 and folate deficiency)
4. Duodenum less commonly involved

X. Whipple Disease: Cause
A. Tropheryma whippelii
B. Systemic tissue damage involving the small bowel lamina propria
C. Macrophages with live and partially destroyed organisms
D. Macrophages compress lacteals
E. Chylomicrons unable to transfer from enterocytes to lymphatics
F. Fat malabsorption and steatorrhea

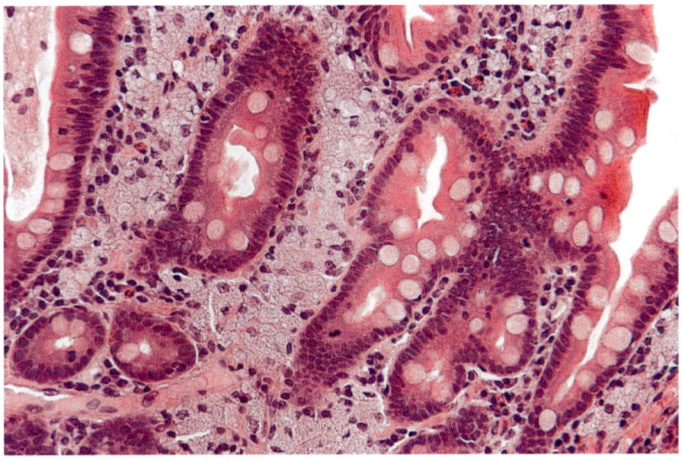

FIGURE 10.8.34 - Whipple Disease

XI. Whipple Disease: Diagnosis and Treatment
A. PAS-positive (glycoprotein)
B. Other common sites include synovium of joints, cardiac valves, lymph nodes, and CNS
C. Treat with antibiotics

XII. Carcinoid Tumor: Cause
A. Malignant proliferation of neuroendocrine cells
B. Tumor cells contain neurosecretory granules that stain for chromogranin
C. Can arise anywhere along the gut (small bowel most common)
D. Can occur in the appendix, usually benign
E. Grows as a submucosal polyp-like nodule

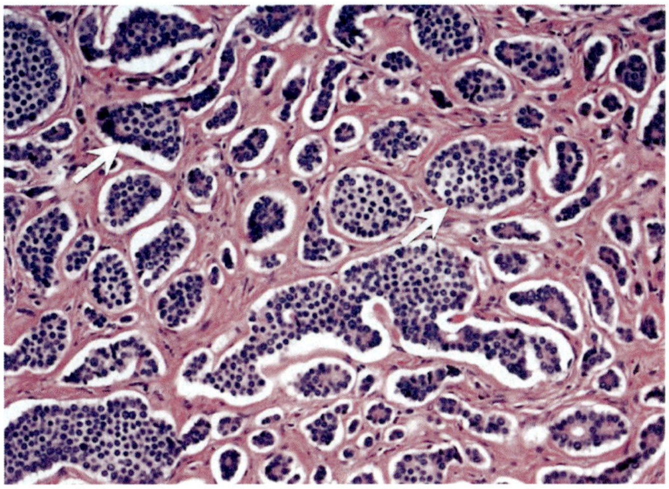

FIGURE 10.8.35 - Carcinoid Tumor

XIII. Carcinoid Tumor: Carcinoid Syndrome
A. Secretes serotonin, which is metabolized by MAO to 5-HIAA and excreted in urine
B. Metastasis (especially to liver) can lead to carcinoid syndrome
1. Bronchospasm, diarrhea, flushing of skin
2. Triggered by alcohol or stress, which stimulate serotonin release from tumor
3. Carcinoid heart disease (right-sided)

REVIEW QUESTIONS

1. An 84-year-old man with a history of smoking and coronary bypass surgery presents to the office for evaluation of abdominal pain. He states that he has been experiencing intense epigastric pain after eating for the past several months and that it has begun affecting his ability to eat. He thinks he has lost several pounds as a result. Upper endoscopy reveals no abnormalities. Which layer of the small intestine is likely to be most affected by this patient's disorder?

   - **The correct answer is the mucosal layer.**
   - We are presented with a patient who has a history of atherosclerotic disease, as evidenced by his coronary bypass surgery, and risk factors of vasculopathy, namely smoking and old age. His symptoms of postprandial epigastric pain, aversion to food, and weight loss are classic for chronic mesenteric ischemia. His upper endoscopy is normal, ruling out GERD.
   - The mechanism of this condition is similar to the mucosal infarction caused by hypotension.
   - In the case of atherosclerotic disease of the mesenteric arteries with diffusely diminished blood flow, the mucosal layer, which is the innermost layer of the intestinal wall and thus furthest from the blood supply, would most likely be affected first by any decrease in blood flow.

2. A 46-year-old man presents to the clinic complaining of diarrhea, abdominal discomfort, and some weight loss for the past 3 months. He travels frequently to the developing world on business and recently returned from South America several months ago. A biopsy of his small bowel is performed and reveals PAS-positive foamy macrophages in the lamina propria. In addition to GI symptoms, what other issues might this patient experience as a result of his condition?

   - **This patient has Whipple's disease and may therefore experience several systemic issues.**
   - Whipple disease is a multi-system disorder that affects tissues throughout the body.
   - The most common additional symptom patients with Whipple disease are likely to experience is arthritis, since the bacteria cause a migratory inflammation in various joints. Whipple disease can also affect the CNS, causing dementia and other central nervous system findings in the later stages of the disease.
   - Finally, Whipple disease can also affect the heart. In addition to endocarditis, *Tropheryma whipplei* infection has also been associated with pericarditis and myocarditis.

3. A 35-year-old Congolese man presents to the clinic complaining of worsening diarrhea, weight loss, and loss of appetite for the past three years. He recently immigrated to the United States and is concerned he might have a dietary intolerance to something in the country. Laboratory results show a vitamin B12 deficiency. A biopsy of the patient's small intestine is obtained. The findings will likely be similar to a condition associated with which of the following?

   A. IgA deficiency
   B. Bronchospasm
   C. Progressive ataxia
   D. Acanthocytosis
   E. Bloody stools

   - **The correct answer is A.**
   - From the question stem you were able to determine that this patient's most likely diagnosis is tropical sprue. His recent immigration status from a tropical region combined with classic symptoms of diarrhea, weight loss, and anorexia all point to this diagnosis.
   - Recall that tropical sprue tends to primarily affect the jejunum and ileum, predisposing patients to B12 and folate deficiencies, and that biopsy of the small intestine shows a flattening of villi similar to that found in patients with celiac disease. Celiac disease is an autoimmune condition closely associated with IgA deficiency.
   - B is incorrect because bronchospasm is a feature of carcinoid syndrome, which would not have a biopsy similar to that of tropical sprue and is not a complication of celiac disease.
   - C and D are incorrect because progressive ataxia and acanthocytosis are features of abetalipoproteinemia, which is not associated with celiac disease. Recall that small bowel biopsies in patients with abetalipoproteinemia tend to show foamy, lipid-laden enterocytes at the tips of villi, not villi flattening.
   - E is incorrect because bloody stools are more closely associated with small bowel infarction and Meckel diverticulum, not celiac disease, which tends to present with abdominal discomfort and loose, non-bloody stools.

Section VI - Appendix

I. Acute Appendicitis
   A. Acute inflammation of the appendix
   B. Appendix gets filled with pus, causing pain
   C. Related to obstruction of the appendix by lymphoid hyperplasia (children) or a fecalith (adults)

II. Acute Appendicitis: Clinical Features
   A. Nonspecific symptoms: fever, nausea
   B. Periumbilical pain (early)
      1. Eventually localizes to right lower quadrant (McBurney point)
   C. If left untreated, rupture of appendix results in peritonitis
      1. Guarding
      2. Rebound tenderness
      3. Complication: periappendiceal abscess

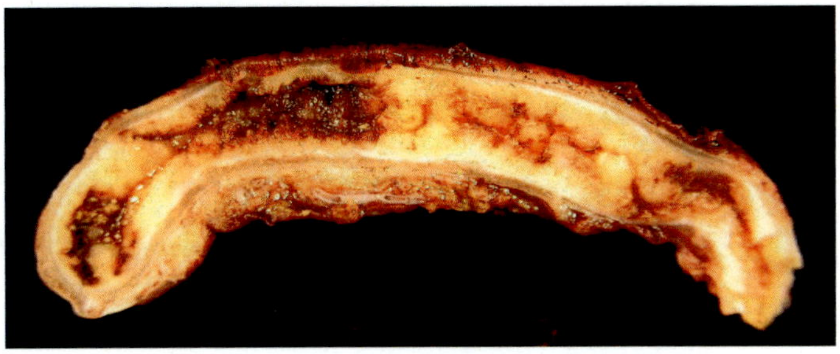

FIGURE 10.8.36 - Inflamed Appendix

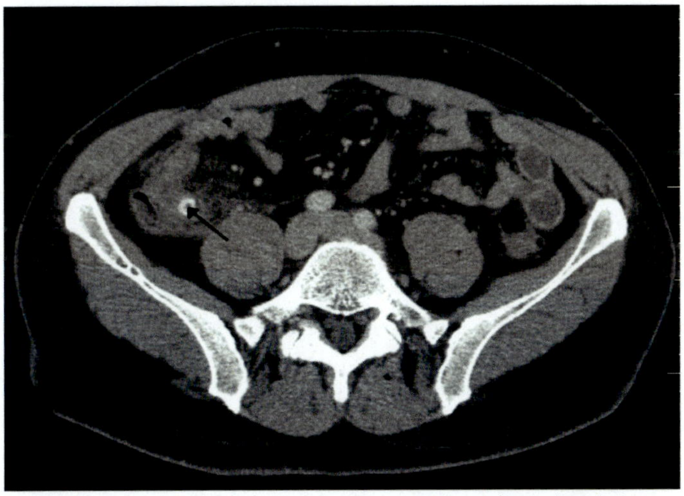

FIGURE 10.8.37 - Axial CT of Acute Appendicitis with Fecalith (Arrow)

REVIEW QUESTIONS ?

1. A 52-year-old male presents to the emergency department with a high-grade fever and abdominal pain. He explains that the pain was initially around his umbilicus but has since moved to the right lower quadrant. His heart rate is 100 beats/minute, blood pressure is 149/82 mmHg, and temperature is 39.4 °C (103 °F). On physical examination, there is tenderness of the right lower quadrant. What most likely initiated this patient's condition?

   A. Telescoping of a proximal segment of the small bowel
   B. Twisting of small bowel along its mesentery
   C. Luminal obstruction
   D. Viral infection

- **The correct answer is C.**
- This is a 52-year-old male who presents with a high-grade fever and abdominal pain. The patient then explains that the pain initially started at the periumbilical area and now moved to the right lower quadrant. On physical exam, the physician notices a tenderness of the right lower quadrant. This is a classic finding in someone with acute appendicitis.
- Since the appendix is a hollow tube, the most common cause of its inflammation is luminal obstruction, which can be caused by lymphoid hyperplasia in children or fecalith, which is a hardened lump of fecal matter, in adults.
- A is incorrect because telescoping of the proximal segment of the small bowel refers to intussusception.
- B is incorrect because the twisting of a small bowel along its mesentery refers to volvulus.
- D is incorrect because although this patient has a high-grade fever, the pain is unlikely to be caused by a viral infection.

Section VII - Inflammatory Bowel Disease

I. Basic Principles
   A. Chronic inflammation of digestive tract
   B. Possible etiology: dysregulated immune response to intestinal flora
   C. Clinical presentation
      1. Young woman
      2. Caucasian or Eastern European Jewish
      3. Recurrent bloody diarrhea and abdominal pain
         a) Diagnosis of exclusion

	Ulcerative Colitis	Crohn Disease
Type of inflammation	- Mucosal and submucosal	- Transmural
Colon involvement	- Begins in rectum and extends up to the cecum - Continuous lesions - The rest of the GI tract is unaffected	- Extending from mouth to anus - Skip lesions - Terminal ileum: most common site - Rectum spared
Symptoms	- Left lower quadrant pain - Bloody diarrhea	- Right lower quadrant pain - Non-bloody diarrhea
Gross	- Pseudopolyps - Loss of haustra ("lead pipe" sign)	- Cobblestone mucosa - Creeping mesenteric fat/strictures
Microscopy	- Crypt abscesses with neutrophils	- Non-caseating granulomas
Complications	- Toxic megacolon - Carcinoma (based on extent of mucosal involvement, duration > 10 years)	- Malabsorption of vitamins/minerals - Formation of renal stones - Formation of fistula - Carcinoma (with preexisting disease)
Smoking	- Protective	- Increases risk

TABLE 10.8.1 - Types of Inflammatory Bowel Disease

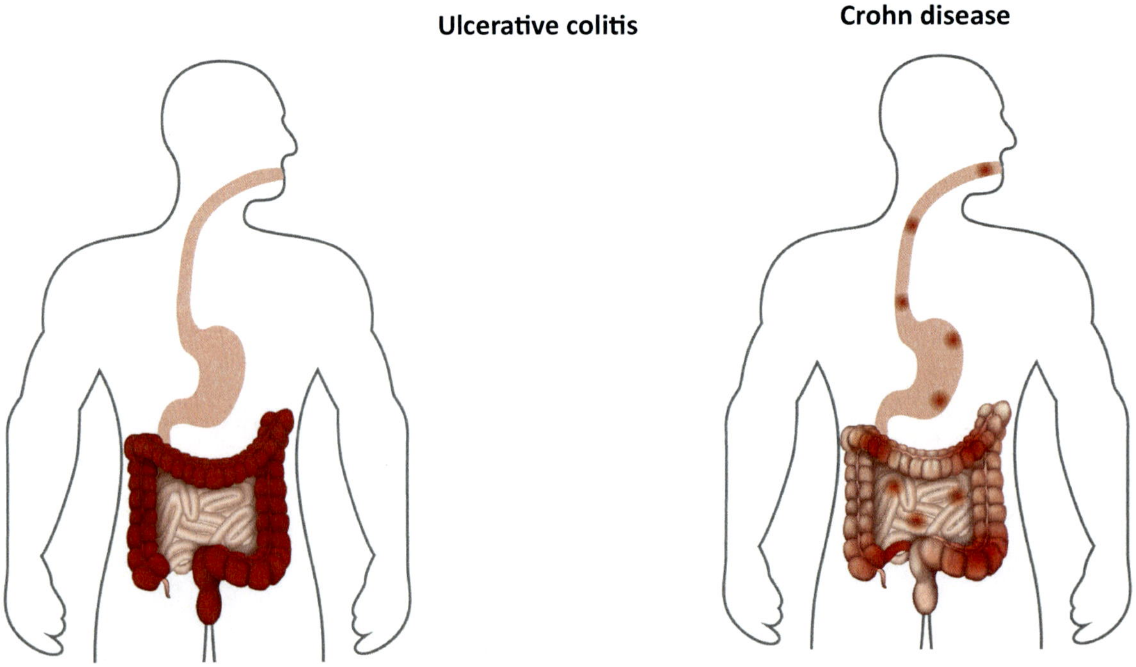

FIGURE 10.8.38 - Lesion Location in Inflammatory Bowel Disease

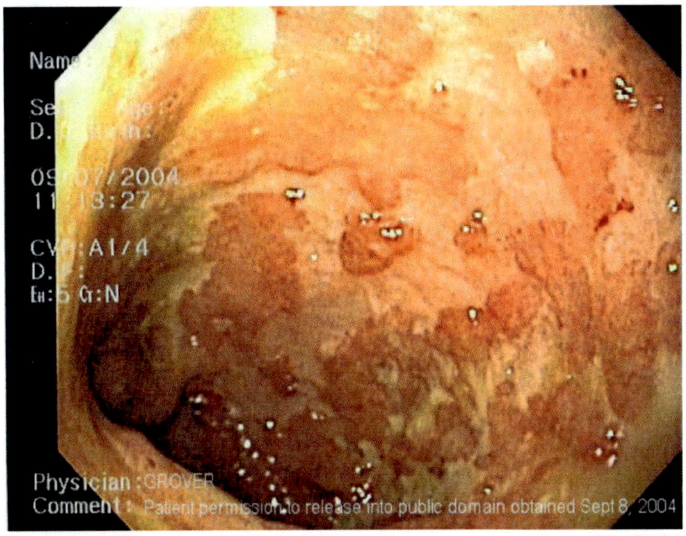

FIGURE 10.8.39 - Ulcerative Colitis

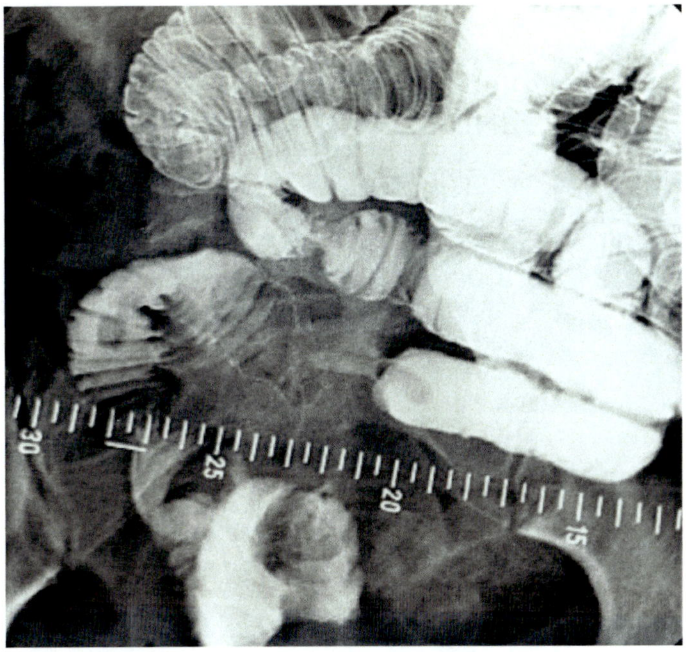

FIGURE 10.8.40 - "Lead Pipe" Sign of Ulcerative Colitis

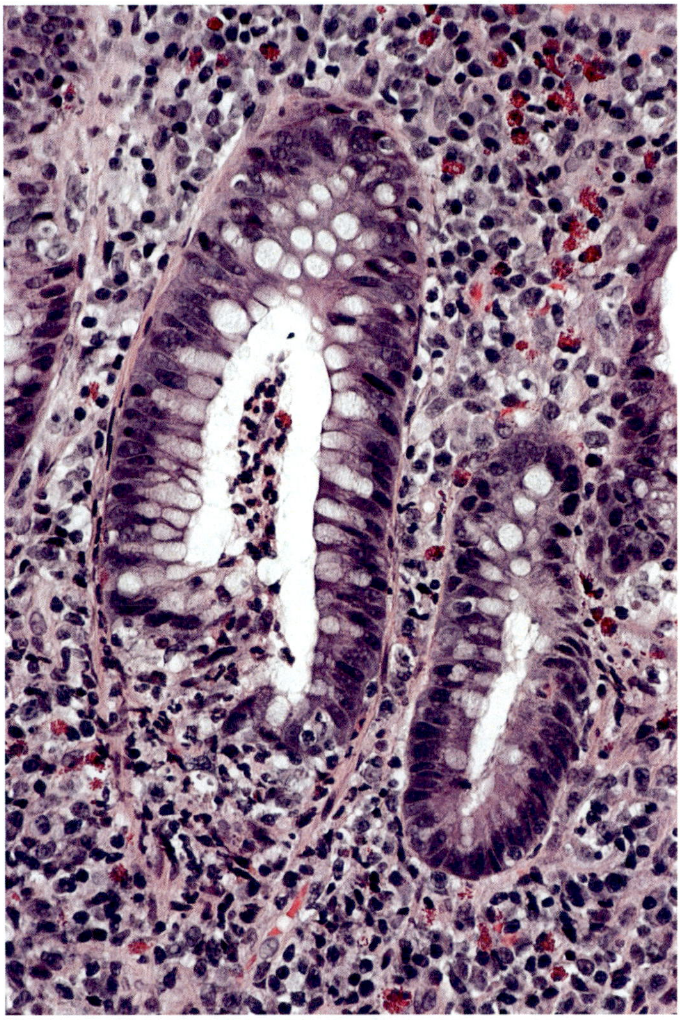

FIGURE 10.8.41 - Crypt Abscess with Neutrophils

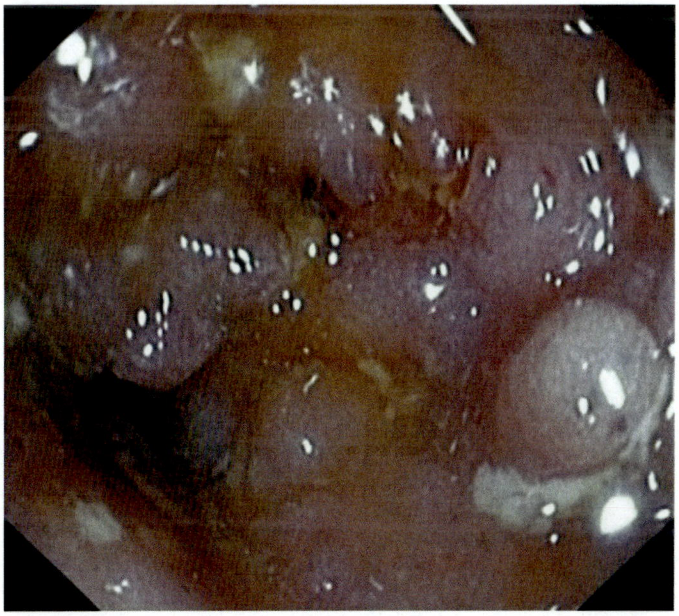

FIGURE 10.8.42 - Cobblestone Mucosa

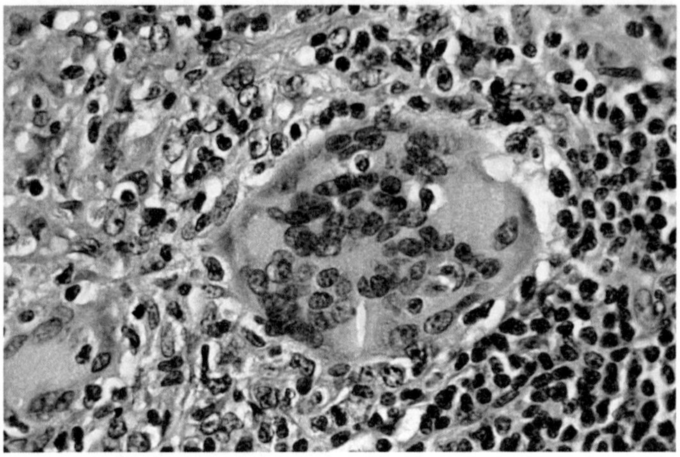

FIGURE 10.8.43 - Non-caseating Granuloma with Giant Cells

REVIEW QUESTIONS

1. A 29-year-old female comes to the clinic for a 5-day history of progressively worsening abdominal pain and bloody diarrhea. She denies any trauma or prior abdominal surgery. On physical examination, she has pain in the lower left quadrant of the abdomen. On microscopic examination following a biopsy, crypt abscesses with neutrophils are observed. What is the most common, life-threatening complication of this disease?

- **The correct answer is toxic megacolon.**
- This is a 29-year-old female presenting with a 5-day history of progressively worsening left lower quadrant abdominal pain and bloody diarrhea. On microscopy, crypt abscesses with neutrophils are observed, which confirms the diagnosis of ulcerative colitis.
- Toxic megacolon is the most common complication of someone with ulcerative colitis. It occurs when ulcerative colitis causes the colon to distend and dilate and the colon is unable to remove gas or feces from the body as a consequence.
- If gas and feces build up in the colon, the colon could eventually rupture, which can be life-threatening.

REVIEW QUESTIONS

2. A 19-year-old female presents to the clinic with non-bloody diarrhea and abdominal pain for the past few weeks. A colonoscopy shows cobblestone mucosa with creeping fat and patchy inflammation of the small intestine and colon. Light microscopy of a biopsy sample shows multinucleated giant cells without central necrosis. Which of the following nutritional deficiencies is most likely to be observed in this patient?

   A. Vitamin C
   B. Vitamin B6
   C. Vitamin B9
   D. Vitamin B12

- **The correct answer is D.**
- This is a 19-year-old female presenting with non-bloody diarrhea and abdominal pain. Colonoscopy shows cobblestone mucosa with creeping fat and patchy inflammation of the small intestine and the colon. Moreover, light microscopy of the tissue sample shows multinucleated giant cells without central necrosis, which confirms the diagnosis of Crohn disease.
- Since Crohn disease most commonly affects the terminal ileum, vitamin B12 deficiency is likely to occur, as it is absorbed in the terminal ileum.
- A is incorrect because vitamin C is unlikely to be deficient in someone with Crohn disease since it is not absorbed in the terminal ileum.
- B is incorrect because although vitamin B6 gets absorbed in the jejunum, vitamin B6 is unlikely to be severely deficient in someone with Crohn disease since the terminal ileum is most heavily involved.
- C is incorrect because although vitamin B9 also gets absorbed in the jejunum, there is a small reserve pool of vitamin B9 stored in the liver. Therefore, vitamin B9 deficiency is unlikely for acute onset of symptoms in someone with Crohn disease.

Section VIII - Diseases of the Colon

I. Hirschsprung Disease: Etiology
   A. Congenital absence of ganglion cells and enteric nervous plexus
   B. Increased risk with Down syndrome

II. Hirschsprung Disease: Pathophysiology
   A. Failure of neural crest cell migration
   B. Defective myenteric and submucosal plexuses
      1. Myenteric plexus: regulates GI motility
      2. Submucosal plexus: regulates glandular activity
   C. Abnormal peristalsis and relaxation of rectum and sigmoid colon

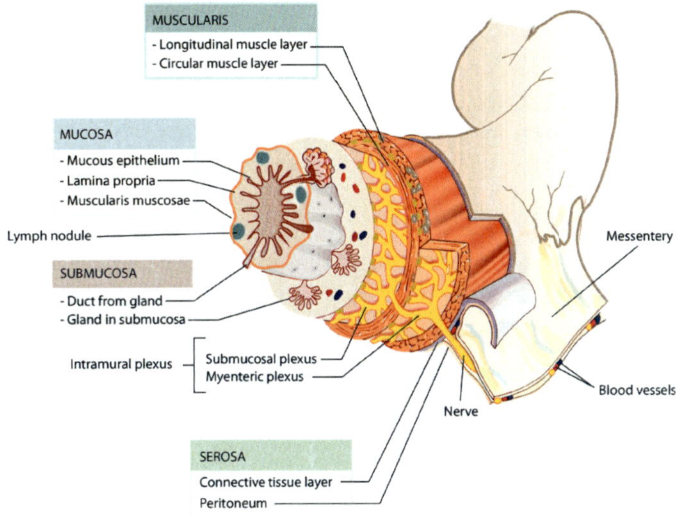

FIGURE 10.8.44 - Layers of the Colonic Wall

III. Hirschsprung Disease: Clinical Features
   A. Failure to pass meconium
   B. Empty rectum on digital exam
   C. Megacolon proximal to aganglionic bowel
   D. Diagnosed via rectal suction biopsy
   E. Treat with bowel resection

IV. Angiodysplasia: Etiology
   A. Acquired dilation of colonic blood vessels
   B. Increased incidence in the elderly

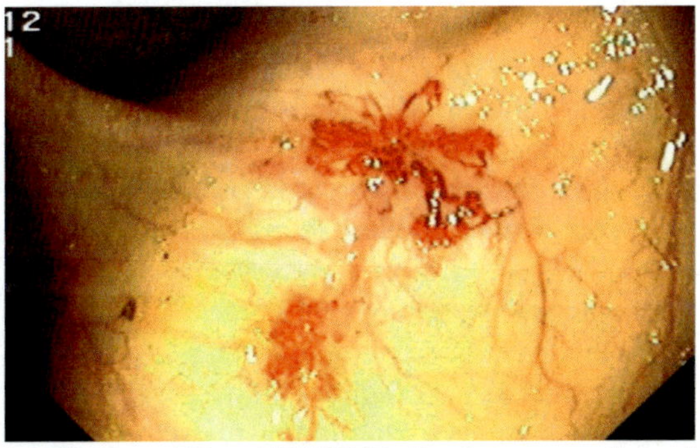

FIGURE 10.8.45 - Colonoscopic Image of Angiodysplasia

V. Angiodysplasia: Clinical Features
   A. Commonly affects the right colon
   B. Patients present with hematochezia

VI. Hereditary Hemorrhagic Telangiectasia: Etiology
   A. Autosomal dominant
   B. Thinning of vasculature

VII. Hereditary Hemorrhagic Telangiectasia: Symptoms
   A. Hematochezia
   B. Telangiectasia
   C. Epistaxis
   D. Arteriovenous malformations

VIII. Ischemic Colitis: Etiology
   A. Most commonly secondary to atherosclerosis
   B. Occurs at the splenic flexure

IX. Ischemic Colitis: Symptoms
   A. Pain with eating
   B. Hematochezia

X. Colonic Diverticula: Etiology
   A. Associated with low fiber diet, constipation, and old age
   B. Commonly occurs on the left-sided colon

XI. Colonic Diverticula: Pathophysiology
   A. Increased colonic wall stress
   B. Causes outpouching of colonic mucosa and submucosa

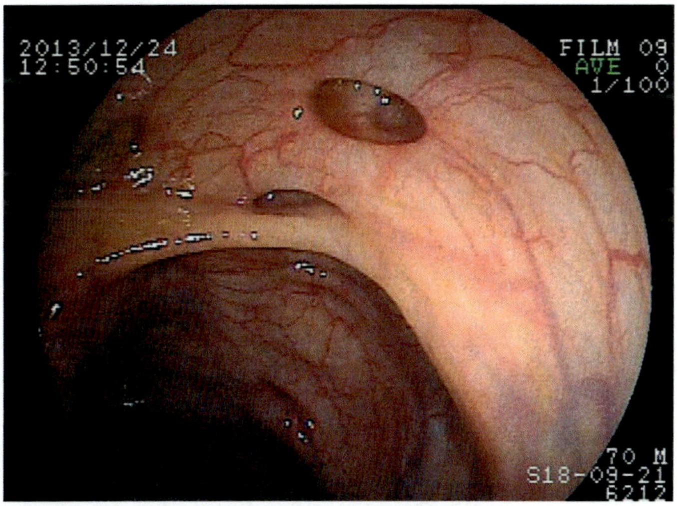

FIGURE 10.8.46 - Colonoscopic Image of Diverticulosis

XII. Colonic Diverticula: Clinical Features
   A. Commonly asymptomatic
   B. May present as painless hematochezia
   C. Can progress to diverticulitis and/or fistulas

XIII. Irritable Bowel Syndrome: Etiology

A. Idiopathic
B. Increased incidence in middle-age females

XIV. Irritable Bowel Syndrome: Clinical Features

A. Relapsing abdominal pain, diarrhea, constipation, and flatulence
B. Abdominal pain improves with bowel movements
C. No pathological abnormalities are seen
D. High-fiber diets may improve symptoms

REVIEW QUESTIONS

1. A 1-day-old female neonate was born via an uncomplicated vaginal birth. The neonate has yet to pass her meconium stool. The digital rectal exam shows an empty rectum. What is the likely cause of this patient's condition?

   - **The correct answer is absence of ganglion cells and enteric nervous plexus.**
   - The patient is suffering from Hirschsprung disease. This disease is caused by a congenital absence of ganglion cells and enteric nervous plexus. This leads to abnormal peristalsis and relaxation of rectum and sigmoid colon.
   - Patients will present with failure to pass meconium in the first 48 hours. The digital rectal exam will show an empty rectum.

2. A 71-year-old female with a past medical history of constipation and poor diet presents with 2 days of painless hematochezia. What is the underlying pathophysiological mechanism behind this patient's condition?

   - **The correct answer is increased colonic wall stress.**
   - The patient is suffering from diverticulosis. Constipation, low-fiber diet (poor diet), and painless hematochezia are commonly associated with diverticulosis.
   - The pathophysiological mechanism is related to increased colonic wall stress. This causes colonic outpouching that consists of the mucosa and submucosa.

3. A 31-year-old female with no past medical history presents to her primary care physician due to 8 months of abdominal pain. The patient's current temperature is 98.7 °F (37 °C), blood pressure is 123/78 mmHg, heart rate is 62 beats/minute, and the respiratory rate is 14 breaths/minute. The patient states she has had intermittent diarrhea and flatulence for the past 8 months. She also states there have been periods where she experiences constipation as well. She says the pain is relieved upon defecation. She denies any weight loss, blood in the stool, or fever. Which of the following is associated with this patient's disorder?

   A. Dilated colonic vasculature
   B. Colonic outpouching
   C. Normal bowel structures
   D. Telangiectasia

   - **The correct answer is C.**
   - This patient is suffering from irritable bowel syndrome. The patient's history of diarrhea, flatulence, constipation and abdominal pain that is relieved by defecation is indicative of irritable bowel syndrome. A colonoscopy will reveal normal bowel structures.
   - This disorder causes abdominal pain, diarrhea, constipation, and flatulence. Patients' abdominal pain improves upon having a bowel movement. There are no pathological abnormalities associated with this disorder. In some patients a high fiber diet may improve their symptoms.
   - A is incorrect because dilated colonic vasculature is seen in angiodysplasia, which most commonly occurs in the elderly. Patients present with hematochezia.
   - B is incorrect because colonic outpouching of the mucosa and submucosa leads to diverticulosis. In some cases this can progress to diverticulitis and fistula formation.
   - D is incorrect because telangiectasias are associated with hereditary hemorrhagic telangiectasia due to thinning of the patient's vasculature.

Section IX - Colon Polyps and Carcinoma

I. Colonic Polyps: Epidemiology
   A. Abnormal tissue growth of colonic mucosa
   B. Can be benign or malignant
   C. Grossly characterized as sessile or pedunculated
   D. Histologically characterized as villous, tubular, or tubulovillous

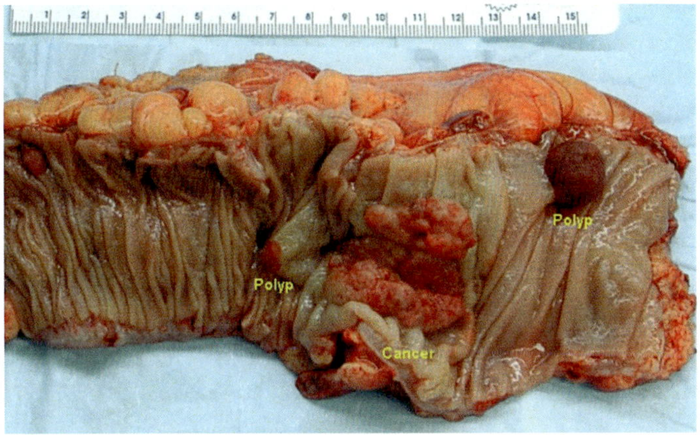

FIGURE 10.8.47 - Gross Pathology of Colon with Adenomatous Polyp and Carcinoma

II. Colonic Polyps: Common Types
   A. Hyperplastic
      1. Most common type
      2. Benign growth of colonic mucosal glands
   B. Adenomatous
      1. Second most common type
      2. Neoplastic growth of colonic mucosal glands
      3. Premalignant lesions may develop into carcinoma

III. Colonic Polyps: Adenoma-Carcinoma Sequence
   A. Genetic mutations in the *APC* gene increase susceptibility for polyp formation
   B. Genetic mutations in the *KRAS* gene lead to polyp formation
   C. Genetic mutations in the *P53* gene and elevated levels of *COX* result in carcinoma formation

IV. Colonic Polyps: Malignant Risk Factors
   A. Sessile growth
   B. Villous histology
   C. Greater than 2 cm in size

V. Colonic Polyps: Screening
   A. Colonoscopy
   B. Fecal occult blood testing

VI. Juvenile Polyps
   A. Benign colonic polyps that occur in children
   B. Juvenile polyposis occurs when multiple polyps arise in the GI tract
   C. Juvenile polyposis poses an increased risk of carcinoma formation

VII. Familial Adenomatous Polyposis: Key Features
   A. Autosomal dominant mutation in the *APC* gene
   B. Thousands of colonic adenomatous polyps
   C. Colorectal carcinoma formation occurs in all patients
   D. Prophylactic colectomy is performed to avoid carcinoma formation

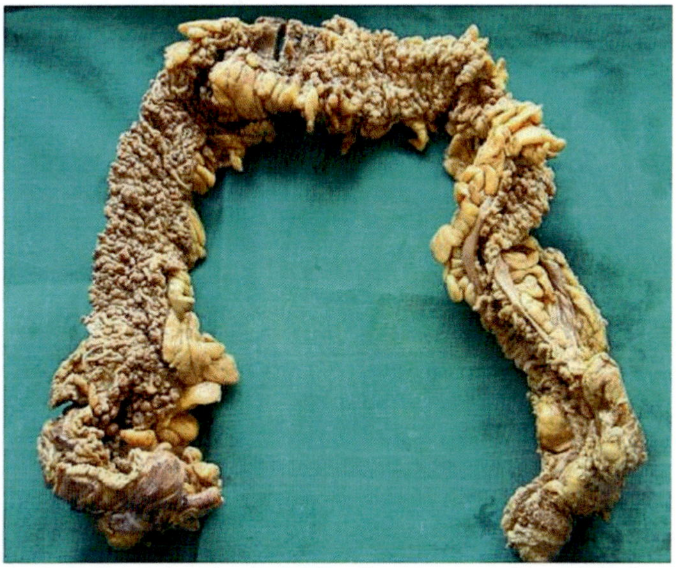

FIGURE 10.8.49 - Gross Pathology of Familial Adenomatous Polyposis

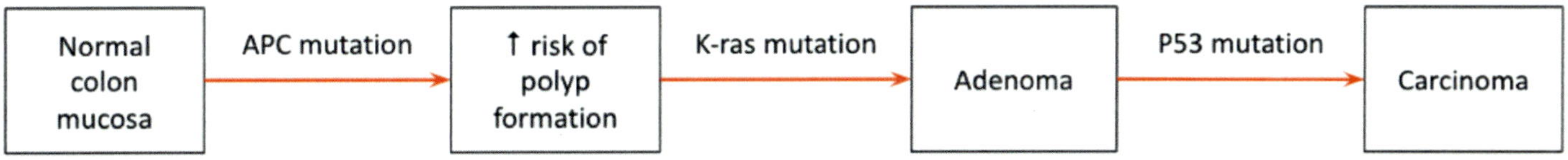

FIGURE 10.8.48 - Adenoma-Carcinoma Sequence

VIII. Familial Adenomatous Polyposis: Associations
   A. Gardner syndrome
      1. Osteomas, fibromatosis, and familial adenomatous polyposis
   B. Turcot syndrome
      1. Malignant CNS tumors and familial adenomatous polyposis

IX. Peutz-Jeghers Syndrome: Key Features
   A. Autosomal dominant
   B. Hamartomatous polyp formation in the GI tract
   C. Hyperpigmented macules on the oral mucosa, genitalia, and hands
   D. Increased risk of developing breast and GI cancer

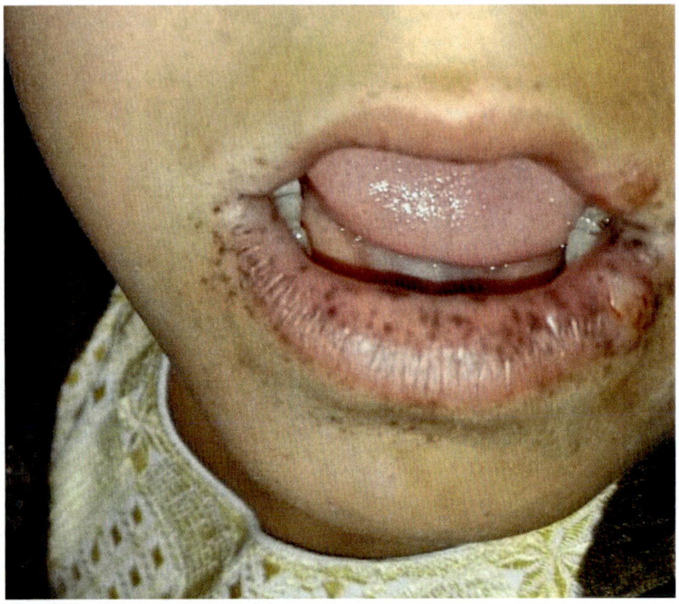

FIGURE 10.8.50 - Hyperpigmented Macules on the Oral Mucosa

X. Colorectal Carcinoma: Epidemiology
   A. Abnormal growth of colonic mucosa
   B. Typically occurs in ages 60 and above
   C. More common in men than women

XI. Colorectal Carcinoma: Pathogenesis
   A. Usually occurs due to the adenoma-carcinoma sequence
   B. Other causes include Lynch Syndrome

XII. Colorectal Carcinoma: Lynch Syndrome
   A. Otherwise known as hereditary nonpolyposis colorectal carcinoma
   B. Autosomal dominant
   C. Due to microsatellite instability
      1. Defective DNA mismatch repair enzymes
   D. Increased risk of early sporadic colorectal carcinoma

XIII. Colorectal Carcinoma: Clinical Features
   A. Screen with colonoscopy and fecal occult blood at 50 years of age
   B. CEA tumor marker is used to assess the risk of recurrence

REVIEW QUESTIONS

1. A 50-year-old male with no past medical history presents to the physician for routine colonoscopy screening. Several polyps are found, and a biopsy shows that they are adenomatous. What genetic mutations likely led to this patient's adenomatous polyp formation?

- **The correct answer is defects in the *APC* and *KRAS* genes.**
- The patient is found to have adenomatous polyp formation on routine colonoscopy. However, there is no mention of carcinoma. Understanding the adenoma-carcinoma sequence is the key to answering this question.
- Recall that defects in the tumor suppressor *APC* gene place colonic mucosa at risk for developing adenomas. Defects in the *KRAS* gene cause adenomatous polyp formation. We can be certain that there is not a *P53* mutation because there was no mention of carcinoma.

2. A 16-year-old female with no past medical history presents to the physician for a routine physical examination. The patient notes that her father and grandfather both passed away from colon cancer at a young age. It is determined that the patient has a rare inherited genetic mutation that makes her at risk for colon cancer. It is advised that the patient undergo a prophylactic colectomy to avoid carcinoma formation. What is the likely genetic mutation responsible for this patient's inherited condition?

- **The correct answer is a defective *APC* tumor suppressor gene.**
- The patient has familial adenomatous polyposis. This is an autosomal dominant disorder that results in a defective *APC* gene. The *APC* gene is a tumor suppressor gene.
- All patients with familial adenomatous polyposis will develop colorectal carcinoma if left untreated. Patients are treated with a prophylactic colectomy to avoid this.

3. A 45-year-old male with no past medical history presents to the physician for concern of blood in his stool for the past 3 weeks. The patient's current temperature is 36.94 °C (98.5 °F), blood pressure is 119/75 mmHg, heart rate is 66 beats/minute, and the respiratory rate is 12 breaths/minute. The patient describes his stool as a dark red color. He denies any fever, weight loss, nausea, or abdominal pain. Upon further questioning, the patient states his mother passed away from colon cancer in her early 50s. The patient undergoes a colonoscopy and adenomatous polyps are discovered in the right colon. Upon genetic testing, the patient is diagnosed with Lynch syndrome. What is the mechanism of this patient's disorder?

   A. Increased levels of CEA
   B. *BRCA1* gene mutation
   C. *APC* gene mutation
   D. Microsatellite instability

- **The correct answer is D.**
- This patient is suffering from Lynch syndrome. The patient's age, melena, family history, and findings on colonoscopy all point to this disorder. This disorder is due to an autosomal dominant defect in DNA mismatch repair enzymes.
- Recall that Lynch syndrome is otherwise known as hereditary nonpolyposis colorectal carcinoma (HNPCC). This disorder is inherited in an autosomal dominant fashion. Lynch syndrome is due to microsatellite instability. This leads to an increased risk of early sporadic colorectal carcinoma.
- A is incorrect because CEA levels are not used to diagnose Lynch syndrome or colorectal carcinoma in general. CEA levels are useful for determining a patient's risk of colorectal carcinoma recurrence.
- B is incorrect because *BRCA1* gene mutations are not associated with Lynch syndrome or colorectal carcinoma. *BRCA1* gene mutations are seen in breast and ovarian cancers.
- C is incorrect because *APC* gene mutations are not associated with Lynch syndrome. *APC* gene mutations are seen in patients with familial adenomatous polyposis.

Section X - Pancreas

I. Acute Pancreatitis
  A. Basics
    1. Acute inflammation of the pancreas
    2. Characterized by autodigestion of pancreatic tissue by pancreatic enzymes
      a) Premature activation of trypsin → activation of other pancreatic enzymes (e.g. pro-phospholipase, proelastase)
  B. Etiology
    1. Most commonly due to alcohol and gallstones
    2. Other causes: trauma, steroids, mumps, scorpion stings, drugs, hypercalcemia, and hypertriglyceridemia
  C. Clinical Features
    1. Nonspecific: nausea and vomiting
    2. Acute epigastric pain radiating to the back
    3. Elevated serum amylase or lipase
      a) Lipase is more specific for pancreatic damage
    4. Hypocalcemia
      a) Calcium is used during saponification in fat necrosis
  D. Complications
    1. Pancreatic pseudocysts on CT scans
      a) Lined by granulation tissue composed of inflammatory debris and pancreatic enzymes
    2. Pancreatic abscess (*E. coli*)
    3. Disseminated intravascular coagulation
    4. Acute respiratory distress syndrome

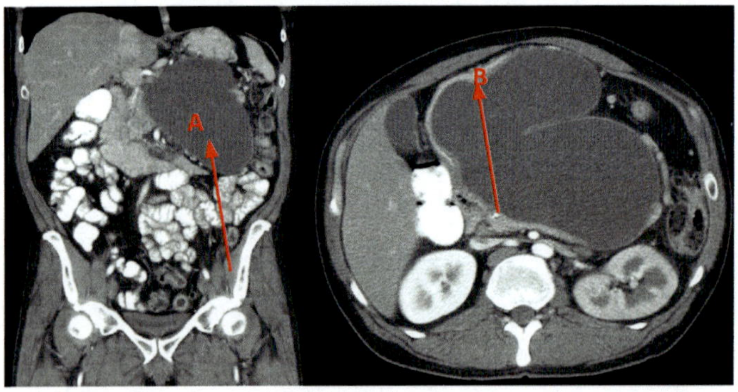

FIGURE 10.8.51 - CT Scans Showing Pancreatic Pseudocysts (A) and Fibrous Tissue with Inflammatory Debris (B)

II. Chronic Pancreatitis
  A. Basics
    1. Chronic inflammation of pancreas
    2. Atrophy and calcification of pancreatic parenchyma
    3. Due to alcohol abuse (adults) and cystic fibrosis (children)
      a) Most cases are idiopathic
  B. Clinical Features
    1. Epigastric pain radiating to the back
    2. Pancreatic insufficiency (typically when < 10% pancreas is functional)
      a) Steatorrhea
      b) Fat-soluble vitamin deficiency
      c) Diabetes mellitus
    3. Pancreatic calcification
    4. Serum amylase and lipase may or may not be elevated

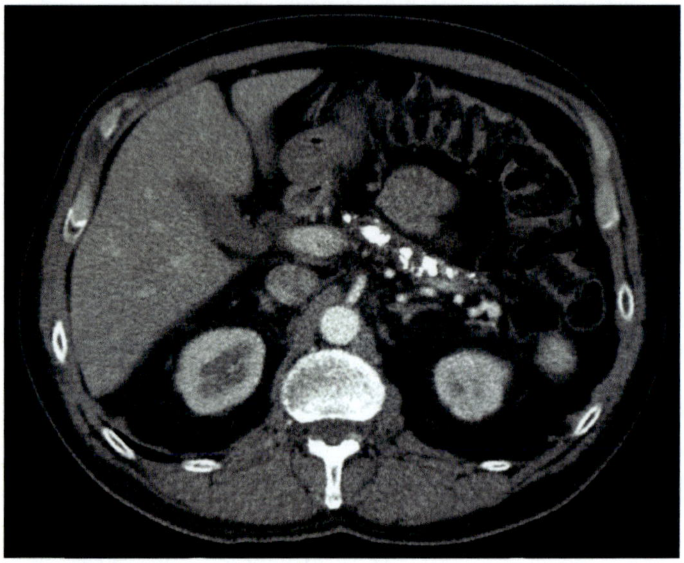

FIGURE 10.8.52 - Chronic Pancreatitis

III. Pancreatic Adenocarcinoma
  A. Very aggressive tumor arising from the pancreatic ducts
  B. Risk factors: smoking, chronic pancreatitis (especially > 20 years), diabetes, age > 50 years, and Jewish and African-American males
  C. Very poor prognosis: average survival < 1 year after diagnosis

IV. Pancreatic Carcinoma: Clinical Features
  A. Epigastric pain radiating to the back and weight loss
  B. Symptoms can vary based on location of tumor
    1. Head of pancreas: obstructive jaundice, pale stools, and a palpable gallbladder
    2. Body or tail of pancreas: secondary diabetes mellitus
  C. Migratory thrombophlebitis (Trousseau syndrome)
  D. Serum tumor marker: CA19-9

REVIEW QUESTIONS

1. A 62-year-old man presents to the emergency department with nausea, vomiting, and epigastric pain radiating to the back. He has a past medical history of hyperlipidemia and type II diabetes mellitus. He has been drinking 15 cans of beer per day for more than 30 years. He also notes that he has never had these symptoms before. On physical exam, he is afebrile but there is tenderness in the epigastric region. His blood is drawn. What would the lab studies most likely show?

   - **The lab studies are likely to reveal significantly elevated serum amylase and lipase.**
   - This is a classic case of someone with acute pancreatitis. This is a 62-year-old chronic alcoholic who presents with epigastric abdominal pain that radiates to the back along with nausea and vomiting.
   - His past medical history is notable for hyperlipidemia and diabetes. He is afebrile but has tenderness in the epigastric region and mentions that he has never had these symptoms before.

2. A 54-year-old man presents to the emergency department with severe abdominal pain. He has had a 30-pound weight loss since last month. He has been smoking two packs of cigarettes for more than 30 years. On physical exam, there is tenderness in the epigastric region. An abdominal CT scan shows a mass at the head of the pancreas. Which of the following complications is most likely seen in this patient?

   A. Reflux of acid from the stomach
   B. Scleral icterus with pale stools and dark urine
   C. Polydipsia, polyuria, and numbness of hands and feet
   D. Elevated serum lipase and amylase

   - **The correct answer is B.**
   - This is a 54-year-old chronic smoker who has abdominal pain and a significant weight loss over the past month. On physical examination, there is tenderness in the epigastric region and the abdominal CT scan shows a mass at the head of the pancreas.
   - This is a classic case of someone with pancreatic carcinoma. When a pancreatic mass arises from the head, patients are likely to experience obstructive jaundice with scleral icterus, pale stools, and dark urine.
   - A is incorrect because acid reflux from the stomach refers to gastroesophageal reflux disease. It is not one of the complications of pancreatic cancer.
   - C is incorrect because polydipsia, polyuria, and numbness of hands and feet refers to the symptoms of type II diabetes mellitus. Although diabetes is one of the complications of pancreatic cancer, it is associated with a mass at the body or the tail of the pancreas, not the head.
   - D is incorrect because elevated serum lipase and amylase can be seen in acute pancreatitis, not in pancreatic cancer. Instead, CA19-9 is a useful serum tumor marker.

Section XI - Gallbladder and Biliary Tract

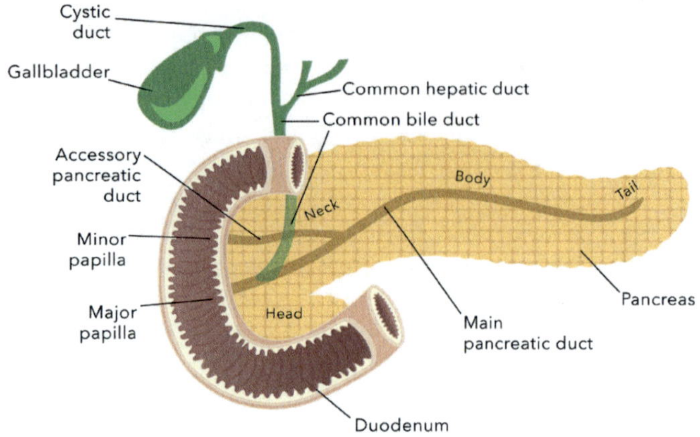

FIGURE 10.8.53 - Gallbladder and Biliary Tract

I. Cholelithiasis (Gallstones)
   A. Stones in the gallbladder
   B. Cholesterol (most common), pigment (bilirubin) stones, or mixed
   C. Increased concentration, decreased ability to break down, or stasis
   D. Symptoms: asymptomatic or RUQ with biliary colic and nausea
   E. Complications: obstruction, inflammation of gallbladder, gallstone ileus (fistula), and gallbladder cancer

II. Cholesterol Stones
   A. Increased cholesterol or hypomobility of the gallbladder (stasis) → biliary sludge → precipitation of crystals
   B. Risk factors include: estrogen (middle-aged female, obesity, OCP); diseases affecting terminal ileum (Crohn disease)
   C. Pale-yellow, radiolucent

III. Pigment Stones
   A. Increased bilirubin
   B. Black or brown stones
   C. Black stones: chronic hemolysis (eg, sickle cell anemia)
   D. Brown stones: infection (β-glucuronidase) → leads to deconjugation of the conjugated bilirubin in bile → increased unconjugated bilirubin
      1. *Clonorchis sinensis*
      2. *Ascaris lumbricoides*

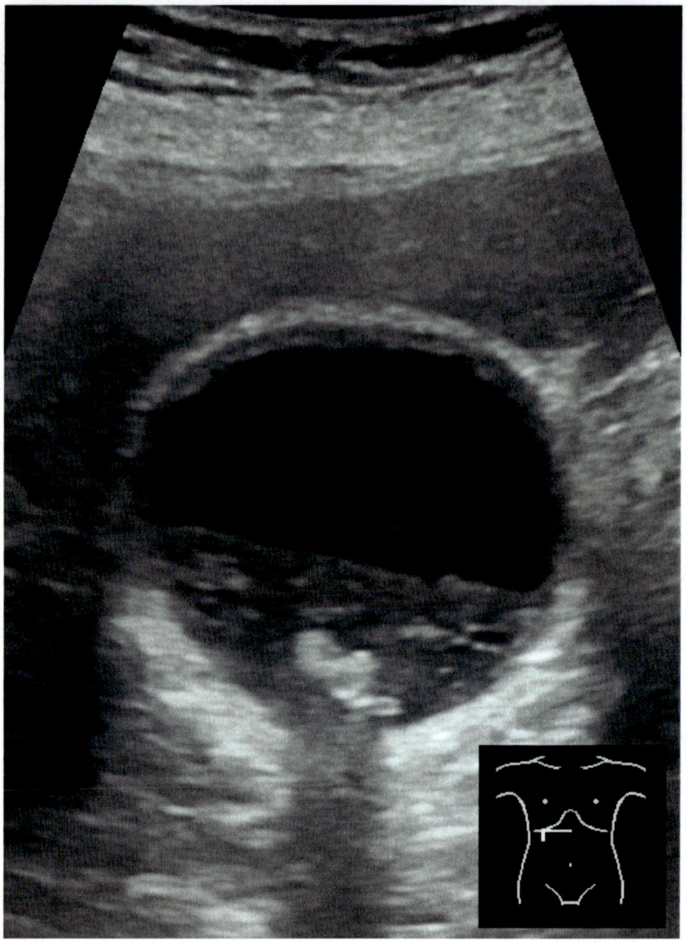

Photo Credit: Mikael Häggström, M.D. - Author info - Reusing imagesWritten informed consent was obtained from the individual, including online publication. / CC0

FIGURE 10.8.54 - Ultrasound Showing Biliary Sludge

IV. Cholecystitis
   A. Inflammation of the gallbladder wall
   B. Acute or chronic

V. Acute Cholecystitis
   A. Acute inflammation of gallbladder wall (calculus or acalculus)
      1. Calculus: due to a stone obstructing the cystic duct → inflammation
      2. Acalculus: in critically ill patients (e.g. major surgery, trauma, burns, sepsis)
   B. Symptoms include: severe RUQ pain radiating to scapula/right shoulder, Murphy's sign, fever, nausea, leukocytosis
   C. Ultrasound is the imaging method of choice
   D. HIDA scan for functional examination of the gallbladder

VI. Chronic cholecystitis
  A. Chronic inflammation of gallbladder wall
  B. Due to long-standing cholelithiasis or recurrent acute cholecystitis
  C. Less severe symptoms (RUQ pain after fatty meals, nausea, vomiting)
  D. Thick, calcified gallbladder (porcelain gallbladder).
  E. Gallstone ileus
  F. Outpouching of mucosa → muscular wall (Rokitansky-Aschoff sinus)

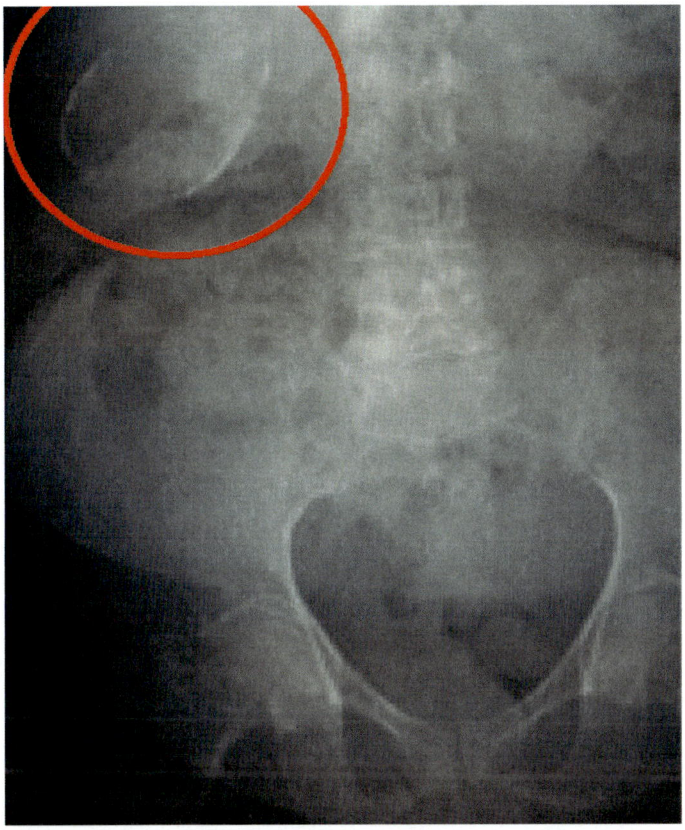

FIGURE 10.8.55 - X-Ray Showing Porcelain Gallbladder

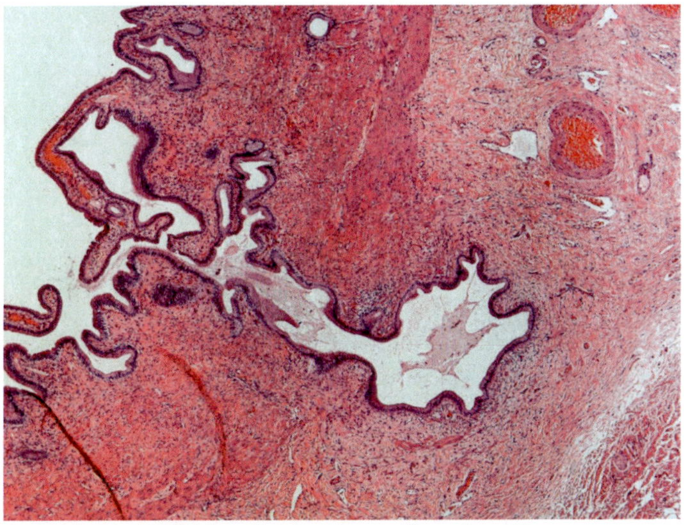

FIGURE 10.8.56 - Rokitansky-Aschoff Sinus

VII. Gallstone Ileus
  A. Complication of chronic cholecystitis
  B. Chronic inflammation due to gallstone → adhesion of the gallbladder to adjacent small intestine (usually duodenum) → fistula formation and passage of gallstones into the lumen → obstruction of bowel
  C. Crampy pain, bloating, vomiting
  D. Terminal ileum is the most commonly affected site
  E. Dilated bowel loops on imaging and air in the biliary tract (pneumobilia)

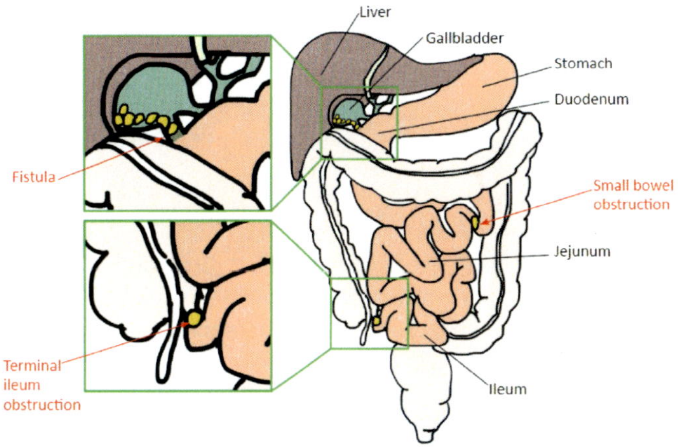

FIGURE 10.8.57 - Gallstone Ileus

VIII. Choledocholithiasis
  A. Presence of stones in the common bile duct
  B. May be asymptomatic or obstruct the ducts
  C. Obstruction can lead to complications such as cholangitis, chronic liver disease, acute cholecystitis and pancreatitis

IX. Cholangitis
  A. Infection and inflammation of the walls of the bile ducts
  B. Mostly due to a bacterial infection by gram negative bacteria (*E.coli*, *Klebsiella*, *Enterococcus*)
  C. Fever, RUQ abdominal pain, and jaundice = Charcot's triad
  D. Charcot's triad + hypotension and altered mental status = Reynold's pentad

X. Biliary Atresia
  A. Destruction or absence of the extrahepatic bile ducts leading to obstruction of bile flow
  B. Presents with jaundice, pale stools, dark urine, and hepatomegaly within the first 2 months of life
  C. Often progresses to cirrhosis
  D. Diagnosis is confirmed with a liver biopsy
  E. Treatment is liver transplantation

XI. Primary Biliary Cirrhosis
   A. Chronic autoimmune destruction of intrahepatic bile ducts leading to cholestasis and eventually cirrhosis
   B. Middle-aged women
   C. Pruritus (especially during the night), fatigue, hepatosplenomegaly, and jaundice (advanced)
   D. Increased ALP, GGT, and serum IgM
   E. Anti-mitochondrial antibodies confirm the diagnosis

XII. Gallbladder Carcinoma
   A. Due to recurrent trauma and chronic inflammation
   B. Most commonly adenocarcinomas
   C. Elderly women
   D. Poor prognosis
   E. Symptoms similar to cholelithiasis and cholecystitis (abdominal pain, nausea and vomiting, jaundice, anorexia)

XIII. Cholangiocarcinoma
   A. Adenocarcinomas from lining of intra- and extrahepatic biliary ducts
   B. Chronic cholestasis and inflammation
   C. Poor prognosis

REVIEW QUESTIONS ?

1. A 30-year-old African American man comes to the emergency department due to upper abdominal pain and nausea. He does not smoke or use tobacco products. His history is significant for multiple hospitalizations due to severe extremity pain that required the administration of opioids. His BMI is 23 kg/m^2. An abdominal X-ray shows multiple small, round radiopaque structures within the gallbladder. How would these structures appear on gross examination?

- **The correct answer is black and pigmented.**
- This African American man has a history of episodes of severe extremity pain that required opioids.
- From this, we can deduce that he very possibly has sickle cell anemia, a chronic hemolytic process.
- Recall that sickle cell anemia is associated with vaso-occlusive crises and when this occurs in the fingers it can cause extremity pain, better known as dactylitis.
- Now, this patient comes in with upper abdominal pain and nausea and his abdominal X-ray shows radiopaque structures in his gallbladder, likely representing gallstones.
- Collectively, these clues are highly suggestive of black pigmented gallstones as a result of chronic hemolysis from sickle cell disease.
- Black pigment stones occur in the setting of chronic hemolysis, are usually numerous and appear radiopaque on X-ray.

REVIEW QUESTIONS ?

2. A 45-year-old woman comes to the emergency department due to upper abdominal pain for the past 2 days. She recalls having similar pain after eating fatty meals in the past, but they never lasted this long before. Her BMI is 32 kg/m^2 and temperature is 38.5 °C (101.3 °F). The right upper quadrant is exquisitely tender to touch and deep palpation under the right costal margin causes the patient to pause her breath while inhaling deeply. Leukocyte count is 20,000/mm^3 (normal: 4,500-11,000/mm^3). What is the most likely initial event that led to these findings?

   A. Fistula formation between the gallbladder and bowel
   B. Obstruction of the cystic duct by a stone
   C. Trauma to the bile ducts
   D. Ischemia of the gallbladder wall

- **The correct answer is B.**
- Hopefully, from this question you noticed a few risk factors that led to this patient's condition.
- First, the patient is a middle-aged female and is obese with a BMI of 32.
- Next, we see that she has signs and symptoms of infection such as fever and leukocytosis.
- RUQ and breathing arrest on deep palpation, also called Murphy's sign, along with all the other symptoms point towards option: B acute cholecystitis due to a stone causing obstruction of the cystic duct.
- This is also supported by the fact that this patient experienced similar pain in the past, probably due to the recurrent lodging of a gallstone in the bile ducts that have spontaneously resolved.
- Recall that acute cholecystitis is the acute inflammation of the gallbladder wall.
- Calculus, which is the case with our patient, or acalculus.
- The diagnosis can be made with an ultrasound.
- A stone in the cystic duct could block off bile trying to leave the gallbladder, resulting in inflammation.
- Option A is not correct because fistula formation occurs due to chronic inflammation and adhesions rather than acute inflammation.
- Option C is incorrect as there was no major history of trauma that could have caused acute acalculus cholecystitis.
- Lastly, option D is incorrect as ischemia of the gallbladder is a later complication of prolonged obstruction of the biliary tract and is not the initial event that caused this patient's symptoms.

Section XII - Jaundice

I. Jaundice
   A. Often an early sign of liver pathology
   B. Causes
      1. Bilirubin > 2.5 mg/dL
      2. Disturbances of bilirubin metabolism

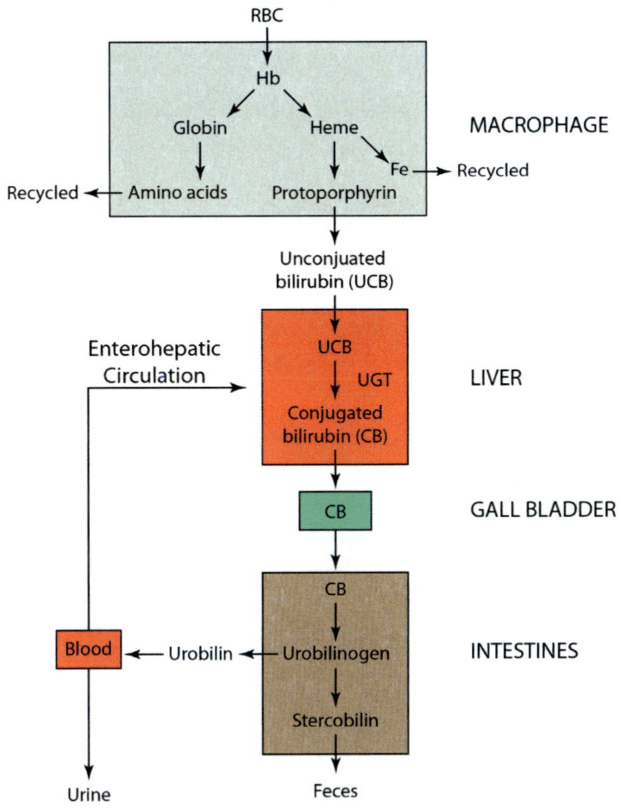

FIGURE 10.8.58 - Bilirubin Metabolism

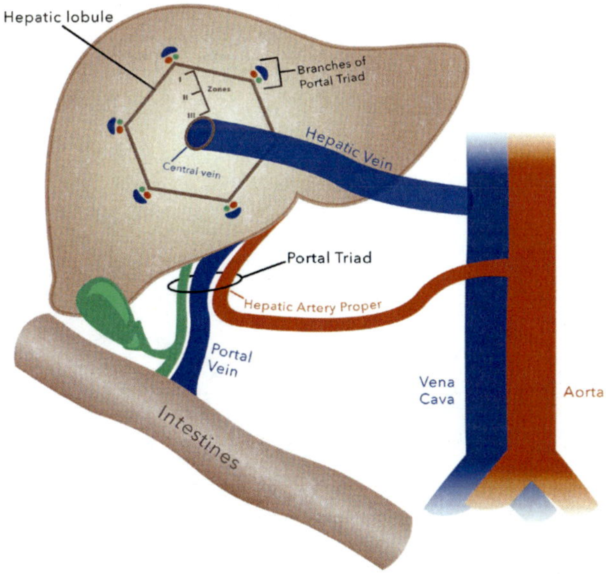

FIGURE 10.8.59 - Hepatic Blood Supply and Functional Anatomy

II. Extravascular Hemolysis
   A. High levels of UCB overwhelm liver capacity
   B. Lab findings
      1. Increased serum UCB
   C. Clinical features
      1. Dark urine due to increased urobilinogen (not UCB)
      2. Increased risk of pigmented gallstones

III. Physiologic Jaundice of the Newborn
   A. Newborn liver has transiently low UGT activity
   B. Lab findings
      1. Increased UCB
   C. Clinical features
      1. UCB is fat-soluble and can therefore deposit in the basal ganglia, leading to kernicterus and death
      2. Treated with phototherapy, which makes UCB water-soluble

IV. Gilbert Syndrome
   A. Autosomal recessive condition causing mildly low UGT activity
   B. Lab findings
      1. Increased UCB
   C. Clinical features
      1. Not generally clinically significant
      2. Causes jaundice during stress

V. Crigler-Najjar Syndrome
   A. Autosomal recessive absence of UGT activity
   B. Lab findings
      1. Increased UCB
   C. Clinical features
      1. Kernicterus
      2. Usually fatal

VI. Dubin-Johnson Syndrome
   A. Autosomal recessive deficiency of bilirubin canalicular transport protein
   B. Lab findings
      1. Increased CB
   C. Clinical features
      1. Liver is dark but otherwise not clinically significant
      2. Rotor syndrome is similar but lacks a dark liver

VII. Biliary Tract Obstruction
   A. Associated with gallstones, pancreatic carcinoma, parasites, cholangiocarcinoma, and liver fluke
   B. Lab findings
      1. Increased CB
      2. Decreased urine urobilinogen
      3. Increased alkaline phosphatase

VIII. Biliary Tract Obstruction: Clinical Features

A. Dark urine (bilirubinuria) and pale stool
B. Pruritis due to increased plasma bile acids
C. Hypercholesterolemia with xanthomas
D. Steatorrhea with malabsorption of fat-soluble vitamins

IX. Viral Hepatitis

A. Inflammation disrupts hepatocytes and small bile ductules
B. Lab findings
   1. Increased CB and UCB
C. Clinical features
   1. Dark urine (bilirubinuria)
D. Urine urobilinogen is normal or decreased

Disease	Pathologic Mechanism	Laboratory Findings	Other Features
Extravascular hemolysis	- High levels of UCB overwhelm the liver's conjugating capacity	- Increased UCB	- Dark urine due to urine urobilinogen - Increased risk for pigmented bilirubin gallstones
Physiologic jaundice of the newborn	- Transiently low UGT activity	- Increased UCB	- UCB is fat-soluble and can deposit in the basal ganglia (kernicterus) -Treatment is phototherapy
Gilbert syndrome	- Mildly reduced UGT activity - Autosomal recessive	- Increased UCB	- Jaundice during stress
Crigler-Najjar syndrome	-A bsence of UGT	- Increased UCB	- Kernicterus - Usually fatal
Dubin-Johnson syndrome	- Deficiency of bilirubin canalicular transport protein - Autosomal recessive	- Increased CB	- Dark liver - Otherwise not clinically significant
Biliary tract obstruction	- Obstruction of the biliary tract (gallstones, pancreatic cancer, etc.)	- Increased CB, decreased urine urobilinogen, and increased alkaline phosphatase	- Dark urine (due to bilirubinuria), pale stool, pruritus, hypercholesterolemia with xanthomas, and steatorrhea
Viral hepatitis	- Inflammation of hepatocytes	- Increased UCB and CB	- Dark urine (increased urine bilirubin) - Urine urobilinogen is normal or decreased

TABLE 10.8.2 - Causes of Jaundice

REVIEW QUESTIONS

1. A 35-year-old man presents to your office with 1 day of yellowish discoloration of his eyes and face. He has otherwise been feeling fine, but does admit that he has been under a great deal of stress lately while finding a contractor to renovate his home. He has had previous episodes of this during college, but has not had any issues since then. What is the most likely color of this patient's urine and why?
   - **The correct answer is that the patient's urine color would be normal.**
   - In this question, we are presented with an otherwise asymptomatic patient experiencing jaundice and an increase of stress. Hopefully, you were able to deduce that this patient most likely has Gilbert syndrome, an autosomal recessive disorder that results in diminished UGT activity.
   - Recall that UGT is responsible for coverting unconjugated bilirubin to conjugated bilirubin in the liver. A decrease in UGT activity results in increased serum unconjugated bilirubin (↑ UCB outside of liver).
   - Unconjugated bilirubin is not water-soluble. Therefore, this patient's urine would likely have no change in color as a result of his condition, as only conjugated bilirubin can be excreted by the kidneys.

2. A 78-year-old male hospitalized for treatment of a pulmonary embolism dies suddenly from a cardiac arrhythmia. Autopsy shows extensive blood clots in the pulmonary vasculature of both lungs and significant atherosclerosis of the coronary arteries. Examination of the patient's liver shows pigmentary changes consistent with a disorder related to canalicular transport. What laboratory changes would have been observed in this patient as compared to the general population prior to his death?

   A. Elevated UCB
   B. Elevated CB
   C. Elevated UCB and CB
   D. Decreased urine urobilinogen
   E. Increased alkaline phosphatase

- **The correct answer is B.**
- This patient had Dubin-Johnson syndrome based on the dark pigmentary changes in his liver with no significant history of liver disease. Recall that Dubin-Johnson syndrome is caused by an autosomal recessive deficiency of bilirubin canalicular transport protein that causes dark pigmentary changes in the liver parenchyma. It is not clinically significant and likely did not contribute to this patient's death.
- Patients with Dubin-Johnson syndrome tend to have elevated levels of conjugated bilirubin, as the transport mechanism for conjugated bilirubin is slightly defective but the conjugating ability of the liver remains intact. Thus, you would expect to see elevated conjugated bilirubin in a patient such as this.
- A is incorrect because elevated unconjugated bilirubin is associated with conditions that either overwhelm the ability of the liver to conjugate bilirubin, such as extravascular hemolysis, or involve deficiencies in the conjugating ability of the liver, such as physiologic jaundice of the newborn, Gilbert syndrome, and Crigler-Najjar syndrome. None of these conditions present with a darkened liver that is otherwise clinically insignificant.
- C is incorrect because an elevation in both unconjugated and conjugated bilirubin is associated with viral hepatitis, which causes general inflammation of the liver.
- D and E are incorrect because both decreases in urine urobilinogen and increases in alkaline phosphatase are associated with biliary tract obstruction, which does not cause dark pigmentary changes in the liver. While Dubin-Johnson syndrome does involve a mild defect in canalicular transport, it is not clinically significant and is not associated with obstruction of the biliary tract.

Section XIII - Cirrhosis and Liver Cancer

I. Cirrhosis
   A. End-stage liver damage
      1. Fibrosis
      2. Regenerative nodules
   B. TGF-β released by stellate cells
   C. Decreased blood flow throughout the liver

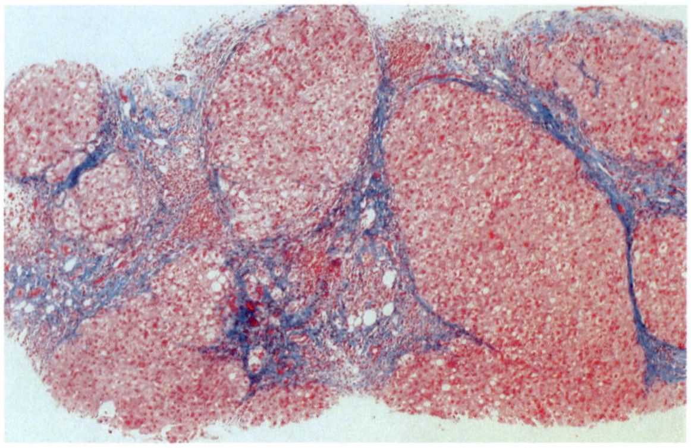

FIGURE 10.8.60 - Cirrhosis

II. Cirrhosis: Presentation
   A. Portal hypertension
   B. Decreased detoxification
   C. Decreased protein synthesis

III. Cirrhosis: Portal Hypertension
   A. Ascites
   B. Congestive splenomegaly/hypersplenism
   C. Hepatorenal syndrome
      1. Liver unable to break down renin
      2. Renal vasoconstriction
      3. Renal failure
   D. Portosystemic shunts
      1. Esophageal varices (left gastric and esophageal veins)
      2. Internal hemorrhoids (superior and middle/ inferior rectal veins)
      3. Caput medusae (paraumbilical veins and superficial epigastric veins)

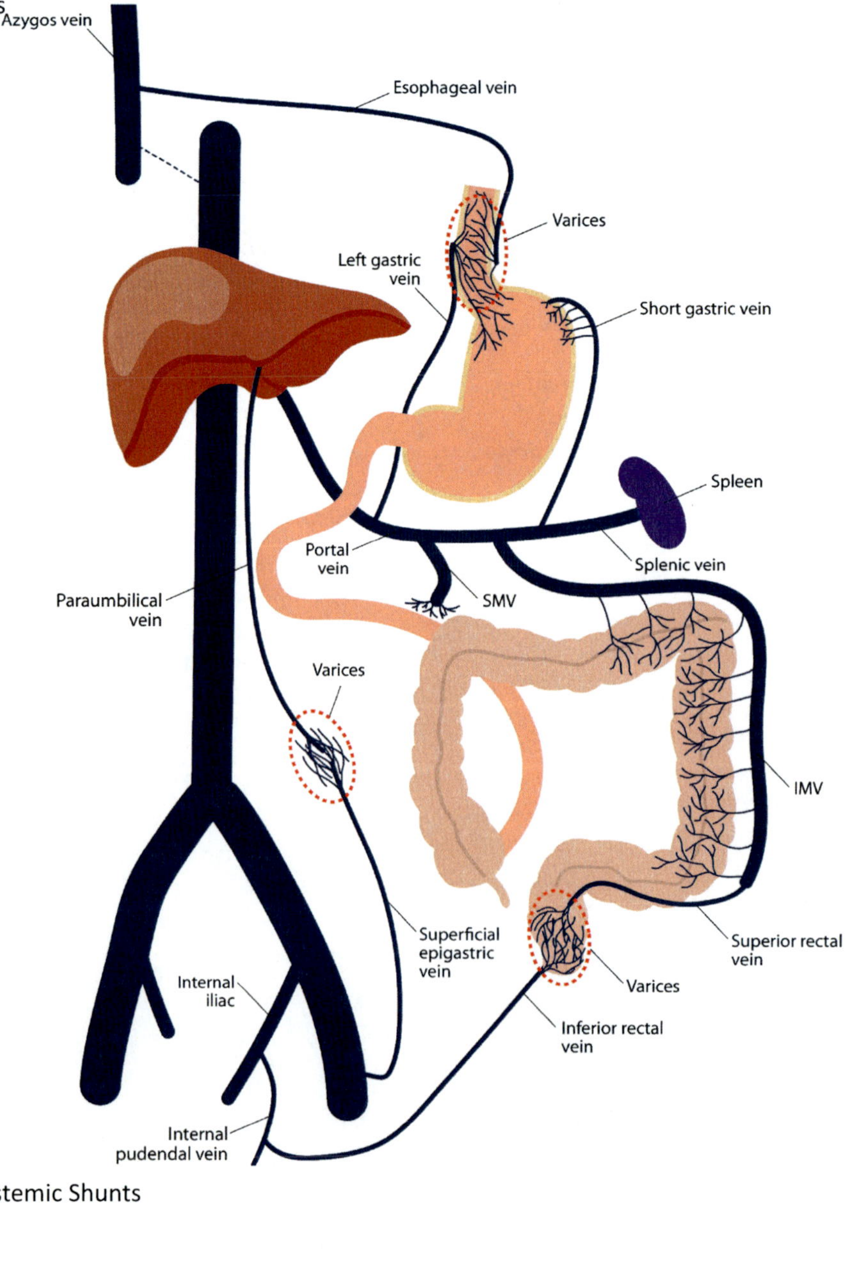

FIGURE 10.8.61 - Portosystemic Shunts

IV. Cirrhosis: Decreased Liver Detoxification
  A. Increased serum ammonia and other toxins
    1. Hepatic encephalopathy, asterixis, and coma
  B. Hyperestrinism
    1. Gynecomastia, spider angiomata, and palmar erythema
  C. Jaundice
    1. Increased serum bilirubin (conjugated and unconjugated)

V. Cirrhosis: Decreased Protein Synthesis
  A. Decreased protein synthesis
    1. Hypoalbuminemia with edema
    2. Coagulopathy due to decreased synthesis of clotting factors
    3. Followed by prothrombin time (PT)

VI. Hepatic Adenoma
  A. Benign tumor of hepatocytes that is usually asymptomatic
  B. Subcapsular
  C. Associated with oral contraceptive use and grows with estrogen exposure
  D. Risk of rupture and intraperitoneal bleeding, especially during pregnancy
  E. Very small risk of malignant transformation

VII. Hepatocellular Carcinoma
  A. Malignant tumor of hepatocytes
  B. Often detected late
  C. Alpha-fetoprotein (AFP)
  D. Risk factors
    1. Chronic hepatitis, cirrhosis, and aflatoxins (*P53* mutations)
  E. Budd-Chiari syndrome
    1. Obstruction of the hepatic vein

VIII. Metastasis to the Liver
  A. More common than primary liver cancer
    1. Fenestrated hepatic sinusoidal epithelium
    2. Dual blood supply
  B. Colon, pancreas, lung, and breast
  C. Multiple liver nodules
  D. Hepatomegaly with nodular free edge

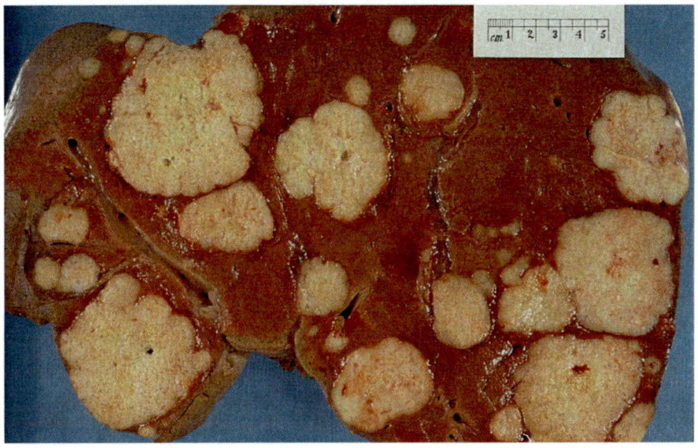

Photo Credit: Haymanj / Public domain

FIGURE 10.8.62 - Metastatic Cancer of Liver

REVIEW QUESTIONS

1. A 65-year-old man with advanced liver cirrhosis presents to the clinic for evaluation of a new rash (shown below). What other findings might you expect to find as a result of the same abnormality responsible for the rash?

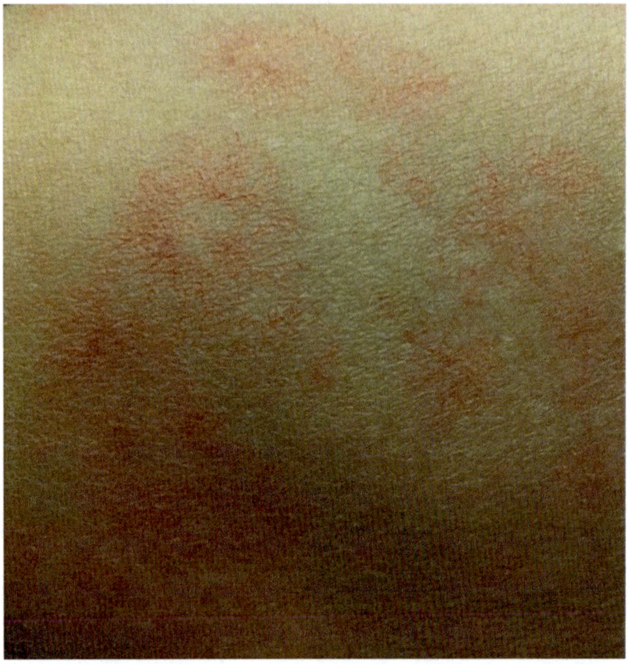

Photo Credit: James Heilman, MD / CC BY-SA (https://creativecommons.org/licenses/by-sa/4.0)

- **The correct answer is gynecomastia and palmar erythema.**
- The rash in this vignette is a spider angioma.
- Note the fine, spider-like spindles visible in each of the erythematous lesions shown.
- Recall that spider angiomas are caused by hyperestrinism due to the inability of the liver to metabolize estrogen.

2. A previously healthy 37-year-old female presents to the emergency department with cramping pain in her right upper quadrant that radiates to her back. She states that she has experienced similar pain several times in the past few months, but that this time it isn't going away. Ultrasound of the abdomen shows evidence of cholecystitis, but also reveals a 3 by 4 cm hyperechoic mass in the left lobe of her liver. This patient's lesion is most likely associated with which of the following?

   A. Elevated alpha-fetoprotein
   B. History of IV drug use
   C. Recent international travel
   D. *BRCA* gene mutation
   E. Oral contraceptive use

- **The correct answer is E.**
- Hopefully, you were able to determine that this patient's most likely diagnosis is hepatic adenoma.
- Hepatic adenomas are most commonly found incidentally on abdominal imaging for some other indication.
- Recall that hepatic adenomas tend to increase in size when exposed to estrogen and are often associated with oral contraceptive use.
- In an otherwise healthy young woman, this is the most likely diagnosis.
- A is incorrect because alpha-fetoprotein is associated with hepatocellular carcinoma.
- While it is not impossible that this patient has a well-differentiated form of HCC, it is far less likely than hepatic adenoma due to a lack of predisposing factors.
- B is incorrect because IV drug use is associated with acute or chronic hepatitis, which would likely either not be detected on abdominal imaging or present as diffuse inflammation.
- C is incorrect because recent international travel would be consistent with acute hepatitis through contraction of hepatitis A, not hepatic adenoma.
- D is incorrect because although a *BRCA* gene mutation could result in breast cancer that might metastasize to the liver, this would present as multiple nodules rather than one small nodule, which is more characteristic of hepatic adenoma.

Section XIV - Other Liver Conditions

I. Reye Syndrome
   A. Fulminant liver failure and encephalopathy in children with a viral illness who take aspirin
   B. Etiology unknown
      1. Mitochondrial damage
         a) Histopathology
   C. Microvesicular steatosis without necrosis or inflammation

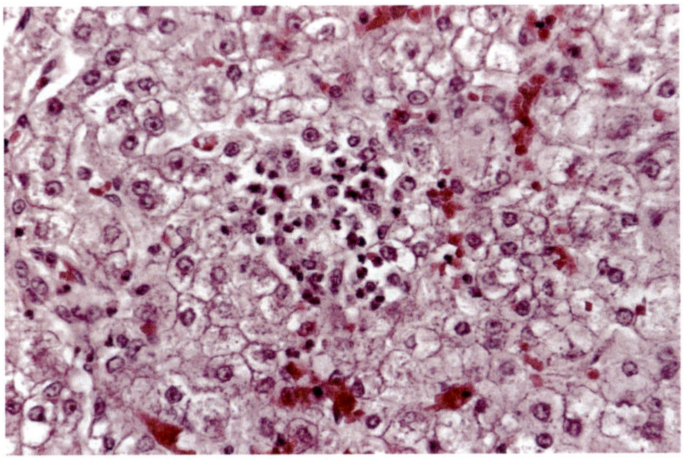

CDC/ Dr. Edwin P. Ewing, Jr. / Public domain

FIGURE 10.8.63 - Histology of Reye Syndrome

II. Reye Syndrome: Presentation
   A. Two major components
      1. Hepatic dysfunction
      2. Encephalopathy (hyperammonemia, cerebral edema)
   B. Hypoglycemia, elevated liver enzymes, hepatomegaly, nausea and vomiting
   C. Coma and death
   D. Supportive therapy

III. Alcohol-Related Liver Disease
   A. Most common cause of liver disease in the developed world
   B. Chemical damage by alcohol metabolites, especially acetaldehyde
   C. Histology
      1. Hepatocyte swelling with damaged cytokeratin filaments (Mallory bodies), necrosis, and inflammation
      2. Fat deposition in hepatocytes
   D. Painful hepatomegaly
   E. Elevated liver enzymes
   F. AST > ALT
   G. GGT
   H. Cirrhosis present in 10-20% of long-term alcoholics
   I. Can be fatal

Disease	Pathologic Mechanism	Laboratory Findings	Other Features
Hepatitis A	- Fecal-oral	- Acute	- IgM indicates active infection - IgG indicates immunity
Hepattis B	- Parental	- Acute and chronic	- Chronic disease occurs in 20% of infections - Complex serology
Hepattis C	- Parental	- Acute and chronic	- Chronic disease occurs in most cases - Can lead ot hepatocellular carcinoma
Hepatitis D	- Parenteral - Requires HBV co-infection	- Superinfection	-Superinfection with hepatitis B causes more severe hepatits
Hepatitis E	- Fecal-oral	- Acute	- Infection of pregnant women associated with liver failure

TABLE 10.8.3 - Hepatitis Overview

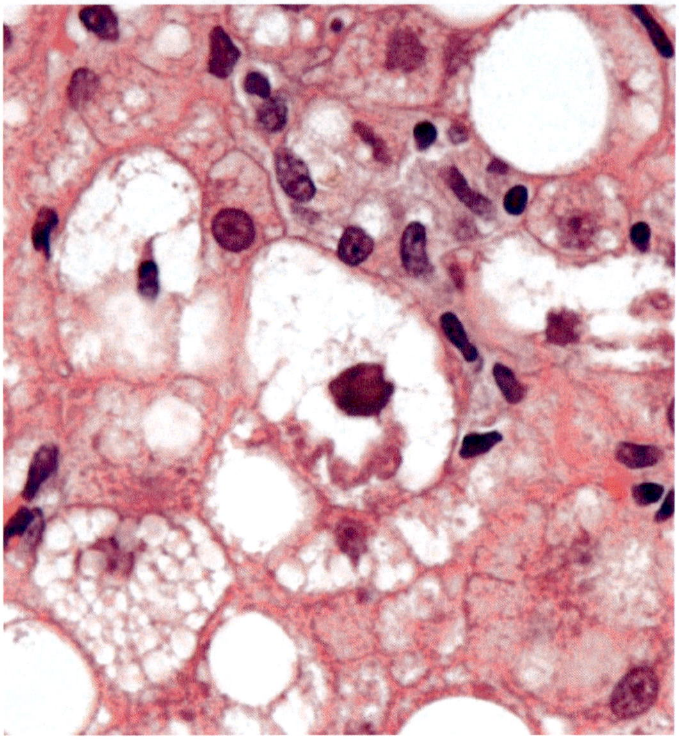

FIGURE 10.8.64 - Histology of Alcohol-Related Liver Disease

IV. Non-Alcoholic Fatty Liver Disease
   A. Fatty changes and hepatitis that take place in the absence of alcohol exposure
   B. Associated with obesity
   C. Diagnosis of exclusion
   D. Histology
      1. Fatty deposition
      2. Mallory bodies

V. Hemochromatosis
   A. Excess iron in the body, leading to deposition in tissues (hemosiderosis) and organ damage
   B. Damage caused by free radical generation

VI. Hemochromatosis: Causes
   A. Primary hemochromatosis
      1. *HFE* gene, *C282Y*
      2. Falsely low iron levels detected
      3. Increased *DMT-1* expression in enterocytes
      4. Decreased hepcidin synthesis
      5. Increased ferroportin expression
   B. Secondary hemochromatosis
      1. Excessive iron transfusions

VII. Hemochromatosis: Presentation
   A. Late adulthood onset
   B. Classic triad: cirrhosis, type 2 diabetes, and bronze skin
   C. Other findings
      1. Dilated cardiomyopathy
      2. Cardiac arrhythmia/conduction blocks
      3. Gonadal dysfunction (testicular atrophy)

VIII. Hemochromatosis: Iron Panel
   A. Ferritin
      1. Stored iron
   B. TIBC
      1. Indirectly measures transferrin
   C. Serum iron
   D. % Saturation (transferrin saturation percentage)
      1. Serum iron / TIBC

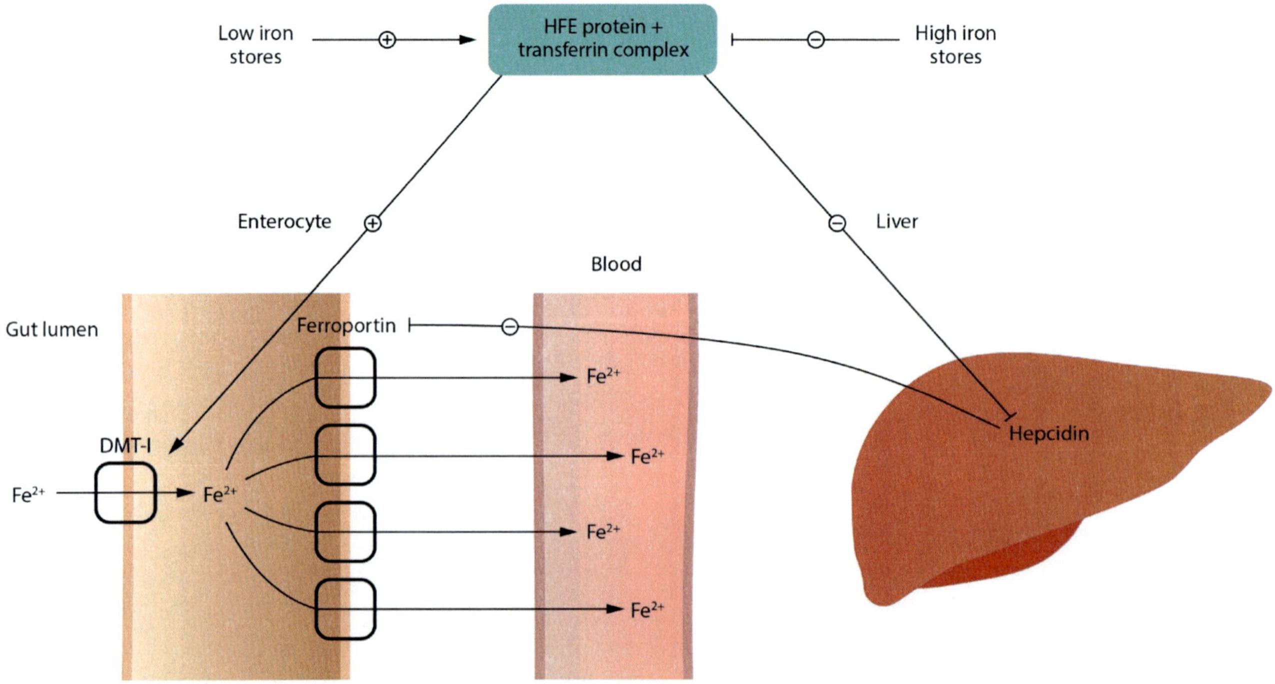

FIGURE 10.8.65 - Iron Signaling Pathway

IX. Hemochromatosis: Labs and Histology
   A. Labs
      1. Increased ferritin, decreased/normal TIBC, increased serum iron, increased % saturation
   B. Histology
      1. Accumulation of brown pigment in hepatocytes
      2. Prussian blue stain

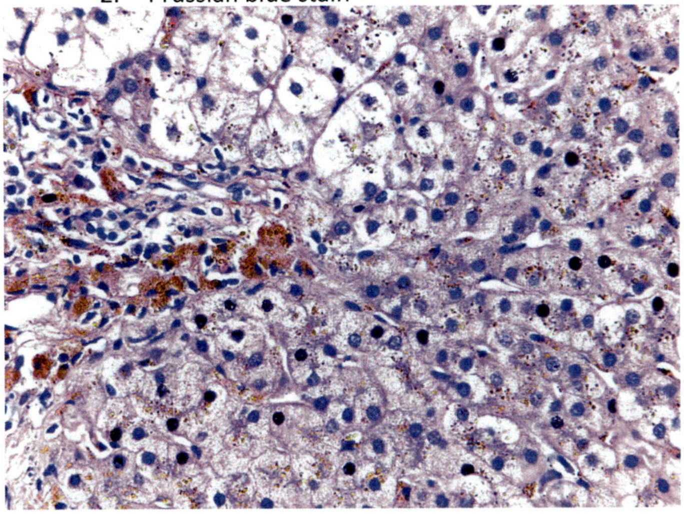

FIGURE 10.8.66 - Histology of Hemochromatosis

X. Hemochromatosis: Complications and Treatment
   A. Increased risk of hepatocellular carcinoma
   B. Treatment
      1. Phlebotomy

XI. Wilson Disease
   A. Excess copper in the body, leading to deposition in the tissues
   B. Causes
      1. Autosomal recessive defect in copper transport (*ATP7B* gene)
      2. Lack of copper transport into bile and lack of copper incorporation into ceruloplasmin
      3. Copper builds up in hepatocytes, leaks into serum, and deposits in tissues producing hydroxyl free radicals that damage tissue

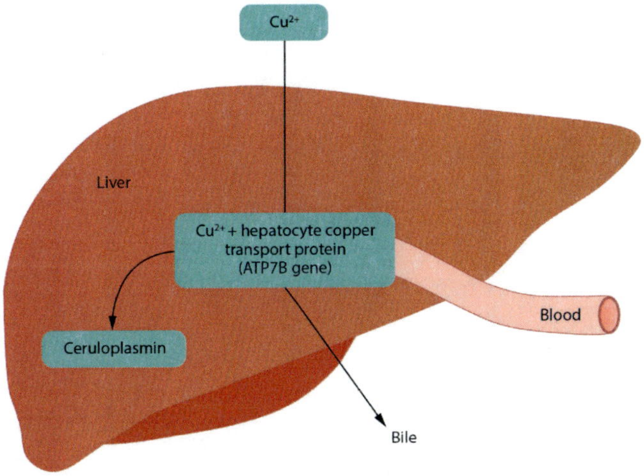

FIGURE 10.8.67 - Copper Transport Pathway

XII. Wilson Disease: Presentation
   A. Presents in childhood
   B. Cirrhosis
   C. Neurologic manifestations
      1. Behavioral changes, dementia, chorea, Parkinsonian symptoms due to deposition in basal ganglia
   D. Kayser-Fleischer rings in the cornea

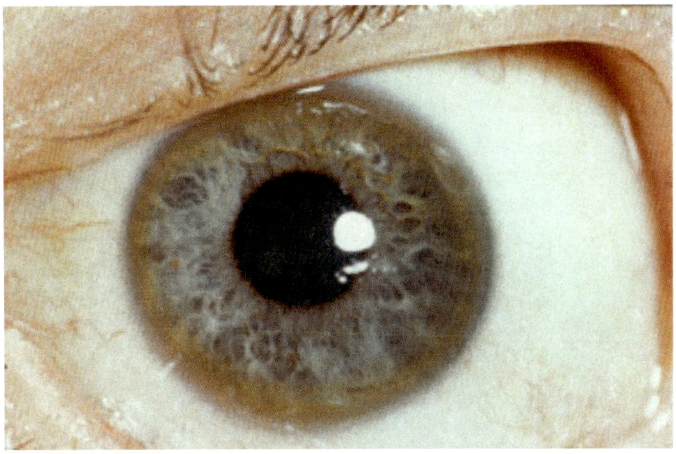

FIGURE 10.8.68 - Kayser-Fleischer Ring in Wilson Disease

XIII. Wilson Disease: Labs, Complications, Treatment
   A. Labs
      1. Increased urinary copper, decreased serum ceruloplasmin, and increased copper on liver biopsy
         a) Increased risk of hepatocellular carcinoma
   B. Treatment
      1. D-penicillamine (chelating agent)

REVIEW QUESTIONS

1. A 44-year-old man with a history of heavy alcohol use presents to your clinic with abdominal pain after a night of binge drinking. He reports that he has had several of these episodes in the past, but that they seem to have gotten better. Physical exam shows diffuse abdominal tenderness with hepatomegaly. His serum lipase is normal, but his liver function tests are elevated. What findings would you expect with regard to his liver enzyme tests?

    - **It is expected to find global liver enzyme elevations with a classic pattern of AST > ALT, often found in a ratio of at least 2:1. You would also expect this patient to have an elevation in GGT.**
    - In this question, the patient presents with alcohol related liver disease.
    - He has classic findings related to this condition including a history of heavy alcohol use, abdominal pain, hepatomegaly, and elevated liver enzymes.

2. A thin 46-year-old man with a history of type 2 diabetes presents with recent-onset jaundice and abdominal swelling consistent with ascites. He states that his symptoms began several days ago and have been getting worse each day. He has no history of alcohol or IV drug use. Biopsy confirms the presence of cirrhosis and pathologic examination shows coarse brown granules in the hepatocytes. Which of the following is most likely diminished in this patient?

    A. Serum ferritin
    B. Serum iron
    C. % saturation
    D. Hepcidin
    E. Ferroportin

    - **The correct answer is D.**
    - A thin, young patient with no risk factors for diabetes or cirrhosis, with coarse brown granules in hepatocytes on liver biopsy, is very likely to have a diagnosis of hemochromatosis.
    - A, B, and C are incorrect because these are referring to hemochromatosis which is a disorder that causes iron overload.
    - By definition, therefore, serum ferritin, serum iron, and % saturation, are all increased, as there is just more iron to go around.
    - The only iron panel result that might be decreased is total iron binding capacity, but this is also commonly normal.
    - E is also incorrect because levels of ferroportin, which is a major iron transporter in the gut, are increased in hemochromatosis. This is because the body attempts to absorb and hold onto as much iron as possible.

Section I - Bone Disorders

I. Osteopetrosis: Etiology
   A. Inherited defect in bone reabsorption
   B. Autosomal dominant or recessive

II. Osteopetrosis: Pathophysiology
   A. Defective carbonic anhydrase II enzyme
   B. Decreased bone reabsorption
   C. Increased bone density

III. Osteopetrosis: Clinical Features
   A. Fractures
   B. Pancytopenia
   C. Hearing and visual defects
   D. Hydrocephalus
   E. Renal tubular acidosis
   F. X-ray: sclerotic bone
   G. May benefit from bone marrow transplant

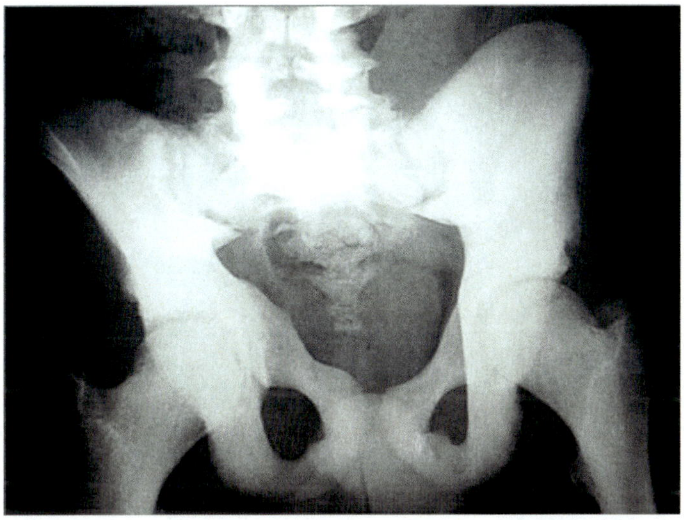

FIGURE 10.9.1 - Osteopetrosis

IV. Rickets/Osteomalacia: Etiology
   A. Vitamin D deficiency
      1. Decreased sun exposure, malabsorption, CKD, and poor diet
   B. Rickets occurs in children
   C. Osteomalacia occurs in adults

V. Rickets/)steomalacia: Pathophysiology
   A. Decreased vitamin D causes a decrease in calcium and phosphate
   B. Defective bone mineralization

VI. Rickets/Osteomalacia: Clinical features
   A. Rickets causes genu varum deformity
   B. Rachitic rosary finding in rickets
   C. Osteomalacia causes bone pain and muscle weakness
   D. Decreased calcium and phosphate
   E. Increased PTH and ALP

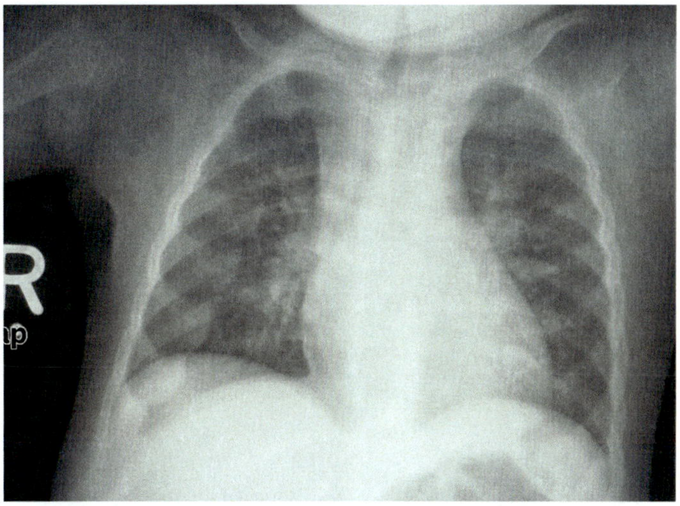

FIGURE 10..8.2 - Rickets: Rachitic Rosary (Pediatric Patient)

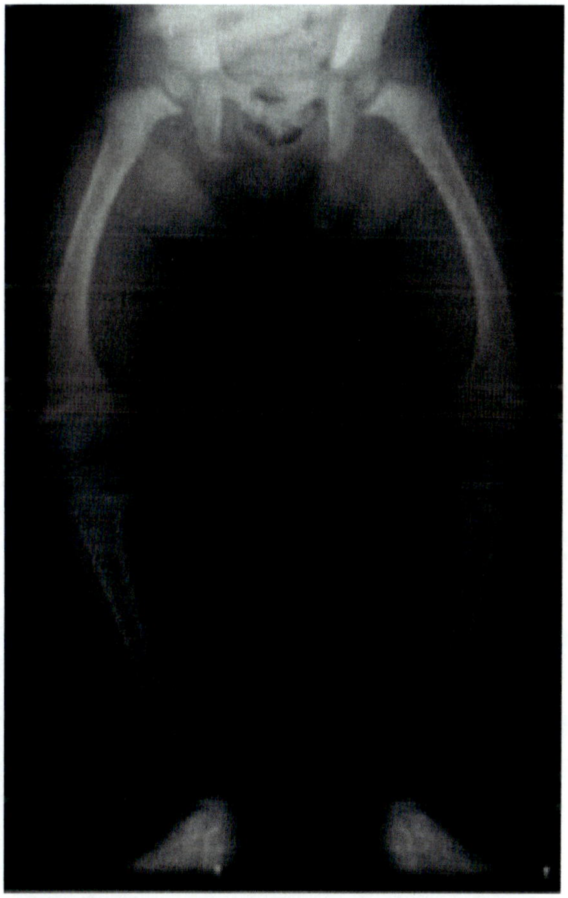

FIGURE 10.9.3 - Rickets: Genu Varum (Pediatric Patient)

VII. Osteoporosis: Etiology
  A. Most common
    1. Advanced age (≥ 65) and postmenopausal
  B. Less common
    1. Hyperparathyroidism, steroids, hyperthyroidism, and multiple myeloma

VIII. Osteoporosis: Pathophysiology
  A. Cortical and trabecular bone loss
  B. Senile osteoporosis is due to decreased osteoblast activity
  C. Postmenopausal osteoporosis is due to decreased estrogen

IX. Osteoporosis: Clinical features
  A. Bone pain and fractures
  B. DEXA T-score ≤ -2.5
  C. Normal calcium, phosphate, PTH, and ALP

X. Osteoporosis: Treatment
  A. Calcium
  B. Vitamin D
  C. Exercise
  D. Estrogen
  E. Bisphosphonates

XI. Paget's Disease of the Bone: Etiology
  A. Unknown etiology
  B. Commonly occurs in older patients

XII. Paget's disease of the Bone: Pathophysiology
  A. Defective bone remodeling causes thick, sclerotic bone
  B. Lytic, mixed, sclerotic, and quiescent phase
  C. Mosaic pattern of lamellar bone

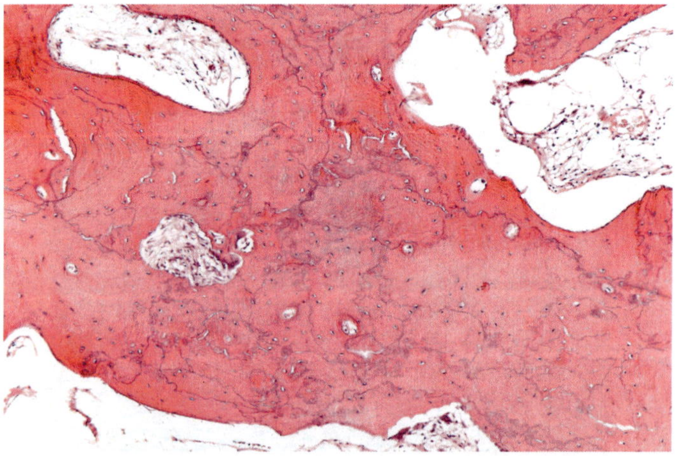

FIGURE 10.9.4 - Bone Biopsy of Paget's Disease of Bone

XIII. Paget's disease of the Bone: Clinical features
  A. Long bone fractures
  B. Increased skull thickness
  C. Hearing loss
  D. Osteosarcoma
  E. High-output cardiac failure
  F. Normal calcium and phosphate and increased ALP

XIV. Osteomyelitis: Etiology
  A. Bacterial infection of the bone and marrow
  B. Most commonly *Staphylococcus aureus*

Organism	Association
Staphylococcus aureus	Most common cause
Salmonella	Sickle cell
Pasteurella	Dog/cat bites and scratches
Pseudomonas	IV drug use and diabetics
Neisseria gonorrhoeae	Sexually active people
Mycobacterium tuberculosis	Pott's disease

TABLE 10.9.1 - Osteomyelitis Etiology

XV. Osteomyelitis: Clinical features
  A. Risk factors include sickle cell, joint replacement, and IV drug use
  B. Diagnosed via blood cultures

REVIEW QUESTIONS

?

1. A 69-year-old male with a past medical history of hypertension and type 2 diabetes mellitus presents to the physician with a primary complaint of hearing loss. The patient states his hearing has gotten worse over the last 2 years and he has noticed that his hat size has increased as well. What is a potential complication of this patient's condition?

    - **A correct answer would be hearing loss, osteosarcoma, or high-output cardiac failure.**
    - The patient is suffering from Paget's disease of bone.
    - Paget's disease of bone is due to defective bone remodeling that leads to thick sclerotic bone.
    - The patient's hat size has increased due to his skull becoming thicker.
    - The patient is also experiencing hearing loss due to cranial nerve impingement secondary to skull thickening.

2. A 9-month-old male with no past medical history is brought to the physician for a routine visit. The mother states that she has been exclusively breastfeeding him. He takes no vitamins or supplements. Physical examination is normal. However, a blood test reveals decreased levels of calcium and phosphate with elevated levels of parathyroid hormone. Which of the following is most likely associated with this patient's current condition?

    A. Defective carbonic anhydrase II
    B. Bony nodularities at the costochondral junction
    C. Thick sclerotic bones
    D. Infection

    - **The correct answer is B.**
    - A 9-month-old patient has been exclusively breastfed. Along with decreased calcium and phosphate as well as elevated parathyroid hormone, this is highly suggestive of rickets.
    - This can occur in young children who are exclusively breastfed without vitamin D supplementation.
    - Therefore, the correct answer is B: bony nodularities at the costochondral junction. This is called rachitic rosary.
    - A is incorrect because defective carbonic anhydrase II is not associated with rickets. It is associated with osteopetrosis and this often presents with other features such as anemia, vision impairment, and hydrocephalus.
    - C is incorrect because it describes defective bone remodeling seen in Paget's disease of bone.
    - D is incorrect as an infection would likely present with fever and pain and would be unlikely considering that this patient doesn't have significant risk factors such as sickle cell disease or IV drug use.

Section II - Bone Tumors

I. Osteoma
   A. Benign outgrowth of bone
   B. Usually found on the bones of the skull
   C. Associated with Gardner syndrome
      1. Familial adenomatous polyposis and osteomas

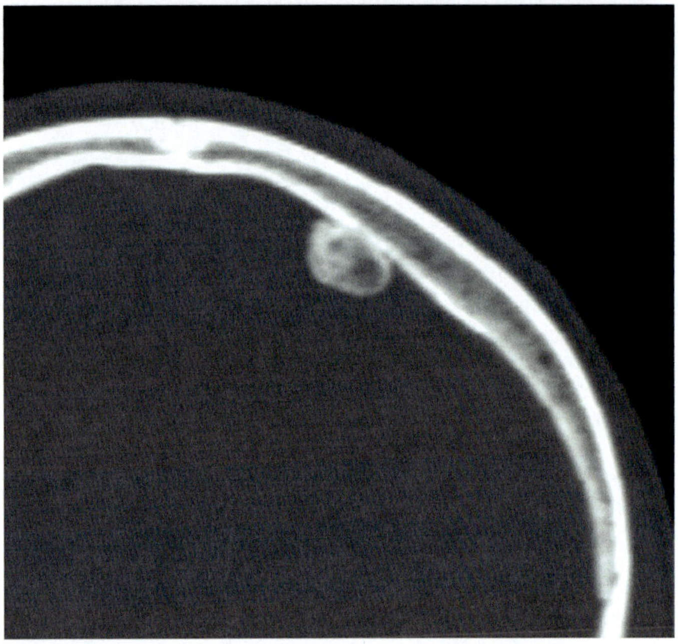

FIGURE 10.9.5 - Head CT of Osteoma (Bone Window)

II. Osteoid Osteoma
   A. Benign bone tumor that develops in the long bones of the leg
   B. Often occurs in young adult males < 25 years of age
   C. Bone pain that resolves with aspirin
   D. Imaging: bony mass < 1.5 cm in size with radiolucent core and radiopaque surrounding rim

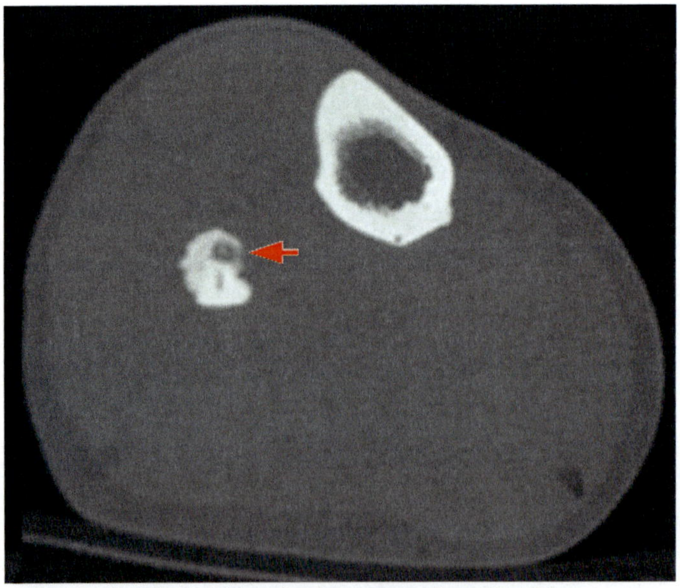

FIGURE 10.9.6 - Leg CT of Osteoid Osteoma of the Fibula

III. Osteoblastoma
   A. Benign bone tumor closely related to osteoid osteoma
   B. Occurs in young adult males < 25 years of age
   C. Tumor develops in the vertebrae
   D. Bone pain that does not respond to aspirin
   E. Imaging: bony mass > 1.5 cm in size with radiolucent core and radiopaque surrounding rim

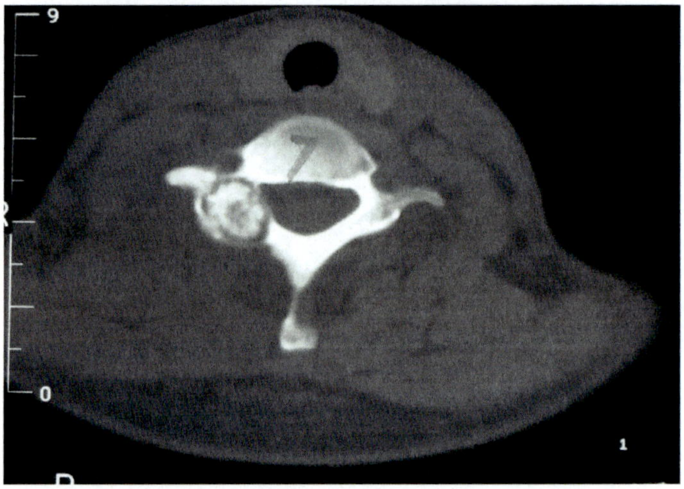

FIGURE 10.9.7 - Spine CT of Osteoblastoma of the Vertebrae

IV. Osteochondroma
   A. Overgrowth of cartilage and bone
   B. Most common benign bone tumor
   C. Lateral bone protuberance with surrounding cartilage cap
   D. Overlying cartilage can transform to chondrosarcoma

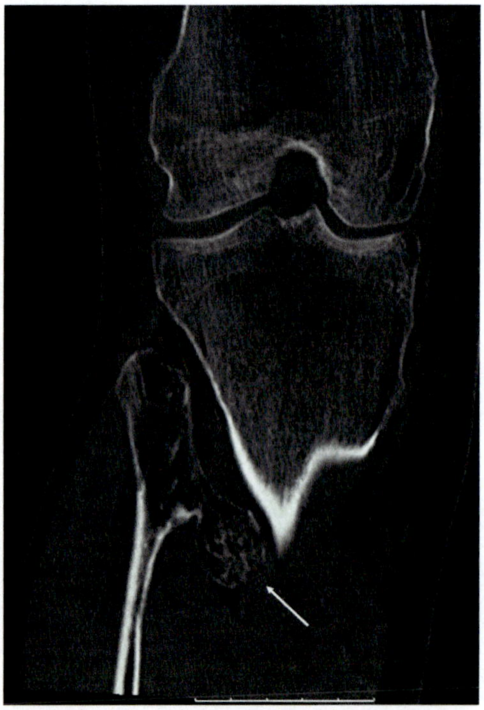

FIGURE 10.9.8 - CT of Osteochondroma

V. Osteosarcoma
  A. Most common malignant bone tumor
  B. Common in teenagers
  C. Risk factors
    1. Radiation to bones, hereditary retinoblastoma, Paget disease of bone, Li-Fraumeni syndrome

VI. Osteosarcoma: Findings
  A. Tumor often found in the metaphyseal region of long bones
    1. Most common around the knee
  B. Occurs in young adult males < 25 years of age
  C. Imaging: "sunburst" patterns and/or Codman triangle
  D. Biopsy: pleomorphic cells that produce osteoid

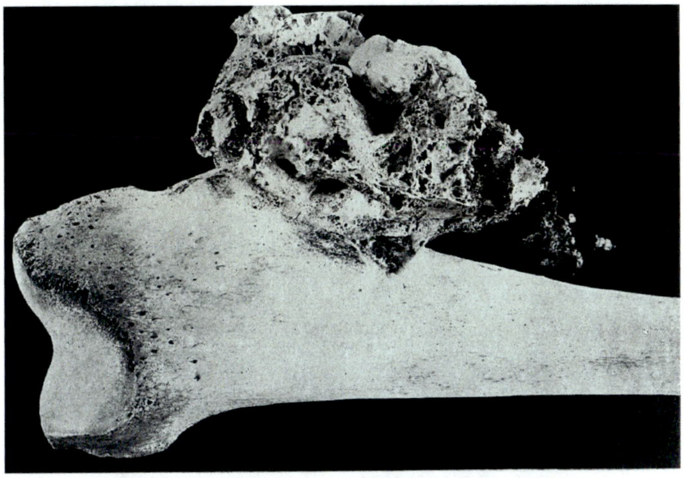

FIGURE 10.9.9 - Gross Image of Osteosarcoma of the Distal Femur

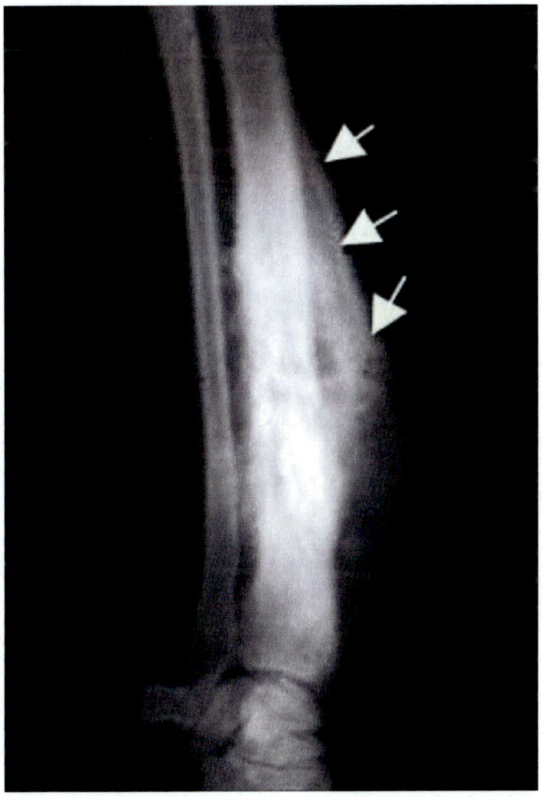

FIGURE 10.9.10 - "Sunburst" Pattern in Tibial Osteosarcoma

VII. Giant Cell Tumor
  A. Benign tumor, but locally aggressive
  B. Tumor develops in the epiphyseal region of long bones
    1. Femur or upper end of the tibia close to the knee joint
  C. "Soap-bubble" pattern on X-ray
  D. Biopsy: multinucleated giant cells and stromal cells

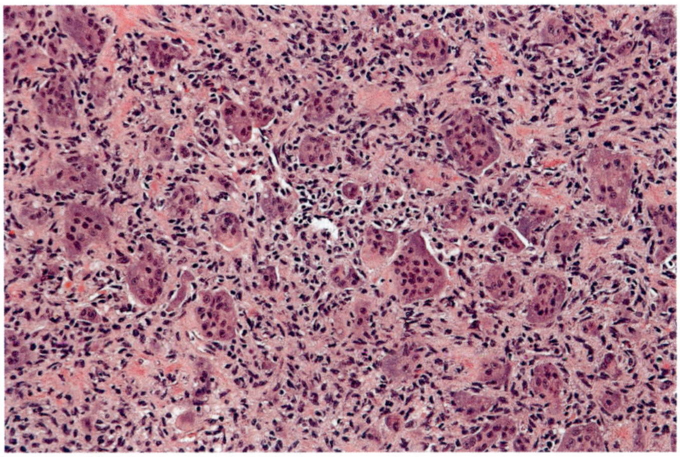

FIGURE 10.9.11 - Multinucleated Giant Cells in Giant Cell Tumor

VIII. Ewing Sarcoma
  A. Malignant bone tumor that often spreads to the lungs and other bones
  B. Common in male children and young adults
  C. Tumor develops in diaphyseal region of long bones
  D. "Onion-skin" pattern on X-ray
  E. Biopsy: small, round blue cells that resemble lymphocytes
  F. (11;22) translocation

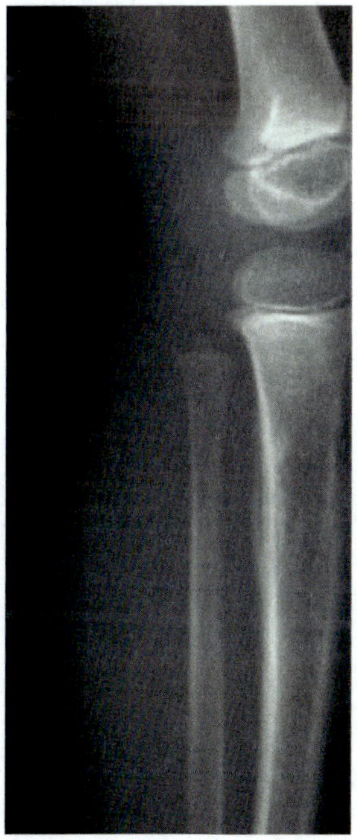

FIGURE 10.9.12 - "Onion-skin" Pattern in Ewing Sarcoma

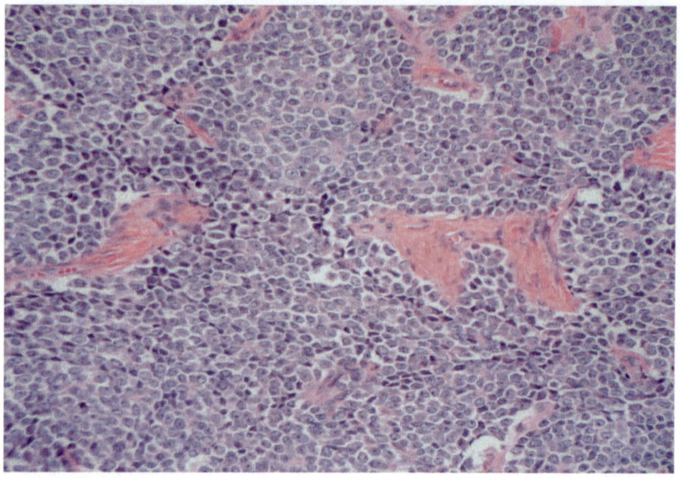

FIGURE 10.9.13 - Biopsy of Ewing Sarcoma

IX. Chondroma
  A. Benign cartilaginous tumor
  B. Tumor arises in small bones of the hands and feet

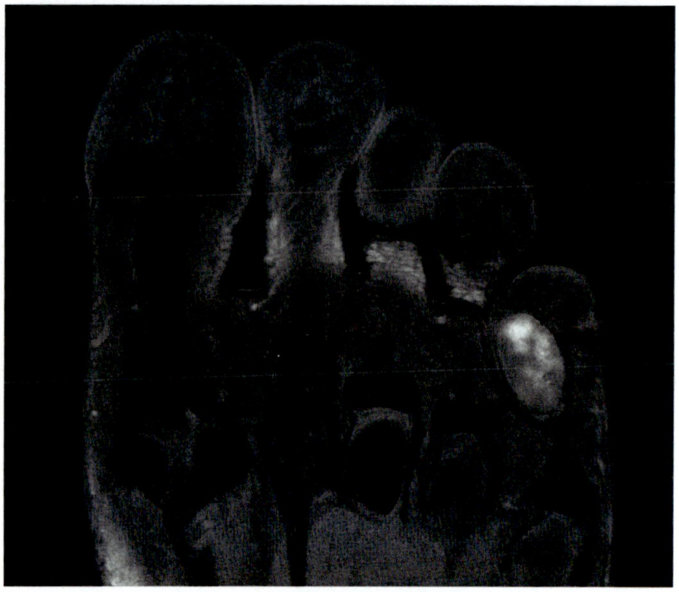

FIGURE 10.9.14 - MRI Foot of Chondroma of Left Little Toe

X. Chondrosarcoma
  A. Malignant cartilaginous tumor
  B. Most common in the pelvis, shoulder, hip

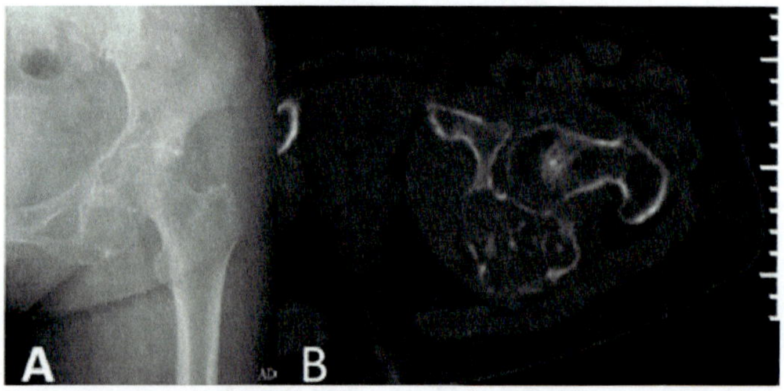

FIGURE 10.9.15 - X-Ray and CT showing Chondrosarcoma of Pelvis and Proximal Femur

XI. Metastatic Tumors
  A. Malignant cells from the primary tumor spread to the bones
  B. "Punched-out" osteolytic lesions
    1. Exception: prostatic carcinoma (osteoblastic lesions in vertebrae)

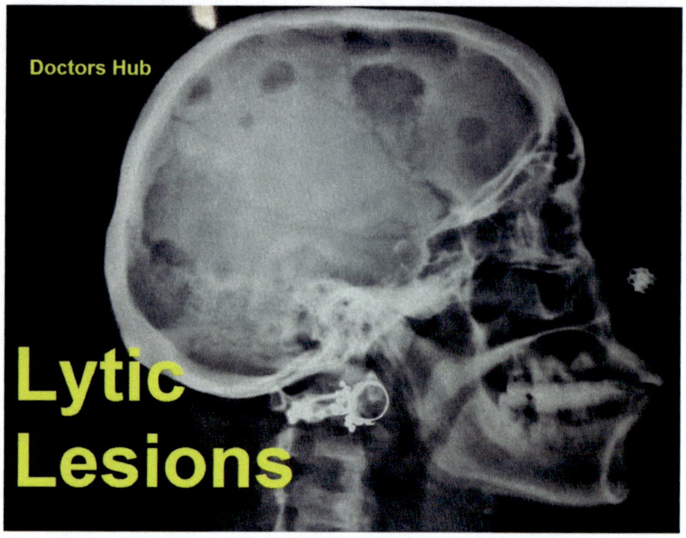

FIGURE 10.9.16 - "Punched-Out" Lesions of Metastatic Tumors

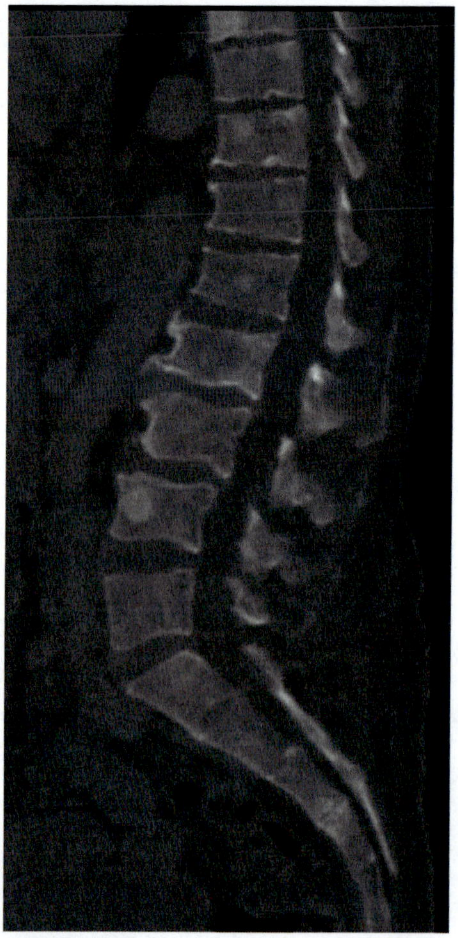

FIGURE 10.9.17 - Multiple Osteoblastic Lesions

REVIEW QUESTIONS

1. An 18-year-old male presents to the clinic with pain in his left leg. Imaging reveals a bony mass that is about 1 cm in size with a radiolucent core in the cortical region of his left femur. Would this patient's pain resolve with the administration of aspirin?

   - **The correct answer is yes, the bone pain would resolve with the administration of aspirin.**
   - This is an 18-year-old male presenting with pain in his left leg with an image revealing a bony mass that is 1 cm in size with a radiolucent core in the cortical region of his left femur.
   - The location of the tumor, the size, and the description of the mass confirm the diagnosis of osteoid osteoma. In someone with osteoid osteoma, the bone pain resolves with aspirin.

2. A 29-year-old female presents to the clinic with persistent pain in her right leg. She denies any fever, rash, swelling, or trauma. On X-ray, there is a radiolucent, lytic "soap-bubble" lesion of the distal femur on the right. The physician orders a confirmatory biopsy. What would the biopsy reveal?

   - **The biopsy would reveal multinucleated giant cells and stromal cells.**
   - This is a 29-year-old female presenting with persistent pain in her right leg with an image revealing a radiolucent, lytic "soap-bubble" lesion of the distal femur.
   - The location and the description of the tumor confirm the diagnosis of giant cell tumor. In someone with a giant cell tumor, the biopsy would reveal multinucleated giant cells and stromal cells.

3. A 10-year-old male presents with his mother to the clinic complaining of progressive right leg pain. He denies any recent trauma to the area. His temperature is 37 °C (98.6 °F), blood pressure is 117/65 mm Hg, and the respiratory rate is 20 breaths/min. On physical examination, there is tenderness over the distal diaphyseal region of the right femur. Biopsy shows small, round blue cells that resemble lymphocytes. Which of the following genetic mutations is most likely associated with this patient's condition?

   A. Inherited *APC* mutation
   B. *JAK2* kinase mutation
   C. t(9;22)
   D. t(11;22)

   - **The correct answer is D.**
   - This is a 10-year-old male who presents with progressive right leg pain and denies any recent trauma to the area. On physical examination, tenderness in the distal diaphyseal region of the right femur is present and the biopsy shows small, round, blue cells that resemble lymphocytes.
   - Based on the age and gender of the patient, the location of the tenderness, and finally the biopsy, the diagnosis of Ewing sarcoma. Ewing sarcoma is associated with (11;22) translocation. Recall that in Ewing sarcoma, the tumor arises in the diaphyseal region of the long bones. On X-ray, these tumors often have an "onion-skin" appearance. Also, small, round blue cells that resemble lymphocytes can be observed on biopsy.
   - A is wrong because inherited *APC* mutation is associated with familial adenomatous polyposis. Someone with an inherited APC mutation has an increased risk of colon polyps and colorectal cancer.
   - B is wrong because *JAK2* kinase mutation is associated with many myeloproliferative disorders, such as polycythemia vera, essential thrombocythemia, and myelofibrosis.
   - C is wrong because (9;22) translocation is associated with chronic myeloid leukemia, which is a neoplastic proliferation of mature myeloid cells.

Section III - Septic Arthritis, Gout, and CPPD Disease

I. Septic Arthritis
   A. Bacterial, fungal, or mycobacterial infection of a joint
   B. Pathogenesis: spread through the bloodstream, direct inoculation, or from neighboring skin infections

II. Septic Arthritis: Etiology
   A. Due to an infectious agent (most commonly *Staph aureus, Streptococcus, Neisseria gonorrhoeae)*
      1. *S. aureus*: older children and adults
      2. *N. gonorrhoeae*: young adults

III. Septic Arthritis: Clinical Presentation
   A. Red, swollen, warm, and painful joint with limited range of motion
   B. Gonococcal arthritis: purulent arthritis (knee), tenosynovitis (wrist and ankles), dermatitis (pustules on wrists or ankles)
   C. Systemic symptoms (e.g. fever)

IV. Septic Arthritis: Diagnosis
   A. Increase in erythrocyte sedimentation rate and C-reactive protein
   B. Increase in white blood cell count, typically > 50,000 cells/μL
   C. Arthrocentesis shows purulent synovial fluid

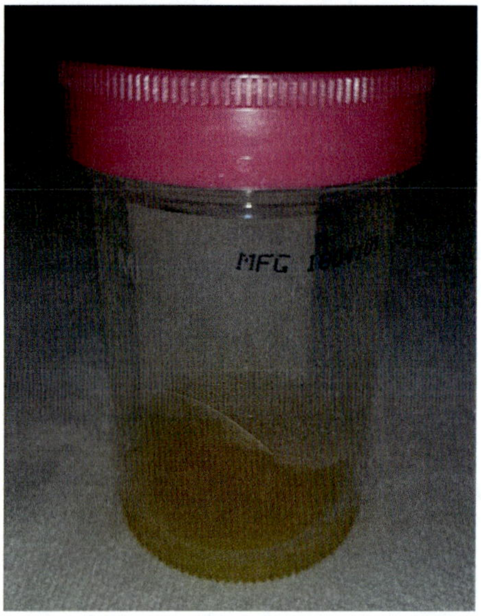

FIGURE 10.9.18 - Purulent Synovial Fluid in Septic Arthritis

V. Gouty Arthritis: Etiology
   A. Accumulation of monosodium urate (MSU) crystals in the joints
   B. Most common is primary gout: hyperuricemia due to unidentifiable cause
   C. Secondary gout is due to a known cause: either underexcretion or overproduction of uric acid → hyperuricemia

VI. Gouty Arthritis: Secondary Causes
   A. Underexcretion (90% of cases): renal failure, lead poisoning, alcoholism, red meat diets, and diuretics (thiazides)
   B. Overproduction (10% of cases): Lesch-Nyhan syndrome, tumor lysis syndrome, leukemia, and myeloproliferative disorders
   C. Risk factors: hypertension, male sex, obesity, dyslipidemia, and alcohol use

VII. Gouty Arthritis: Lab Findings
   A. Hyperuricemia
   B. Joint aspiration will show crystals that are needle-shaped and negatively birefringent under polarized light
   C. Yellow crystals when parallel to the polarizer

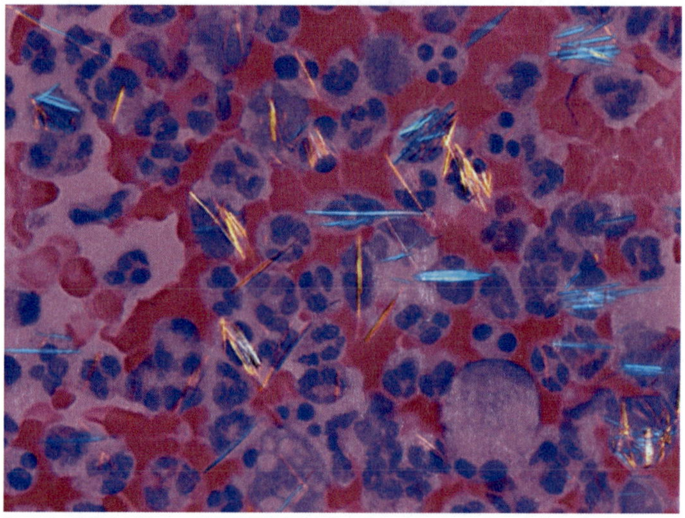

FIGURE 10.9.19 - Blue and Yellow Crystals of Gout Under Polarized Light Microscopy

VIII. Gouty Arthritis: Acute Attacks
   A. Presentation: first toe (podagra), painful to touch, and joint appears swollen and red
   B. Risk factors: alcohol, large meal with red meat, seafood, illness, exercise, stress, trauma, and surgery

IX. Gouty Arthritis: Chronic
   A. Presentation: uric acid crystals accumulate forming tophi (white, chalky aggregates of uric acid in the joints), arthritis, and renal failure
   B. Risk factors: uncontrolled gout without proper treatment or lifestyle modification

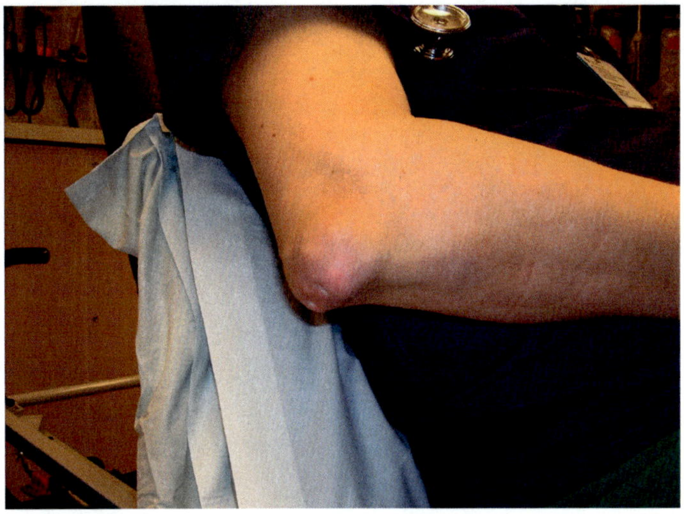

Photo Credit: NickGorton / CC BY-SA (http://creativecommons.org/licenses/by-sa/3.0/)

FIGURE 10.9.20 - Tophi in Chronic Gout

X. CPPD Disease
  A. Due to calcium pyrophosphate deposition, typically in large joints
  B. Presentation is similar to gout
  C. Affects both sexes equally (age is usually > 50)
  D. Usually idiopathic
  E. ↑ incidence with hemochromatosis, hemosiderosis, primary hyperparathyroidism, and joint trauma

XI. CPPD Disease: Lab Findings
  A. Rhomboid-shaped crystals
  B. Positively birefringent under polarized light (blue when parallel)

REVIEW QUESTIONS

1. A 62-year-old male presents to the emergency room with a complaint of knee pain that has been getting worse since the morning. He has a past medical history of hypertension and hyperparathyroidism. On examination, the knee is painful to touch, warm and erythematous. The patient denies recent changes in his diet or medications. Arthrocentesis of the joint is performed. What is most likely to be seen under polarized microscopy of the aspiration?

   A. Needle-shaped, negatively birefringent monosodium urate crystals
   B. Needle-shaped, positively birefringent monosodium urate crystals
   C. Rhomboid-shaped, negatively birefringent CPPD crystals
   D. Rhomboid-shaped, positively birefringent CPPD crystals

- **The correct answer is D.**
- From the patient's presentation of a painful knee, we should be considering gout, pseudogout, or a possible infectious etiology.
- His age (62) as well as the history of hyperparathyroidism should clue us into pseudogout being more likely, especially since the knee is typically affected.
- In acute gouty arthritis, the great toe is more likely affected.
- Recall that the crystals of patients with CPPD disease are rhomboid-shaped and are positively birefringent under polarized light and so they will appear blue when parallel.
- A and B are wrong because pseudogout involves the deposition of CPPD crystals and not monosodium urate crystals.
- Monosodium urate crystals are seen in patients with gouty arthritis.
- C is wrong because patients with CPPD disease have positively birefringent crystals, not negatively birefringent crystals.

Section IV - Osteoarthritis and Rheumatoid Arthritis

I. Osteoarthritis: Etiology
   A. Due to degeneration of articular cartilage
   B. Most common type of joint disease resulting from "wear and tear" on weight-bearing joints
   C. Non-inflammatory degenerative bone disease
   D. Pathogenesis: cytokines activate metalloproteinases that cause breakdown of proteoglycans and collagen

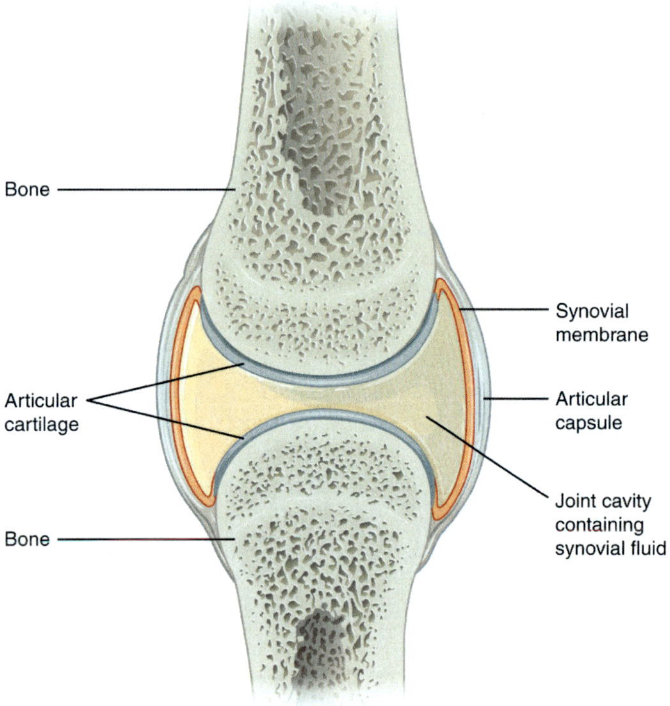

Photo Credit: OpenStax College / CC BY (https://creativecommons.org/licenses/by/3.0)

FIGURE 10.9.21 - Anatomy of a Joint

II. Osteoarthritis: Clinical Presentation
   A. Joint stiffness that worsens later in the day
   B. Pain typically gets worse with movement and better with rest
   C. Crepitus with movement
   D. Limited range of motion
   E. Usually in patients > 60 years old, obese, history of trauma, or repetitive stress
   F. Asymmetric involvement of a few joints without systemic symptoms
      1. Hips: pain in the groin area
      2. Lower lumbar spine: disc disease and neuropathies
      3. Hands: osteophytes in finger joints
      4. DIP joint - Heberden's nodes
      5. PIP joint - Bouchard nodes
      6. Knees: bow-legged from medial degeneration

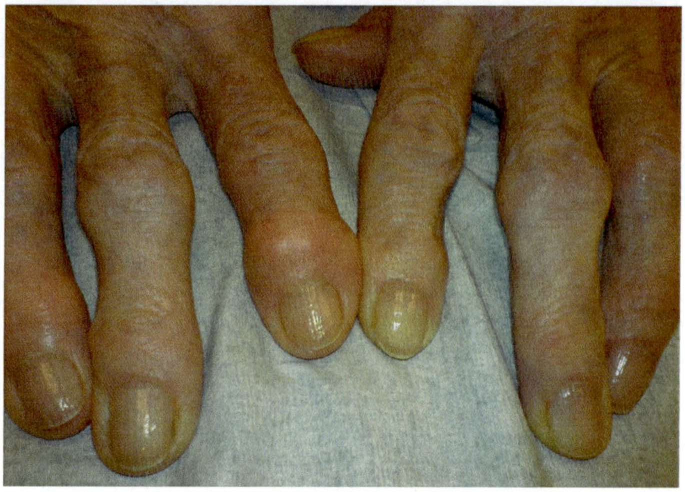

Photo Credit: Drahreg01 / CC BY-SA (http://creativecommons.org/licenses/by-sa/3.0/)

FIGURE 10.9.22 - Osteophytes in Osteoarthritis

III. Osteoarthritis: Joint Findings
   A. Joint space narrowing
   B. Bone rubs on bone, causing it to become dense and sclerotic
   C. Fissuring and flaking of articular cartilage
   D. Fragments of cartilage floating in the joint space
   E. Osteophytes at the margins
   F. Subchondral sclerosis and cyst formation

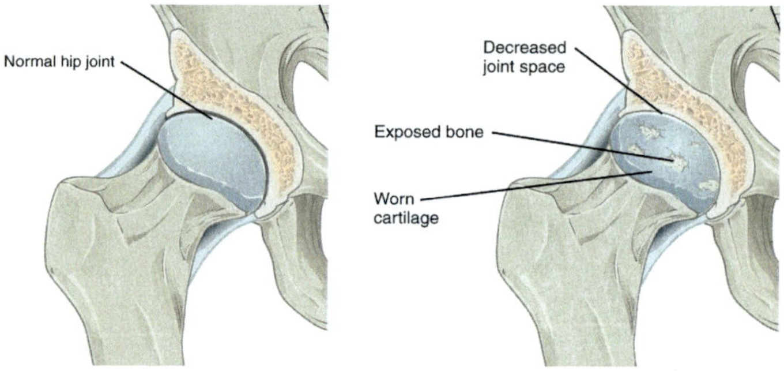

Photo Credit: https://commons.wikimedia.org/wiki/File:0910_Oateoarthritis_Hip_A.png

FIGURE 10.9.23 - Effects of Osteoarthritis on the Hip Joint

IV. Rheumatoid Arthritis
   A. Chronic autoimmune joint disease with the possibility of systemic involvement (extra-articular)
   B. Can involve more than one organ/system including lungs, heart, eyes, skin, kidneys, GI and nervous systems

V. Rheumatoid Arthritis: Pathogenesis
   A. Synovial inflammation → formation of a pannus (granulation tissue)
   B. Activation of T lymphocytes in response to rheumatoid antigens → cytokine release causing synovial hyperplasia
   C. Accelerated metabolic rate of synovium leads to local hypoxia → synovial angiogenesis (neovascularization)
   D. Proteinases cause destruction of cartilage matrix → ankylosis

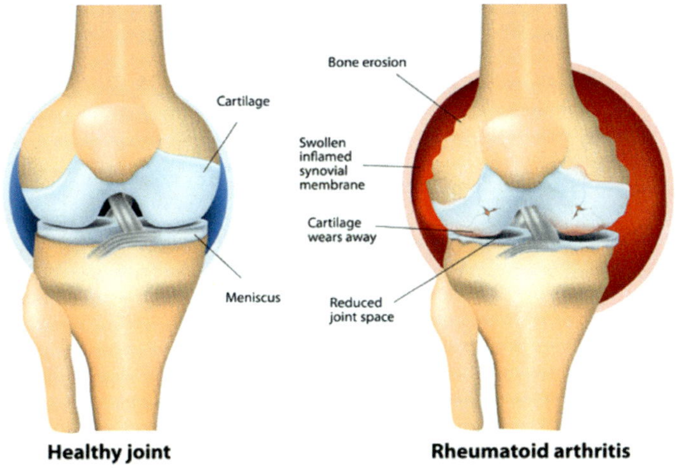

Photo Credit: https://commons.wikimedia.org/wiki/File:Severe_(T%C3%B6nnis_grade_3)_osteoarthritis_of_the_hip.jpg

FIGURE 10.9.24 - Effects of Rheumatoid Arthritis

VI. Rheumatoid Arthritis: Clinical Presentation
   A. Pain, swelling, and morning stiffness > 1 hr that improves with activity
   B. Joints are soft/spongy and warm
   C. Fever, malaise, weight loss, and body aches
   D. Most commonly affects middle-aged and older females (60-85 years)
   E. Associated with HLA-DR4
   F. Symmetric involvement of second/third metacarpophalangeal and PIP joints, DIP usually spared
   G. Radial deviation of wrist and ulnar deviation of fingers
   H. Swan neck deformity: flexed DIP joints and extended PIP joints
   I. Boutonniere deformity: extend DIP joints and flexed PIP joints
   J. Cervical spine: subluxation of atlantoaxial joint

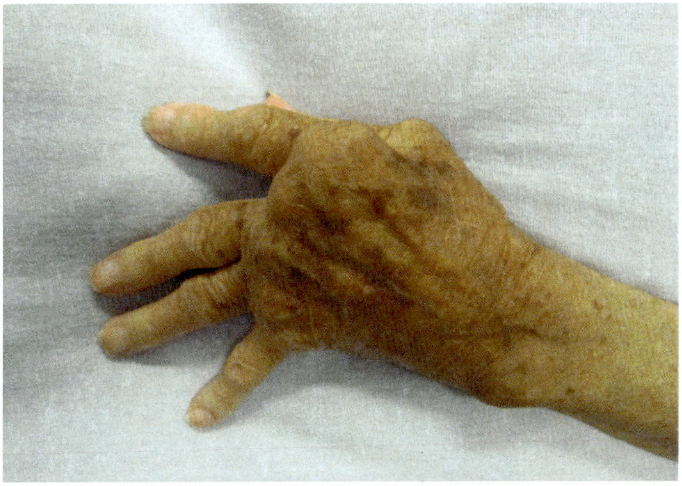

Photo Credit: James Heilman, MD / CC BY-SA (https://creativecommons.org/licenses/by-sa/3.0)

FIGURE 10.9.25 - Ulnar Deviation of the Fingers and Radial Deviation of the Wrist in Rheumatoid Arthritis

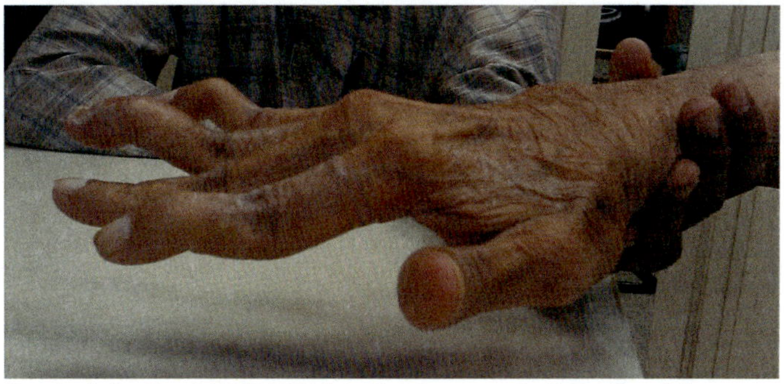

Photo Credit: User:Phoenix119 / CC BY-SA (https://creativecommons.org/licenses/by-sa/3.0)

FIGURE 10.9.26 - Swan Neck Deformity in Rheumatoid Arthritis

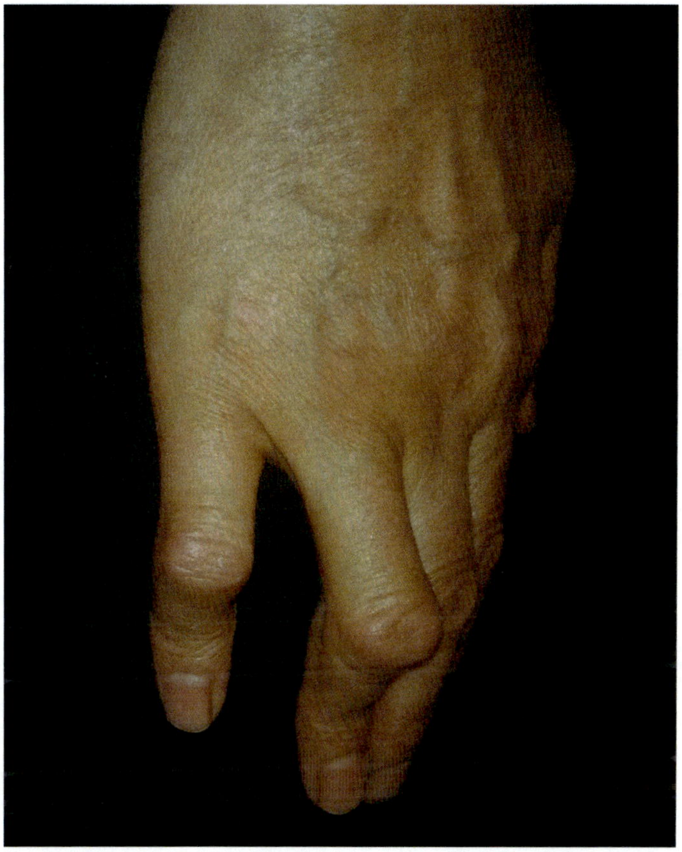

Photo Credit: Alborz Fallah / CC BY-SA (https://creativecommons.org/licenses/by-sa/3.0)

FIGURE 10.9.27 - Boutonniere Deformity in Rheumatoid Arthritis

   K. Lung disease: pleuritis with effusions and interstitial lung fibrosis
   L. Rheumatoid nodules: central zone of fibrinoid necrosis with palisading epithelioid histiocytes
   M. Cardiovascular disease: fibrinous pericarditis and small vessel vasculitis
   N. Popliteal (Baker) cyst: outpouching of bursa behind the knee
   O. Hematologic disease: anemia of chronic disease

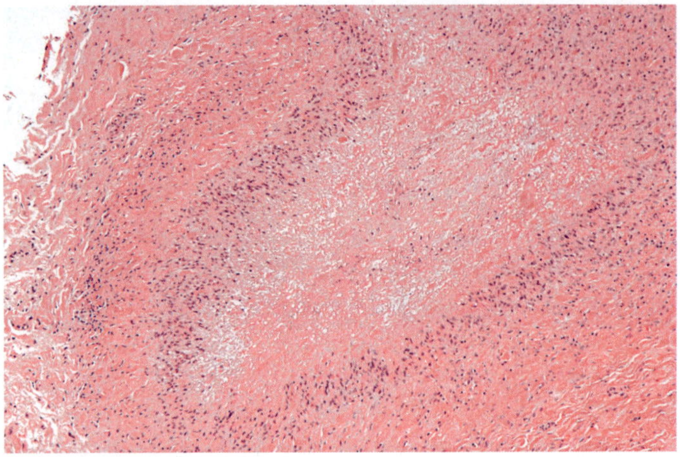

FIGURE 10.9.28 - Central Zone of Fibrinoid Necrosis with Palisading Epithelioid Histiocytes in Rheumatoid Nodules

VII. Rheumatoid Arthritis: Lab Findings
   A. Positive rheumatoid factor
      1. IgM antibody that targets the Fc portion of IgG
   B. Anti-cyclic citrullinated peptide antibody (more specific)
   C. Positive serum ANA in about 30% of cases
   D. Increased neutrophils and high protein in synovial fluid

REVIEW QUESTIONS

1. A 54-year-old female presents to the clinic with increasing pain in her back and hips. She states that the pain is worse after her afternoon walk. She describes the pain as achy and dull. Physical examination reveals limited range of motion at the hip and crepitus with movement. An X-ray of the patient's hip is obtained. What abnormal joint findings would most likely be observed with this imaging modality?

- **X-ray would likely show joint space narrowing, osteophytes, and bone fragments in the joint space.**
- If we want to imagine the X-ray of a patient with osteoarthritis, we need to think about what changes to the bone structure will become apparent.
- One of the first things that would stand out would be the joint space narrowing. We can also anticipate seeing osteophytes at the margins of the joint due to the frequent rubbing of bone on bone and the bone remodeling that would occur. Finally, we might see the fragments of bone that eventually float in the joint space.
- These are helpful to keep in mind as radiography along with the physical clues mentioned and the history can aid in making a diagnosis.

REVIEW QUESTIONS

2. A 50-year-old male presents to the clinic with shortness of breath and a cough that has gotten worse over the past week. He states that the cough is particularly bad when he is at work. On physical exam, fine crackles are heard in the upper lungs. The patient's fingers are flexed at the DIP joints and extended at the PIP joints with ulnar deviation of the wrist. What additional finding is most likely associated with this patient's joint condition?

   A. Positive HLA-B27
   B. Heberden nodes
   C. Negatively birefringent crystals under microscopy
   D. Anti-cyclic citrullinated peptide antibody

- **The correct answer is D.**
- We can piece together from the physical exam, as well as the lung complaints, that the patient has a joint condition that can also affect organs outside the joint (extra-articular manifestations), or extra-articular manifestations. The description of flexed DIP joints and extended PIP joints should remind us of the swan neck deformity seen in rheumatoid arthritis; the ulnar deviation of the wrist adds another clue.
- Now, going back to the question, we have what we need to find the right association. Knowing that anti-cyclic citrullinated peptide antibody is a specific marker for rheumatoid arthritis will help us pick D as the right answer. Interestingly, when a patient has the combination of rheumatoid arthritis and a pneumoconiosis, it is called Caplan syndrome.
- A is incorrect because HLA-B27 is associated with seronegative spondyloarthropathies and not RA. HLA-DR4 is more likely in RA patients.
- B is incorrect because it describes distal nodes that appear in osteoarthritis, not rheumatoid arthritis.
- C is incorrect because we would expect to see these crystals in gouty arthritis.

Section V - Spondyloarthropathies

I. Basic Principles
  A. Family of overlapping syndromes causing arthritis without rheumatoid factor
  B. Axial skeleton involvement, HLA-B27 positive, usually males, sacroiliitis with or without peripheral arthritis
  C. Types: ankylosing spondylitis, reactive arthritis, and psoriatic arthritis

II. Ankylosing Spondylitis
  A. Affects sacroiliac joint and spine in young men
  B. Presents with low back pain and morning stiffness
  C. Can involve the entire spine → fusion of the vertebrae ("bamboo spine") → kyphosis → restrictive lung disease
  D. Extra-articular manifestations: aortitis with aortic regurgitation and anterior uveitis

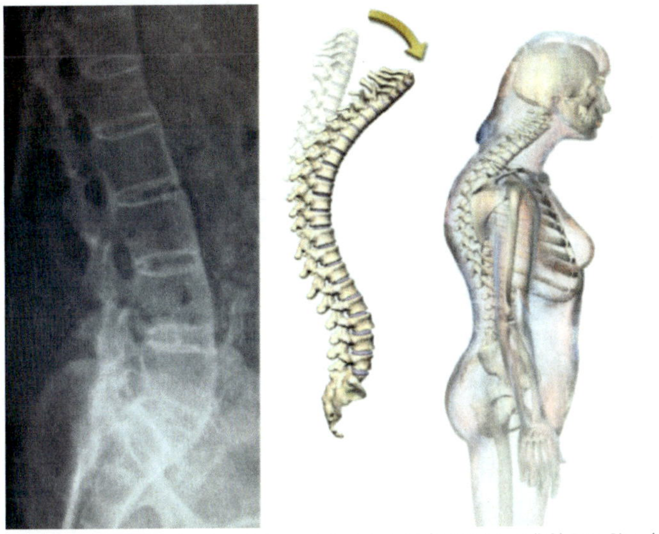

Photo Credit: http://en.wikipedia.org/wiki/User:Glitzy_queen00 / Public domain (left), BruceBlaus / CC BY-SA (https://creativecommons.org/licenses/by-sa/4.0) (right)

FIGURE 10.9.29 - Lateral Lumbar Spine X-ray of a Patient with Ankylosing Spondylutus

III. Reactive Arthritis
  A. Triad of conjunctivitis, urethritis, and arthritis
    1. "can't see, can't pee, can't climb a tree"
  B. Usually occurs one week following a *Chlamydia trachomatis* infection
  C. Arthritis: can cause bone formation near Achilles tendon attachment
  D. Other implicated bacteria: *Shigella, Yersinia, Campylobacter,* and *Salmonella*

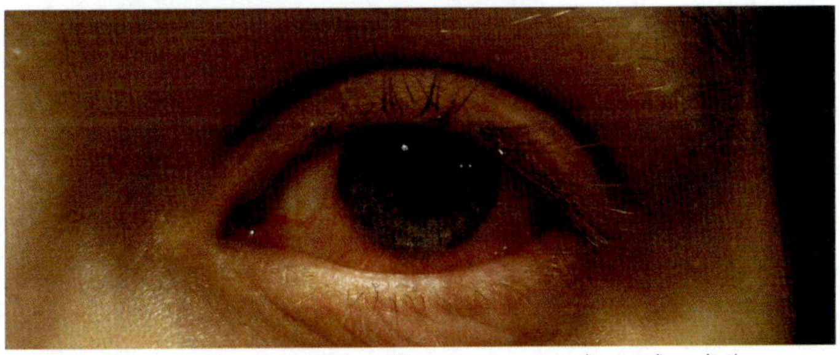

Photo Credit: Daemonanyndel / CC BY-SA (https://creativecommons.org/licenses/by-sa/3.0)

FIGURE 10.9.30 - Conjunctivitis

IV. Psoriatic Arthritis
  A. Seen in 10% of psoriasis cases
  B. "Sausage-shaped" distal interphalangeal joints
  C. Asymmetric involvement of the skin with extensive nail pitting
  D. Radiographs will show "pencil in cup" deformity due to eroding bone

REVIEW QUESTIONS

1. A 39-year-old male presents to the clinic with low back pain and morning stiffness. He states that the stiffness improves after he works out at the gym. He mentions that he has also recently noticed abnormal heart beats. On exam, an early diastolic decrescendo murmur is heard along the left side of the chest near the third intercostal space. What initial test would be most helpful in establishing a specific diagnosis?

    A. HLA-B27
    B. Echocardiogram
    C. X-ray of the sacroiliac region
    D. Rheumatoid factor

- **The correct answer is C.**
- Using the patient's physical complaints of low back pain and morning stiffness that improves with exercise, we can consider ankylosing spondylitis on our differential. His abnormal heart beats and the murmur point us to possible cardiac abnormalities like aortic regurgitation, which we know is associated with ankylosing spondylitis.
- Ankylosing spondylitis primarily affects the sacroiliac joint. Our initial test should assess for a change that only occurs in this subtype of spondyloarthropathies. An X-ray of the sacroiliac joint would assess the underlying cause of the patient's low back pain, visualize the characteristic joint changes of this disease, and help us best make the diagnosis before further evaluation.
- A is incorrect as an initial test because HLA-B27 would be positive in all the subtypes of this family of diseases, like psoriasis and reactive arthritis, and not just in ankylosing spondylitis, so it may not be as helpful in establishing an exact diagnosis.
- B is incorrect as an initial test because it doesn't look for the root cause of the extra-articular manifestation of aortic regurgitation. We want to eventually do an echocardiogram on this patient to assess for the valvular disease that may be present.
- D is incorrect because seronegative arthritis is a family of joint diseases that are negative for rheumatoid factor.

Section VI - Skeletal Muscle Disorders

I. Dermatomyositis
   A. Inflammatory disease of the muscles and skin
   B. Unknown etiology
   C. Sometimes associated with adenocarcinoma
      1. Ovarian cancer
      2. Gastric cancer

II. Dermatomyositis: Clinical Features
   A. Bilateral proximal muscle weakness
   B. Heliotrope rash
   C. Malar (butterfly) rash
   D. Gottron papules

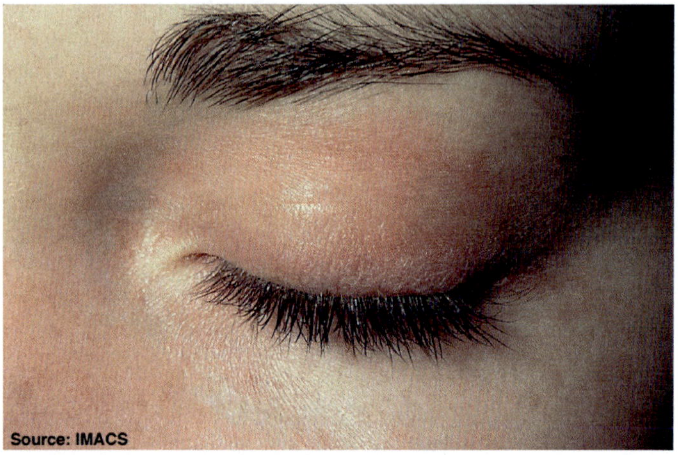

Photo Credit: Elizabeth M. Dugan, Adam M. Huber, Frederick W. Miller, Lisa G. Rider [CC BY-SA (https://creativecommons.org/licenses/by-sa/3.0)]

FIGURE 10.9.31 - Heliotrope Rash in Dermatomyositis

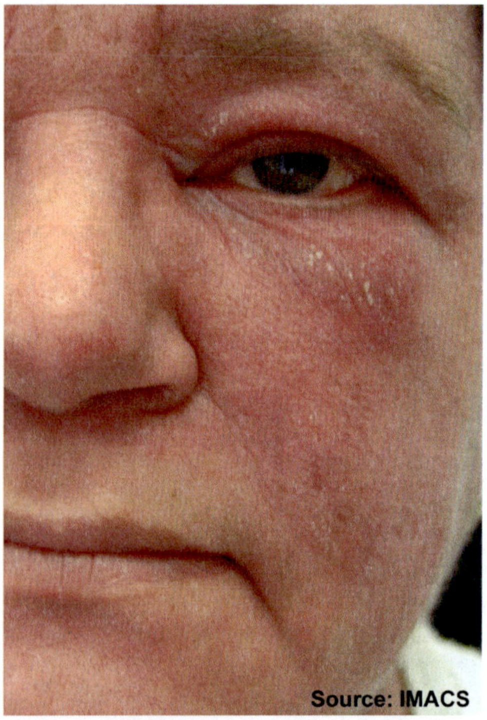

Photo Credit: Elizabeth M Dugan, Adam M Huber, Frederick W Miller, Lisa G Rider [CC BY-SA (https://creativecommons.org/licenses/by-sa/3.0)]

FIGURE 10.9.32 - Malar Rash in Dermatomyositis

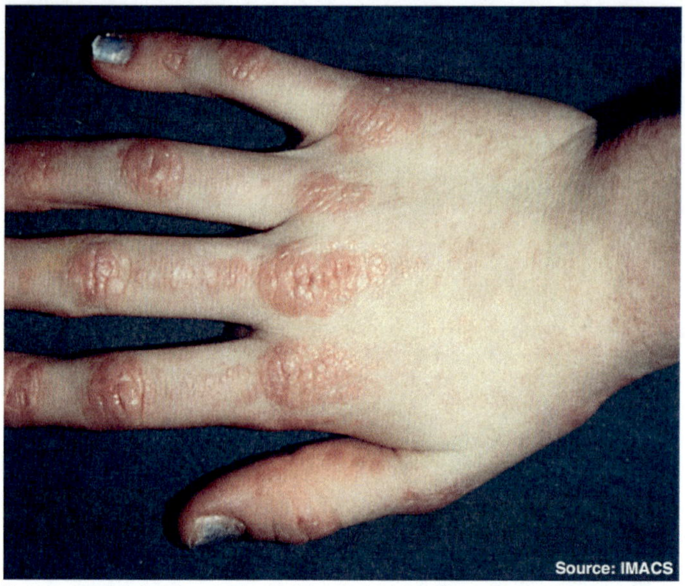

Photo Credit: Elizabeth M. Dugan, Adam M. Huber, Frederick W. Miller, Lisa G. Rider [CC BY-SA (https://creativecommons.org/licenses/by-sa/3.0)]

FIGURE 10.9.33 - Gottron's Papules in Dermatomyositis

III. Dermatomyositis: Laboratory Findings
   A. Nonspecific markers: ANA and increased creatine kinase
   B. Specific markers: antisynthetase (anti-Jo-1), anti-SRP (signal recognition particle), and anti-helicase (anti-Mi-2) antibodies
   C. Perimysial inflammation ($CD4^+$ T cells) seen on biopsy

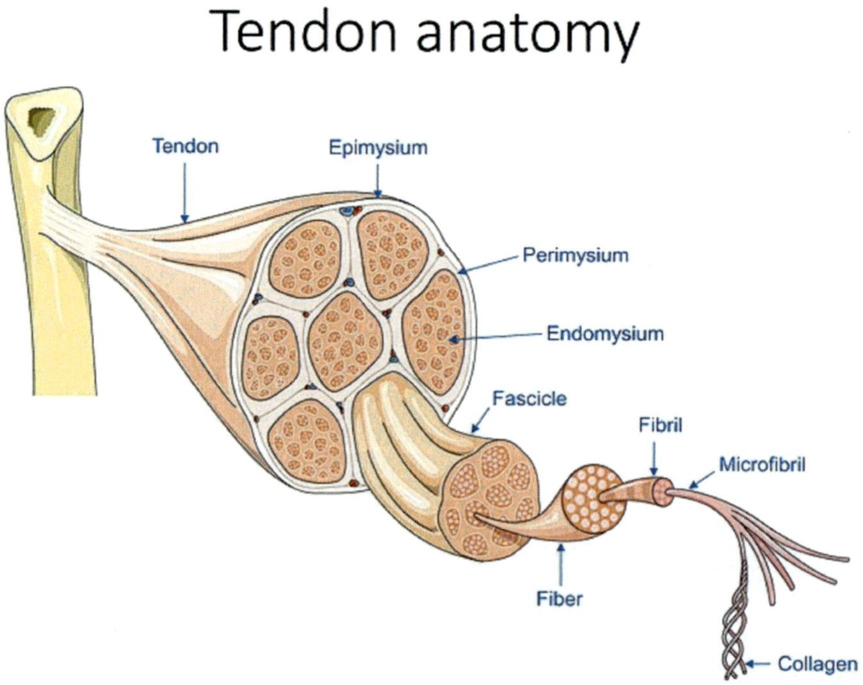

Photo Credit: Laboratoires Servier / CC BY-SA (https://creativecommons.org/licenses/by-sa/3.0)

FIGURE 10.9.34 - Skeletal Muscle Cross Section

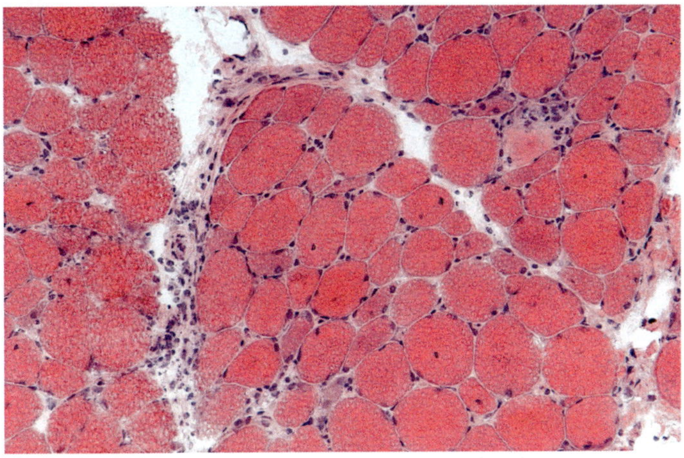

Photo Credit: Nephron [CC BY-SA (https://creativecommons.org/licenses/by-sa/3.0)]

FIGURE 10.9.35 - Perimysial Inflammation in Dermatomyositis

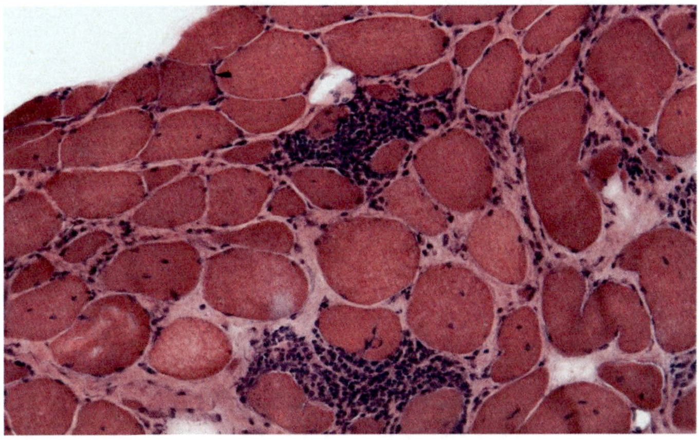

Photo Credit: Jensflorian [CC BY-SA (https://creativecommons.org/licenses/by-sa/3.0)]

FIGURE 10.9.36 - Endomysial Inflammation in Polymyositis

IV. Dermatomyositis: Treatment
   A. Corticosteroids

V. Polymyositis
   A. Inflammatory muscle disease
   B. Skin is not involved

VI. Polymyositis: Clinical Features
   A. Bilateral proximal muscle weakness

VII. Polymyositis: Laboratory Findings
   A. Nonspecific markers: ANA and increased creatine kinase
   B. Specific markers: antisynthetase (anti-Jo-1), anti-SRP (signal recognition particle), and anti-helicase (anti-Mi-2) antibodies
   C. Endomysial inflammation ($CD8^+$ T cells) seen on biopsy

VIII. Polymyositis: Treatment
   A. Corticosteroids

IX. X-linked muscular dystrophy
   A. Inherited X-linked disorder characterized by muscle degeneration
   B. More common in boys

X. X-linked muscular dystrophy: Types
   A. Duchenne muscular dystrophy
   B. Becker muscular dystrophy

XI. X-linked muscular dystrophy: Etiology
   A. Defects in dystrophin gene
      1. Connects cytoskeleton of muscle fiber to extracellular matrix
   B. Duchenne muscular dystrophy: deletion of dystrophin
   C. Becker muscular dystrophy: mutation of dystrophin

XII. Duchenne Muscular Dystrophy: Clinical Features
   A. Proximal muscle weakness → progresses to distal muscle weakness
   B. Calf pseudohypertrophy
   C. Gower's sign
   D. Cardiac or respiratory failure

XIII. Becker Muscular Dystrophy: Clinical Features
   A. Proximal muscle weakness
   B. Clinically milder disease with later onset
   C. Cardiac or respiratory failure

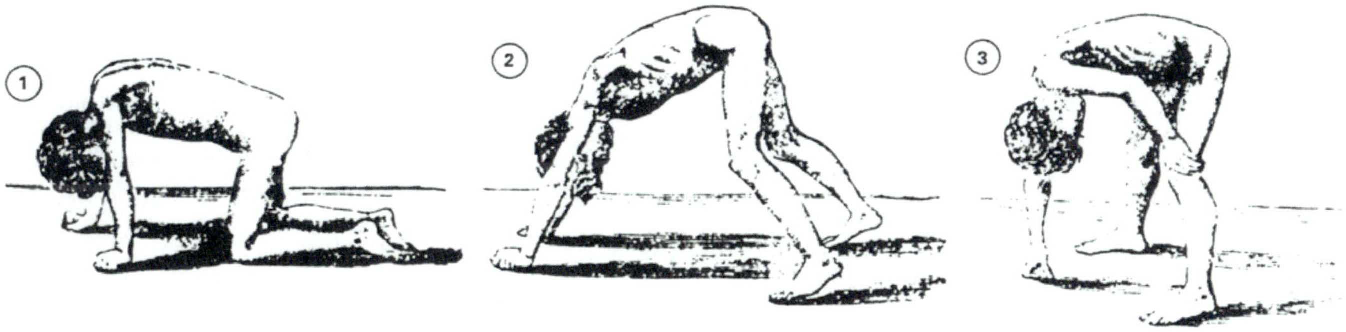

Photo Credit: William Richard Gowers (1845–1915) / Public domain

FIGURE 10.9.37 - Gower's Sign in Duchenne Muscular Dystrophy

REVIEW QUESTIONS

1. A 49-year-old woman presents with progressive weakness. She complains that she has difficulty climbing the stairs and combing her hair every morning. Physical exam shows decreased strength, especially in the quadriceps and shoulders. She has facial erythema and macular erythema confined to her upper eyelids. What would the muscle biopsy show?

    - **The muscle biopsy would show perimysial inflammation that is composed of CD4+ T cells.**
    - Here is a 49-year-old woman presenting with progressive weakness and decreased strength in the quadriceps and shoulders.
    - Also, she has facial erythema as well as macular erythema confined to her upper eyelids, which is a heliotrope rash.
    - The mentioned findings strongly suggest dermatomyositis.

2. A 4-year-old boy is brought to the clinic due to difficulty getting up from a chair and muscle fatigue. His parents have noticed he uses his hands to walk up his own body from a squatting position. His heart rate is 92 beats/minute, blood pressure is 92/50 mmHg, and the temperature is 37 °C (98.6 °F). On physical examination, his calves appear enlarged. Which of the following is the most likely cause of his symptoms?

    A. Endomysial inflammation composed of $CD8^+$ T cells
    B. Perimysial inflammation composed of $CD4^+$ T cells
    C. Defect in genes responsible for anchoring the muscle cytoskeleton to the extracellular matrix
    D. Mutation of genes responsible for a glycoprotein that forms a sheath around elastin

    - **The correct answer is C.**
    - This is a 4-year-old boy with difficulty getting up from a chair and muscle fatigue.
    - He also uses his hands to walk up his own body from a squatting position, which is the Gower sign. On examination, his calves are enlarged, resembling calf pseudohypertrophy.
    - These findings indicate Duchenne muscular dystrophy.
    - X-linked muscular dystrophy, including Duchenne and Becker muscular dystrophy, is due to defects of the dystrophin gene.
    - Dystrophin connects the cytoskeleton of a muscle fiber to the surrounding extracellular matrix, which is critical for maintaining muscle integrity.
    - As a consequence of deletion of dystrophin gene, someone with Duchenne muscular dystrophy experiences muscle weakness, especially in the proximal muscles.
    - A is wrong because endomysial inflammation composed of CD8+ T cells is found in someone with polymyositis on muscle biopsy.
    - B is wrong because perimysial inflammation composed of CD4+ T cells is found in someone with dermatomyositis on muscle biopsy.
    - D is wrong because mutation of genes responsible for a glycoprotein that forms a sheath around elastin (*FBN1* gene) causes Marfan syndrome, which is a connective tissue disorder affecting the skeleton, heart, and eyes.

Section VII - Diseases of the Neuromuscular Junction

I. Myasthenia Gravis
   A. Autoimmune disease
   B. More common in women
   C. Associated with thymic hyperplasia or thymoma
   D. Autoantibodies against postsynaptic nicotinic acetylcholine receptors at the neuromuscular junction
      1. Decreased muscle signaling
      2. Muscle cell destruction

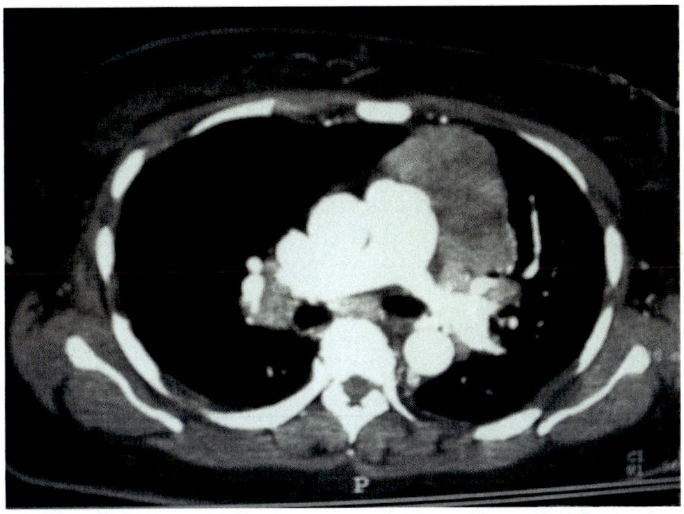

FIGURE 10.9.38 - Chest CT Showing a Thymoma

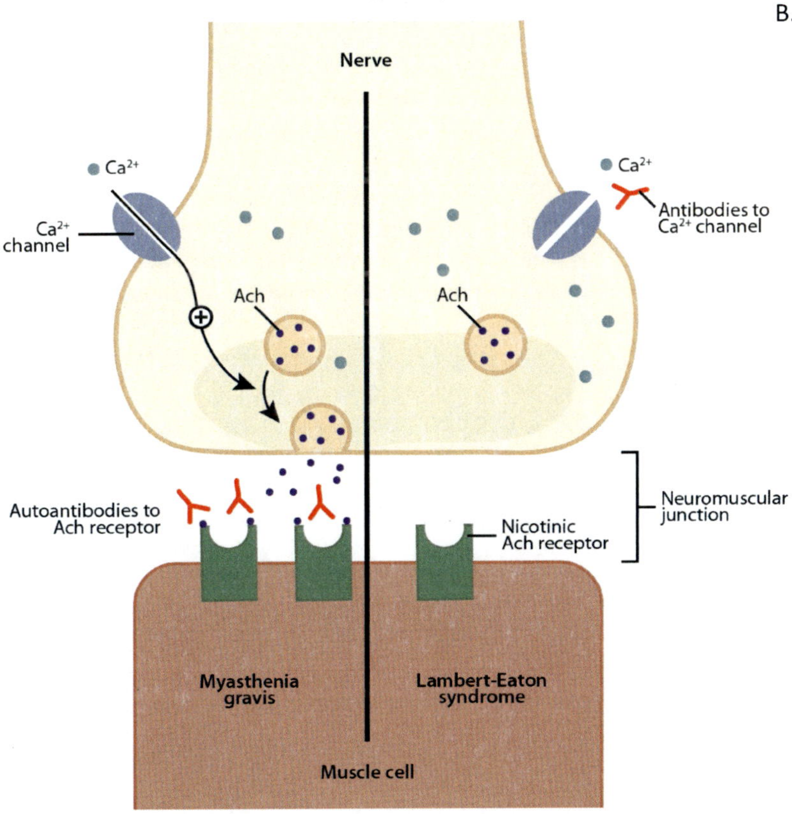

FIGURE 10.9.39 - Pathophysiology of Myasthenia Gravis and Lambert-Eaton Syndrome

II. Myasthenia Gravis: Clinical Features
   A. Muscle weakness that worsens with activity and improves with rest
      1. Classically involves extraocular muscles → diplopia/ptosis
   B. Myasthenic crisis: life-threatening
      1. Respiratory muscle weakness → severe dyspnea

III. Lambert-Eaton Syndrome
   A. Antibodies against presynaptic calcium channels of the neuromuscular junction → impaired acetylcholine release
   B. Paraneoplastic syndrome (small cell carcinoma of the lung)

IV. Lambert-Eaton syndrome: Clinical features
   A. Proximal muscle weakness that improves with activity
   B. Extraocular muscles are spared

V. Myasthenia Gravis: Treatment
   A. Anticholinesterase agents (e.g. neostigmine, pyridostigmine)
   B. Thymectomy

VI. Lambert-Eaton Syndrome: Treatment
   A. Anticholinesterase agents have no effects in improving symptoms
   B. Resection of cancer

REVIEW QUESTIONS

1. A 42-year-old female presents to the emergency department due to progressive fatigue and weakness in the arms for the past 3 months. These symptoms are better in the morning and worsen throughout the day. Physical exam shows diplopia and ptosis. What type of autoantibodies are most likely present in this patient?

    - **The correct answer is autoantibodies against postsynaptic nicotinic acetylcholine receptors at the neuromuscular junction.**
    - Progressive fatigue and weakness in the arms that worsen throughout the day along with diplopia and ptosis are indicative of myasthenia gravis.

2. A 56-year-old man presents to the clinic with difficulty getting up from a chair and raising his arms. He denies any blurry vision. He has been smoking 2 packs of cigarettes daily for the past 33 years. His heart rate is 92 beats/minute, blood pressure is 135/72 mmHg, and the temperature is 37 °C (98.6 °F). A chest X-ray shows a centrally located mass in the hilar region of the right lung. Which of the following is the most likely cause of his symptoms?

    A. Autoantibodies against postsynaptic acetylcholine receptors at the neuromuscular junction
    B. Antibodies against phospholipase A2 receptors
    C. Antibodies against presynaptic calcium channels at the neuromuscular junction
    D. Antibodies against TSH receptors

    - **The correct answer is C.**
    - This is a 56-year-old man presenting with weakness in the proximal muscles of the legs and arms.
    - While he denies any blurry vision, he has a 33-year smoking history, and a centrally located mass in the hilar region of the right lung is found.
    - This patient has Lambert-Eaton syndrome that arose as a paraneoplastic syndrome due to small cell lung cancer.
    - Lambert-Eaton syndrome is characterized by antibodies against presynaptic calcium channels at the neuromuscular junction that impair the acetylcholine release.
    - A is wrong because myasthenia gravis is due to autoantibodies against postsynaptic acetylcholine receptors at the neuromuscular junction.
    - Although it has similar symptoms, myasthenia gravis does not arise due to paraneoplastic syndrome and classically involves the extraocular muscles, resulting in ptosis and diplopia.
    - B is wrong because antibodies against phospholipase A2 receptors are characterized by membranous nephropathy.
    - D is wrong because antibodies against TSH receptors are characterized by Graves' disease.

Section VIII - Soft Tissue Tumors

I. Lipoma
   A. Benign adipose tissue tumor
   B. Most common benign soft tissue tumor in adults

II. Lipoma: Findings
   A. Gross: benign tumor of adipose tissue with fibrous capsules
   B. Microscopy: mature adipocytes arranged in lobules and fibrous septa
   C. Painless, soft mobile mass that slowly enlarges over time
   D. Commonly seen in the upper back, neck, abdomen, and proximal extremities

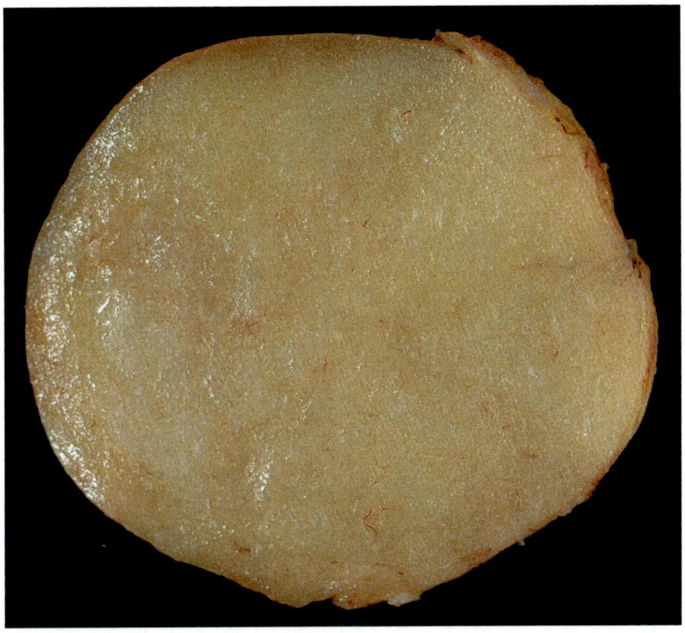

Photo Credit: https://commons.wikimedia.org/wiki/File:Lipoma_gross.jpg

FIGURE 10.9.40 - Cross-Section of a Lipoma

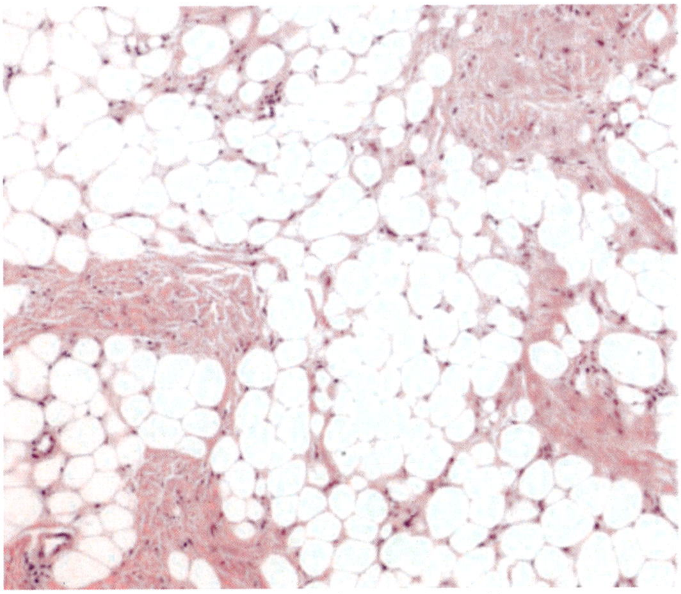

Photo Credit: https://commons.wikimedia.org/wiki/File:Histopathology_of_lipoma.jpg

FIGURE 10.9.41 - Histopathology of a Lipoma

III. Lipoma: Treatment
   A. Surgical excision

IV. Liposarcoma
   A. Malignant tumor of adipose tissue
   B. Lipoblast is the characteristic cell
      1. Immature fat cells with fat vacuoles
      2. Abundant mitoses
   C. Atypical spindle cells

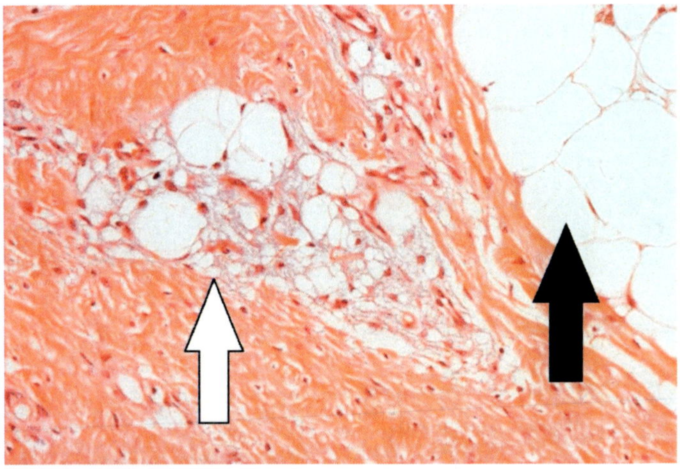

Photo Credit: https://commons.wikimedia.org/wiki/File:Lipoblasts_and_lipocytes.jpg

FIGURE 10.9.42 - Lipoblasts (White Arrow) and Lipocytes (Black Arrow) in a Lipoblastoma

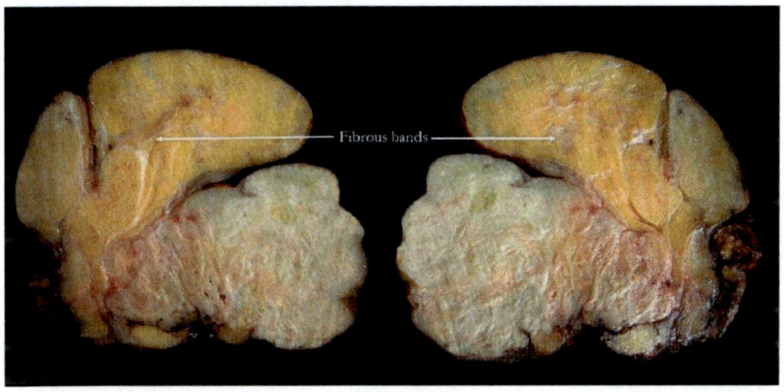

Photo Credit: https://commons.wikimedia.org/wiki/File:Dedifferentiated_liposarcoma.jpg

FIGURE 10.9.43 - Cross-Section of a Liposarcoma

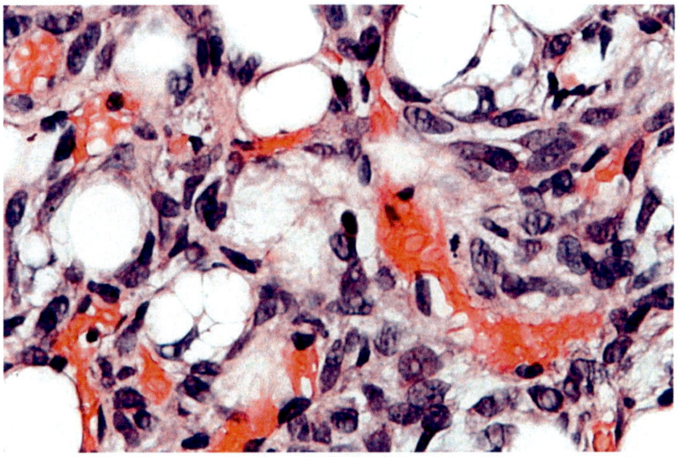

Photo Credit: https://commons.wikimedia.org/wiki/File:Dedifferentiated_liposarcoma_-_cropped_-_very_high_mag.jpg

FIGURE 10.9.44 - Lipoblasts in a Liposarcoma

V. Liposarcoma: Findings
  A. Commonly seen in middle-age or older adults (> 40)
  B. Painful and rapidly growing
  C. Found on thigh or retroperitoneum
    1. Deep in the tissue

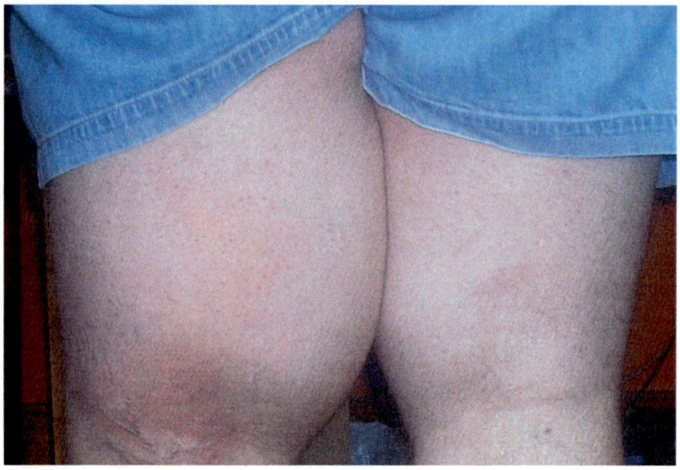

Photo Credit: https://commons.wikimedia.org/wiki/File:Edemaliposarcoma.jpg

FIGURE 10.9.45 - Liposarcoma

VI. Liposarcoma: Treatment
  A. Surgical excision
  B. Radiation
  C. Chemotherapy

VII. Rhabdomyoma
  A. Benign tumor of skeletal muscle
  B. Well-circumscribed
  C. Spider cells
  D. No mitotic activity observed
  E. Commonly seen on the tongue, head, neck region, and heart

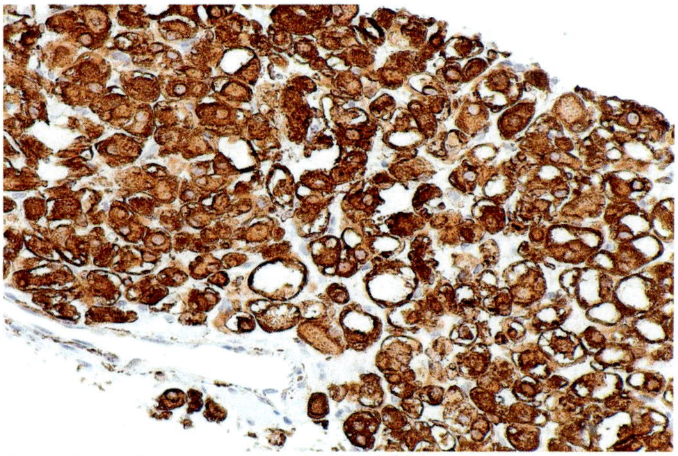

Photo Credit: https://commons.wikimedia.org/wiki/File:Rhabdomyoma_-_desmin_--_high_mag.jpg#/media/File:Rhabdomyoma_-_desmin_--_high_mag.jpg

FIGURE 10.9.46 - Rhabdomyoma with Desmin Stain

VIII. Rhabdomyoma: Cardiac Type
  A. Primary tumor of the heart in infants and children
  B. Associated with tuberous sclerosis
  C. Ventricles primarily affected
  D. May obstruct valves and inflow or outflow tracts
  E. Murmur

IX. Rhabdomyoma: Treatment
  A. Surgical excision
  B. Open heart surgery for cardiac rhabdomyomas

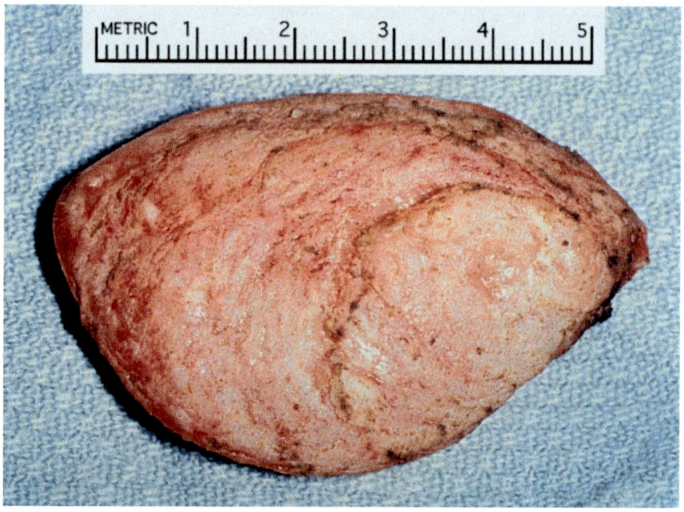

Photo Credit: https://commons.wikimedia.org/wiki/File:Cardiac_rhabdomyoma.jpg

FIGURE 10.9.47 - Biopsy of Rhabdomyosarcoma

X. Rhabdomyosarcoma
  A. Malignant skeletal muscle tumor
  B. Rhabdomyoblast is the characteristic cell
    1. Tadpole cells with eosinophilic granular cytoplasm
  C. Desmin and myogenin positive

XI. Rhabdomyosarcoma: Findings
  A. Presents as a mass in children and adolescents (< 20 years of age)
  B. Affects the head and neck
  C. Sarcoma botryoides is seen in young girl presenting with a gelatinous, grape-like mass protruding from vagina

XII. Rhabdomyosarcoma: Treatment
  A. Surgery
  B. Chemotherapy
  C. +/- radiation

Tumor	Location	Age group	Morphology
Lipoma	- Upper back - Trunk - Extremities	- Adults	- Subcutaneous mass - Yellow tumor - Well-differentiated mature fat cells
Liposarcoma	- Thighs - Retroperitoneum	- 50-60	- Deep tissue mass - Lipoblasts (immature fat cells)
Rhabdomyoma	- Heart - Head - Neck	- Infants - Children	- Ventricular myocardial mass - Associated with tuberous sclerosis - Spider cells
Rhabdomyosarcoma	- Nasopharyngeal sinuses - Vagina	- Children - Adolescents	- Grape-like, gelatinous, necrotic mass - Rhabdomyoblasts (immature cells also known as tadpole cells due to oval shape)

TABLE 10.9.2 - Types of Soft Tissue Tumors

REVIEW QUESTIONS

1. A 29-year-old medical student presents with a mass on his upper back. He first noticed the mass approximately 2 years ago. Since that time the mass has only grown slightly. A CT scan is performed and reveals a mass that is beginning to compress adjacent structures. The surgeon recommends that the mass be excised to alleviate potential complications. A biopsy of the mass is obtained. What will most likely be observed microscopically?

   - **The correct answer is mature adipocytes.**
   - This patient is experiencing a mass on his upper back that has not changed much in size in a couple of years. This mass seems to be very slowly enlarging and is not affecting normal life.
   - Knowing the age group and location of the mass can help you narrow down the diagnosis, which is a benign lipoma.

2. An 8-year-old girl is brought to her primary care physician by her mother. The mother informs the physician that there is a mass visible from her daughter's vagina. On physical exam, there is a gelatinous mass protruding from the vagina. A biopsy of the specimen reveals oval elongated immature muscle cells in different stages of maturation. What is the most likely diagnosis?

   - **The correct answer is sarcoma botryoides.**
   - This patient is a female child who is coming in with a protruding mass from the vagina.
   - Again, knowing the age group and location of the mass along with biopsy results can help you narrow down the diagnosis.

3. A 2-year-old girl with mental impairment and a history of seizures is brought to the clinic. Physical exam shows an irregular area of white skin in a leaf-like pattern on the back as well as a systolic murmur. An echocardiogram shows a mass blocking the left ventricular outflow tract. A CT scan shows calcifications in the subependymal region. What is the most likely diagnosis?

   A. Cardiac myxoma
   B. Embryonal rhabdomyosarcoma
   C. Carcinoid tumor
   D. Cardiac rhabdomyoma

   - **The correct answer is D.**
   - This is a female infant who has a history of mental impairment with seizures. The rash seen on the back during physical exam is the classic ash leaf pattern of a shagreen patch seen in tuberous sclerosis. Echocardiography revealing a mass in the ventricle also helps narrow down the diagnosis. The age group and the location of the mass, along with the history of mental impairment and seizures, are suggestive of tuberous sclerosis.
   - Recall that rhabdomyoma occurs in infants and children who have tuberous sclerosis and the tumor mostly affects the ventricles of the heart.
   - A is wrong because cardiac myxoma is not associated with tuberous sclerosis and it does not affect the ventricles. Cardiac myxoma affects adults and is found in the left atrium.
   - B is wrong because embryonal rhabdomyosarcoma mostly affects mucosa lining the hollow structures, such as the nasopharyngeal sinuses and vagina. Sarcoma botryoides, the major variant of embryonal rhabdomyosarcoma, presents as a gelatinous mass protruding from the vagina of young girls. It is not associated with Tuberous sclerosis, nor does it affect the ventricles of the heart.
   - C is wrong because carcinoid tumor mostly affects the right heart and is associated with diarrhea, flushing and pulmonary manifestations. This is a female infant who has a mass blocking the left ventricle. Hence, we can rule out carcinoid tumor.

Section IX - Dermatitis and Acne

I. Atopic Dermatitis
   A. Also known as eczema
   B. Affects children < 5 years old
   C. Associated with asthma and allergic rhinitis association
   D. ↑ risk among those with a family history of atopy

II. Atopic Dermatitis: Pathophysiology
   A. Mutation of epidermal barrier protein → impaired skin barrier → type I hypersensitivity reaction

III. Atopic Dermatitis: Findings
   A. Pruritic rash with erythema, vesicles, edema, and oozing fluid
      1. Scratching of rash may cause it to leak clear fluid or bleed
   B. Affects the face and flexor surfaces (diaper area spared)
   C. High IgE and eosinophilia

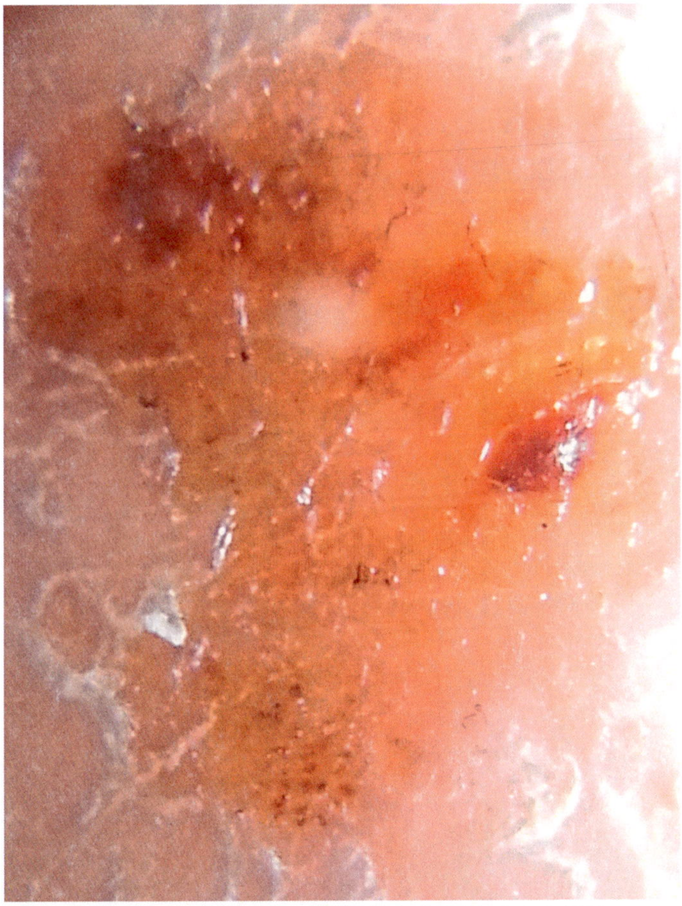

Photo Credit: https://commons.wikimedia.org/wiki/File:Atopic_dermatitis_close_up_ad.jpeg

FIGURE 10.9.48 - Atopic Dermatitis Rash

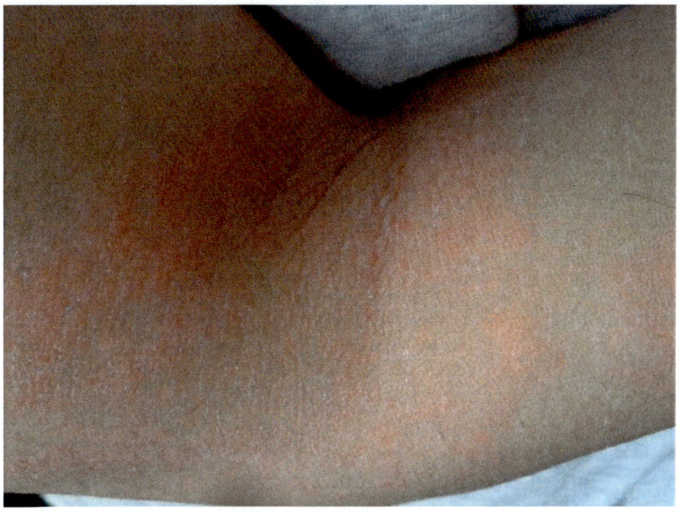

Photo Credit: https://commons.wikimedia.org/wiki/File:Dermatitis_atopica_04.JPG

FIGURE 10.9.49 - Atopic Dermatitis Rash

IV. Atopic Dermatitis: Treatment
   A. Moisturizer
   B. Topical steroids

V. Contact Dermatitis
   A. A form of eczema caused by type IV hypersensitivity reaction
   B. Drugs (penicillin), chemicals (soaps), poison ivy (urushiol), nickel, and jewelry act as allergens

VI. Contact Dermatitis: Findings
   A. Pruritic rash with erythema, vesicles, edema, and oozing fluid
   B. Intraepidermal vesicles and spongiosis

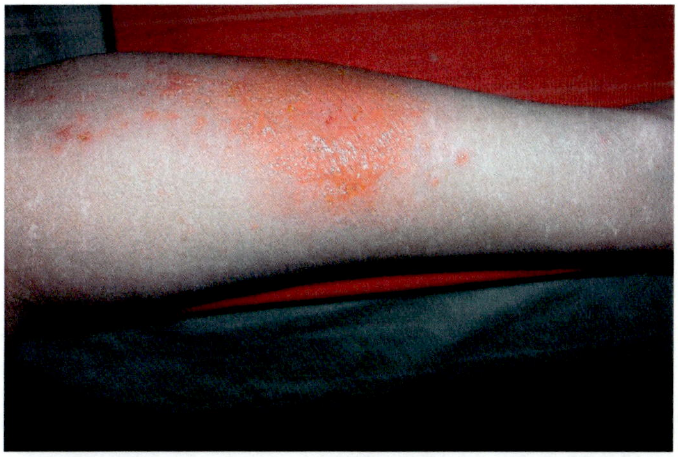

Photo Credit: https://commons.wikimedia.org/wiki/File:Urushiol-induced_contact_dermatitis_7_days_after_contact.jpg

FIGURE 10.9.50 - Contact Dermatitis

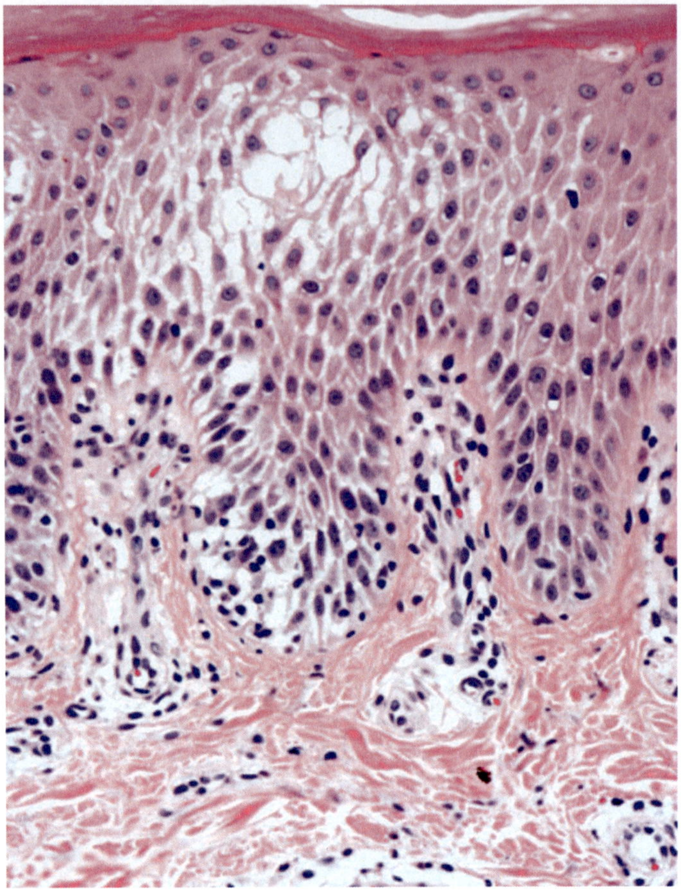

Photo Credit: https://commons.wikimedia.org/wiki/File:Spongiotic_dermatitis_(2)_Dyshidrotic.JPG

FIGURE 10.9.51 - Histological Image of Spongiosis

VII. Contact Dermatitis: Treatment
   A. Removal of allergen
   B. Topical steroids

VIII. Acne Vulgaris
   A. Inflammatory skin disorder of adolescents
   B. Presents as comedones (whiteheads and blackheads), pustules (pimples), and nodules (nodulocystic acne)
   C. Seen mostly on the face, chest, and back

IX. Acne Vulgaris: Etiology
   A. Increase in androgenic hormones (e.g. puberty, PCOS)
   B. Obstruction of sebaceous glands (e.g. oil-based beauty products)
   C. Mechanical irritation (e.g. tight-fitting clothing, protective gear)
   D. Heat
   E. Obesity
   F. Poor hygiene (e.g. unclean having blades, post-workout shower)

X. Acne Vulgaris: Pathophysiology
   A. Sebum production and hyperkeratinization → comedones
   B. Cutibacterium acnes (*Propionibacterium*) infection
   C. Follicular and perifollicular inflammation → pustules and nodules

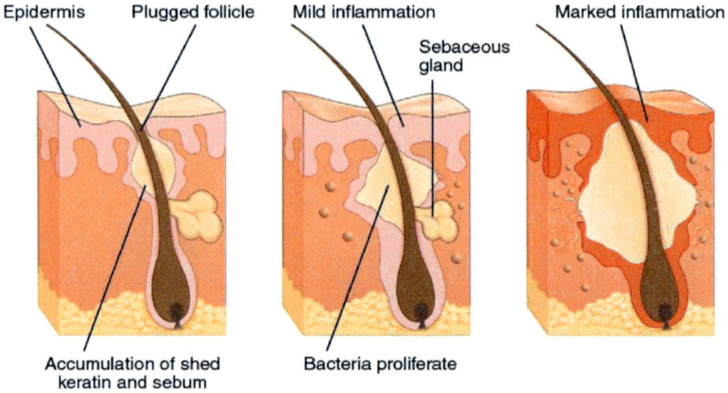

Photo Credit: https://commons.wikimedia.org/wiki/File:515_Acne_formation.jpg

FIGURE 10.9.52 - Pathophysiology of Acne Formation

Type	Manifestations
Comedonal	- Open skin pore (blackhead) - Closed skin pore (whitehead) - Chin, forehead, nose
Inflammatory	- Erythematous papules and pustules (pimples) - Small in size
Nodular	- Painful subcutaneous nodules, scar formation - Large in size

TABLE 10.9.2 - Acne Vulgaris Manifestations

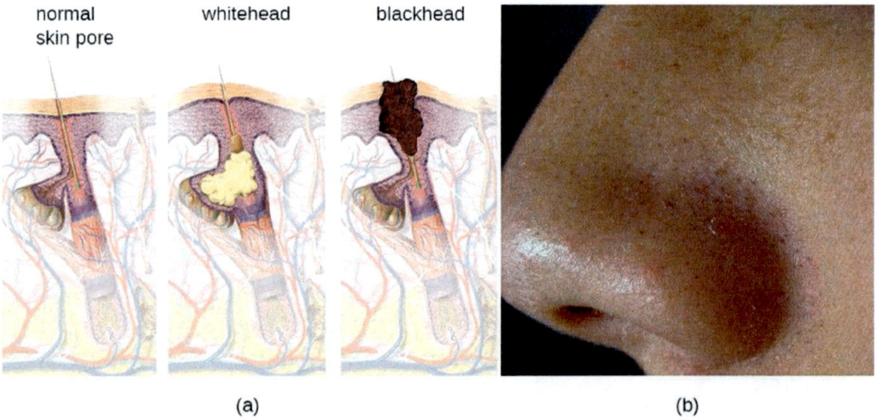

Photo Credit: https://commons.wikimedia.org/wiki/File:OSC_Microbio_21_02_acne.jpg

FIGURE 10.9.53 - Comedonal Acne Vulgaris

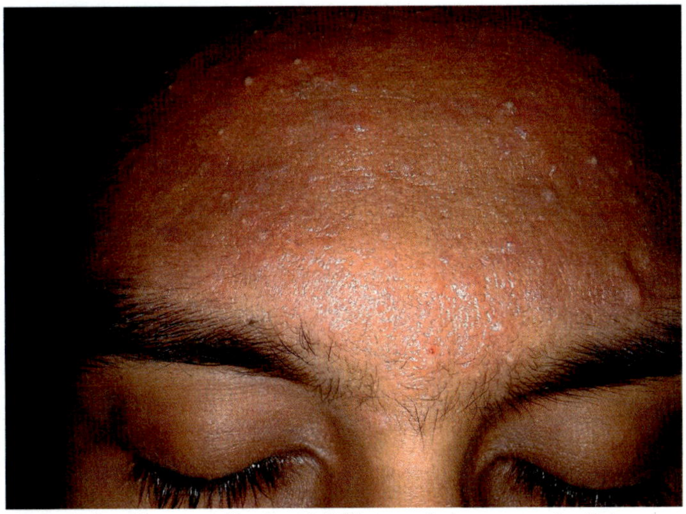

Photo Credit: https://commons.wikimedia.org/wiki/File:Acne_vulgaris_on_a_very_oily_skin.jpg

FIGURE 10.9.54 - Acne Vulgaris

XI. Acne Vulgaris: Treatment
   A. Benzoyl peroxide: antimicrobial
   B. Salicylic acid: removes oil and dead skin cells clogging the pores
   C. Isotretinoin: reduces keratin production

REVIEW QUESTIONS

1. A 4-year-old girl with a history of asthma is brought to the clinic by her mother due to a rash on her forearms that began 4 days ago. The mother denies a history of recent travel. Physical exam shows erythematous, dry, and itchy skin on the elbows bilaterally. The physician recommends applying a moisturizer on a daily basis. Based on the information provided, what is the most likely diagnosis?

    - **The correct answer is atopic dermatitis.**
    - The patient has a history of asthma and she is presenting with an itchy dry rash. Recall that asthma along with family history of atopy puts patients at risk for allergic skin rash that may resolve with the use of moisturer.

2. A 16-year-old boy presents to the clinic with a history of facial acne. He complains of a non-pruritic red papulopustular rash on his upper back. He reports that he recently began summer soccer training camp and received a new training kit that fits him very tightly. He denies eating junk or spicy food and reports that he showers religiously. What is the most likely cause of his acne flare-up?

    A. Performance-enhancing steroids
    B. Mechanical irritation
    C. Poor hygiene
    D. Hypersensitive dermal reaction to a new jersey

    - **The correct answer is B.**
    - The patient has a history of facial acne with a flare-up to his upper back.
    - Considering he started a soccer training camp, there could be possible risk factors that could have exacerbated his acne. Heat, poor hygiene, and tight-fitting clothing worn during sports activities can cause mechanical irritation of hair follicles, resulting in acne.
    - A is incorrect because there is no indication that the boy took performance-enhancing steroids. Even though taking steroids is common in athletes, his adolescent age and history of facial acne strongly suggest an endogenous phenomenon instead of an exogenous one.
    - C is incorrect because even though poor hygiene is a possible etiology for acne, the patient states he showers religiously.
    - D is incorrect because a hypersensitive dermal reaction to a new jersey, although possible, would not cause an acne flare-up.

Section X - Psoriasis and Lichen Planus

I. Psoriasis
   A. Autoimmune inflammatory skin disorder
   B. Associated with HLA-C
   C. Scaly rash with erythematous plaques on extensor surfaces
   D. Arises in areas with past trauma or exposed to pressure/friction (Koebner phenomenon)

II. Psoriasis: Pathophysiology
   A. Damage to skin epithelial barrier → inflammatory response
   B. Keratinocyte proliferation → hyperkeratosis and parakeratosis
   C. Epidermal hyperplasia (acanthosis) and elongation of rete ridges
   D. Neutrophils in stratum corneum → Munro abscesses
   E. Elongation of dermal papilla and epidermal thinning → pinpoint bleeding (Auspitz sign)

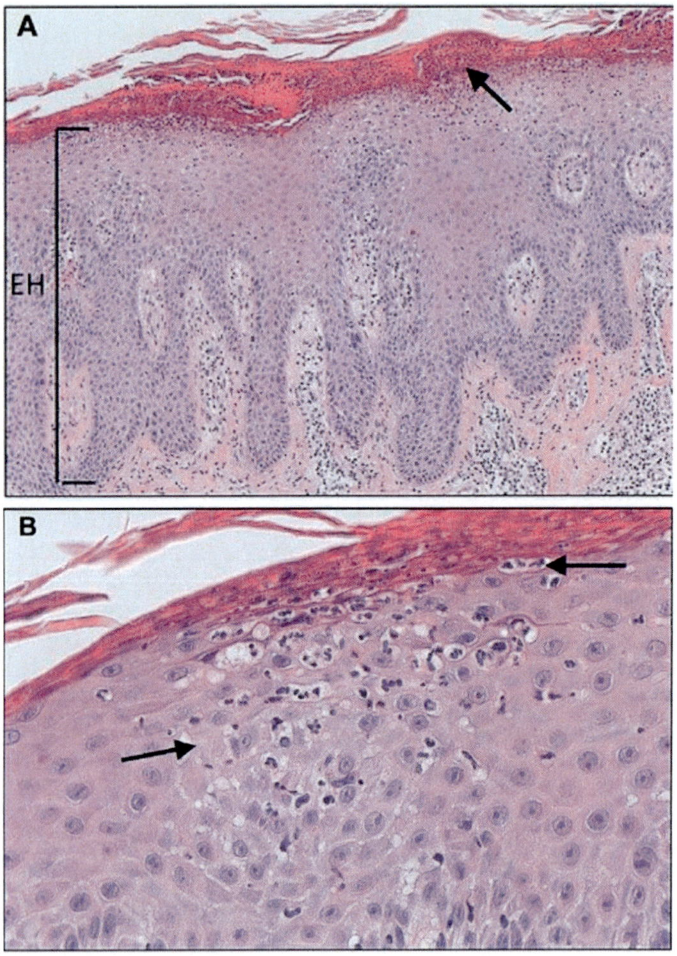

Photo Credit: https://commons.wikimedia.org/wiki/File:Micrograph_of_psoriasis_vulgaris.jpg

FIGURE 10.9.55 - Hyperkeratosis and Acanthosis (A) and Munro Abscesses (B) in Psoriasis

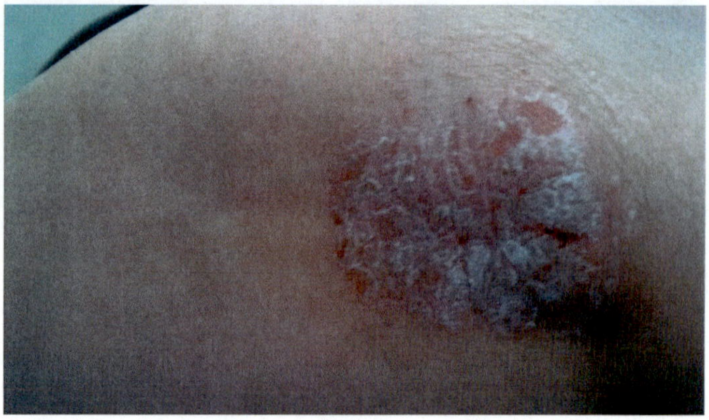

Photo Credit: https://commons.wikimedia.org/wiki/File:Psoriasis_in_elbow.jpg

FIGURE 10.9.56 - Auspitz Sign

III. Psoriasis: Findings
   A. Salmon-colored, well-circumscribed plaques
   B. Silver scales
   C. Extensor surfaces and scalp
   D. Nail changes (e.g. yellow discoloration, pitting)
   E. Associated with psoriatic arthritis, uveitis, conjunctivitis, and blepharitis

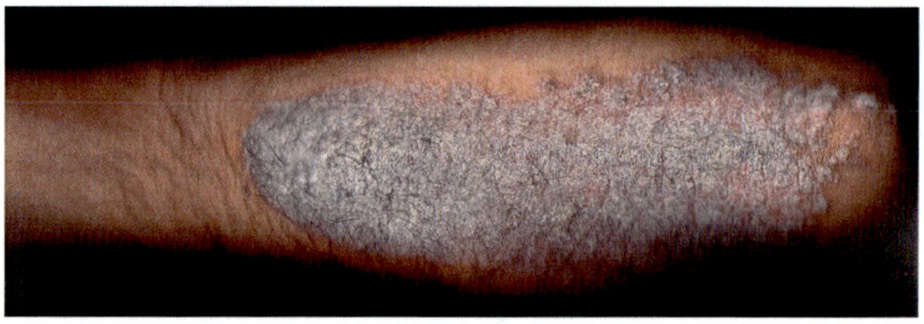

Photo Credit: https://commons.wikimedia.org/wiki/File:An_Arm_Covered_With_Plaque_Type_Psoriasis.jpg

FIGURE 10.9.57 - Silver Scaly Plaque

IV. Psoriasis: Treatment
   A. Corticosteroids
   B. UV light
   C. Immunotherapy

V. Lichen Planus
   A. Purple, polygonal, planar, and pruritic papules (5 Ps) seen in middle-aged adults
   B. Associated with hepatitis C virus

VI. Lichen Planus: Etiology
   A. Unknown etiology
   B. CD8+ T cell mediated response

VII. Lichen Planus: Pathology
   A. Chronic thickening of the stratum corneum (hyperkeratosis)
   B. Inflammation of the dermal-epidermal junction (interface dermatitis)
   C. Colloid (civatte) bodies in the papillary dermis
   D. Sawtooth appearance of rete ridges

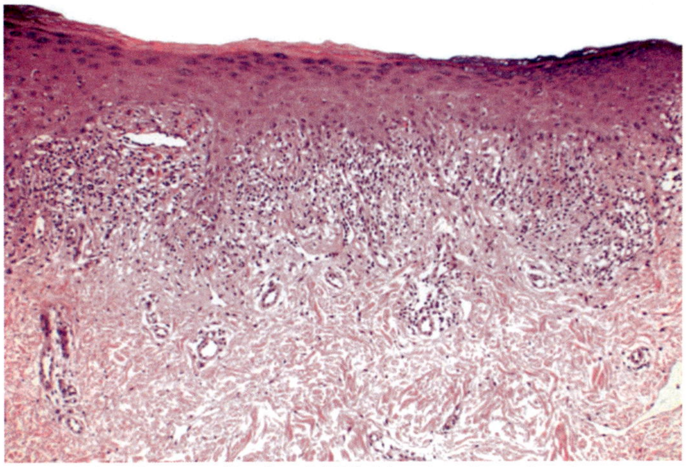

Photo Credit: https://commons.wikimedia.org/wiki/File:Lichen_planus_intermed_mag.jpg

FIGURE 10.9.58 - Lichen Planus

VIII. Lichen Planus: Findings
   A. Papules seen on the wrists, elbows, nails, oral mucosa, shin, ankles, and genitalia
   B. Wickham striae (reticular white lines)

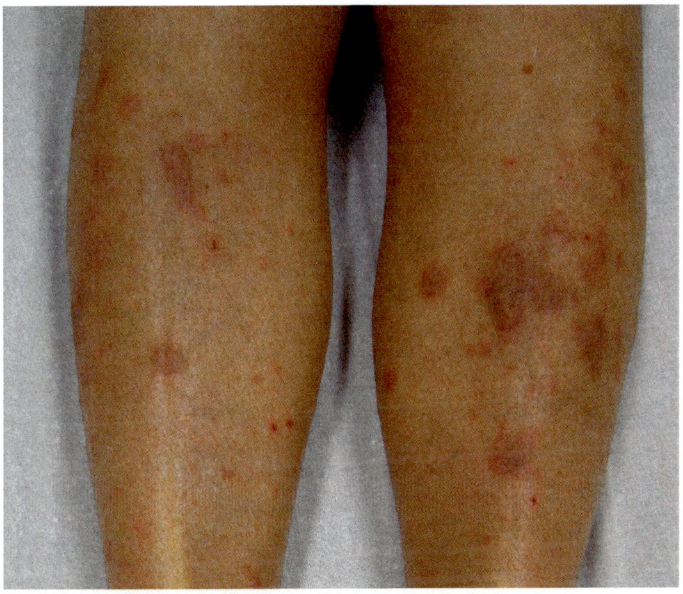

Photo Credit: https://commons.wikimedia.org/wiki/File:Lichen_Planus_(2).JPG

FIGURE 10.9.59 - Purple Planar Papules

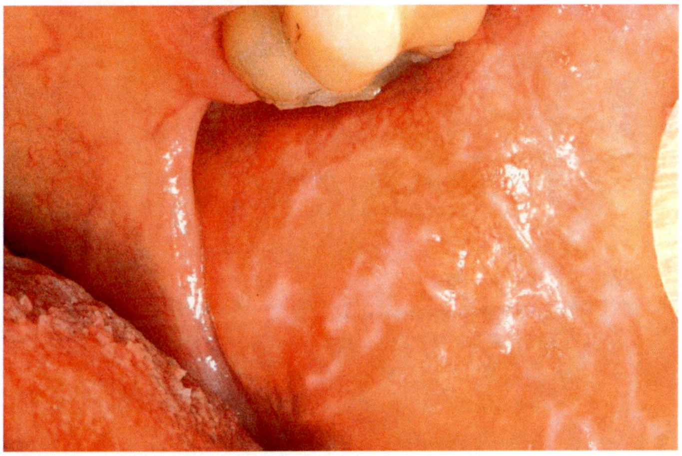

Photo Credit: https://commons.wikimedia.org/wiki/File:Lichen_planus.jpg

FIGURE 10.9.60 - Wickham Striae

IX. Lichen Planus: Treatment
   A. Resolves on its own over months to years
   B. Corticosteroids

REVIEW QUESTIONS

1. A 28-year-old male with a 2-day history of a self-resolving diarrheal episode presents with a rash on the extensor surface of his right elbow. He plays football and often gets wounds on his elbows and knees. He states that he likes to itch the rash, which sometimes causes it to bleed. Physical examination reveals an erythematous rash with rough silver scales and pinpoint bleeding of the scratched areas. Biopsy of the lesion would most likely show which of the following?

   A. IgA deposition in dermal papillae
   B. Neutrophils causing abscesses
   C. Spongiosis
   D. Colloid bodies

- **The correct answer is B.**
- Hopefully from the question stem you noticed that this is a young male who has a history of itchy rash on the extensor surface of his right elbow.
- Physical exam shows erythematous rash with rough silver scales. This patient is suffering from psoriasis.
- Remember that keratinocyte proliferation causing hyperkeratosis and parakeratosis results in formation of silver scales.
- Acanthosis and elongation of rete ridges contribute to formation of erythematous plaques.
- Neutrophils in the stratum corneum form microabscesses known as Munro abscesses.
- Elongation of dermal papilla and epidermal thinning exposes underlying blood vessels.
- This causes pinpoint bleeding when scales are removed, which is known as the Auspitz sign.
- A is wrong because even though the patient has a rash on his elbow coupled with diarrhea, the rash does not look like dermatitis herpetiformis. Hence, biopsy will not show IgA deposition in dermal papillae.
- C is wrong because spongiosis of epidermis is seen in contact dermatitis.
- D is wrong because colloid bodies are apoptotic keratinocytes that are seen in lichen planus.

Section XI - Blistering Skin Disorders

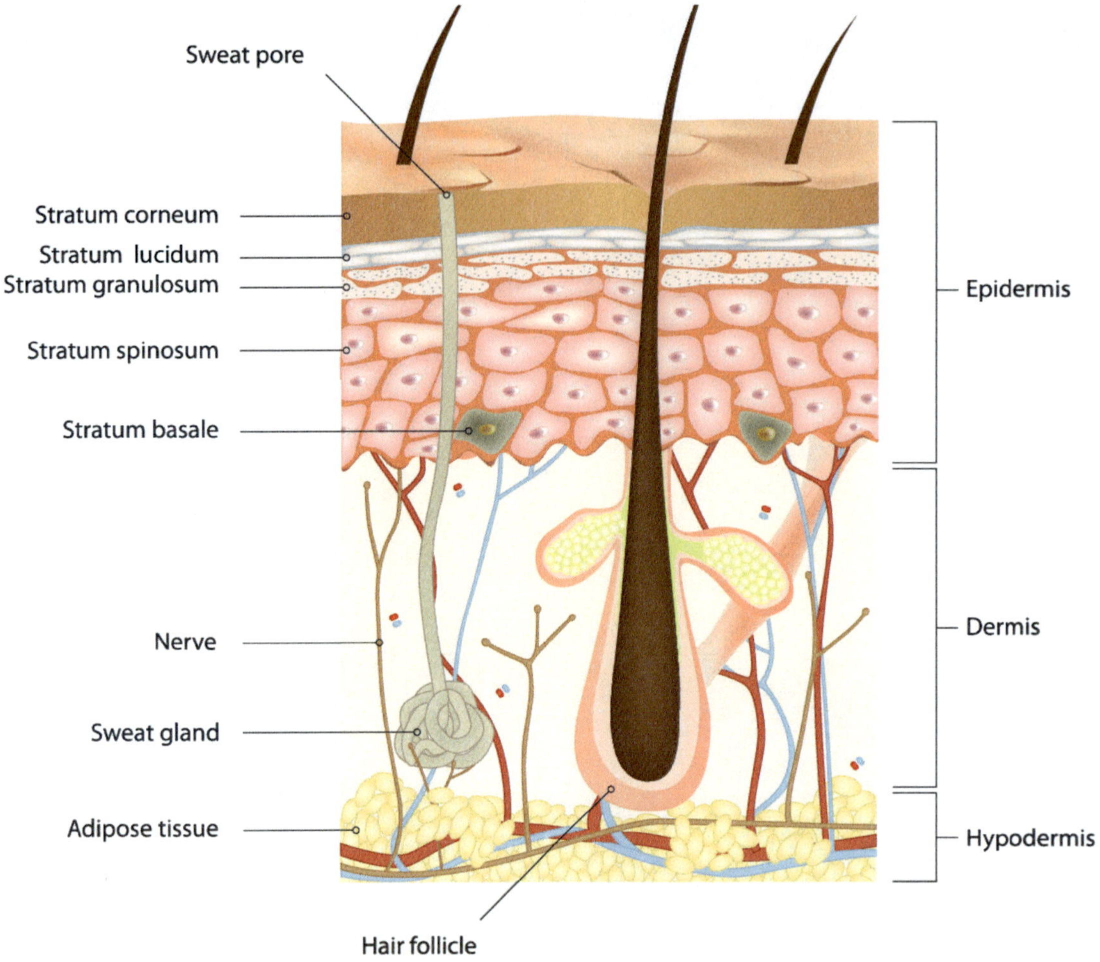

FIGURE 10.9.61 - Layers of the Skin

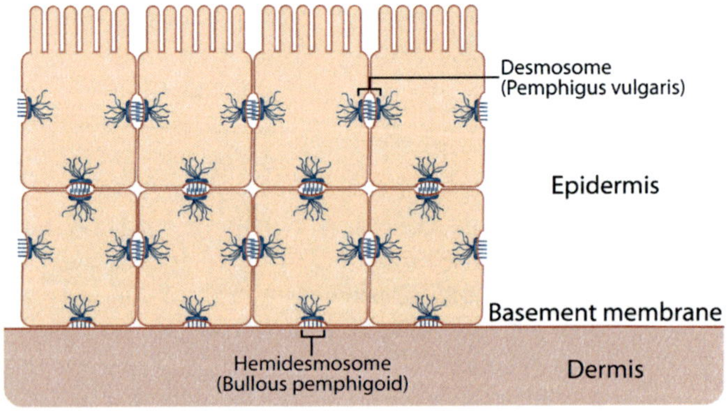

FIGURE 10.9.62- Desmosomes and Hemidesmosomes

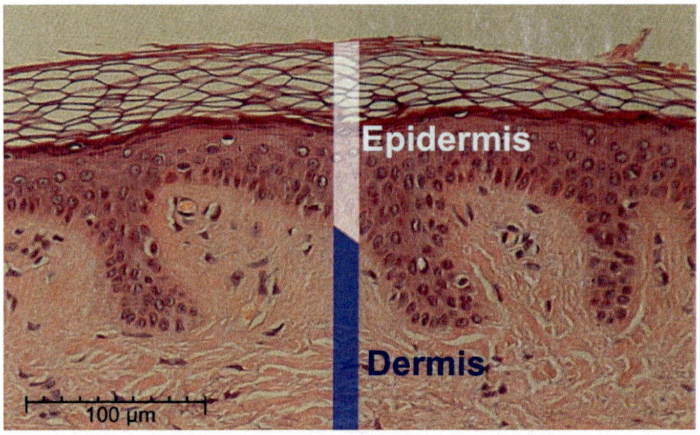

Photo Credit: Normal Epidermis and Dermis with Intradermal Nevus 10x.JPG: KilbadCropped and labeled by Fama Clamosa (talk) and Mikael Häggström, respectively / Public domain

FIGURE 10.9.63 - Dermoepidermal Junction

I. Bullous Pemphigoid
   A. Antibodies against hemidesmosome protein: BP180
   B. Separation of epidermis and dermis with presence of eosinophils
   C. Tense bullae with sparing of the oral mucosa
   D. (-) Nikolsky sign
   E. Linear pattern on immunofluorescence due to IgG deposition

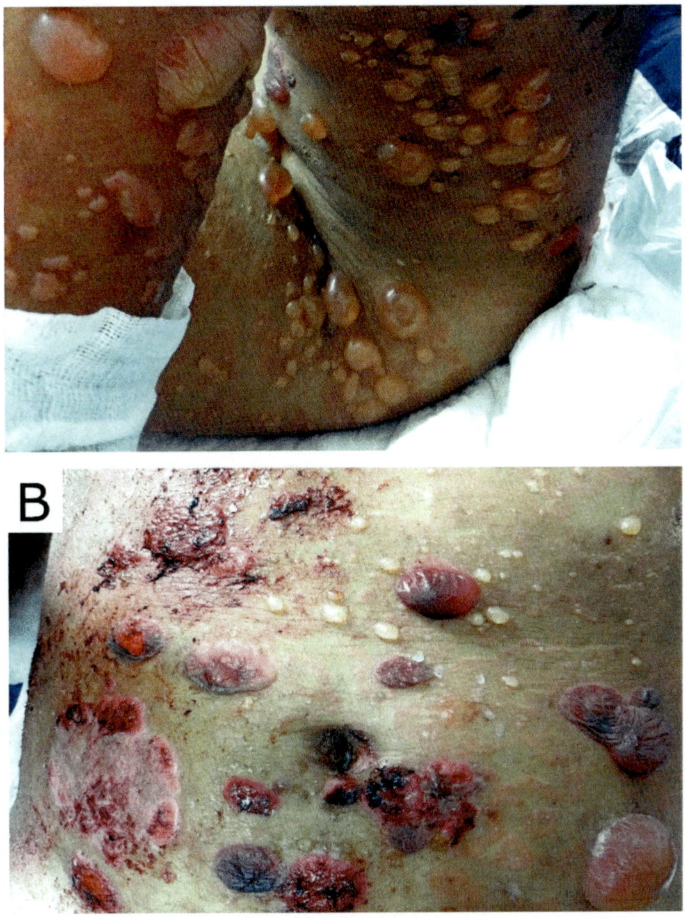

Photo Credit: Turra, Acosta, Alvarez. "Bullous pemphigoid: can it occur in any pediatric age?" [CC BY-SA 4.0 https://creativecommons.org/licenses/by-sa/4.0/)]. This image may have been modified by cropping, labeling, or captions.

FIGURE 10.9.64 - Bullous Pemphigoid

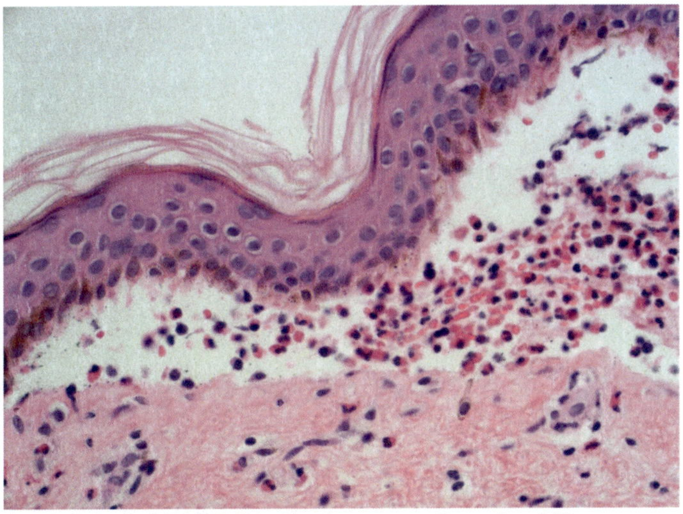

Photo Credit: Sarahkayb / CC BY-SA [(https://creativecommons.org/licenses/by-sa/4.0)]

FIGURE 10.9.65 - Skin Biopsy in Bullous Pemphigoid

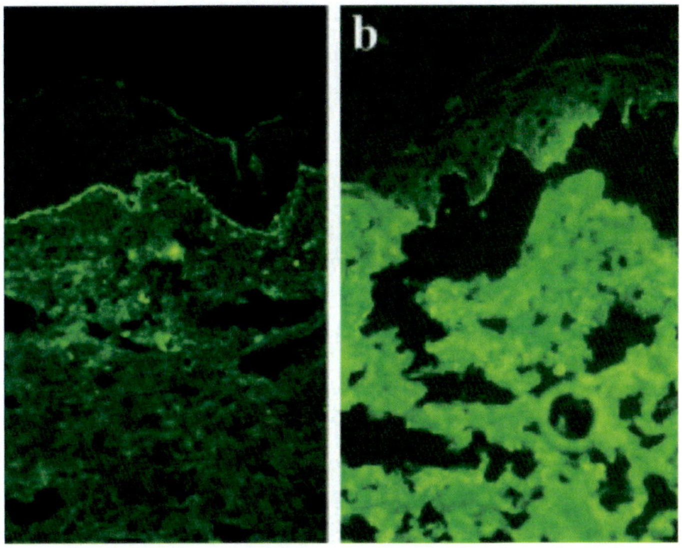

Photo Credit: Si, Ge, Li. "Erythrodermic psoriasis with bullous pemphigoid: Combination treatment with methotrexate and compound glycyrrhizin" [CC BY 2.0 (https://creativecommons.org/licenses/by/2.0/)]. This image may have been modified by cropping, labeling, or captions.

FIGURE 10.9.66 - Bullous Pemphigoid Under Immunofluorescence

II. Pemphigus Vulgaris
   A. Antibodies against desmosome proteins: desmoglein-1 and desmoglein-3
   B. Flaccid bullae with involvement of oral mucosa
   C. (+) Nikolsky sign
   D. Immunofluorescence: reticular pattern with a "fishnet" appearance

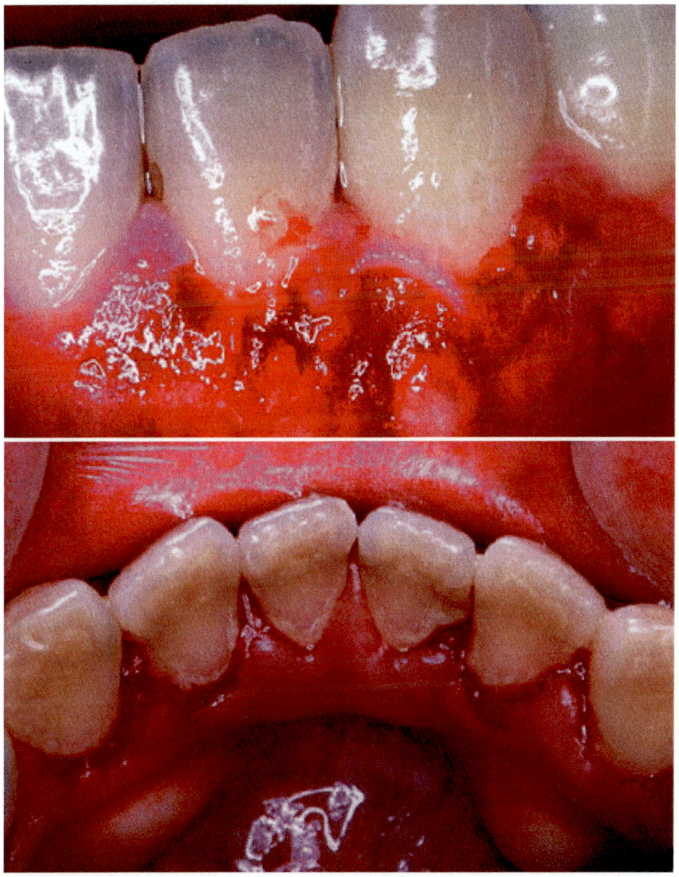

Photo Credit: Endo, Rees, To. "Gingival Nikolsky's Sign: A Valuable Tool in Identifying Oral manifestations of Mucous Membrane Pemphigoid and Pemphigus Vulgaris." [CC BY 3.0 (https://creativecommons.org/licenses/by/3.0/)]

FIGURE 10.9.67 - Gingival Lesions in Pemphigus Vulgaris

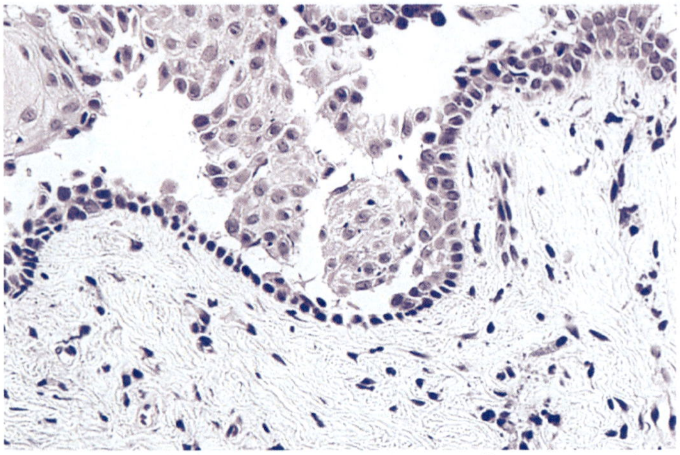

Photo Credit: Endo, Rees, To. "Desquamative Gingivitis." [CC BY 3.0 https://creativecommons.org/licenses/by/3.0/)]

FIGURE 10.9.68 - Acantholysis in Pemphigus Vulgaris

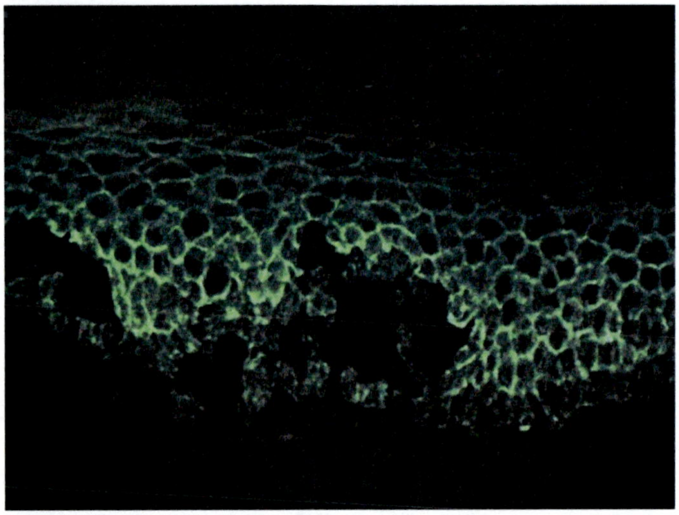

Photo Credit: Emmanuelm at English Wikipedia / CC BY 3.0 [(https://creativecommons.org/licenses/by/3.0)]

FIGURE 10.9.69 - Pemphigus Vulgaris Under Immunofluorescence

III. Dermatitis Herpetiformis
   A. Pruritic vesicles and grouped bullae
   B. Typically located on elbows, knees, scalp, or buttocks
   C. Associated with celiac disease
   D. Deposits of IgA at dermal papillae
   E. Treatment: gluten-free diet and dapsone

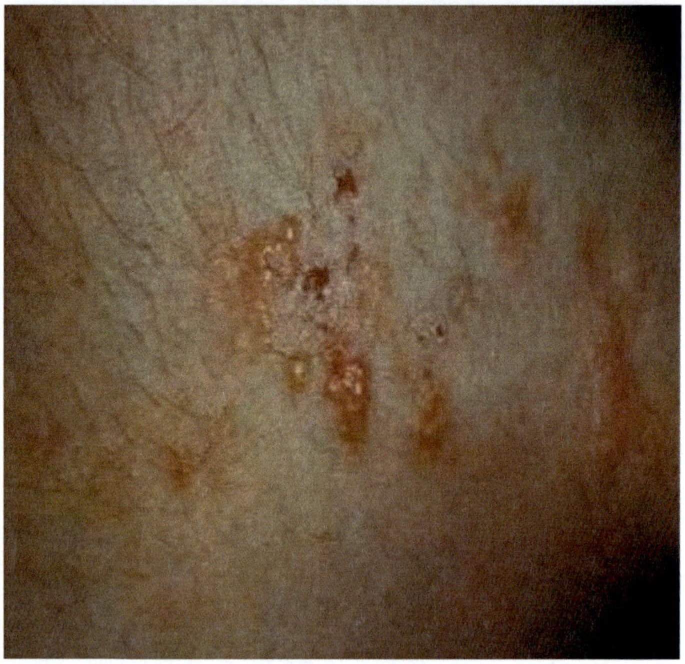

Photo Credit: Weinstock, Myers, Smith. "Successful Treatment of Adult-Onset Dermatitis Herpetiformis with Low Dose Naltrexone" [CC BY 4.0 (https://creativecommons.org/licenses/by/4.0/deed.en)]

FIGURE 10.9.70 - Dermatitis Herpetiformis

IV. Erythema Multiforme
   A. Hypersensitivity reaction with targetoid lesions
   B. Infection: *Mycoplasma pneumoniae* or herpes simplex virus
   C. Drugs: penicillin, sulfa drugs, and phenytoin

Feature	Bullous Pemphigoid	Pemphigus Vulgaris
Antibody target	- Hemidesmosomes - BP180	- Desmosomes - Desmoglein-1/desmoglein-3
Hypersensitivity type	- Type 2	- Type 2
Gross morphology	- Tense blisters	- Flaccid intraepidermal bullae
Oral mucosa involvement	- Spared	- Involved
Appearance on H&E	- No acantholysis - Presence of eosinophils	- Acantholysis - "Row of tombstones" appearance
Immunofluorescence pattern	- Linear pattern	- Reticular pattern
Nikolsky sign	(-)	(+)

TABLE 10.9.4 - Bullous Pemphigoid vs. Pemphigus Vulgaris

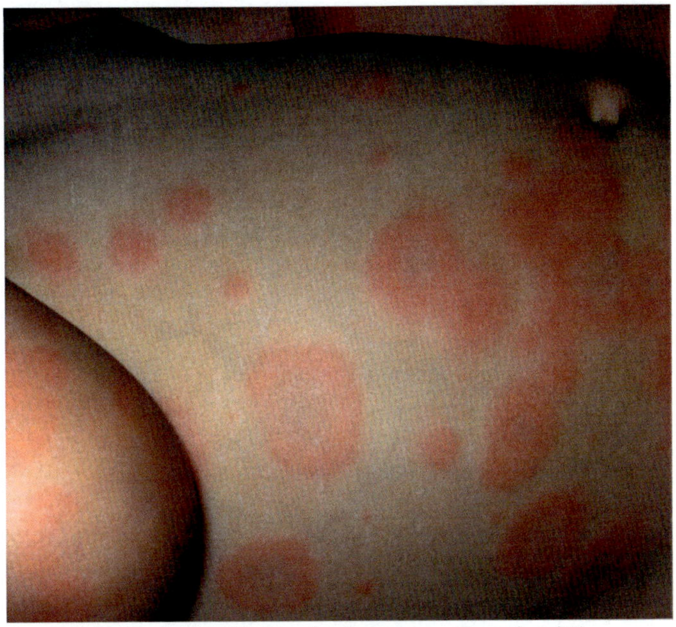

FIGURE 10.9.71 - Erythema Multiforme

REVIEW QUESTIONS ?

1. A 50-year-old male presents to his dermatologist with numerous skin lesions. A skin biopsy shows complete separation of the epidermis from the underlying dermis. What is the likely diagnosis and antibody target?

- **The correct diagnosis is bullous pemphigoid, and this condition involves antibodies against hemidesmosomes.**
- The Nikolsky sign will be negative.

REVIEW QUESTIONS ?

2. A 21-year-old female comes to the office complaining of a fever and a dry, non-productive cough that began one week ago. Additionally, she says she has a new rash on her right arm. Physical examination of the lungs reveals bilateral crackles. Further workup reveals diffuse interstitial infiltrates on chest X-ray. Which of the following is the most likely diagnosis?

   A. Erythema migrans
   B. Erythema infectiosum
   C. Erythema multiforme
   D. Erythema nodosum

- **The correct answer is C.**
- From this question, you must recognize that this is talking about *Mycoplasma pneumoniae* infection. This is due to the typical history of "walking pneumonia" in a college student. Additionally, you will hear crackles and classically see interstitial infiltrates on CXR. Further, this patient is also presenting with a rash. Recall that *Mycoplasma pneumoniae* is commonly associated with erythema multiforme.
- When considering the incorrect answer choices, you must recall what each of these lesions is and what they are associated with.
- Choice A, erythema migrans, is the "bulls-eye" rash you will see in Lyme disease. The patient has no history of camping or travel to areas in the Northeast like Connecticut. Additionally, the patient would not present with pulmonary findings in Lyme disease.
- Choice B, erythema infectiosum, is the rash associated with parvovirus B19. This is classically a "slapped-cheek" rash that starts on the face (not the arm like this in vignette) and then spreads downwards to the rest of the body. Additionally, it is typically a rash seen in childhood.
- Choice D, erythema nodosum, is a type of inflammation with nodules typically on the anterior shins. It's usually seen in chronic inflammatory states like sarcoidosis and inflammatory bowel disease, as well as fungal infections like histoplasmosis. Although technically the clinical history could support pulmonary findings found in histoplasmosis, erythema nodosum usually is found on the anterior shins rather than the arms.

Section XII - Epithelial Tumors

I. Seborrheic Keratosis
   A. Flat, brown lesion with a "stuck on" appearance
   B. Found on head, trunk, and extremities
   C. Benign proliferation of immature keratinocytes
   D. Leser-Trélat sign

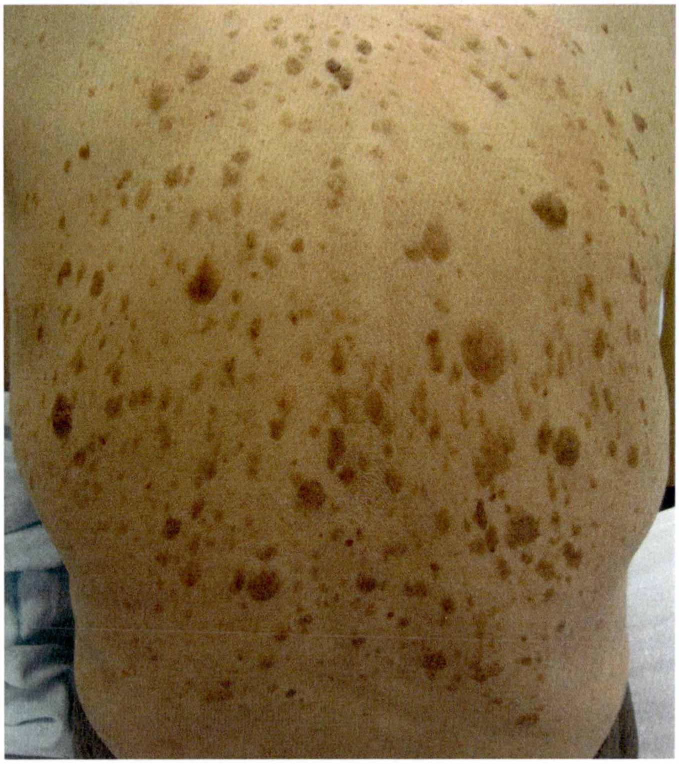

FIGURE 10.9.72 - Leser-Trélat Sign

II. Acanthosis Nigricans
   A. Velvety, hyperpigmented plaque on the skin
   B. Typically found on the neck and axillae
   C. Associated with diabetes mellitus

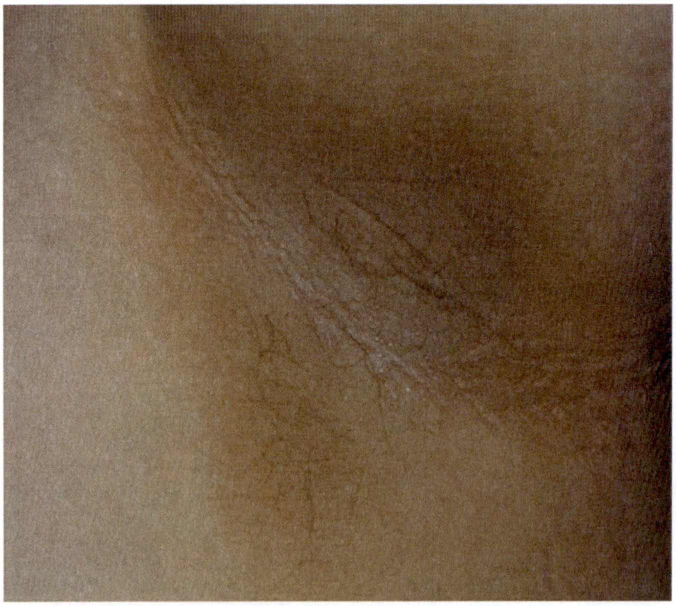

FIGURE 10.9.73 - Acanthosis Nigricans

III. Basal Cell Carcinoma
   A. Most common form of skin cancer
   B. Risk factors: UV radiation
   C. Waxy, pink, and pearly nodules
   D. Typically located above the lip
   E. Histology: basaloid cells that show nuclear palisading

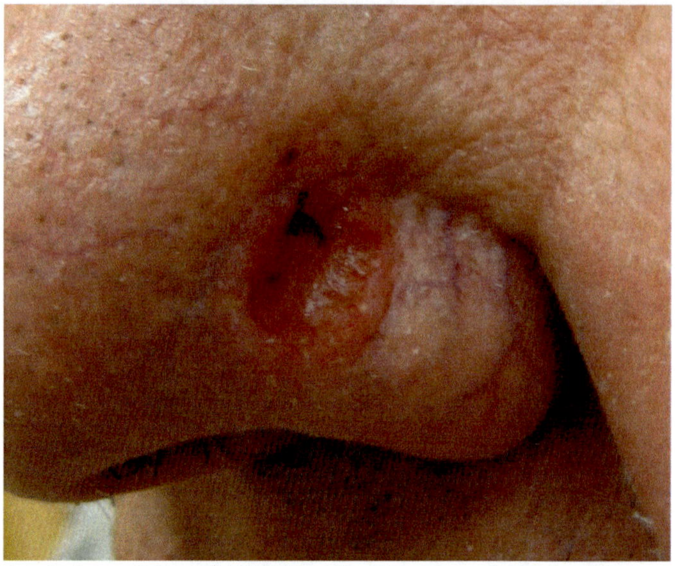

FIGURE 10.9.74 - Basal Cell Carcinoma

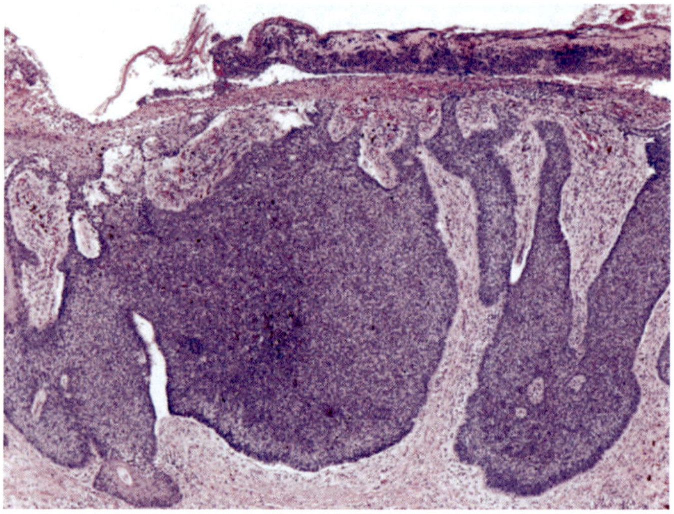

FIGURE 10.9.75 - Histological Image of Basal Cell Carcinoma

IV. Squamous Cell Carcinoma
   A. Ulcerative red plaque in sun-exposed areas
   B. Risk factors: chronic sun exposure, immunosuppression, chronic inflammation, and arsenic
   C. Develops from precursor lesion (actinic keratosis)
   D. Typically located below the lip, ears, or hands
   E. Histology: malignant proliferation of epithelial squamous cells involving the formation of "keratin pearls"

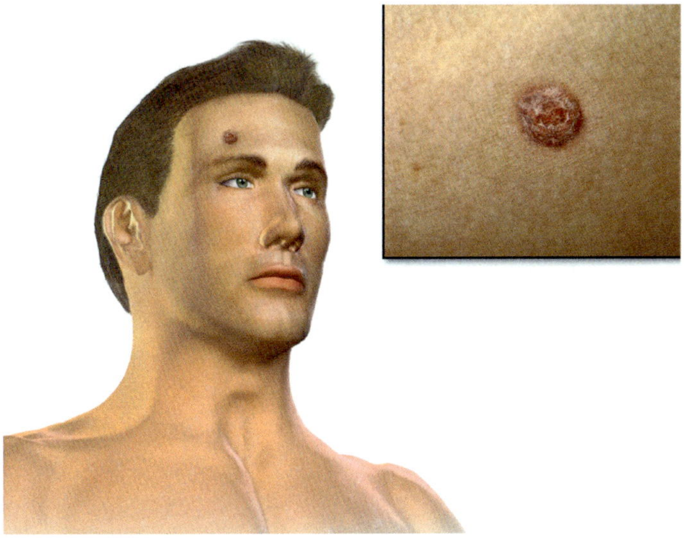

FIGURE 10.9.76 - Squamous Cell Carcinoma

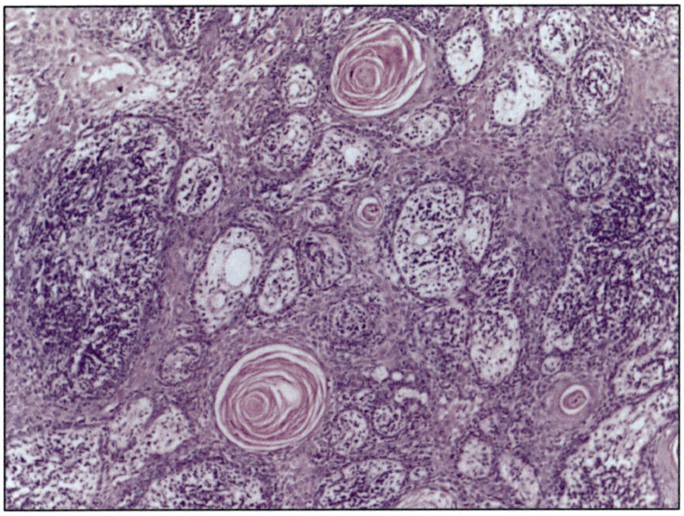

FIGURE 10.9.77 - Histological Image of Squamous Cell Carcinoma

REVIEW QUESTIONS

1. A 57-year-old man presents to the clinic with several lesions on his right hand that he noticed while tending to his farm. Despite trying topical ointments, the lesions have gotten bigger in size. He denies any pruritus associated with them. What malignancy is he most likely at risk of developing?

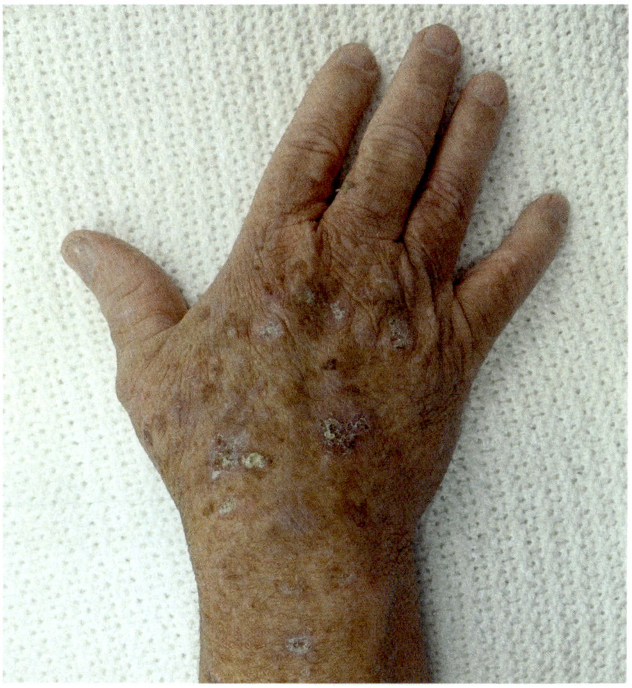

A. Keratoacanthoma
B. Basal cell carcinoma
C. Squamous cell carcinoma
D. Melanoma

- **The correct answer is C.**
- The patient has many actinic or solar keratoses, which are precursor lesions to squamous cell carcinoma. This would fit the clinical presentation since the patient is a farmer who is likely spending lots of time in the sun. Additionally, he has some other risk factors, such as being a male and advanced age.
- Choice A is incorrect because keratoacanthoma is a lesion that is generally dome-shaped (unlike in this image) with a keratin-filled center.
- Choice B is incorrect because basal cell carcinoma is generally on the upper lip. These lesions also look more pink, pearly, and waxy.
- Choice D is incorrect. Recall the ABCDE criteria. Melanomas would generally be asymmetrical with irregular borders, varying in color, large in diameter (> 6 mm), and evolving or rapidly changing in appearance.

Section XIII - Disorders of Pigmentation

I. Biochemistry
   A. Melanocytes are derived from neural crest cells
   B. Melanocytes produce melanin
   C. Melanin provides skin pigmentation
   D. Melanin is stored in melanosomes
   E. Melanin is transported to keratinocytes to provide pigmentation

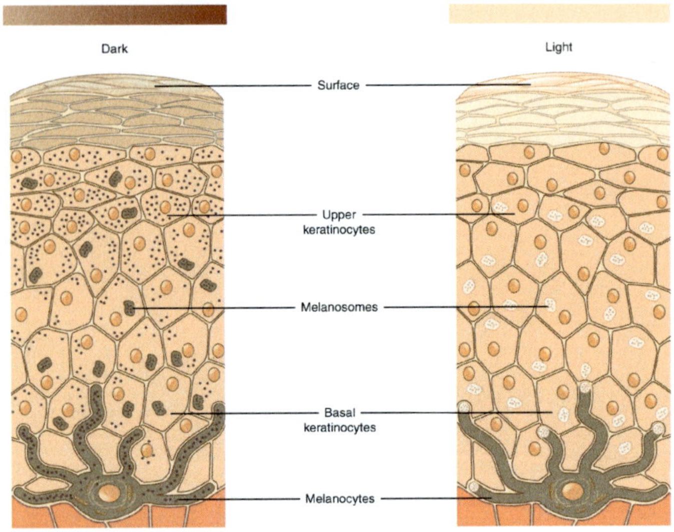

FIGURE 10.9.78 - Distribution of Melanocytes, Melanosomes, and Melanin

II. Vitiligo: Etiology
   A. Autoimmune destruction of melanocytes

III. Vitiligo: Pathophysiology
   A. Destruction of melanocytes leads to a loss of melanin
   B. Decreased melanin results in patchy skin pigmentation

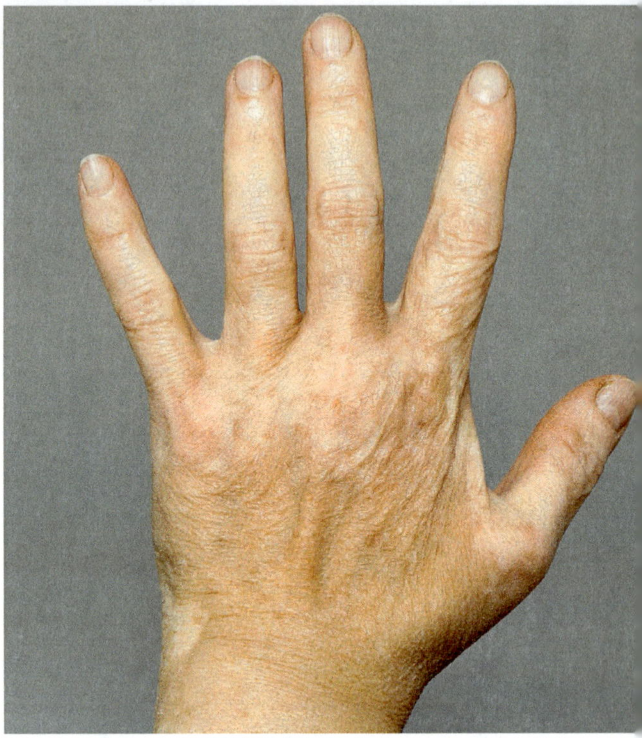

FIGURE 10.9.79 - Vitiligo

IV. Albinism: Etiology
   A. Autosomal recessive
   B. Congenital absence of skin pigmentation

V. Albinism: Pathophysiology
   A. Lack of melanin due to defective tyrosinase enzyme
   B. Dihydroxyphenylalanine (DOPA) is converted to melanin via tyrosinase enzyme

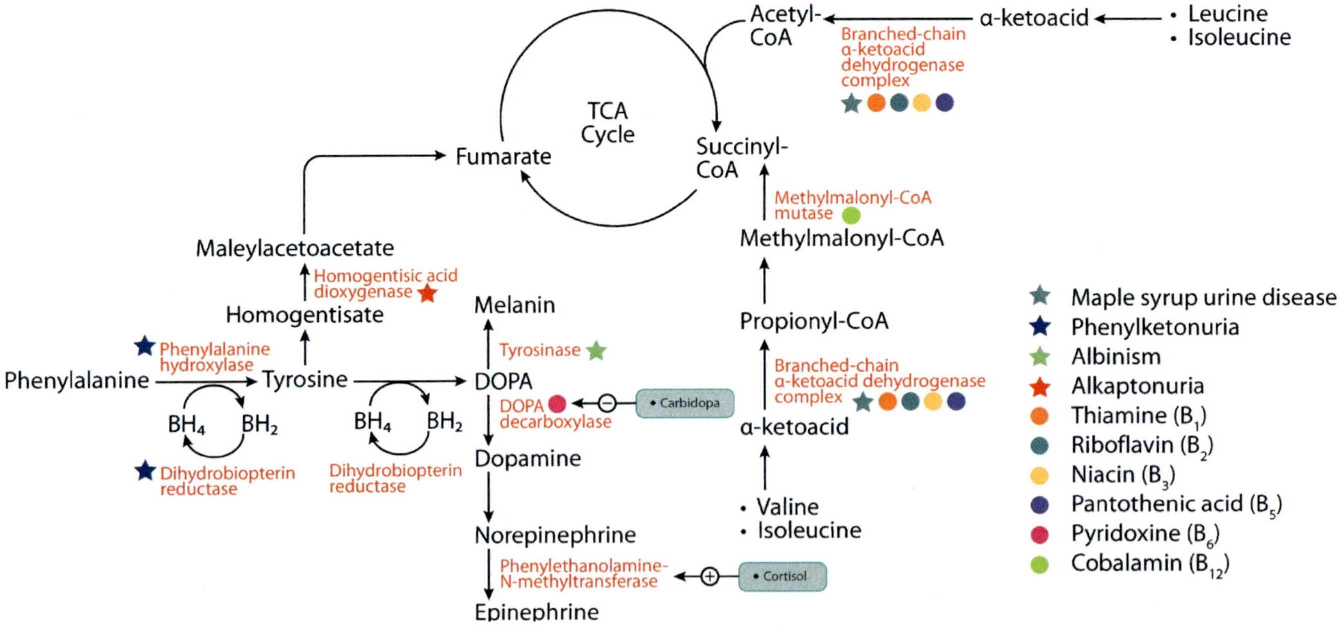

FIGURE 10.9.80 - Melanin Biochemistry

VI. Albinism: Complications
   A. Must avoid excessive sunlight exposure due to an increased risk of skin cancer
   B. May cause ocular impairment

VII. Ephelide
   A. Otherwise known as a freckle
   B. Small tan or brown macule that tends to darken with sun exposure
   C. A result of an increase in the number of melanosomes

VIII. Melasma
   A. Patchy areas of facial hyperpigmentation
   B. Associated with pregnancy or oral contraceptive use
   C. Referred to as a "mask of pregnancy"

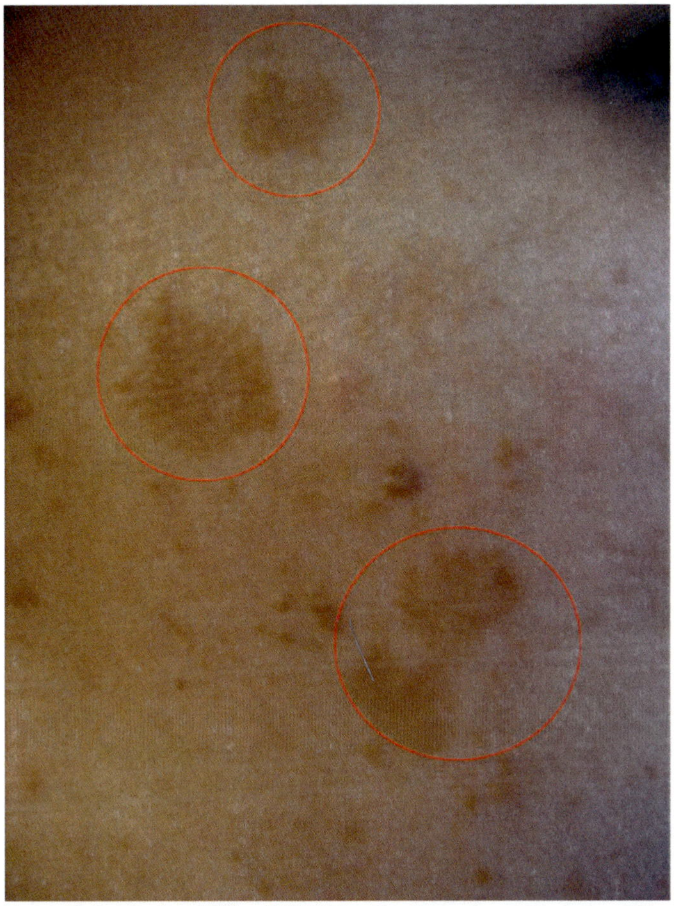

FIGURE 10.9.81 - Melasma

IX. Nevus: Etiology
   A. Congenital
   B. Acquired

X. Nevus: Pathophysiology
   A. Benign proliferation of melanocytes

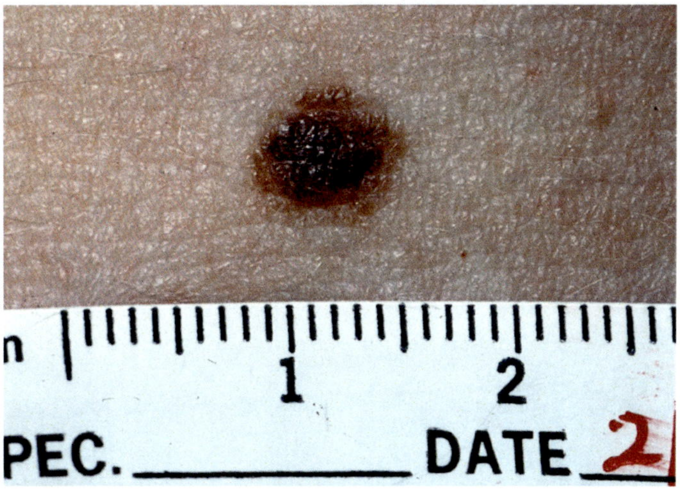

FIGURE 10.9.82 - Congenital Nevus

XI. Melanoma: Etiology
   A. Excessive sunlight exposure
   B. Dysplastic nevus
   C. Xeroderma pigmentosum
   D. Albinism

XII. Melanoma: Pathophysiology
   A. Malignant proliferation of melanocytes
   B. Activating mutation of BRAF kinase

XIII. Melanoma: Clinical Features
   A. Asymmetrical
   B. Irregular borders
   C. Color variation
   D. Diameter is greater than 6 mm
   E. Evolving

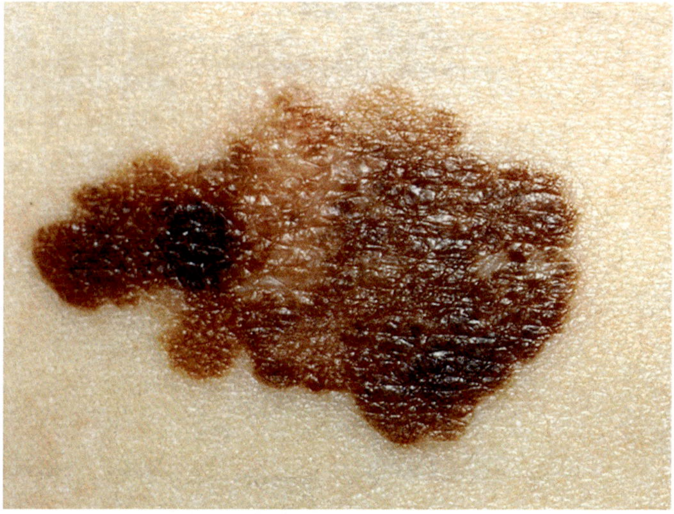

FIGURE 10.9.83 - Melanoma

XIV. Melanoma: Growth
   A. Horizontal growth is generally lower risk
   B. Vertical growth increases the risk of metastasis

XV. Melanoma: Types
  A. Superficial
  B. Nodular
  C. Lentigo maligna
  D. Acral lentiginous

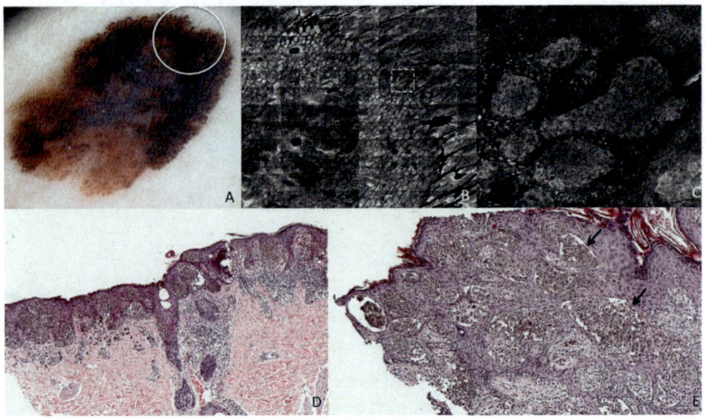

FIGURE 10.9.84 - Melanoma Types

REVIEW QUESTIONS

1. A 42-year-old African American female with a past medical history of Crohn's disease and rheumatoid arthritis presents to the physician for her annual physical examination. The patient has large areas of patchy skin depigmentation on her face, hands, shoulders, and legs. What is the mechanism behind this patient's skin condition?

- **The correct answer is the autoimmune destruction of melanocytes.**
- The patient is suffering from Crohn's disease, rheumatoid arthritis, and a skin condition called vitiligo.
- The pathophysiological mechanism behind vitiligo is the autoimmune destruction of melanocytes.
- Melanocytes create melanin, which in turn gives the skin pigmentation.
- The destruction of melanocytes results in a loss of melanin; therefore, patchy depigmentation occurs.

REVIEW QUESTIONS

2. A 55-year-old female with a past medical history of hypertension and depression presents to the physician for her annual physical examination. The patient's current temperature is 97.9 °C (36.6 °F), blood pressure is 122/76 mmHg, heart rate is 69 beats/minute, and the respiratory rate is 13 breaths/minute. The patient states she is concerned about skin cancer. Further questioning reveals that her father and brother both have been diagnosed with melanoma. She spends ample time swimming in an outdoor pool several times per week and does not wear sunscreen. The patient is concerned about her risk of melanoma. Which of the following is the best indicator of metastatic potential of this disorder?

   A. Horizontal growth
   B. CA 19-9 marker
   C. Vertical growth
   D. Melasma

- **The correct answer is C.**
- The important thing to recognize here is that this patient has an increased risk for melanoma, which is a form of skin cancer.
- Vertical growth of melanoma is the best indicator of metastatic potential.
- Growth of melanoma is monitored both vertically and horizontally.
- Horizontal growth generally has lower risk and does not spread into the deep dermis.
- Vertical growth is the most important prognostic factor for melanoma. Vertical growth into the deep dermis increases the risk of metastasis.
- A is incorrect because horizontal growth is not a predictor of metastatic potential.
- B is incorrect because serum CA 19-9 marker levels are not associated with melanoma. CA 19-9 levels are associated with pancreatic tumors.
- D is incorrect because melasma is a hyperpigmentation disorder and is not related to melanoma. Melasma is associated with pregnancy and oral contraceptive use.

Section I - Primary Hemostasis

I. Basic Principles
   A. Hemostasis = control of bleeding
   B. Primary hemostasis → platelet plug
   C. Secondary hemostasis → coagulation cascade → stabilization

II. Overview
   A. Primary hemostasis physiology
   B. Findings: symptoms, physical exam, and labs
   C. Platelet disorders
      1. Quantitative disorders: immune thrombocytopenic purpura (ITP) and microangiopathic hemolytic anemia (MAHA)
      2. Qualitative disorders: Bernard-Soulier, Glanzmann, and uremic platelet dysfunction

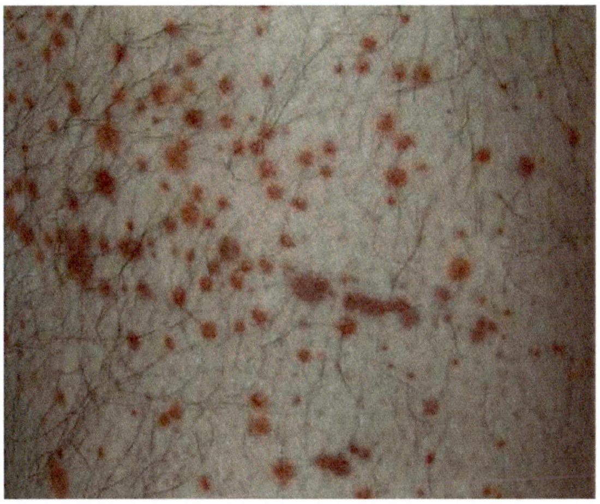

FIGURE 10.10.1 - Petechiae

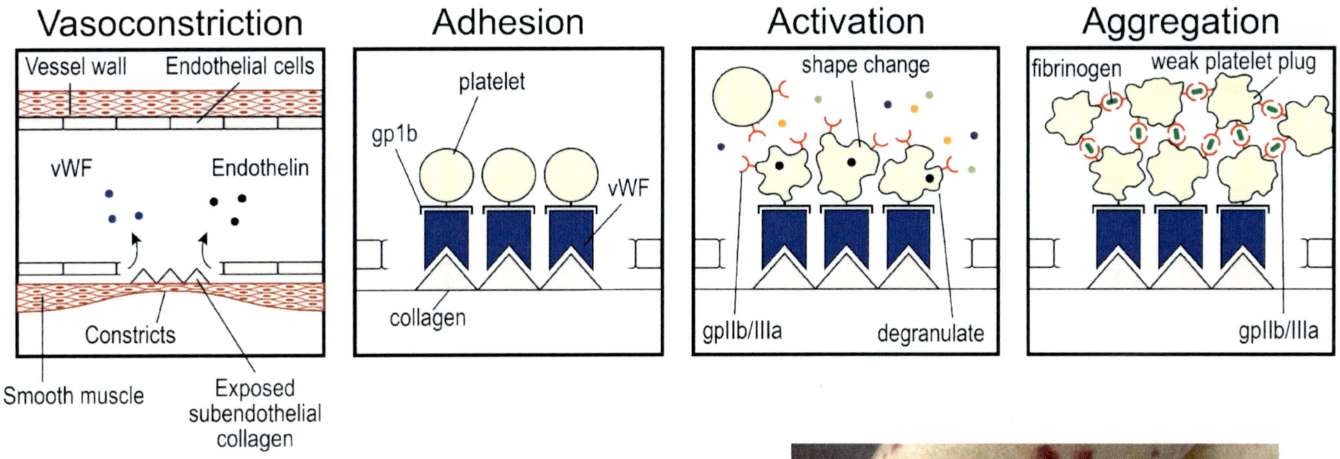

FIGURE 10.10.2 - Steps of Primary Hemostasis

III. Primary Hemostasis Physiology
   A. Vasoconstriction
   B. Adhesion
   C. Activation
   D. Aggregation

IV. Findings in Platelet Disorders: Symptoms
   A. Epistaxis
   B. Hemoptysis
   C. Gastrointestinal bleeding
   D. Hematuria
   E. Menorrhagia

V. Findings in Platelet Disorders: Physical Examination
   A. Petechiae
   B. Purpura

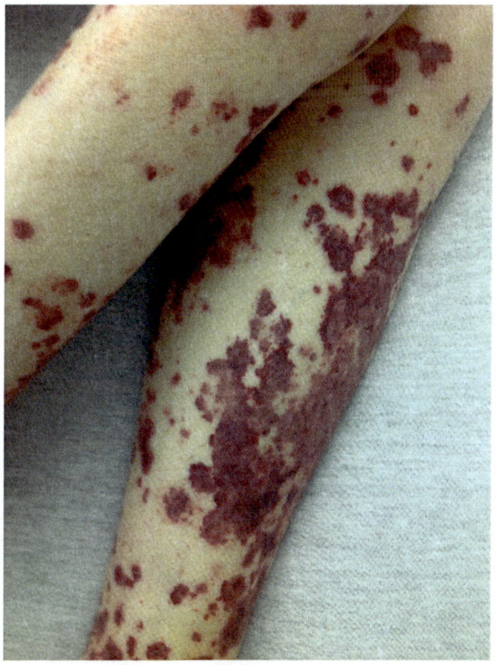

FIGURE 10.6.14 - Purpura

VI. Findings in Platelet Disorders: Lab Workup
   A. Complete blood count (CBC)
      1. Platelet count: low (quantitative) or normal (qualitative)
   B. Coagulation studies
      1. Bleeding time: increased
      2. Prothrombin time (PT), international normalized ratio (INR), and partial thromboplastin time (PTT) are normal
   C. Peripheral blood smear

VII. Immune Thrombocytopenic Purpura
   A. May be idiopathic or due to autoimmune disease, virus, drugs, cancer
   B. Autoantibodies against GPIIb/IIIa → platelets destroyed by splenic macrophages → thrombocytopenia
   C. Acute: seen in children, often occurs after a virus, self-limited
   D. Chronic: seen in reproductive-age women, may relapse
   E. Treatment: steroids, IVIG, monoclonal antibodies, and splenectomy

VIII. Microangiopathic Hemolytic Anemia
   A. Thrombotic thrombocytopenic purpura (TTP)
   B. Hemolytic uremic syndrome
   C. Disruption of ADAMTS13 → ↑ vWF multimers → ↑ thrombus formation
   D. Platelet consumption → thrombocytopenia
   E. RBC fragmentation → schistocytes → hemolytic anemia (↓ Hb, ↑ LDH)
   F. Acute kidney injury (↑ Cr)

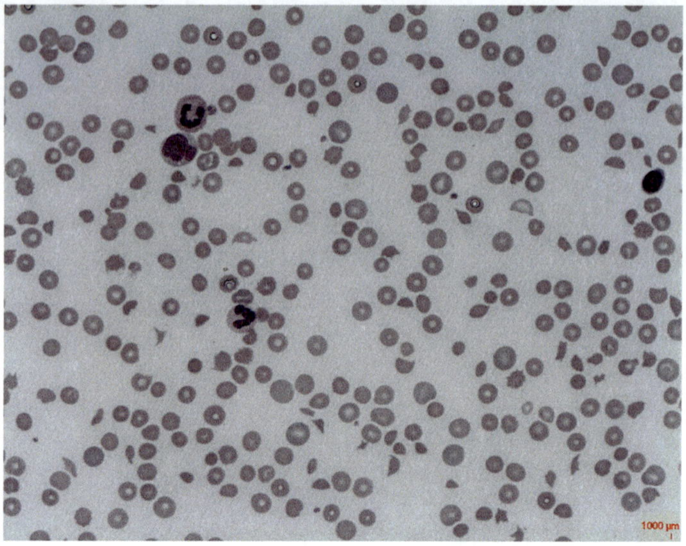

FIGURE 10.10.4 - Schistocytes of Microangiopathic Hemolytic Anemia (MAHA)

IX. Thrombotic Thrombocytopenic Purpura
   A. Absent or low ADAMTS13
      1. Less vWF cleavage → platelet microthrombi → TTP → triad and neurologic problems
   B. Treatment: corticosteroids and plasmapheresis

X. Hemolytic Uremic Syndrome
   A. *E. coli* O157:H7 → Shiga-like toxin → decreased protein synthesis → disruption of ADAMTS13 → endothelial damage → platelet thrombi
   B. Triad plus progressive renal failure, uremia, and bloody diarrhea
   C. Treatment: supportive care

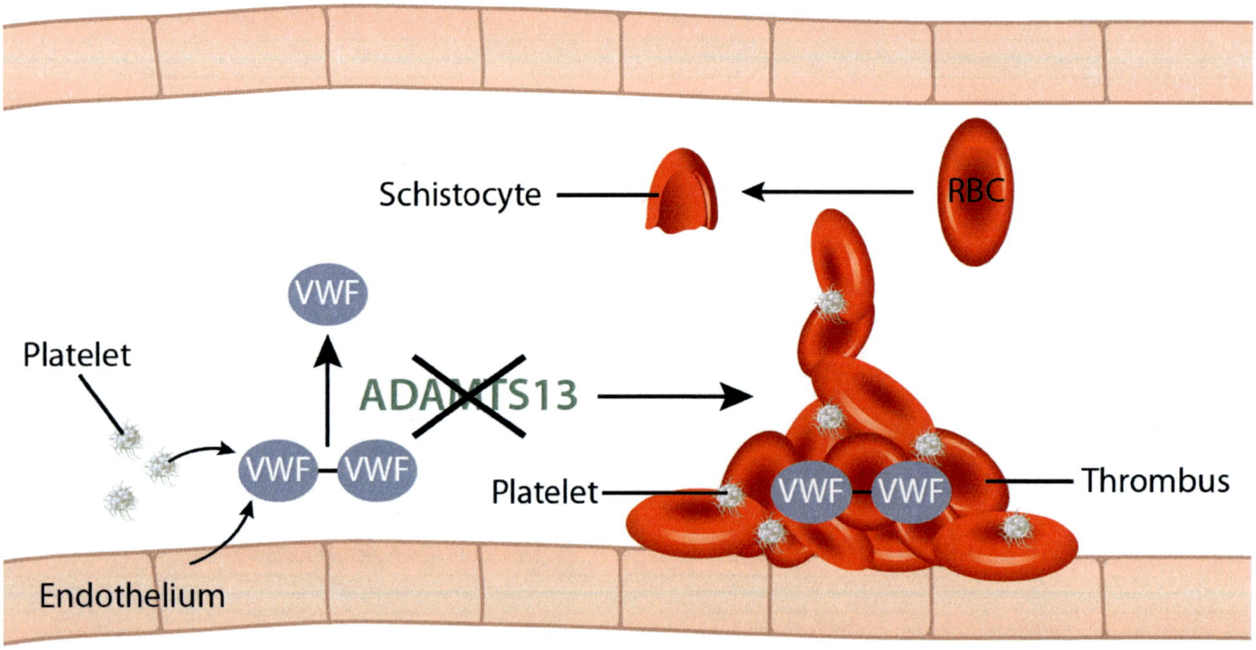

FIGURE 10.10.3 - Pathophysiology of Microangiopathic Hemolytic Anemia (MAHA)

XI. Qualitative Platelet Disorders
  A. Acquired
    1. Uremic platelet dysfunction
  B. Genetic
    1. Bernard-Soulier syndrome
    2. Glanzmann thrombasthenia

XII. Uremic Platelet Dysfunction
  A. End-stage renal disease
  B. Uremia causes platelet dysfunction (adhesion and aggregation)
  C. Improves with dialysis

XIII. Genetic Qualitative Platelet Disorders
  A. Bernard-Soulier syndrome → decreased GPIb → impaired platelet adhesion
  B. Glanzmann thrombasthenia → decreased GPIIb/IIIa → impaired platelet aggregation

REVIEW QUESTIONS

1. A 27-year-old woman presents to the urgent care clinic with a nosebleed. She has had a few nosebleeds recently that seem to last quite long. On physical exam, she has a tissue against her nose that is soaked in blood and scattered small purple spots on her legs and arms. ITP is suspected. What lab findings would be expected if a CBC, bleeding time, PT, and PTT are ordered?

- **The correct answer is thrombocytopenia on CBC, prolonged bleeding time, and normal PT and PTT.**
- The platelets would be low because of the autoantibodies against GPIIb/IIIa causing destruction of platelets by splenic macrophages. She is a young woman of reproductive age, which increases her risk for autoimmune problems.
- Her bleeding time would be prolonged because of the thrombocytopenia.
- Her PT and PTT would be normal,because her clotting factors aren't affected.

2. A 7-year-old boy comes to the physician with a cough, runny nose, fever, and malaise. He is diagnosed with an upper respiratory tract infection. Two weeks later, he returns with bleeding from his gums after brushing his teeth and bruises on his arms and legs. A CBC shows a platelet count of 12,000 per microliter (normal: 150,000-400,000 per microliter). Bleeding time is prolonged at 9 minutes (normal: 2-7 minutes). What would be an appropriate first line treatment for this patient?

   A. IVIG
   B. Aspirin
   C. Rituximab
   D. Corticosteroids
   E. Vitamin D

- **The correct answer is D.**
- While there are a few medications on this list that can treat ITP, the first-line treatment is corticosteroids.
- This is a 7-year-old boy who has symptoms consistent with an upper respiratory tract infection. He returns to the physician with signs of mucosal bleeding in the form of bleeding from his gums. He also has bruises on his arms and legs.
- CBC shows a low platelet count of 12,000. Bleeding time is prolonged at 9 minutes. This is consistent with ITP after a viral upper respiratory illness.
- A is incorrect because IVIG is not the first-line and should only be used when the patient is actively bleeding at a high rate.
- B is incorrect because aspirin is an antiplatelet agent that would worsen bleeding.
- C is incorrect because monoclonal antibodies are not the first-line.
- E is incorrect because Vitamin D has no indication in the treatment of ITP.

Section II - Secondary Hemostasis

I. Disorders of Secondary Hemostasis
    A. Clinical features
    B. Lab values
    C. Disorders: hemophilia (A, B, and C), coagulation factor inhibitor, von Willebrand disease, vitamin K deficiency, other abnormalities

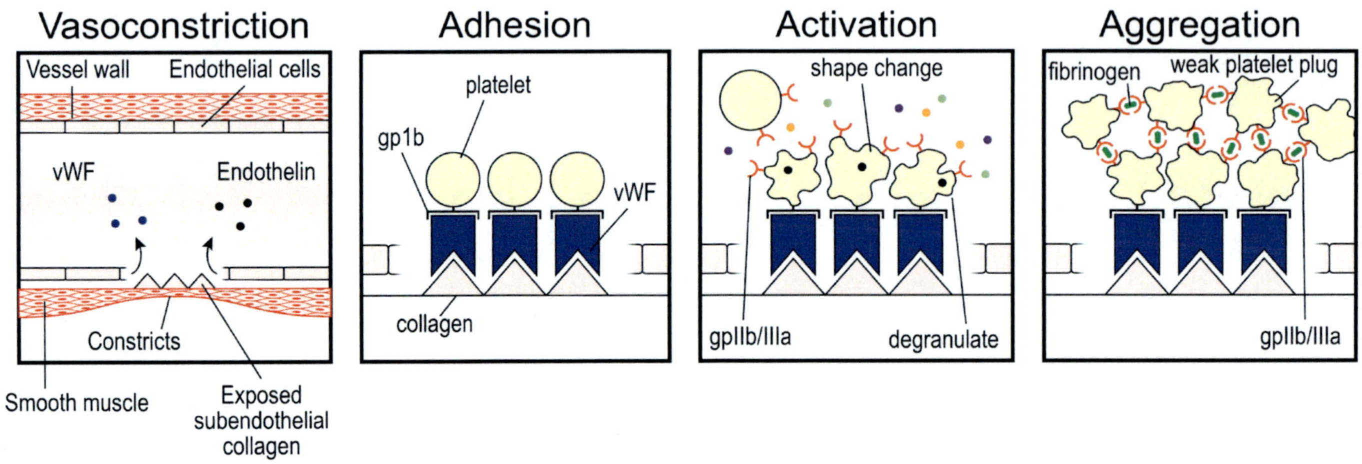

FIGURE 10.10.2 - Steps of Primary Hemostasis

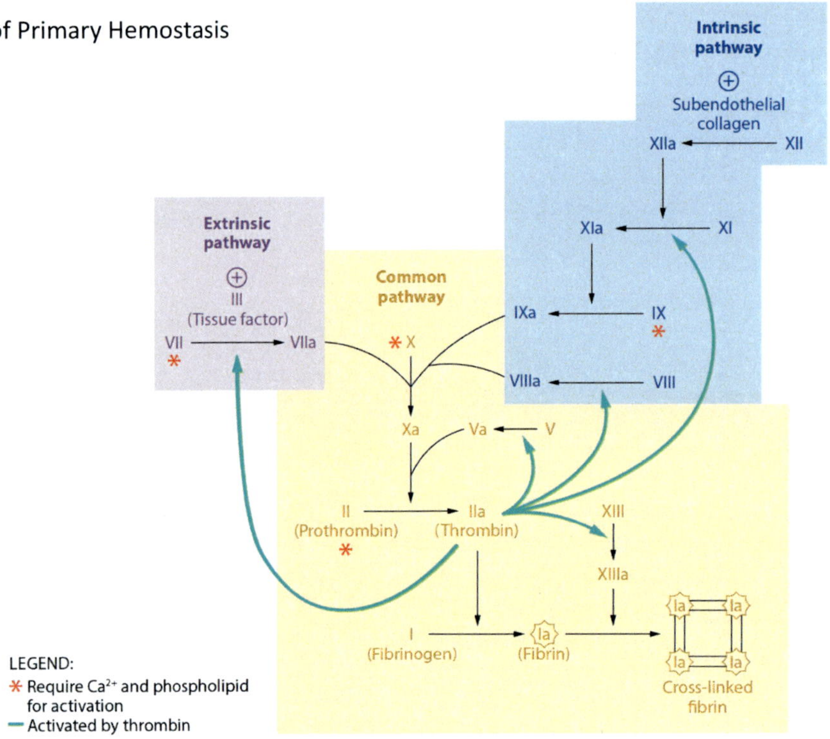

FIGURE 10.10.5 - Coagulation Cascade

II. Clotting Factors
    A. Proteins made in liver (factor III and VIII made in endothelial cells)
    B. Require activation
        1. Activating substance: tissue factor or subendothelial collagen
        2. Preceding factor
        3. Thrombin
        4. Calcium & phospholipid layer (platelets or tissue factor)
            a) Factors II, VII, IX, and X

III. Common Clinical Features
   A. Bleeding into deep layers (muscles and joints)
      1. Hemarthrosis
   B. Rebleeding following surgical procedure (e.g. tooth extraction)
   C. Elevated PT or PTT

IV. Lab Values
   A. PTT (partial thromboplastin time)
      1. Integrity of intrinsic and common pathway (normal: 25-40 sec)
      2. Monitored during heparin treatment
   B. PT (prothrombin time)
      1. Integrity of extrinsic and common pathway (normal: 11-15 sec)
      2. Monitored during warfarin treatment
   C. TT (thrombin time)
      1. Measures conversion rate of fibrinogen to fibrin
   D. Bleeding time
      1. Measures function of platelets

Hemophilia	Deficiency	Mode of Inheritance	Lab Findings	Treatment
A	- Factor VIII	- X-linked (usually males)	- ↓ factor VIII - ↑ PTT - Normal PT - Normal bleeding time	- Recombinant factor VIII - Thrombin
B (Christmas disease)	- Factor IX	- X-lined (usually males)	- ↓ factor IX - ↑ PTT - Normal PT - Normal bleeding time	- Recombinant factor IX - Thrombin
C	- Factor XI	- Autosomal recessive	- ↓ factor XI - ↑ PTT - Normal PT - Normal bleeding time	- Recombinant factor XI - Thrombin

TABLE 10.10.1 Types of Hemophilia

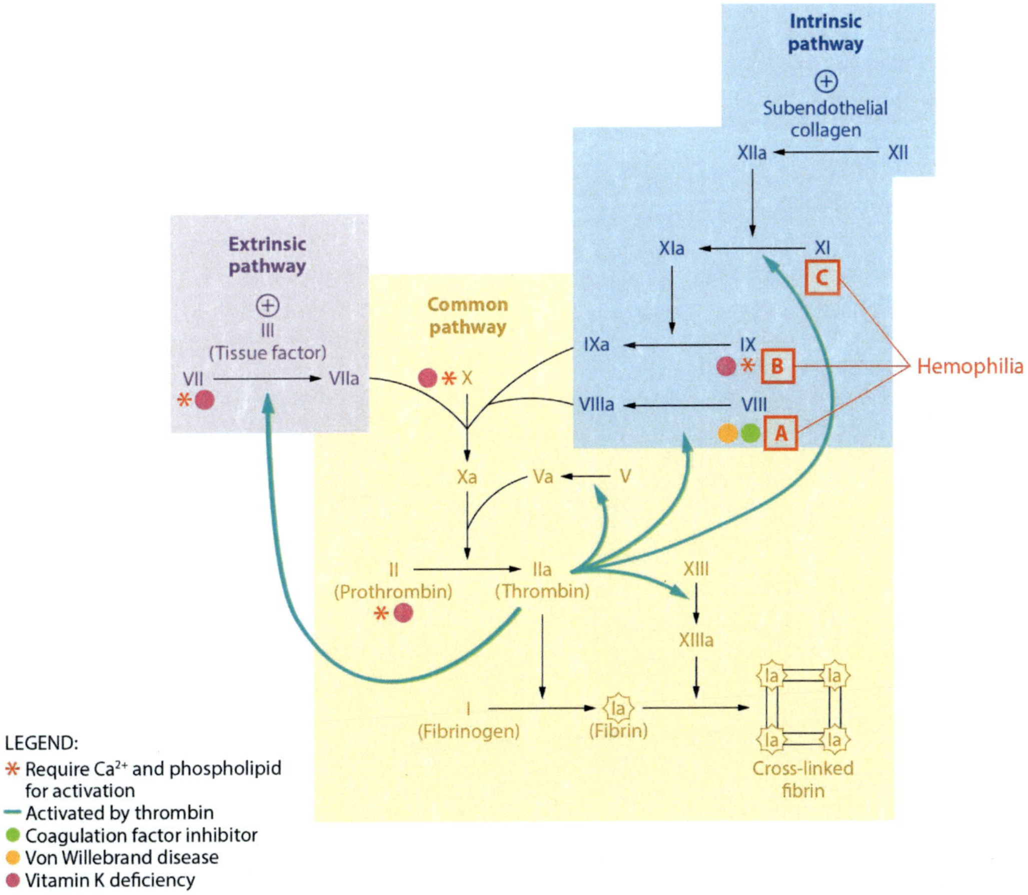

FIGURE 10.10.6 - Overview of Secondary Hemostasis

V. Coagulation Factor Inhibitor
   A. Antibodies develop against factors (most commonly factor VIII)
   B. Similar lab findings to hemophilia A
      1. ↑ PTT, ↓ Factor VIII, normal PT
   C. Differentiate with a "mix study"
      1. Hemophilia A : PTT will normalize
      2. Coagulation factor inhibitor: PTT will not normalize

VI. Von Willebrand Disease
   A. Autosomal dominant von Willebrand factor (vWF) deficiency
      1. Most common inherited coagulation disorder
   B. Low levels of vWF
      1. Decreased factor VIII → ↑ PTT
      2. Impaired platelet adhesion → ↑ bleeding time
      3. Abnormal ristocetin test
   C. Treatment: desmopressin

VII. Vitamin K Deficiency
   A. Vitamin K activated by epoxidase reductase
      1. Gamma-carboxylates factors II, VII, IX, and X and proteins C & S
   B. Deficiency seen in
      1. Newborns
      2. Long-term antibiotic use
      3. Malabsorption (cystic fibrosis)

VIII. Other Abnormalities
   A. Blood transfusion
      1. Coagulation factors diluted
   B. Liver failure
      1. Measure PT

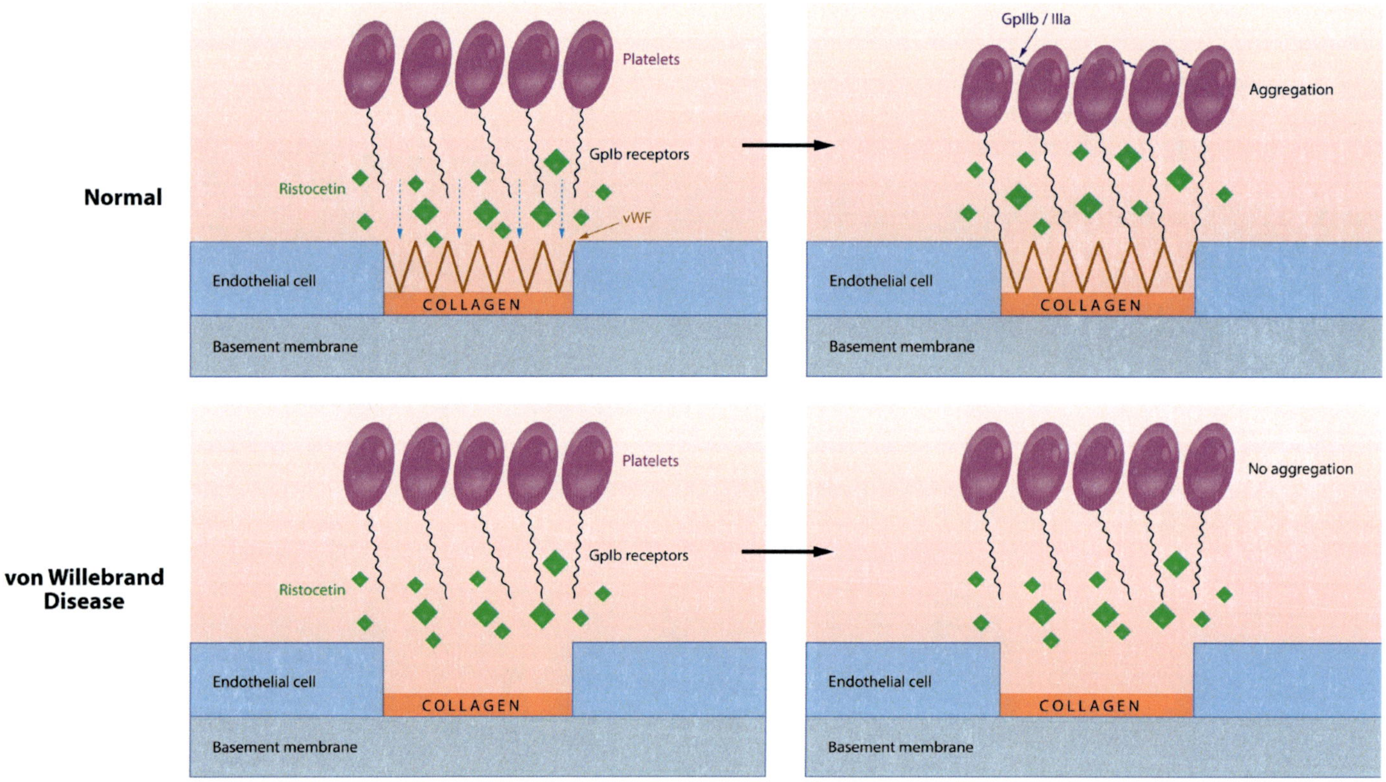

FIGURE 10.10.7 - Ristocetin Test

REVIEW QUESTIONS

1. A 5-year-old boy is brought to the emergency department due to bleeding that has persisted since a dental extraction earlier in the day. On physical examination, he has a slow oozing of blood at the site of extraction. The mother mentions her brother had a similar pattern of bleeding after dental procedures, as well as recurrent bleeding into his joints. What hematologic lab value is expected to be elevated in this patient?

- **The correct answer is PTT.**
- This patient most likely has a bleeding disorder as evidenced by the uncontrollable bleeding following a tooth extraction. This disorder may be inherited because the patient's maternal uncle has a history of hemarthrosis, or bleeding into the joint cavity.
- Since hemophilia A and B are X-linked disorders, they predominantly present in males. Both disorders cause a deficiency of clotting factors in the intrinsic pathway, so we would expect an increase in PTT. PT and bleeding time will be normal in hemophilia A and B.

2. An 8-year-old girl is brought to the emergency department with a nosebleed that has persisted for 30 minutes despite applying pressure. There are no signs of physical trauma. Her parents said that she has a history of frequent nosebleeds that last > 15 minutes. Laboratory results indicate a prolonged bleeding time, prolonged PTT, normal PT, normal TT, and normal D-dimer. Which of the following is most likely the diagnosis?

   A. Disseminated intravascular coagulopathy
   B. Vitamin K deficiency
   C. Von Willebrand disease
   D. Hemophilia A

- **The correct answer is C.**
- The patient has a history of frequent and prolonged nosebleeds, creating a clinical suspicion of an ongoing bleeding disorder. From the lab findings, both the bleeding time and the PTT are abnormal, which indicates a problem in both primary and secondary hemostasis. Von Willebrand disease presents with a complication in both primary and secondary hemostasis.
- This disorder causes low levels of von Willebrand factor and leads to impaired platelet adhesion in primary hemostasis and therefore increases the bleeding time. Low levels of von Willebrand factor also causes factor VIII levels to decrease because von Willebrand factor is responsible for stabilizing factor VIII and increasing its half-life. This explains the prolonged PTT seen in our patient.
- A is incorrect because coagulopathy is commonly seen in septic shock. Also, D-dimers are usually elevated in DIC, which is not seen in this patient.
- B and D are incorrect because although they could cause a rise in PTT, there would be no increase in the bleeding time as they only affect secondary hemostasis, not primary.

Section III - Other Disorders of Hemostasis

I. Heparin-Induced Thrombocytopenia
   A. Platelet destruction due to treatment with heparin
      1. Most common with unfractionated heparin
      2. Occurs 5-10 days following exposure
   B. Thrombocytopenia
   C. Arterial or venous thrombus

II. Heparin-Induced Thrombocytopenia: Pathophysiology
   A. Heparin binds to platelet factor 4 (PF4)
   B. Targeted by IgG antibodies for destruction in the spleen
   C. IgG-PF4-platelet complex causes platelet aggregation

III. Heparin-Induced Thrombocytopenia: Treatment
   A. Stop heparin
   B. Give any other anticoagulant except warfarin

IV. Disseminated Intravascular Coagulation
   A. Inappropriate, widespread activation of the coagulation cascade
   B. Clinical presentation
      1. Microthrombi formation
      2. Bleeding from mucosal surfaces and IV sites

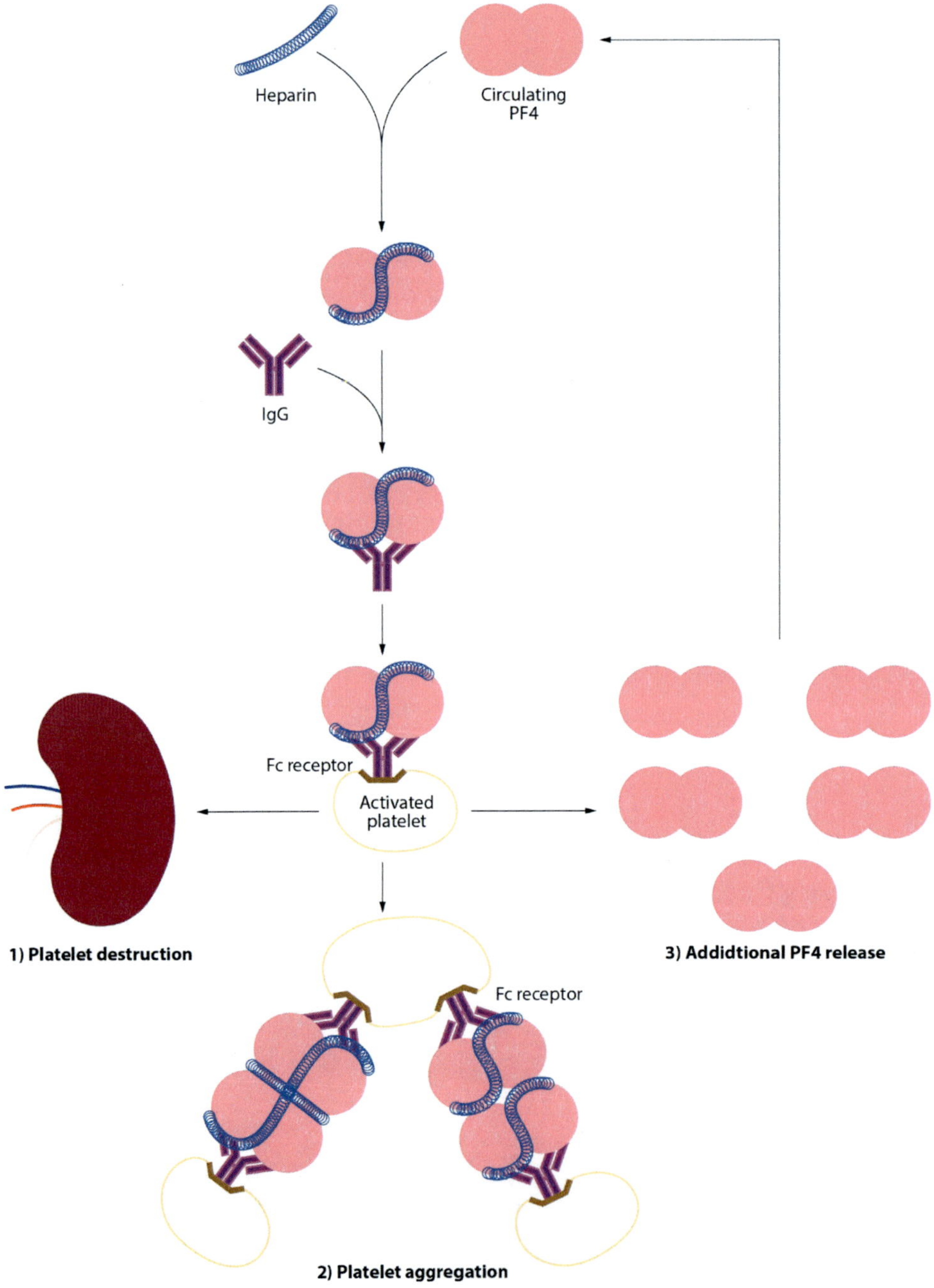

FIGURE 10.10.8 - Consequences of Antibody-Platelet Complexes

V. Disseminated Intravascular Coagulation: Etiology
   A. Trauma → exposes tissue factor
   B. Obstetric issue → tissue factor mixes with maternal circulation
   C. Sepsis (*E. coli* and *N. meningitidis*) → TNF and IL-1
   D. Rattlesnake bite → venom
   E. Malignancy
      1. Adenocarcinoma → mucin
      2. Acute promyelocytic leukemia → primary granules

VI. Disseminated Intravascular Coagulation: Lab Findings
   A. ↑ PT/PTT
   B. ↓ Platelet count
   C. ↑ Bleeding time
   D. ↑ D-dimer
   E. Microangiopathic hemolytic anemia
      1. Schistocytes on blood smear

VIII. Fibrinolysis
   A. Removes formed clot
   B. Plasminogen → plasmin by tPA
   C. Plasmin
      1. Breaks down fibrin and fibrinogen
      2. Degrades clotting factors
      3. Inhibits platelet aggregation
      4. Inactivated by α2-antiplasmin

IX. Disorders of Fibrinolysis
   A. Plasmin overactivity → excessive fibrinogen breakdown
      1. Fibrinogen is depleted
   B. Etiology
      1. Liver cirrhosis → decreased level of α2-antiplasmin
      2. Prostatectomy → urokinase activates plasmin

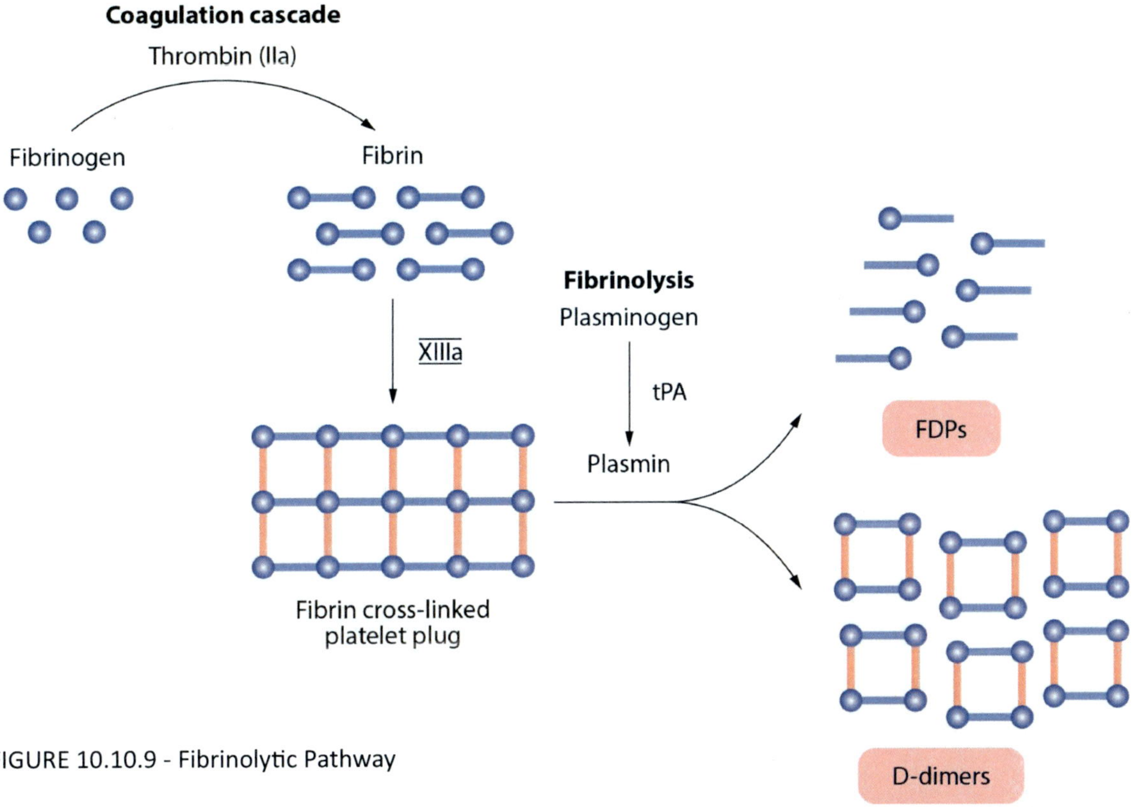

FIGURE 10.10.9 - Fibrinolytic Pathway

VII. Disseminated Intravascular Coagulation: Treatment
   A. Treat underlying pathology
   B. In the case of severe bleeding
      1. Blood product transfusion (platelets or fresh frozen plasma)
         a) Cryoprecipitate (fibrinogen and factor VIII)

X. Disorders of Fibrinolysis: Lab Findings
   A. ↑ PT/PTT
   B. ↑ bleeding time
   C. Normal platelet count
   D. ↑ FDPs
   E. No D-dimers

XI. Disorders of Fibrinolysis: Treatment
   A. Aminocaproic acid: inhibits conversion of plasminogen to plasmin

REVIEW QUESTIONS

1. A 28-year-old man is brought to the emergency department after a car accident. He has a pneumothorax and is in critical condition. A chest tube is placed. The next day, there is bleeding from the chest tube and around IV lines. How would the levels of fibrinogen and factor VIII most likely be altered in this patient?

    - **The correct answer is that the fibrinogen and factor VIII levels are both decreased.**
    - This patient was in a car accident. The trauma from this accident resulted in endothelial damage and overactivated the coagulation cascade, resulting in DIC. The bleeding from the chest tube and around the IV lines is a major clue that there is uncontrolled bleeding and DIC.
    - Recall that the end goal of the coagulation cascade is to form a stable, cross-linked fibrin clot. In order for this to happen, fibrinogen must be converted into fibrin. Therefore, fibrinogen levels are consumed and are therefore decreased.
    - In DIC, clotting factors such as factor VIII are also consumed, so factor VIII levels would also be decreased.

2. A 53-year-old male comes to the physician due to pain in his left leg. Venous duplex ultrasonography shows thrombosis of the left femoral vein. Lab studies show a platelet count of 200,000/mm^3 (normal: 150,000-400,000/mm^3), PT of 12 seconds (normal: 10-12 seconds), and PTT of 32 seconds (normal: 25-35 seconds). Treatment with heparin is initiated. Five days later, the platelet count is 120,000/mm^3. Which of the following factors predisposed this patient to this condition?

    A. Anti-platelet factor 4/heparin antibodies
    B. GPIb deficiency
    C. Acquired protein C deficiency
    D. Decreased ADAMTS13 level

- **The correct answer is A.**
- This man with pain in his left leg has a DVT, which has been confirmed by radiography. At this time, his platelet count is within normal limits. His PT and PTT are also normal. Five days after heparin is given, his platelet count drops to 120,000/mm^3. So we can conclude that the heparin probably induced this patient's thrombocytopenia, or in other words, he has heparin-induced thrombocytopenia.
- We are asked which of the following abnormalities contributes to the development of HIT. Recall that IgG antibodies are targeted against both heparin and platelet factor 4, which contributes to the development of thrombocytopenia as seen in this patient. More specifically, IgG-tagged platelets are targeted for destruction by the spleen. Another consequence of these antibody-platelet-heparin complexes is the tendency to cause platelet aggregation. This is what led to the development of this man's DVT.
- Choice B is referring to Bernard-Soulier syndrome. Bernard-Soulier syndrome is due to a GP1b deficiency, which impairs platelet adhesion. In this disorder, you would find mild thrombocytopenia because platelets that don't get used up in platelet plug formation get degraded and turned over. However, there is no association with heparin in Bernard-Soulier syndrome. Also, it wouldn't cause a DVT as seen in this patient.
- Choice C is incorrect because an acquired protein C deficiency would occur in the setting of warfarin therapy, not heparin. It would also most likely result in warfarin skin necrosis rather than what is being described in the question stem.
- Choice D is incorrect because it is referring to thrombotic thrombocytopenic purpura or TTP. TTP occurs with decreased levels of von Willebrand factor-cleaving protease enzyme ADAMTS13. Although thrombocytopenia is seen in this disorder, it more commonly presents alongside fever, microangiopathic hemolytic anemia, renal insufficiency, and neurologic dysfunction, all of which are absent in this patient.

Section IV - Red Blood Cell Morphology

I. Introduction
   A. RBC variants
   B. Associated diseases

RBC type	Key Features	Diseases
Acanthocytes	- "Spur cells" - Projections with various sizes and spacing	- Liver disease - Abetalipoproteinemia
Echinocytes	- "Burr cells" - Projections with small, uniform size and spacing	- Liver disease - End-stage rental disease - Pyruvate kinase deficiency
Dacrocytes	- "Tear drop cells"	- Bone marrow infiltrative/fibrotic diseases
Macro-ovalocytes	- Large - Oval-shaped	- Megaloblastic anemia
Schistocytes	- "Helmet cells" or "fragmented cells"	- Microangiopathic hemolytic anemias (TTP, HUS) - Mechanical damage (prosthetic heart valve) - HELLP syndrome - DIC
Degmacytes	- "Bite cells"	- Glucose-6-phosphate dehydrogenase deficiency
Elliptocytes	- Elipsis-shaped	- Hereditary elliptocytosis
Spherocytes	- Sphere-shaped	- Hereditary spherocytosis
Target cells	- Red dot in center - Resembles a target	- Thalassemia - Asplenia - Liver disease - Hemoglobin C disease
Sickle cells	- Sickle -haped - Half-moon	- Sickle cell disease

FIGURE 10.10.2 - Variants of RBCs

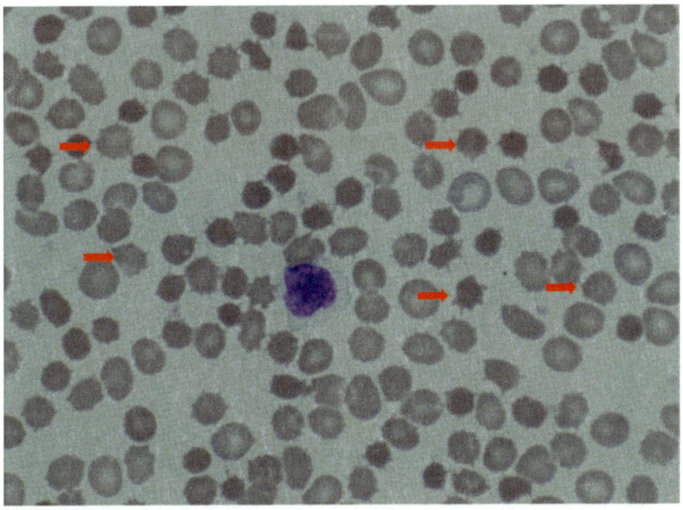

FIGURE 10.10.10 - Blood Smear Showing Spur Cells (Red Arrows)

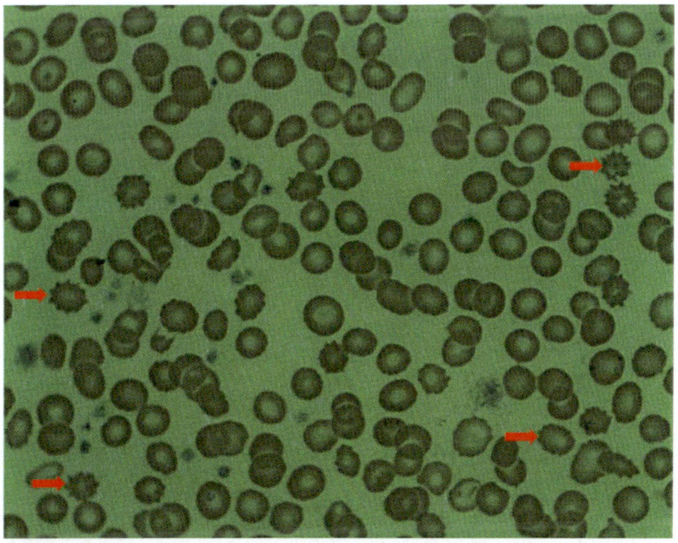

FIGURE 10.10.11 Blood Smear Showing Echinocytes and Burr Cells (Red Arrows)

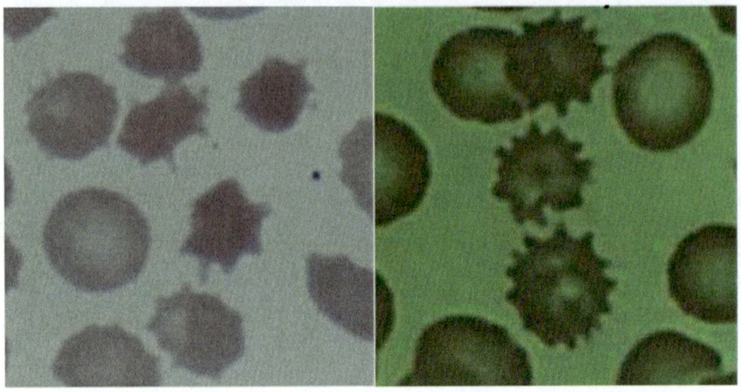

Photo Credit: Cropped: Rola Zamel, Razi Khan, Rebecca L Pollex and Robert A Hegele / CC BY (https://creativecommons.org/licenses/by/2.0) (left) Cropped: Osaretin / CC BY-SA (https://creativecommons.org/licenses/by-sa/4.0) (right)

FIGURE 10.10.12 - Acanthocyte (Left), Echinocyte (Right)

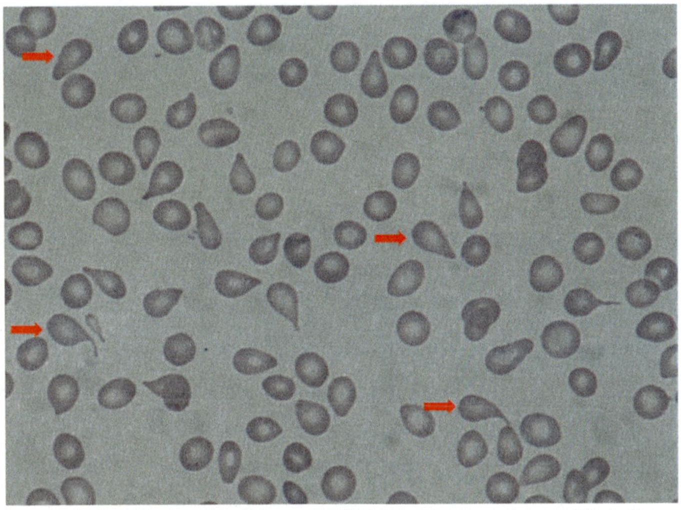

Photo Credit: Paulo Henrique Orlandi Mourao / CC BY-SA (https://creativecommons.org/licenses/by-sa/3.0). This image may have been modified by cropping, labeling, and/or captions.

FIGURE 10.10.13 - Blood Smear Showing Dacrocytes (Tear Drop Cells)

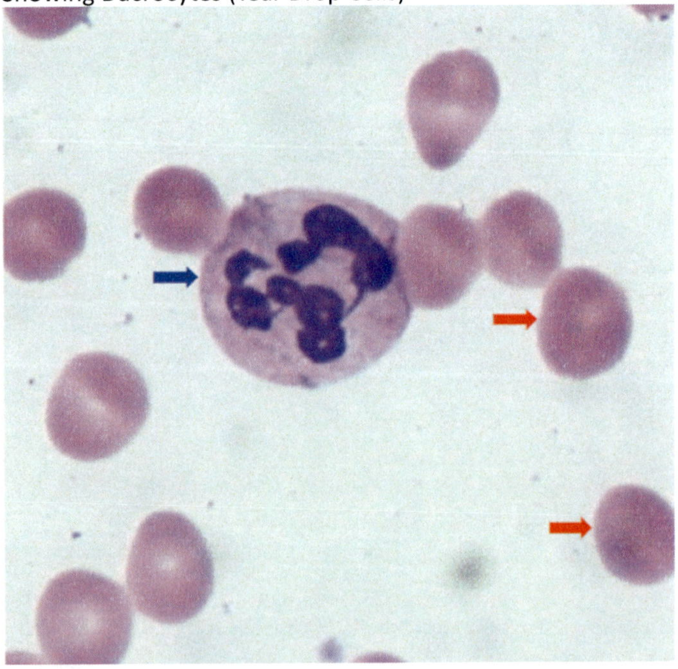

Photo Credit: https://www.flickr.com/photos/euthman/8612790151. This image may have been modified by cropping, labeling, and/or captions.

FIGURE 10.10.14 - Blood Smear Showing Macro-Ovalocytes (Red Arrows) and Hypersegmented Neutrophils (Blue Arrow)

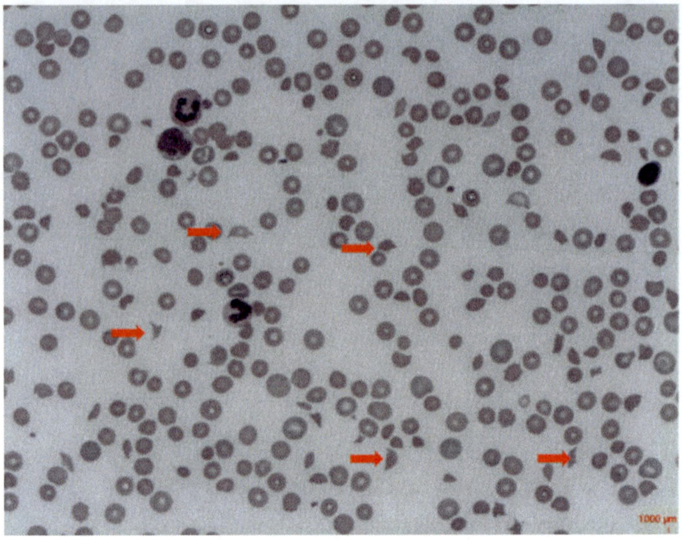

Photo Credit: Erhabor Osaro (Associate Professor) / CC BY-SA (https://creativecommons.org/licenses/by-sa/3.0). This image may have been modified by cropping, labeling, and/or captions.

FIGURE 10.10.15 - Blood Smear Showing Schistocytes (Fragment Cells)

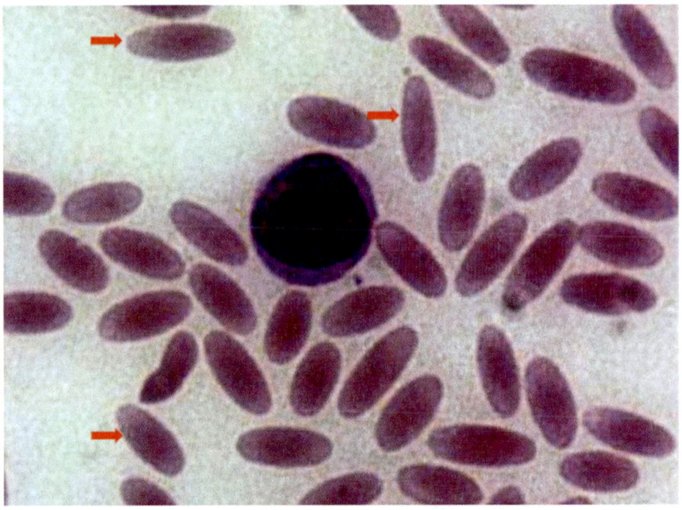

Photo Credit: TheNewMessiah at English Wikipedia / Public domain. This image may have been modified by cropping, labeling, and/or captions.

FIGURE 10.10.16 - Blood Smear Showing Elliptocytes

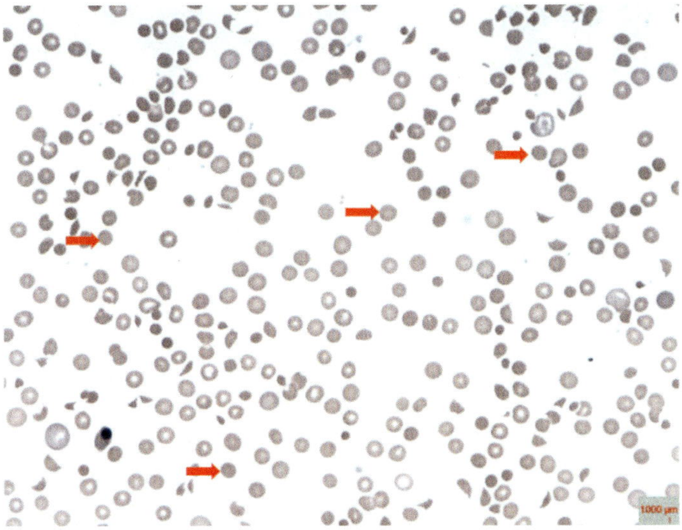

Photo Credit: Prof. Osaro Erhabor / CC0. This image may have been modified by cropping, labeling, and/or captions.

FIGURE 10.10.17 - Blood Smear Showing Spherocytes

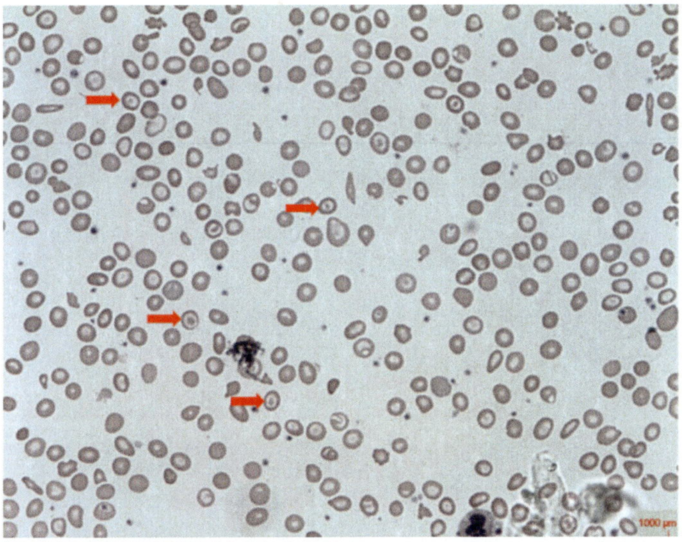

Photo Credit: Prof. Osaro Erhabor / CC0. This image may have been modified by cropping, labeling, and/or captions.

FIGURE 10.10.18 - Blood Smear showing Target Cells

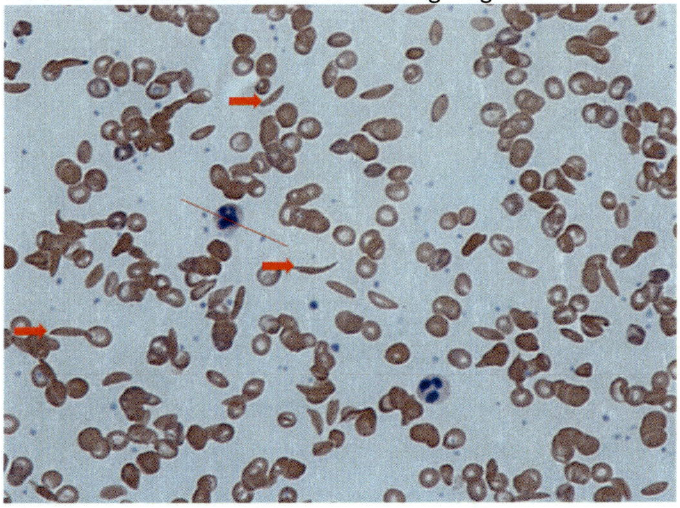

Photo Credit: Prof. Osaro Erhabor / CC0. This image may have been modified by cropping, labeling, and/or captions.

FIGURE 10.10.19 - Blood Smear Showing Sickle Cells

REVIEW QUESTIONS

1. A 66-year-old man with a history of rheumatic heart disease and subsequent mitral valve replacement with a prosthetic valve complains of fatigue, weakness, and shortness of breath. On physical exam he has conjunctival pallor. A CBC shows a hemoglobin of 9.0 g/dL (normal: 13-17 g/dL) but is otherwise normal. What will most likely be seen on peripheral blood smear?

   - **The correct answer is schistocytes.**
   - This is a 66-year-old man with a history of rheumatic heart disease who has had a mitral valve replacement with a prosthetic valve. His symptoms include fatigue, weakness, and shortness of breath which can be symptoms of anemia.
   - His hemoglobin is 9, which confirms he is anemic. On peripheral blood smear, we would expect to find schistocytes, which are also called fragmented cells or helmet cells. We expect this because he has a history of a prosthetic valve, which can cause mechanical damage to RBCs and cause anemia.

2. A 7-year-old African American boy comes to the physician with shortness of breath and severe bone pain most prominent near the left femur. His mom says that he was diagnosed with a blood disorder at birth. They recently moved to New Mexico and this is the second time this has happened to him since moving. What cell type would most likely be seen on peripheral blood smear?

   A. Dacrocytes
   B. Acanthocytes
   C. Spur cells
   D. Sickled cells
   E. Echinocytes

   - **The correct answer is D.**
   - This is a 7-year-old boy who has symptoms consistent with a sickle cell crisis. He was diagnosed with sickle cell disease at birth. He recently moved to an area of high altitude (New Mexico) that caused another sickle cell crisis. On peripheral blood smear, you would expect to see sickled cells.
   - A is incorrect because you would not see tear drop cells in sickle cell disease.
   - B and C are incorrect because they are the same cell type and you see them in liver disease and abetalipoproteinemia.
   - E is incorrect because you do not see echinocytes in sickle cell disease.

Section V - Microcytic Anemias

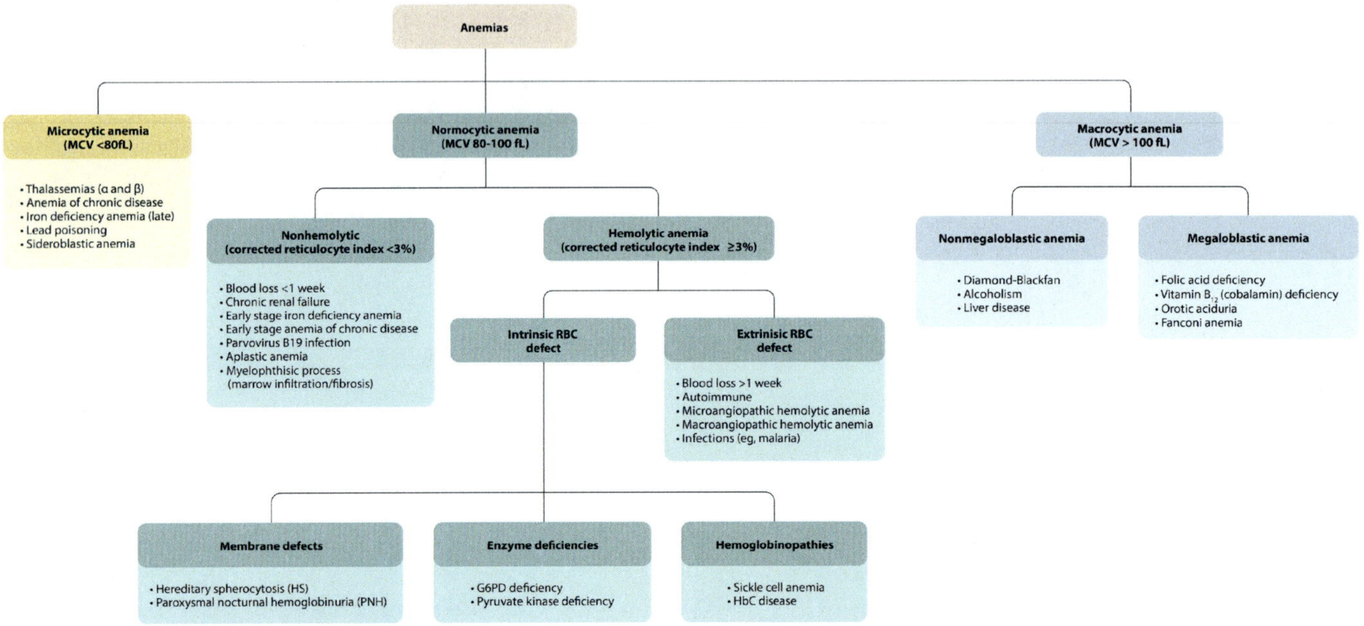

FIGURE 10.10.20 - Anemia Flowchart

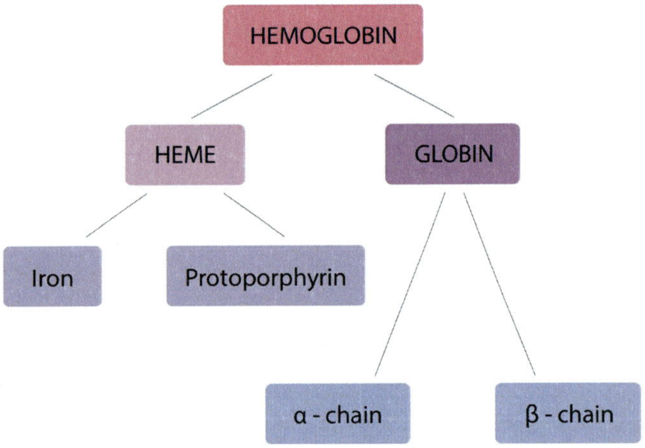

FIGURE 10.10.21 - Breakdown of Hemoglobin

I. Pathophysiology
   A. Decreased hemoglobin production → increased RBC division → microcytosis

II. Key Terms
   A. Serum iron: iron in blood
   B. Total iron-binding capacity (TIBC): transferrin molecules in blood
   C. % saturation: percentage of transferrin molecules bound by iron
   D. Serum ferritin: iron stores in macrophages and liver
   E. Red cell distribution width (RDW): variation in size of RBCs

III. Iron Deficiency Anemia: Causes
   A. Chronic bleeding
   B. Malnutrition, absorption disorders, or GI surgery
   C. Increased demand (pregnancy)

IV. Iron Deficiency Anemia: Clinical Findings
   A. Anemia: fatigue and conjunctival pallor
   B. Koilonychia
   C. Pica

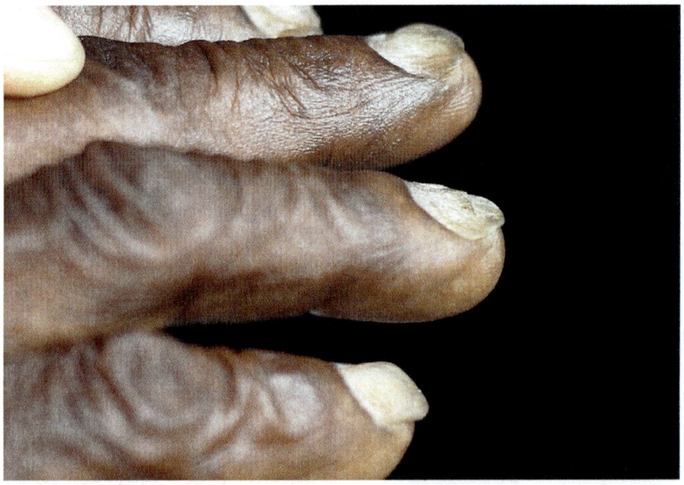

FIGURE 10.10.22 - Koilonychia (Spoon Nails)

V. Iron Deficiency Anemia: Lab Findings
   A. Microcytic, hypochromic RBCs
   B. Increased RDW
   C. Increased free erythrocyte protoporphyrin

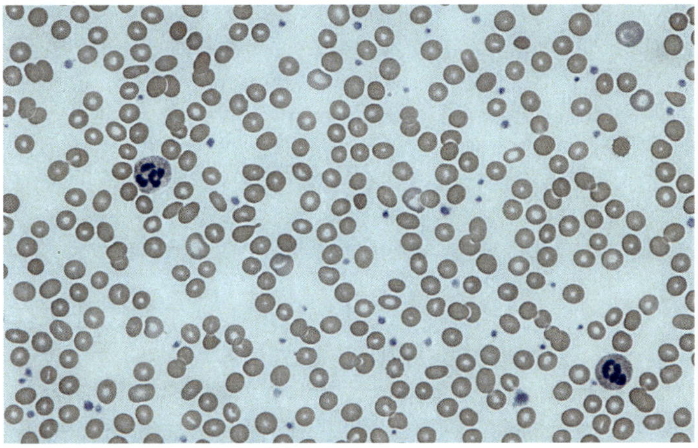

FIGURE 10.10.23 - Micrograph of Iron Deficiency Anemia

Type	Serum Iron	TIBC	% Saturation	Ferritin
Iron deficiency anemia	↓	↑	↓	↓
Anemia of chronic disease	↓	↓	↓	↑
Sideroblastic anemia	↑	↓	↑	↑

FIGURE 10.10.3 - Lab Findings for Various Anemias

VI. Anemia of Chronic Disease: Pathophysiology
   A. Increased production of hepcidin in liver
      1. Hepcidin sequesters iron → decrease in available iron → decreased heme → decreased hemoglobin
   B. Causes: chronic inflammation and cancer
   C. Treatment: treat underlying condition

VII. Sideroblastic Anemia: Pathophysiology
   A. Defective protoporphyrin synthesis → decreased heme → decreased hemoglobin
   B. Causes
      1. Congenital defect in aminolevulinic acid synthase (ALAS)
      2. Alcoholism
      3. Vitamin B_6 deficiency
      4. Lead poisoning

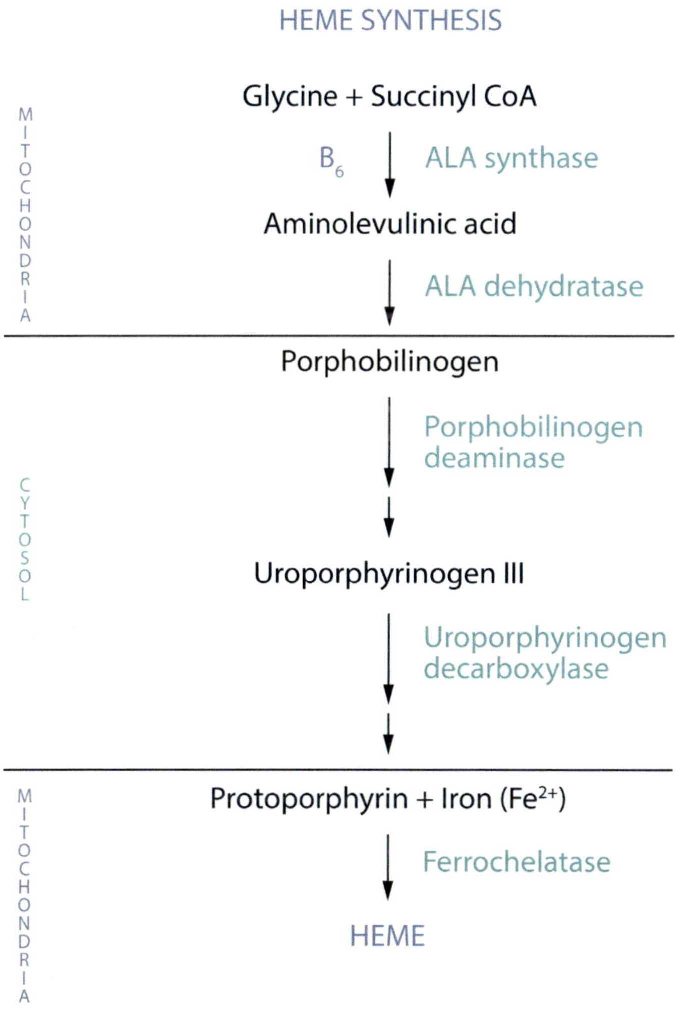

FIGURE 10.10.24 - Heme Synthesis Pathway

VIII. Lead Poisoning
  A. Inhibition of aminolevulinic acid dehydratase and ferrochelatase → decreased heme production
  B. Inhibition of rRNA degradation → basophilic stippling of RBCs

IX. Lead Poisoning: Clinical findings
  A. Lead lines on gingiva (Burton lines) and metaphysis of long bones
  B. Encephalopathy
  C. Abdominal colic
  D. Wrist and foot drop

X. Lead Poisoning: Treatment
  A. Dimercaprol and EDTA
  B. Succimer used for iron chelation in kids

XI. Sideroblastic Anemia: Lab Findings
  A. Bone marrow: ringed sideroblasts
    1. Nucleated RBCs with ring of iron-laden, Prussian blue-stained mitochondria around nucleus
  B. Peripheral blood smear: basophilic stippling of RBCs

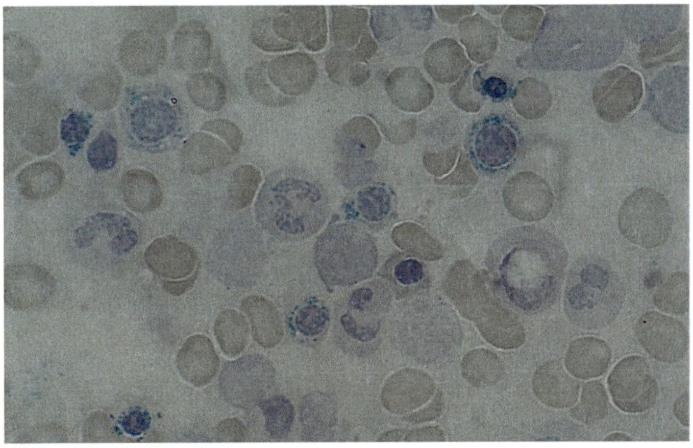

FIGURE 10.10.25 - Bone Marrow Micrograph of Patient with Sideroblastic Anemia

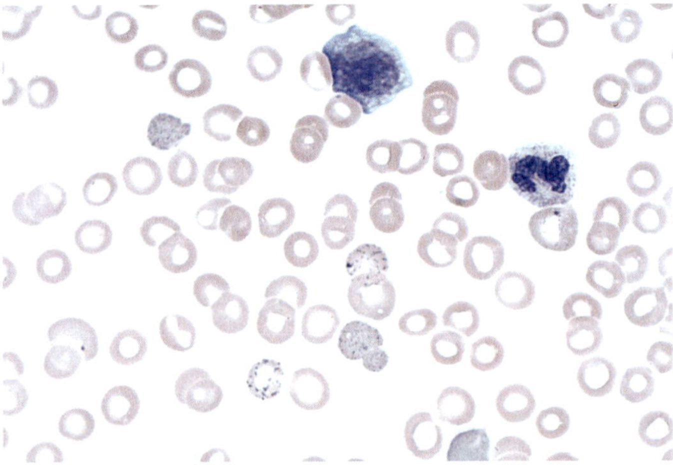

FIGURE 10.10.26 - Sideroblastic Anemia

XII. Sideroblastic Anemia: Treatment
  A. Pyridoxine (vitamin B_6)

REVIEW QUESTIONS

1. A 43-year-old woman presents with fatigue, cold intolerance, and heavy menstrual bleeding. Physical exam reveals conjunctival pallor. Laboratory studies show a hemoglobin of 7 g/dL (normal: 12-15.5 g/dL) and an MCV of 70 μm^3 (normal: 80-100 μm^3). What is the most likely underlying cause of this patient's symptoms?

- **The correct answer is iron deficiency anemia due to chronic blood loss.**
- The patient presents with fatigue, cold intolerance and conjunctival pallor. Her hemoglobin count of 7 g/dL and symptoms are most in line with anemia. Her MCV of 70 µm3 is consistent with microcytic anemia. Because she presented with heavy menstrual bleeding, the most likely cause of her anemia is iron deficiency anemia due to chronic blood loss.

2. A 33-year-old woman presents with a 3-day history of abdominal pain, muscle twitching in her upper extremities, and difficulty concentrating. Physical exam reveals conjunctival pallor, a high-step gait on the right side, decreased sensation in the right foot, and gingival Burton lines. She reveals that her roommate of 10 years is experiencing similar symptoms. What additional findings will most likely be discovered upon further evaluation?

   A. ↑ iron; ↑ TIBC; ↑ %saturation; ↑ ferritin
   B. ↓ iron; ↑ TIBC; ↓ %saturation; ↓ ferritin
   C. ↑ iron; ↓ TIBC; ↑ %saturation; ↑ ferritin
   D. ↓ iron; ↓ TIBC; ↓ %saturation; ↑ ferritin

- **The correct answer is C.**
- The patient presents with abdominal pain, muscle twitching, and difficulty concentrating, which are signs of encephalopathy. She has foot drop, Burton lines on her gingivae, and conjunctival pallor. The patient most likely has sideroblastic anemia due to lead poisoning.
- Sideroblastic anemia presents with elevated serum iron, % saturation, and ferritin. It is caused by a decrease in protoporphyrin synthesis. Protoporphyrin typically binds iron to form heme, so if protoporphyrin is low, then iron has nothing to bind to, resulting in high serum iron, elevated ferritin, and elevated % saturation. TIBC is low because there is so much iron that the transferrin becomes saturated, leading to a decreased total iron-binding capacity.
- A is incorrect because sideroblastic anemia is associated with a low TIBC.
- B is incorrect because these lab findings are associated with iron deficiency anemia.
- D is incorrect because these lab findings are associated with anemia of chronic disease.

Section VI - Thalassemias

I. Hemoglobin Development
   A. Embryonic globin (ε and ζ): first few months of development
   B. HbF ($\alpha_2\gamma_2$): 6 weeks (fetus) to 9 weeks (postpartum)
   C. HbA ($\alpha_2\beta_2$): 9 weeks (postpartum) to adulthood
   D. HbA_2 ($\alpha_2\delta_2$): present in small amounts in adults

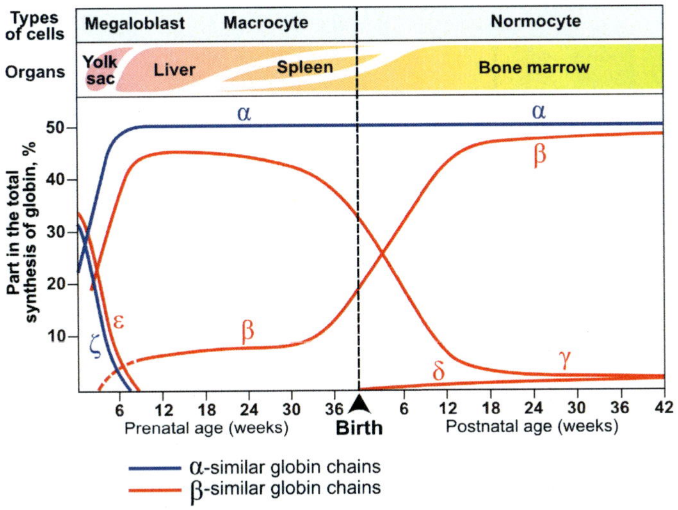

Photo Credit: Postnatal_genetics.svg: original: Furfur, File:Haemoglobin-Ketten.svg, derivation/translation:Leonid 2derivative work: Leonid 2 / CC BY-SA (https://creativecommons.org/licenses/by-sa/3.0)

FIGURE 10.10.27 - Hemoglobin Development

II. Definition
   A. Anemia due to decreased synthesis of globin chains of hemoglobin
   B. Inherited mutations

III. α-thalassemia
   A. Due to an α-globin gene deletion.
   B. Four α genes are normally present on chromosome 16.
   C. Types
      1. α-thalassemia minima
      2. α-thalassemia minor
      3. Hemoglobin H disease (HbH)
      4. Hemoglobin Bart's disease

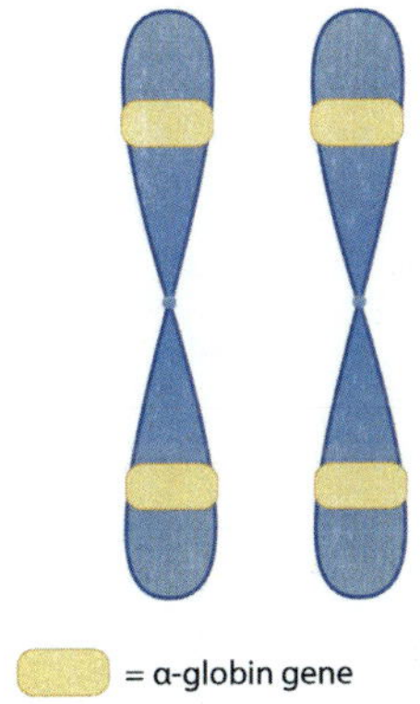

FIGURE 10.10.28 - Normal Chromosome 16

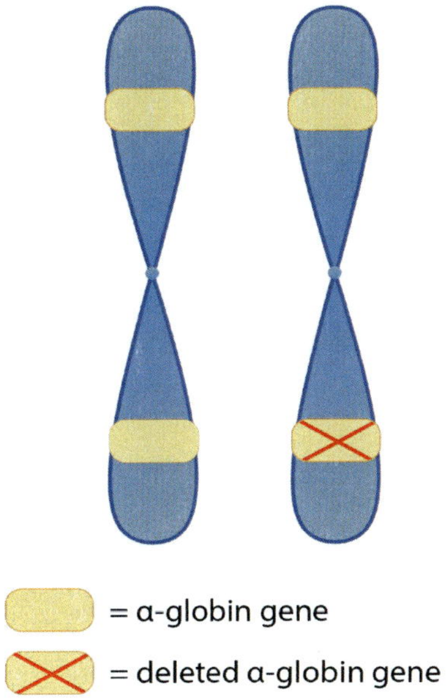

FIGURE 10.10.29 - Chromosome 16 in Thalassemia Minima

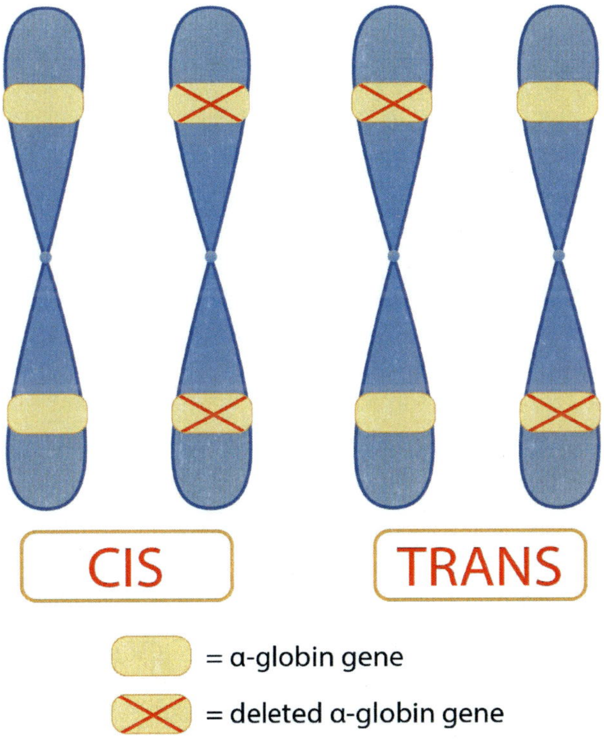

FIGURE 10.10.30 - Chromosome 16 in α-Thalassemia Minor

IV. α-thalassemia Minor
   A. Mild anemia with elevated RBC count
   B. *Cis* deletion: Asian descent
   C. *Trans* deletion: African descent

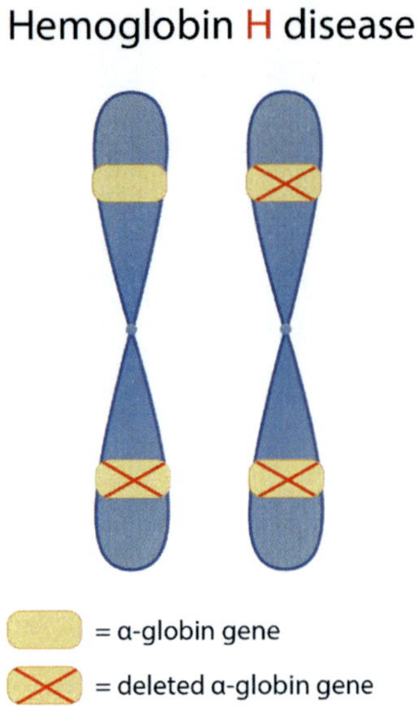

FIGURE 10.10.31 - Chromosome 16 in HbH Disease

V. Hemoglobin H Disease (HbH)
   A. One functional α-globin gene
      1. Excess β-globin forms $β_4$ (HbH) → RBC damage
   B. Moderate to severe microcytic hypochromic anemia
   C. HbH seen on hemoglobin electrophoresis

VI. Hemoglobin Bart's Disease
   A. No α-globin production
   B. Excess γ-globin forms $γ_4$ → RBC damage
   C. Lethal in utero (hydrops fetalis)

VII. β-Thalassemia
   A. Two β-globin genes on chromosome 11
   B. Point mutations in promoter or splicing sites affect β-globin production
      1. Absent β-globin = $β^0$
      2. Diminished β-globin = $β^+$

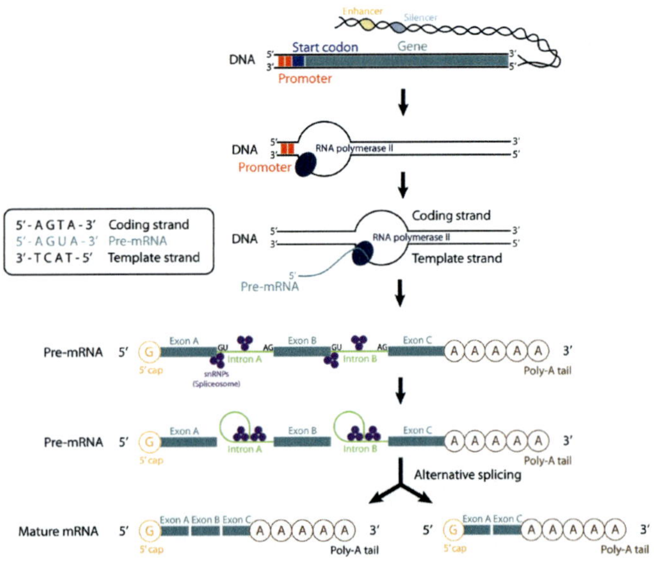

FIGURE 10.10.32 - Splicing in DNA Transcription

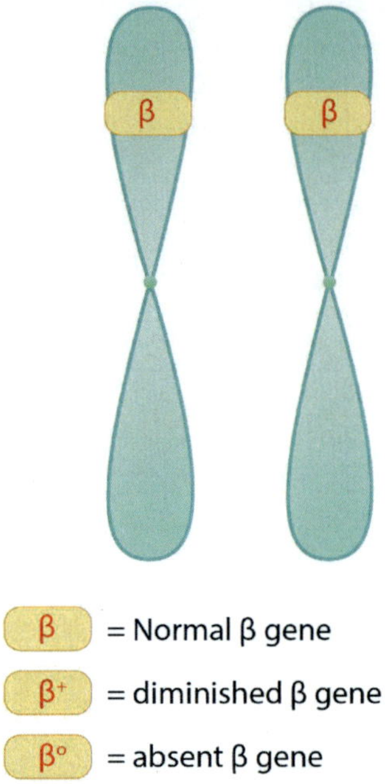

FIGURE 10.10.33 - Normal Chromosome 11

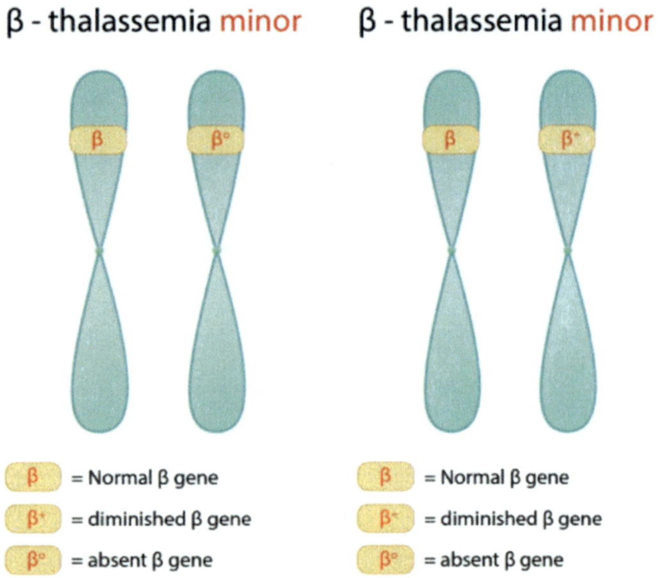

FIGURE 10.10.34 - Chromosome 11 in β-Thalassemia Minor

VIII. β-Thalassemia
   A. Types
      1. β-thalassemia minor ($β/β^+$ or $β/β^0$)
      2. β-thalassemia major ($β^0/β^0$)
      3. HbS/β-thalassemia heterozygote

IX. β-thalassemia Minor: Clinical Findings
   A. Asymptomatic with elevated RBC count
   B. Peripheral blood smear: microcytic hypochromic RBCs and target cells
   C. Electrophoresis: decreased HbA (normal adult Hb), increased HbA_2 (> 3.5%), and HbF
   D. Severe anemia six months after birth
   E. Peripheral blood smear: microcytic hypochromic RBCs, target cells, and nucleated RBCs
   F. Electrophoresis: elevated HbA_2 and HbF with little/no HbA (normal adult Hb)

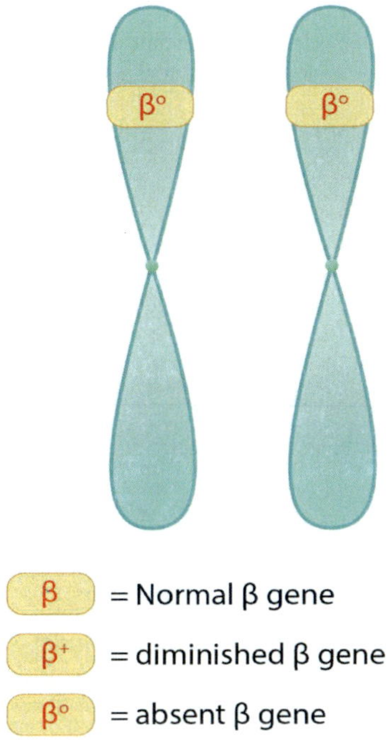

FIGURE 10.10.35 - Chromosome 11 in β-Thalassemia Major

X. β-Thalassemia Major: Pathophysiology
   A. Absent β-globin chain → α chains deposit → damage RBC membrane
      1. Extravascular hemolysis
      2. Ineffective erythropoiesis
         a) Crewcut skull on X-ray
         b) Chipmunk facies
         c) Hepatosplenomegaly

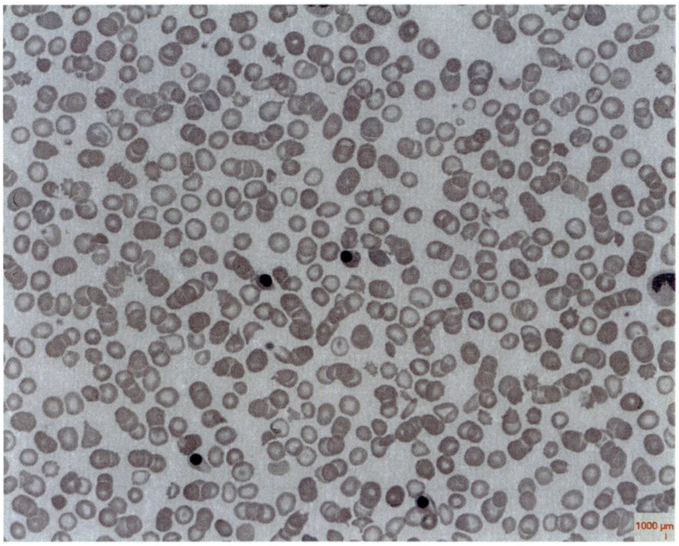

FIGURE 10.10.36 - Peripheral Blood Smear in β-Thalassemia Major

XI. β-Thalassemia Major: Treatment and Complications
   A. Treatment: chronic blood transfusion
   B. Complications
      1. Secondary hemochromatosis
      2. Parvovirus B19 infection → aplastic crisis

XII. HbS/β-Thalassemia Heterozygote
   A. Mild to moderate sickle cell disease

REVIEW QUESTIONS

1. A 25-year-old Asian American man presents for a routine physical exam. Laboratory results reveal a mild, microcytic anemia. A peripheral blood smear shows small, hypochromic red blood cells. He has concerns about having children with his condition. He states that his wife has α-thalassemia minima. What is the worst possible outcome for their future child?

- **The correct answer is hemoglobin H disease, which has three α-globin gene deletions.**
- We have an Asian American man with mild, microcytic anemia with small hypochromic red blood cells. It's most likely that this man has α-thalassemia minor.
- As an Asian American man, he most likely has the *cis* deletion form of α-thalassemia minor. This means that both gene deletions are on the same chromosome.
- We are told that he is planning to have a child with a woman who has α-thalassemia minima.
- The father can pass down either a completely normal chromosome or a chromosome with no α-chains.
- The mother can pass down either a completely normal chromosome or a chromosome with one alpha chain deletion.

2. An 11-month-old boy is brought in by his mother due to failure to thrive. His hemoglobin level is extremely low. Peripheral blood smear reveals very small red blood cells with marked central pallor. Electrophoresis reveals low levels of HbA with elevated levels of HbA_2 and HbF. Which of the following underlying mechanisms is most likely responsible for the findings seen in this patient?

   A. An amino acid substitution in β-globin
   B. An antibody against fetal blood cells
   C. Insufficient production of α-globin
   D. Insufficient production of β-globin

- **The correct answer is D.**
- A baby boy presents with failure to thrive with an extremely low hemoglobin count.
- His peripheral blood smear reveals microcytosis (very small red blood cells) with target cells (marked central pallor).
- Electrophoresis reveals very low levels of HbA with elevated HbA_2 and HbF.
- This patient likely has β-thalassemia.
- Remember that electrophoresis for β-thalassemia major shows elevated HbA_2 and HbF with little or no HbA.
- Also, notice that the boy didn't present with symptoms until after 6 months, which is consistent with β-thalassemia major.
- A is incorrect because an amino acid substitution in β-globin occurs in sickle cell anemia, not thalassemia. Sickle cell anemia is also a normocytic anemia, not a microcytic anemia as described here.
- B is incorrect because an antibody against fetal blood cells describes hemolytic disease of the newborn.
- C is incorrect because insufficient production of α-globin occurs in α-thalassemia. α-thalassemia does not present with target cells.

Section VII - Nonhemolytic Anemia

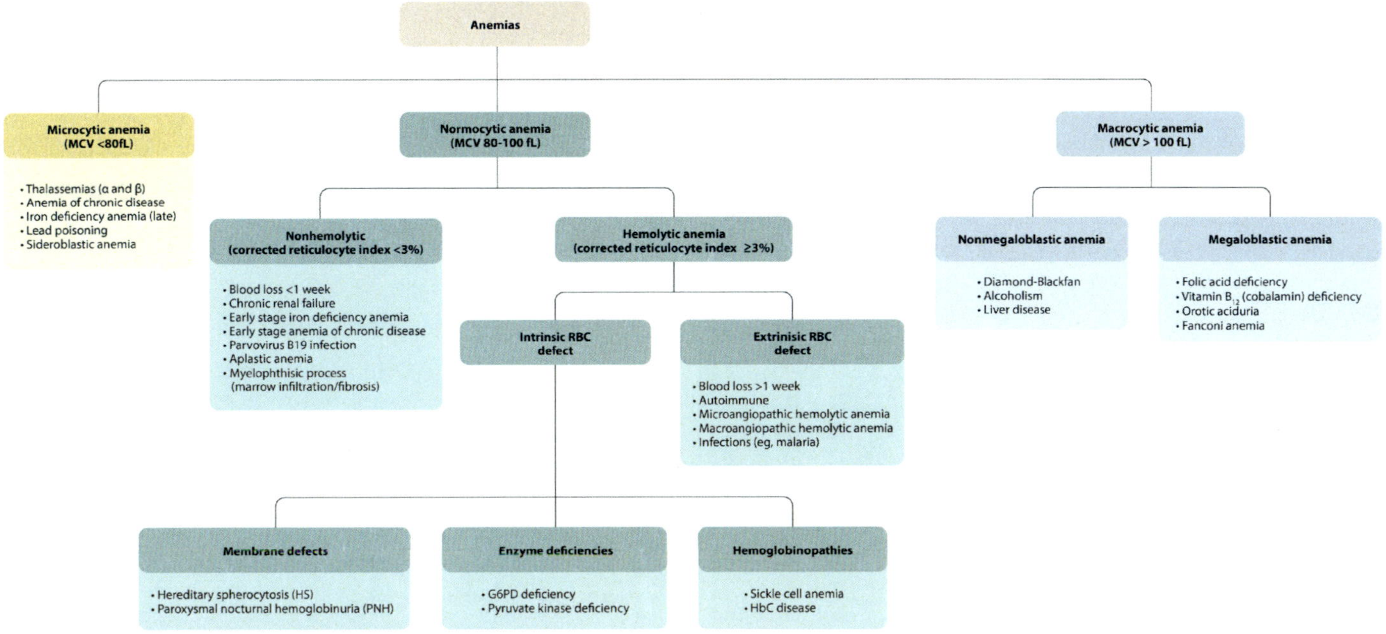

FIGURE 10.10.20 - Anemia Flowchart

I. Reticulocytes
   A. Immature RBCs containing residual RNA
   B. Reticulocyte count: 1-2%
      1. Reduced in nonhemolytic anemias
      2. Elevated in hemolytic anemias
   C. Reticulocyte count can be erroneously elevated on lab tests in anemia
   D. Nonhemolytic anemia: < 3% corrected reticulocyte index

II. Corrected reticulocyte index
   A. Corrected Reticulocyte Index = r(reticulocyte %) * (actual Hct) ÷ (normal Hct)
      1. Normal Hct = 45%
      2. Corrected reticulocyte index = (reticulocyte %) * (actual Hct) ÷ 45
      3. > 3 % → appropriate response
      4. < 3 % → inappropriate response

III. Etiologies of Nonhemolytic Anemia
   A. Acute blood loss
   B. Chronic renal failure
   C. Parvovirus B19 infection
   D. Aplastic anemia
   E. Myelophthisic process

IV. Acute Blood Loss
   A. Acute blood loss (< 1 week)
   B. Hemorrhage → Hgb, Hct and RBC are normal
   C. Compensation → dilution of RBCs → ↓ Hgb, ↓ Hct and ↓ RBC

V. Chronic Renal Failure
   A. Chronic renal failure (decreased erythropoietin)
   B. Decreased RBC production by bone marrow

VI. Parvovirus B19
   A. Non-enveloped DNA virus
   B. Affects the erythroid progenitor cells → halts the production of RBCs
   C. Usually self-limiting
   D. Aplastic crises in hemolytic anemias (e.g. sickle cell anemia)
   E. Supportive treatment

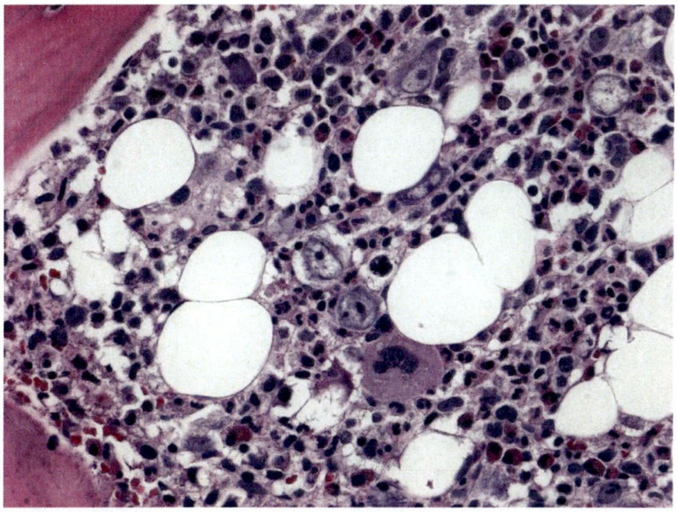

Photo Credit: https://www.flickr.com/photos/drbloodmoney/108793743

FIGURE 10.10.37 - Bone Marrow Biopsy Showing Parvovirus B19

VII. Aplastic Anemia
- A. Hematopoietic failure and associated pancytopenia.
- B. Anemia: fatigue, pallor, lethargy, weakness and exertional dyspnea
- C. Thrombocytopenia: petechiae and ecchymoses
- D. Leukopenia: sudden onset of chills, fever, recurrent infections
- E. Splenomegaly is absent

Causes	Comments
Idiopathic	- Most cases of aplastic anemia are idiopathic (65 %)
Drugs (MNEMONIC: 3 CS)	- Chemotherapy - Carbamazepine - Chloramphenicol - Sulfonamides
Toxins and radiation	- Benzene - Gasoline - Tobacco smoke
Infections	- Hepatitis - Parvovirus B19 infections - EBV

TABLE 10.10.4 - Causes of Aplastic Anemia

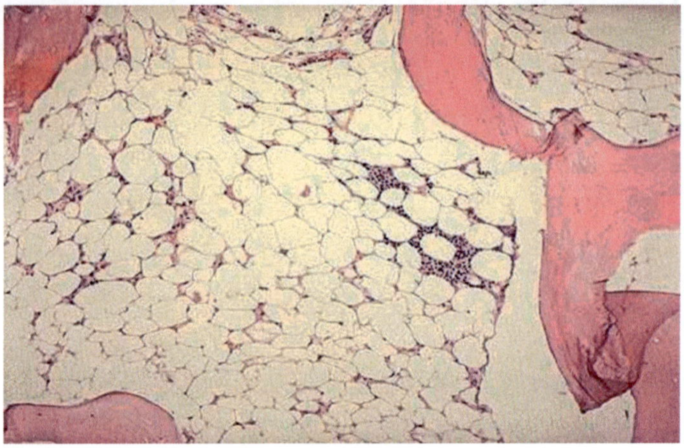

Photo Credit: https://www.flickr.com/photos/92708411@N07/8549744703

FIGURE 10.10.38 - Bone Marrow Biopsy Showing Aplastic Anemia

VIII. Aplastic Anemia: Treatment
- A. Supportive
- B. Blood transfusions
- C. Bone marrow stimulation (G-CSF, GM-CSF)
- D. Discontinue drugs or other causatives
- E. Bone marrow transplantation

IX. Myelophthisic Process
- A. Space-occupying lesions replace normal marrow elements leading to marrow failure
- B. Causes: any infiltrative process, metastatic cancer (e.g. breast, lung, prostate)
- C. Hematopoietic failure leads to pancytopenia.

REVIEW QUESTIONS

1. A medical student is given a complete blood count report. The report shows a hematocrit of 29% and a reticulocyte count of 1.5%. Calculate the corrected reticulocyte index.

- **The correct answer is 0.96%**
- If we recall the formula, we can calculate the corrected reticulocyte index by multiplying the reticulocyte % with the ratio of actual hematocrit and 45.
- The reticulocyte % in this question is 1.5% and the hematocrit is 29%.
- Plugging in the values 1.5% x (29/45), we get a corrected reticulocyte index of 0.96%.
- This is a decreased value and the patient's bone marrow response to anemia is poor and inadequate.
- This question also shows that reticulocyte % is falsely elevated and that is why the corrected reticulocyte index is a more informative parameter.

2. A 32-year-old female with a history of a recent urinary tract infection presents to the clinic with complaints of fatigue, lethargy and generalized weakness for the past 2 weeks. Her temperature is 37.1 °C (98.78 °F), blood pressure is 115/80 mmHg, respiratory rate is 18/min, and pulse is 97/min. Physical examination reveals conjunctival pallor and multiple bruises on her arms. A complete blood count shows normochromic normocytic anemia. A bone marrow biopsy is performed, which reveals a hypocellular marrow filled with fat cells and marrow stroma. Which of the following conditions is most likely?

   A. Vitamin B12 deficiency
   B. Myelodysplastic syndrome
   C. Folate deficiency
   D. Aplastic anemia

- **The correct answer is D.**
- Fatigue, lethargy and generalized weakness are symptoms of anemia. Pallor is a sign of anemia.
- Multiple bruises point towards thrombocytopenia.
- Hypocellular bone marrow filled with fat cells and marrow stroma is a classical finding of aplastic anemia.
- The patient has a recent history of UTI, which implies that she may have been treated with sulfonamides like trimethoprim-sulfamethoxazole, which are a cause of aplastic anemia.
- B is incorrect. Myelodysplastic syndrome is characterized by a defect in stem cell maturation. This defect leads to abnormal cell line production and pancytopenia.
- Myelodysplastic syndrome is marked by a hypercellular marrow with increased blast forms.
- A and C are incorrect. B12 deficiency and folate deficiency are both characterized by macrocytic anemia, not normocytic anemia.

Section VIII - Hemolytic Anemia (Intrinsic Causes)

I. Sickle Cell Disease
   A. Autosomal recessive
      1. Point mutation in β-globin gene: Glu → Val (HbS)
      2. Heterozygotes asymptomatic, homozygotes have disease
   B. Two defective β-globin genes → HbS
   C. HbS forms tetramers that polymerize and sickle when deoxygenated
   D. In US, predominantly seen in African Americans
   E. Protective role against malaria

II. Sickle Cell Disease: Clinical Findings
   A. Pallor
   B. Fatigue
   C. Extravascular hemolysis:
      1. Jaundice
      2. Hepatosplenomegaly
   D. Vaso-occlusive crises: due to dehydration, hypoxemia, or acidosis
      1. Dactylitis, avascular necrosis, and priapism
      2. Acute chest syndrome
      3. Parvovirus B19 → aplastic crisis
      4. Splenic sequestration
      5. End organ damage: renal papillary necrosis and autosplenectomy
   E. ↑ risk of infection from encapsulated organisms following splenectomy
      1. H. influenzae
      2. S. pneumoniae
      3. Salmonella osteomyelitis

III. Sickle Cell Disease: Lab Findings
   A. Hemoglobin electrophoresis
      1. Normal: > 90% HbA, < 5% HbA2
      2. Sickle cell disease: > 90% HbS
      3. Sickle cell trait: < 50% HbS, ↓ HbA
   B. Blood smear: sickled RBCs, target cells, Howell-Jolly bodies
   C. Intravascular hemolysis: ↓ haptoglobin, hemoglobinemia, and hemoglobinuria
   D. X-ray: crew-cut skull
   E. Metabisulfite screen: RBC sickling if HbS is present

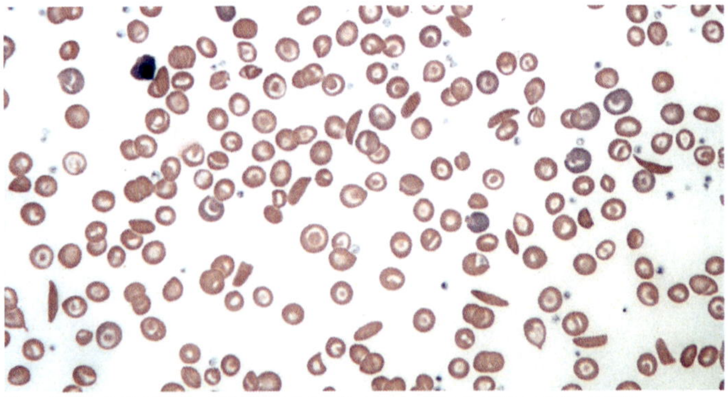

FIGURE 10.10.39 - Blood Smear of Sickle Cell Anemia

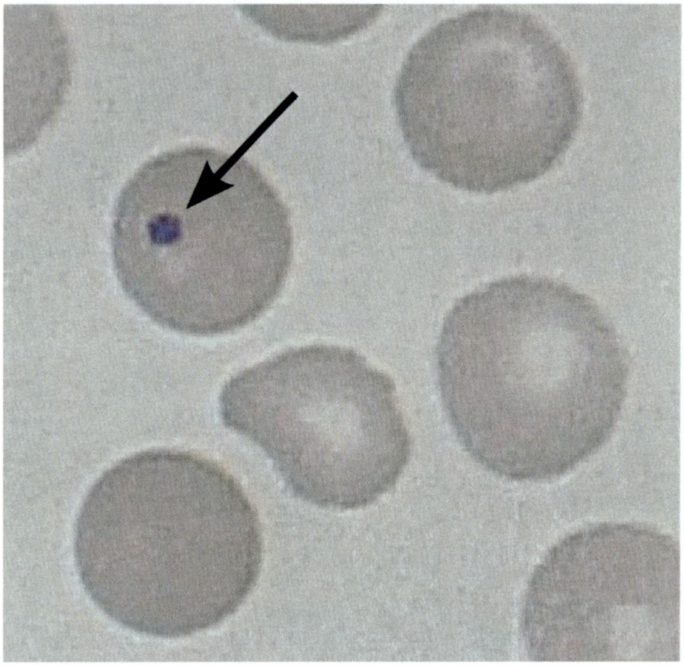

FIGURE 10.10.40 - Howell-Jolly Bodies in Sickle Cell Anemia

IV. Sickle Cell Disease: Treatment
   A. Vaso-occlusive crises: oxygen, hydration, and analgesics
   B. Long-term management
      1. Hydroxyurea: increases HbF levels
      2. Pneumococcal vaccine

V. Hereditary Spherocytosis
   A. Defects in RBC cytoskeleton-membrane binding proteins
      1. Ankyrin, spectrin, band 3, and protein 4.2
      2. Autosomal dominant
      3. Northern European descent
   B. Cells are spherical (spherocytes) instead of biconcave
      1. Consumed by splenic macrophages → extravascular hemolysis

VI. Hereditary Spherocytosis: Clinical/Lab Findings
   A. Extravascular hemolysis: splenomegaly, jaundice, and ↑ unconjugated bilirubin
   B. Parvovirus B19 → aplastic crisis
   C. Blood smear: spherocytes, ↑ MCHC, and ↑ RDW
   D. Osmotic fragility test: RBCs swell and burst
   E. Eosin 5-maleimide binding test

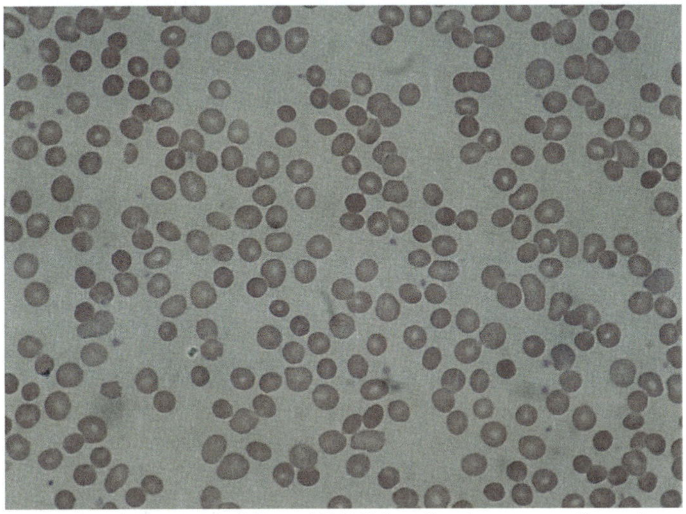

FIGURE 10.10.41 - Blood Smear of Hereditary Spherocytosis

VII. Hereditary Spherocytosis: Treatment
- A. Splenectomy
  1. Anemia resolves
  2. Spherocytes persist
  3. Howell-Jolly bodies emerge

VIII. G6PD Deficiency
- A. X-linked recessive
- B. African and Mediterranean populations
- C. Decreased G6PD → decreased reduction of glutathione
  1. ↓ NADPH → ↓ reduced glutathione → ↑ RBC oxidative injury
  2. Intravascular hemolysis
- D. Protection against malaria

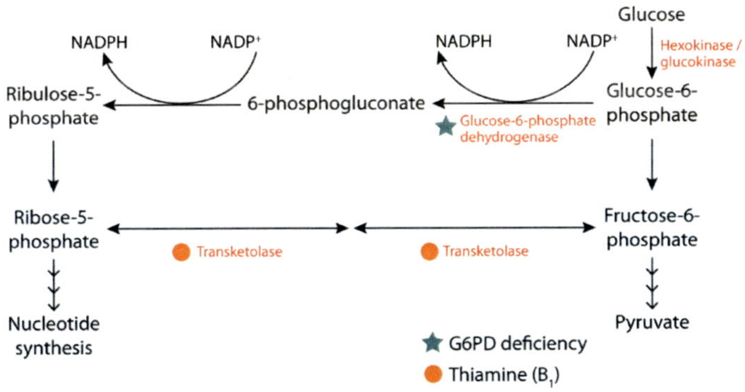

FIGURE 10.10.42 - HMP Shunt

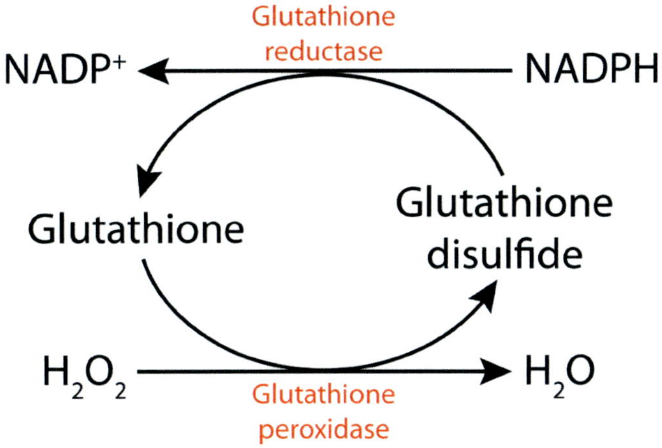

FIGURE 10.10.43 - Glutathione Oxidation and Reduction Reaction

IX. G6PD Deficiency: Clinical/Lab Findings
- A. Fatigue, back pain, and dark urine after oxidative stress
  1. Infection, fava beans, sulfa drugs, primaquine, dapsone
- B. Intravascular hemolysis: ↓ haptoglobin, hemoglobinuria, ↑ LDH, and ↑ unconjugated bilirubin
- C. Blood smear: Heinz bodies and bite cells

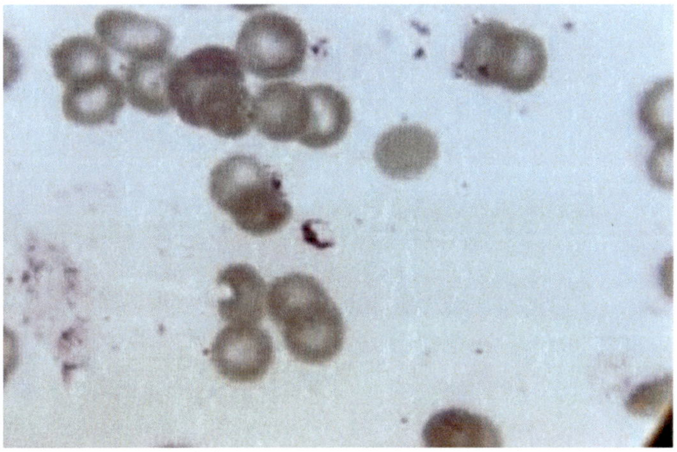

Photo Credit: Author: N. J. Wheeler, Jr, USCDCP

FIGURE 10.10.44 - Blood Smear of G6PD Deficiency

X. Pyruvate Kinase Deficiency
- A. Autosomal recessive
- B. Defective pyruvate kinase enzyme
  1. Irreversible step in glycolysis
- C. ↓ glycolysis = ↓ ATP
  1. Rigid RBCs → extravascular hemolysis

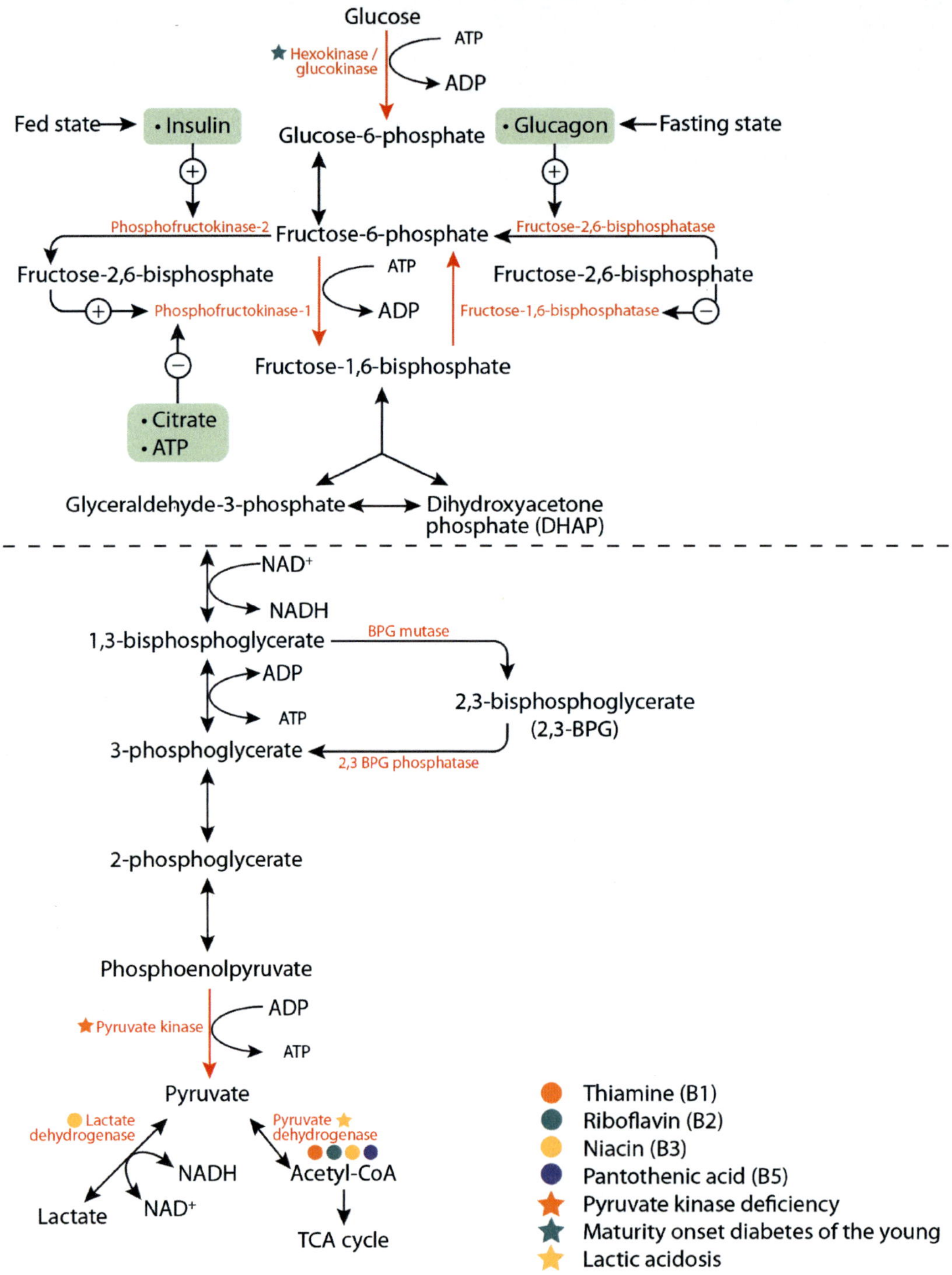

FIGURE 10.10.45 - Glycolysis

XI. Pyruvate Kinase Deficiency: Clinical/Lab Findings
   A. Hemolytic anemia in newborns
   B. Extravascular hemolysis: jaundice and hepatosplenomegaly
   C. ↑ 2,3-BPG
   D. Blood smear: echinocytes (burr cells)

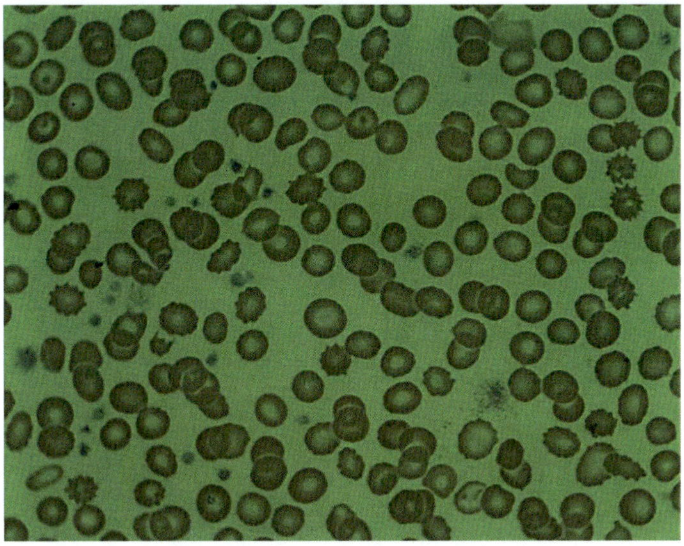

FIGURE 10.10.46 -Blood Smear of Pyruvate Kinase Deficiency

XII. Paroxysmal Nocturnal Hemoglobinuria
   A. Hematopoietic stem cell mutation in *PIGA* gene
      1. Impaired glycosylphosphatidylinositol (GPI) synthesis
   B. DAF (CD55) and MIRL (CD59) anchor to RBC membrane via GPI
      1. ↓ GPI → ↓ DAF and MIRL → ↑ complement destruction
   C. Episodic intravascular hemolysis
      1. Occurs at night due to mild respiratory acidosis
      2. Presents with dark urine in morning

XIII. Paroxysmal Nocturnal Hemoglobinuria: Clinical Findings and Treatment
   A. Classic triad: Coombs negative hemolytic anemia, pancytopenia, and venous thrombosis
   B. Intravascular hemolysis: hemoglobinuria, hemoglobinemia, and hemosiderinuria
   C. Positive sucrose lysis test
   D. Negative CD55/CD59 on flow cytometry
   E. Treatment: eculizumab

XIV. HbC Disease
   A. Autosomal recessive
      1. Mutation of β chain of hemoglobin: Glu → Lys (HbC)
   B. Extravascular hemolysis
   C. Blood smear: HbC crystals and target cells

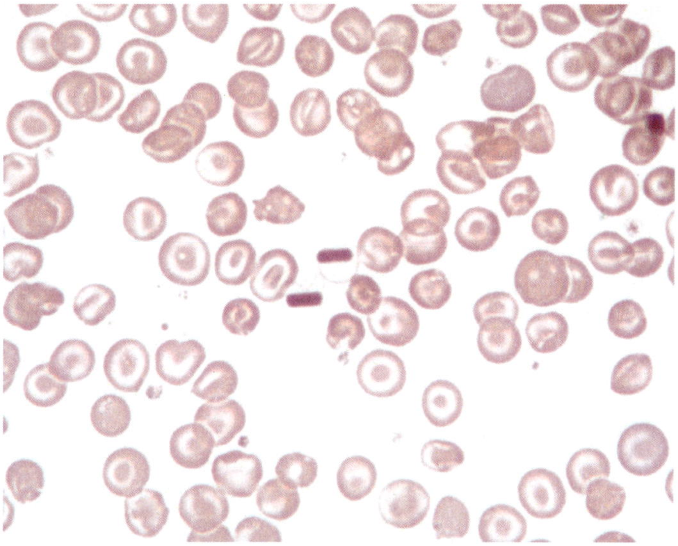

FIGURE 10.10.47 - Blood Smear of HbC Disease

REVIEW QUESTIONS

1. A 28-year-old previously healthy male presents to the physician with fatigue and left upper quadrant pain and swelling for the past day. Upon further investigation, he admits to multiple, transient episodes similar to this one. He states that his "skin turns yellow" during these episodes. His father has had similar episodes his entire life, and had to have his spleen removed as a result. The patient recently immigrated from Norway and started a new job last week that has caused him to be highly emotionally stressed. On physical exam, his skin is jaundiced with scleral icterus, and his abdomen is full and tender in the left upper quadrant. Based on his history and physical exam findings, what is the likely mode of inheritance of this condition, and what would you expect to see on a blood smear?

- **The correct answer is autosomal dominant inheritance with spherocytes on blood smear.**
- The important thing to recognize here is that this patient is presenting with the classic symptoms of hereditary spherocytosis: northern European descent, anemic symptoms, jaundice, and splenomegaly. Additionally, this patient is under high stress from his new job, which is known to trigger extravascular hemolysis in these patients.
- Hereditary spherocytosis is an autosomal dominant disorder. Blood smear will reveal spherocytes.

2. An 18-year-old African American male presents with 3 hours of swelling and pain in his hands. He has had multiple similar episodes, all of which required administration of oxygen and morphine until symptoms subsided. He was previously prescribed a medication for long-term management, but ran out last week. A previous blood smear revealed crescent-shaped red blood cells and target cells. Which of the following is the most likely cause for this patient's underlying condition?

   A. Underproduction of red blood cells
   B. Hydrophobic amino acid substitution in β-globin
   C. Diminished β-globin production
   D. Oxidative injury to red blood cells due to enzymatic deficiency

- **The correct answer is B.**
- The important thing to recognize here is that this patient is presenting with dactylitis, one of the most common presentations of sickle cell disease. Furthermore, his history supports this diagnosis: African American with recurrent pain episodes requiring O_2 and analgesia. His prior blood smear is supportive of the diagnosis of sickle cell anemia: crescent-shaped cells, also known as sickle cells, and target cells.
- Recall that sickle cell disease is caused by an autosomal recessive point mutation in the β-globin gene. This results in glutamate, a hydrophilic amino acid, being substituted with valine, a hydrophobic amino acid. This forms a type of hemoglobin called HbS, which forms tetramers and causes RBC sickling when deoxygenated.
- A is incorrect because underproduction of red blood cells is the cause of aplastic anemia, not sickle cell disease.
- C is incorrect because this is describing β-thalassemia, in which β-globin genes are either diminished or absent. Target cells are seen in β-thalassemia, but not sickle cells, which this patient demonstrates.
- D is incorrect because this is describing G6PD deficiency, in which red blood cells are unable to reduce oxidative stress due to the lack of G6PD.

Section IX - Hemolytic anemia (Extrinsic Causes)

Type	Onset	Mechanism	Type of Hemolysis	Etiology
Warm autoimmune hemolytic anemia	- Chronic	- IgG binds RBCs → agglutination	- Extravascular	- SLE - CLL - Penicillin - Cephalosporins - α-methyldopa
Cold autoimmune hemolytic anemia	- Acute	- IgM binds RBCs and complement in cold temperatures → agglutination	- Extravascular and intravascular	- CLL - *M. pneumoniae* - EBV

TABLE 10.10.5 - Types of Autoimmune Hemolytic Anemia

I. AIHA: Clinical/Lab Findings
   A. Extravascular hemolysis: fatigue, pallor, jaundice, and splenomegaly
   B. Cold AIHA: acrocyanosis
      1. ± intravascular hemolysis (hemoglobinuria/hemoglobinemia)
   C. Coombs test: positive
      1. Direct → detects if Ig and/or complement is coating RBCs
      2. Indirect → detects anti-RBC surface Ig in patient's serum
   D. Blood smear: agglutinated RBCs and spherocytes

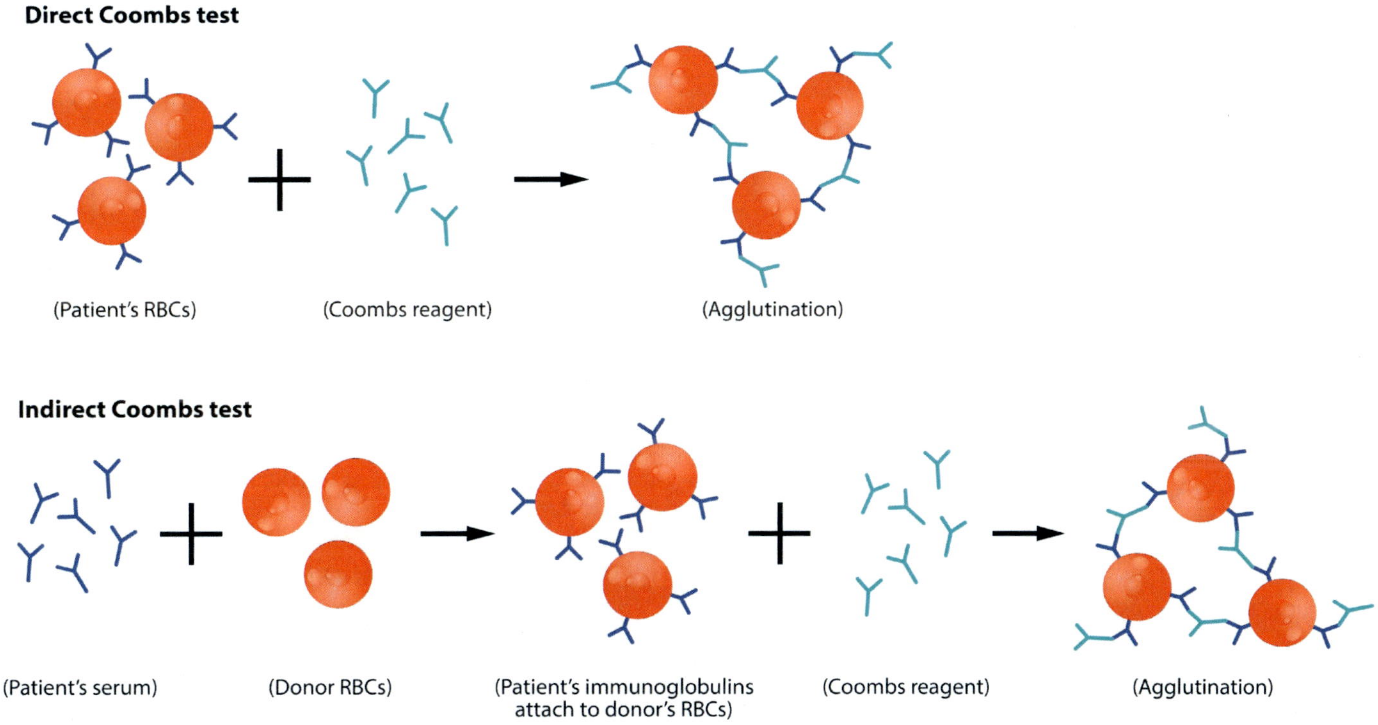

FIGURE 10.10.48 - Direct vs. Indirect Coombs Test

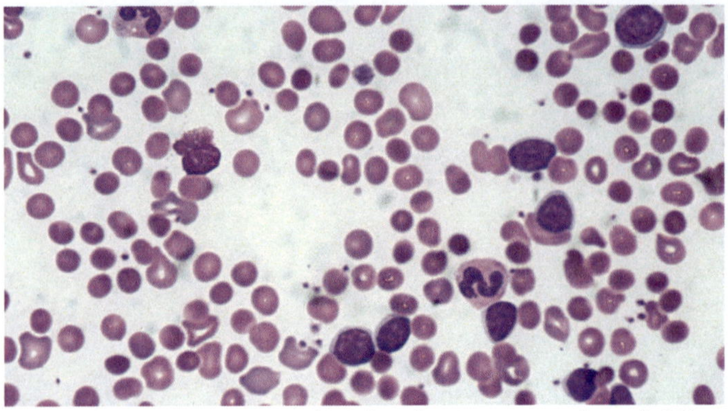

FIGURE 10.10.49 - Blood Smear in Autoimmune Hemolytic Anemia due to CLL

II. AIHA: Treatment
   A. Warm AIHA: steroids, rituximab, and splenectomy
   B. Cold AIHA: rituximab and avoidance of cold temperatures

III. Microangiopathic Hemolytic Anemia
   A. Intravascular hemolysis due to obstructed or narrowed vessels
      1. Possible causes: microthrombi, prosthetic heart valves, aortic stenosis, DIC, TTP/HUS, SLE, HELLP syndrome, and hypertensive emergency
   B. Blood smear: schistocytes

IV. Hemolytic Anemia from Infection
   A. Destruction of RBCs by toxins
      1. P. falciparum, P. vivax, P. ovale, and *Babesia* spp.
   B. Intravascular and extravascular hemolysis
   C. Treatment: address underlying infection

REVIEW QUESTIONS

1. A 44-year-old female with a past medical history significant for SLE and hyperlipidemia presents with 4 days of fatigue, dyspnea, yellow skin, and left upper quadrant pain. She was administered penicillin 1 week ago to treat an infection. On exam, her skin is jaundiced and splenomegaly is present. Her hands and feet are without acrocyanosis. Her hemoglobin level is 10.1 g/dL (normal: 12.0-15.5g/dL). Based on this patient's history and exam, what is the most likely diagnosis?

   - **The correct answer is warm AIHA.**
   - The important thing to recognize here is that this patient is presenting with signs and symptoms characteristic of autoimmune hemolytic anemia, such as history of SLE and penicillin treatment, jaundice, splenomegaly, and anemia. Jaundice and splenomegaly are good indicators of extravascular hemolysis.
   - With no other factors given, it is most likely an autoimmune hemolytic anemia. Based on her history of SLE and the lack of acrocyanosis, it is most likely warm AIHA.

REVIEW QUESTIONS

2. A 22-year-old male presents to the emergency department with fatigue, changes in skin color, and dark urine for the past day. He had a lower respiratory infection two weeks ago, for which he was treated with azithromycin. Physical exam demonstrates jaundiced skin and pale conjunctiva. Labs reveal a hemoglobin of 9.8 g/dL (normal: 13.5-17.5 g/dL), hematocrit of 29.4% (normal: 40-54%), MCV of 83 μm^3 (normal: 80-100 μm^3), indirect bilirubin of 3 mg/dL (normal: 0.3-1.0 mg/dL), and direct bilirubin of 0.1 mg/dL (normal: 0-0.3 mg/dL). A direct Coombs test is positive, and urinalysis reveals hemoglobinuria. What is the most likely mechanism behind this patient's presentation?

   A. Oxidative injury due to enzyme deficiency
   B. IgG-mediated cold agglutinin hemolysis
   C. IgM-mediated cold agglutinin hemolysis
   D. Medication-induced autoimmune hemolytic anemia

   - **The correct answer is C.**
   - It's important to recognize that this patient is presenting with hemolytic anemia based on his low hemoglobin, normal MCV, elevated indirect bilirubin, and hemoglobinuria. Hemoglobinuria specifically is indicative of extravascular hemolysis. Additionally, we can determine that it is an autoimmune hemolytic anemia based on the positive Coombs test.
   - Now we have to determine which type of autoimmune hemolytic anemia it is: warm or cold. The patient was recently treated for a lower respiratory tract infection with azithromycin, which would most likely be due to *Mycoplasma pneumoniae*. We know that *Mycoplasma pneumoniae* is a common etiology for cold AIHA. Additionally, the duration of symptoms is indicative of acute pathology, and we know that cold AIHA is an acute anemia.
   - Recall that cold AIHA is an acute hemolytic anemia caused by IgM binding to RBCs and complement in cold temperatures. This can result in signs of both extravascular and intravascular hemolysis. Causes of cold AIHA include CLL, Mycoplasma pneumoniae infection, and infectious mononucleosis.
   - A is incorrect because this is describing G6PD deficiency, in which red blood cells are unable to reduce oxidative stress due to the lack of G6PD.
   - B is incorrect because this is describing warm AIHA, which IgG binds RBCs and causes hemolysis.
   - D is incorrect because medications are most likely to induce warm AIHA.

Section X - Macrocytic Anemia

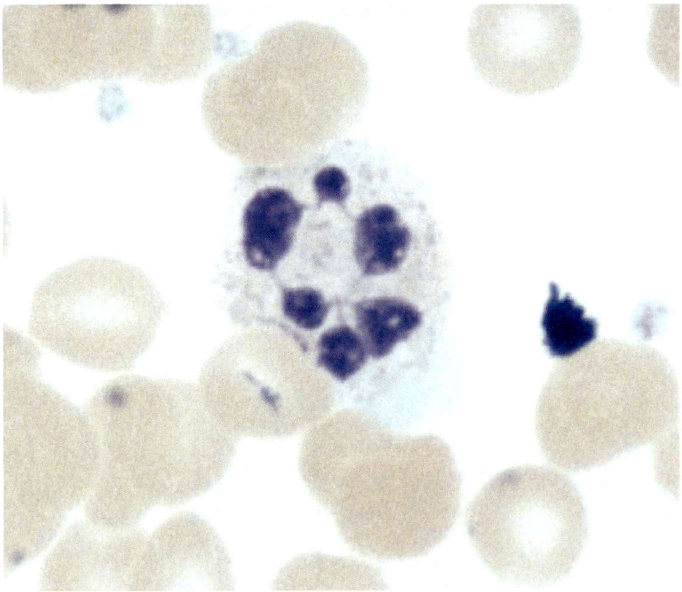

FIGURE 10.10.50 - Megaloblastic Change Causing Hypersegmented Neutrophils

I. Megaloblastic Anemia: Causes
   A. Folate deficiency
   B. B12 (cobalamin) deficiency

II. Megaloblastic Anemia: Pathophysiology
   A. Folate or B12 (cobalamin) deficiency → defect in DNA synthesis → release of immature cells from the bone marrow
      1. Immature RBCs → anemia
      2. Immature granulocytes → hypersegmented neutrophils

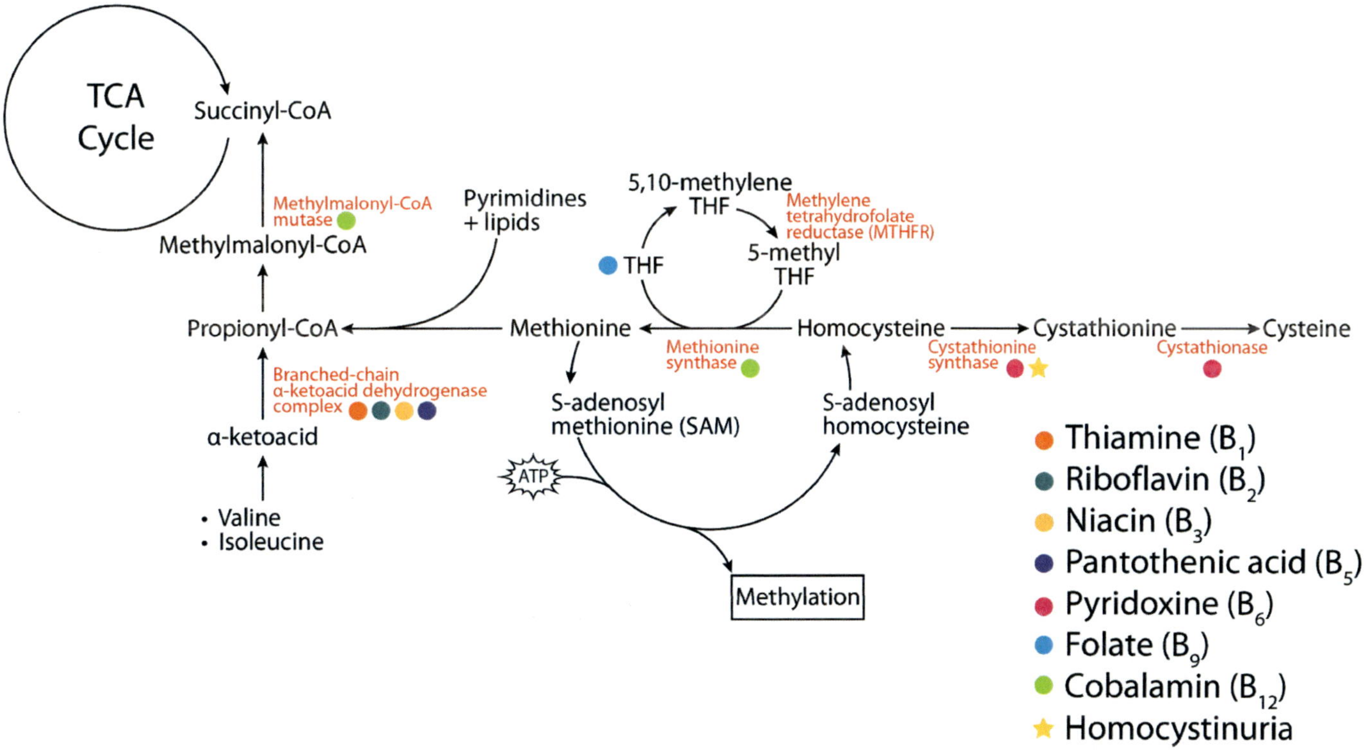

FIGURE 10.10.51 - Homocysteine Metabolic Pathway

Defciency	Causes	Clinical Findings	Absorption Site
Folate	- Poor diet (Alcholics and elderly) - Increased demand - Folate antagonists	- Decreased serum folate - Increased serum homocysteine - Glossitis	- Jejunum
B12 (Cobalamin)	- Pernicious anemia - Pancreatic insufficiency - Damage to terminal ilern - Dietary deficiency (rare)	- Decreased B12 - Increased homocysteine - Increased methylmalonic acid - Glossitis	Ileum

TABLE 10.10.6 - Folate and B12 Deficiency

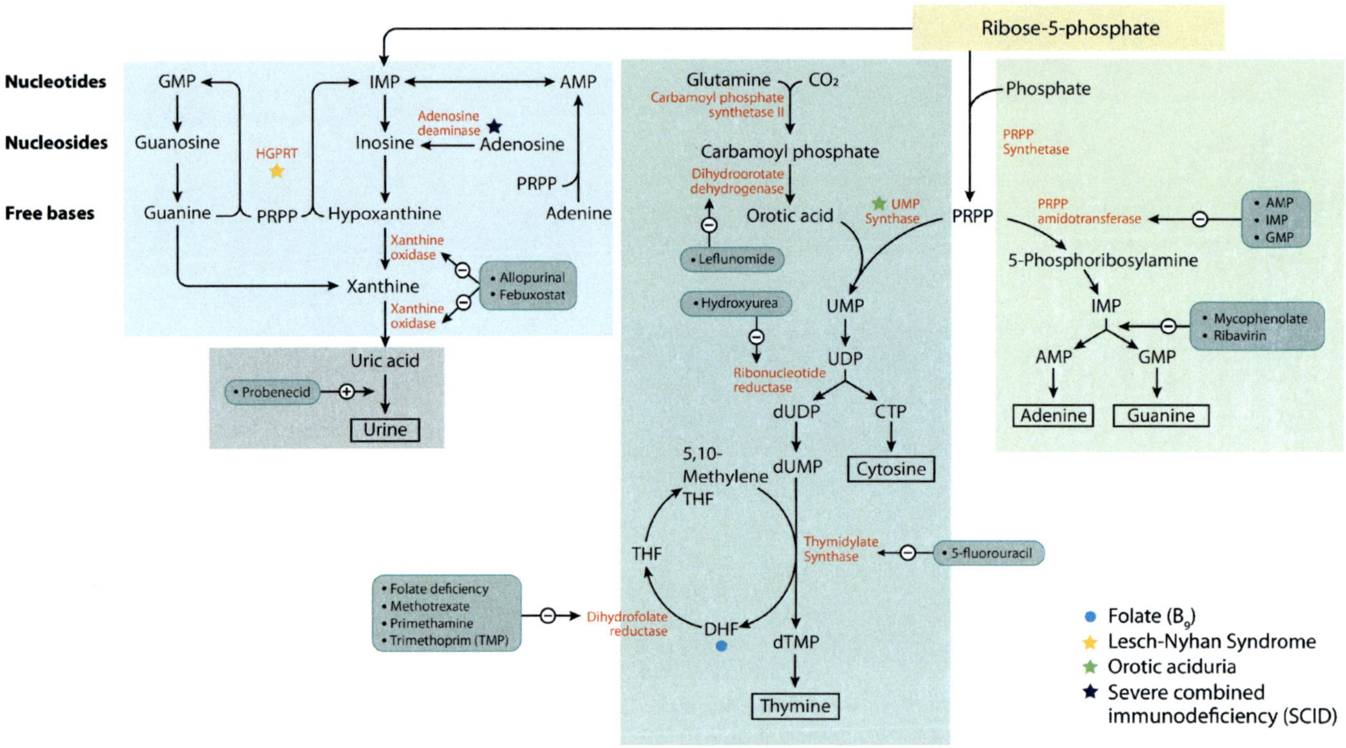

FIGURE 10.10.52 - Purine Salvage Pathway

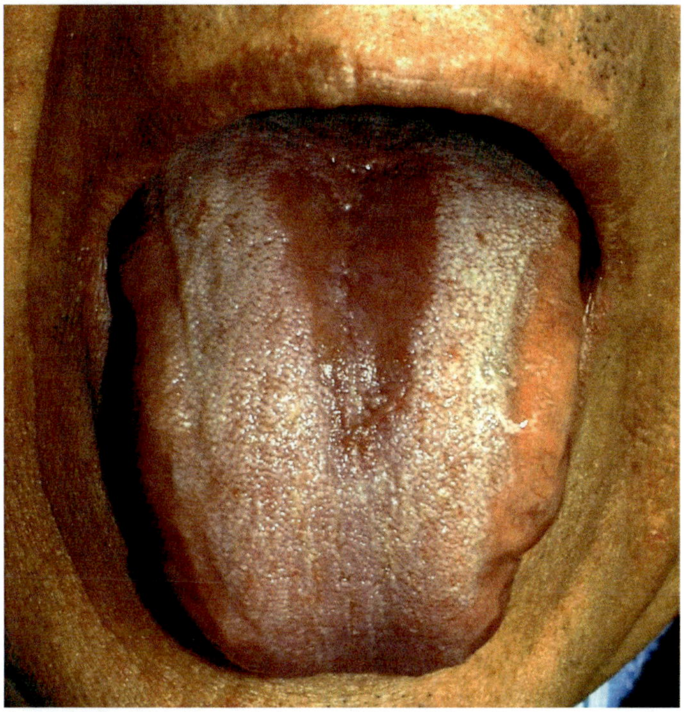

FIGURE 10.10.53 - Glossitis

III. Non-Megaloblastic Anemia
   A. Alcoholism
   B. Liver disease
   C. Drugs

REVIEW QUESTIONS

1. A 34-year-old woman presents with diarrhea, weight loss, and weakness. Testing reveals fecal fat and vitamin deficiencies. She is placed on a special diet, which includes no bread, wheats, or grains; after following this diet for some time, her symptoms improve. What blood smear findings would be expected in this patient before she started treatment?

   - **The correct answer is hypersegmented neutrophils and macrocytosis.**
   - This patient presents with diarrhea, weight loss, and weakness. Physical exam reveals fecal fat and vitamin deficiencies which are symptoms of malabsorption syndrome. After bread, wheat and grains are removed from her diet her symptoms improve. This should make you think of celiac disease, which affects the jejunum. Since folate is absorbed in the jejunum, the patient may have a folate deficiency, which results in hypersegmented neutrophils and macrocytosis on blood smear.

REVIEW QUESTIONS

2. A 23-year-old woman with a history of systemic lupus presents with pain, swelling, and morning stiffness in both hands. Blood analysis reveals anti-cyclic citrullinated peptide antibody. She is prescribed a drug to treat her symptoms. Two weeks later, she presents with easy fatigability. A blood smear shows hypersegmented neutrophils. What additional findings would be expected in this patient?

   A. MCV < 100
   B. Increased methylmalonic acid
   C. Decreased serum folate
   D. Schistocytes

   - **The correct answer is C.**
   - This patient has a history of systemic lupus, pain, swelling and morning stiffness in both hands. Blood analysis reveals anti-cyclic citrullinated peptide antibody. This information should show that the patient has rheumatoid arthritis. After the drug is prescribed to manage the symptoms, the patient presents with easy fatigability and hypersegmented neutrophils, which points to megaloblastic anemia.
   - Methotrexate can be given to a patient with rheumatoid arthritis. Methotrexate inhibits dihydrofolate reductase which causes a folate deficiency leading to megaloblastic anemia.
   - A is incorrect because folate deficiency causes megaloblastic anemia, which presents with a MCV > 100.
   - B is incorrect because an increase in methylmalonic acid is associated with B12 deficiency, not folate deficiency.
   - D is incorrect because this is a characteristic of a microcytic anemia.

Section XI - Leukopenia and Leukocytosis

I. Definition
   A. Normal leukocyte count is between 4,400-11,000 cells/L
      1. Leukopenia < 4,400 cells/L
      2. Leukocytosis > 11,000 cells/L
   B. A change in the normal count is due to increased or decreased production of a specific cell lineage
      1. CD34+ hematopoietic stem cells responsible for production
      2. Develop in bone marrow and released into the blood

II. Neutropenia
   A. Abnormally low number of circulating neutrophils
      1. Increased risk of infection
   B. Causes
      1. Drug toxicity: chemotherapy with alkylating agents
      2. Sepsis
      3. Aplastic anemia
   C. Treatment: GM-CSF or G-CSF to upregulate granulocyte production

III. Lymphopenia
   A. Abnormally low number of circulating lymphocytes
   B. Causes
      1. Immunodeficiency: DiGeorge syndrome, SCID and HIV/AIDS
      2. Excess cortisol: Cushing's syndrome, exogenous steroid use
      3. Autoimmune destruction: SLE
      4. Radiation therapy

IV. Eosinopenia
   A. Decreased circulating eosinophils
   B. Most commonly due to a high cortisol state
      1. Corticosteroids sequester eosinophils in lymph nodes and remove them from circulation

V. Neutrophilia
   A. Abnormally high number of circulating neutrophils
   B. Causes
      1. Bacterial infection or necrosis → acute inflammation
         a) Left shift: increase in immature neutrophils (band cells, metamyelocytes)
         b) Leukoerythroblastic reaction: left shift with immature RBCs
      2. Excess cortisol: impaired migration out of vasculature

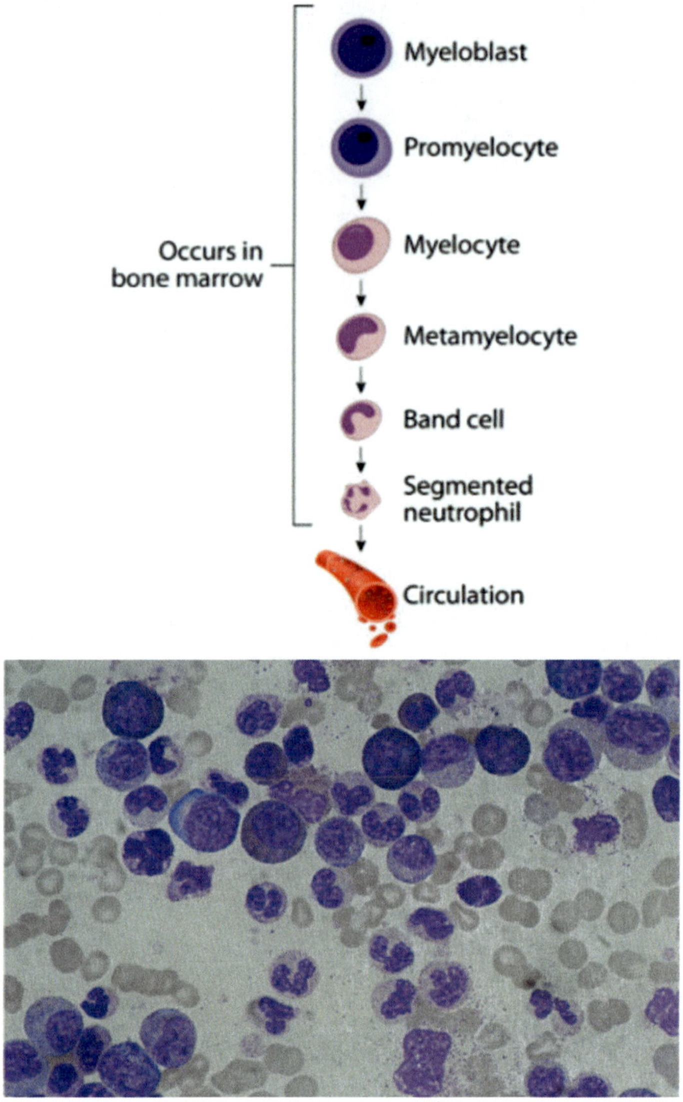

FIGURE 10.10.54 - Structural Changes of Neutrophil Development (Top); Peripheral Blood Smear with Left Shift (Bottom)

VI. Monocytosis, Basophilia, and Eosinophilia
   A. Abnormally high number of the respective cell lineages
   B. Monocytosis: chronic inflammatory state and malignancy
   C. Basophilia: chronic myeloid leukemia
   D. Eosinophilia: anaphylactic reactions, parasitic infections, and Hodgkin lymphoma

VII. Lymphocytosis
   A. Abnormally high number of circulating lymphocytes
   B. Causes
      1. Viral infection → $CD8^+$ T cell hyperplasia
      2. *Bordetella pertussis*
      3. Toxin inhibits chemokine receptor on lymphocytes
      4. Infectious mononucleosis

REVIEW QUESTIONS

1. A 16-year-old male is brought to the clinic with complaints of a fever and feeling extremely tired. Upon physical examination there is symmetrical and nontender cervical lymphadenopathy. Abdominal examination further reveals splenomegaly. The patient's blood is drawn and the presence of EBV viral capsid antigens is noted. Which of the following types of cells is most likely to be seen in abundance?

   A. Lymphocytes
   B. Neutrophils
   C. Basophils
   D. Eosinophils

- **The correct answer is A.**
- Hopefully from the question stem you realized that this 16-year-old boy has infectious mononucleosis due to EBV. We know that he has mono because he has all of the clinical findings we'd suspect: lethargy, sore throat, fever, cervical lymphadenopathy, and splenomegaly. Serologic testing even confirms the presence of EBV.
- The question is asking which cell type is most likely to be seen in excess on a peripheral blood smear of this patient. Recall that EBV mononucleosis leads to a lymphocytosis consisting of atypical or reactive $CD8^+$ T cells.
- B is incorrect because an abundance of neutrophils, or neutrophilia, is seen in conditions that would cause acute inflammation, such as bacterial infection or tissue necrosis, as well as a high cortisol state, none of which are exhibited in this patient.
- Choices C and D are wrong because they would also not likely be seen in abundance on the peripheral blood smear of EBV. Recall that basophils are commonly seen during allergic reactions, while eosinophils are seen during allergic reactions or parasitic infections.

Section XII - Acute Leukemia

I. Definition
   A. Accumulation of > 20% blasts in the bone marrow
   B. Blasts enter the bloodstream → high WBC count

II. Pathophysiology
   A. Mutation results in failure of white blood cells to mature
   B. Increased blasts prevent normal hematopoiesis from occurring
      1. Decreased RBCs → anemia
      2. Decreased megakaryocytes → thrombocytopenia
      3. Decreased myelocytes → neutropenia

III. Clinical Findings
   A. Anemia → fatigue
   B. Thrombocytopenia → bleeding
   C. Neutropenia → infection

IV. Types and Subtypes
   A. Acute lymphoblastic leukemia
      1. B-cell acute lymphoblastic leukemia (B-ALL)
      2. T-cell acute lymphoblastic leukemia (T-ALL)
   B. Acute myelogenous leukemia
      1. Acute promyelocytic leukemia
      2. Acute monocytic leukemia
      3. Acute megakaryoblastic leukemia

V. Acute Lymphoblastic Leukemia (ALL)
   A. Neoplastic collection of lymphoblasts (> 20%) in the bone marrow
   B. Most commonly seen in children
   C. Associated with Down syndrome (over age of 5)
   D. Subtypes
      1. B-cell ALL (B-ALL)
      2. T-cell ALL (T-ALL)

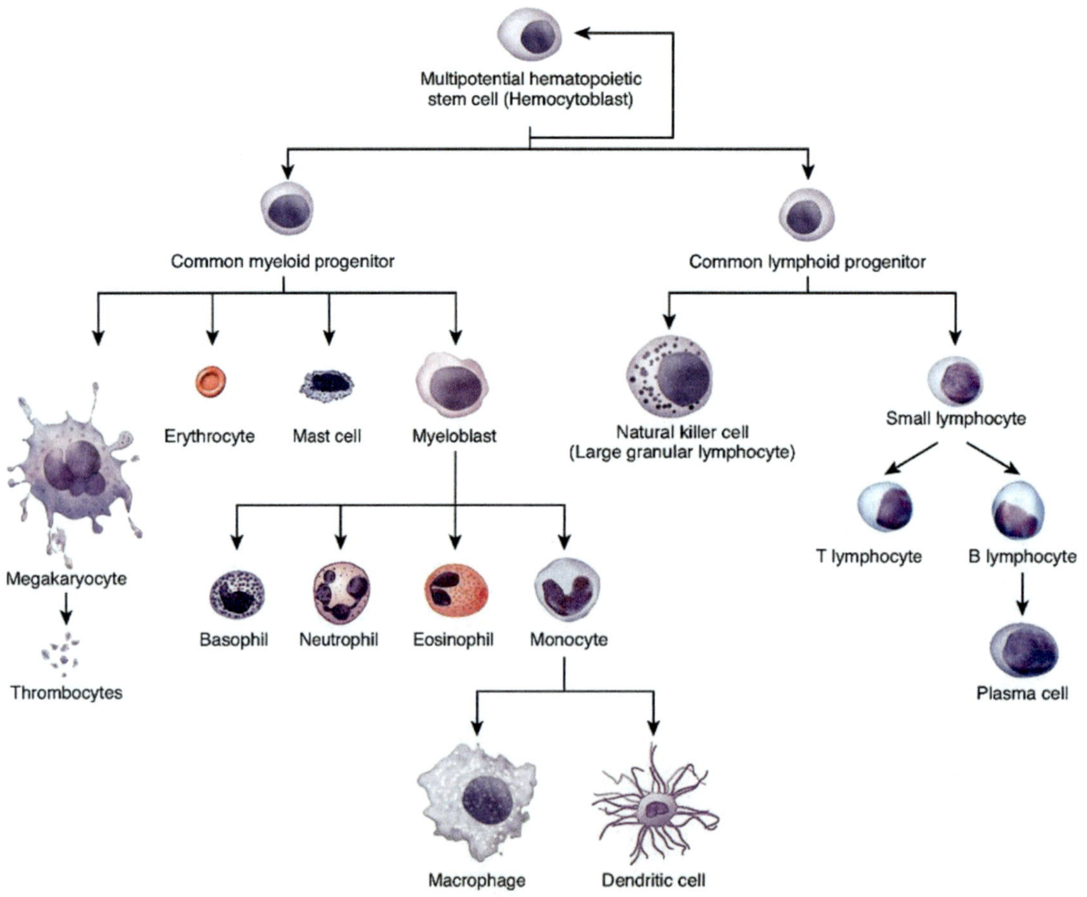

FIGURE 10.10.55 - Differentiation of Hematopoietic Stem Cells

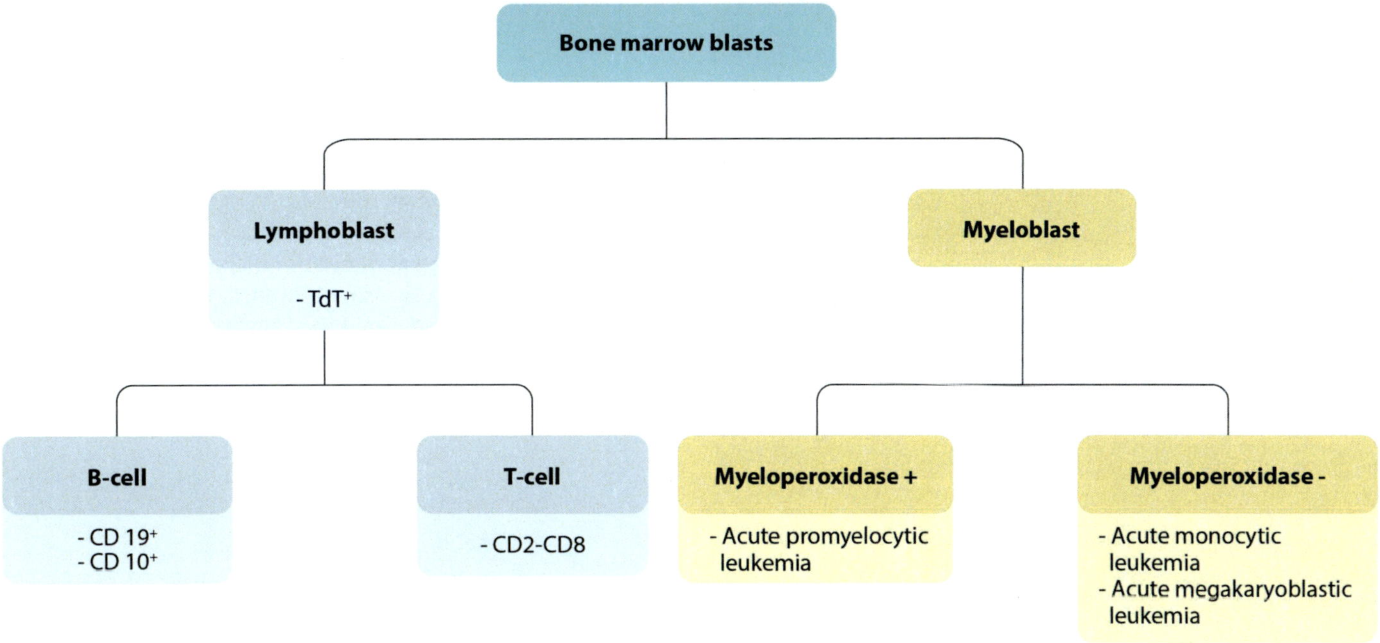

FIGURE 10.10.56 - Genetic Markers in Bone Marrow Blasts

VI. B-Cell Acute Lymphoblastic Leukemia (B-ALL)
   A. Characterized by lymphoblasts that express TdT, CD10, CD19, and CD20
   B. Highly responsive to chemotherapy; requires prophylaxis to scrotum and CSF
   C. Prognosis
      1. t(12;21) - good prognosis; children
      2. t(9;22) - poor prognosis; adults

VII. T-Cell Acute Lymphoblastic Leukemia (T-ALL)
   A. Lymphoblasts that express TdT and CD2 through CD8
   B. Presents in teenagers as a mediastinal (thymic) mass
      1. Compression of esophagus → dysphagia
      2. Compression of the trachea → dyspnea and stridor
      3. Inflammation → pleural effusions

VIII. Acute Myelogenous Leukemia (AML)
   A. Accumulation of immature myeloid cells (> 20%) in the bone marrow
   B. Demographic: 50-60 years old
   C. Crystal aggregates of MPO (Auer rods) on histology
   D. Subtypes
      1. Acute promyelocytic leukemia
      2. Acute monocytic leukemia
      3. Acute megakaryoblastic leukemia

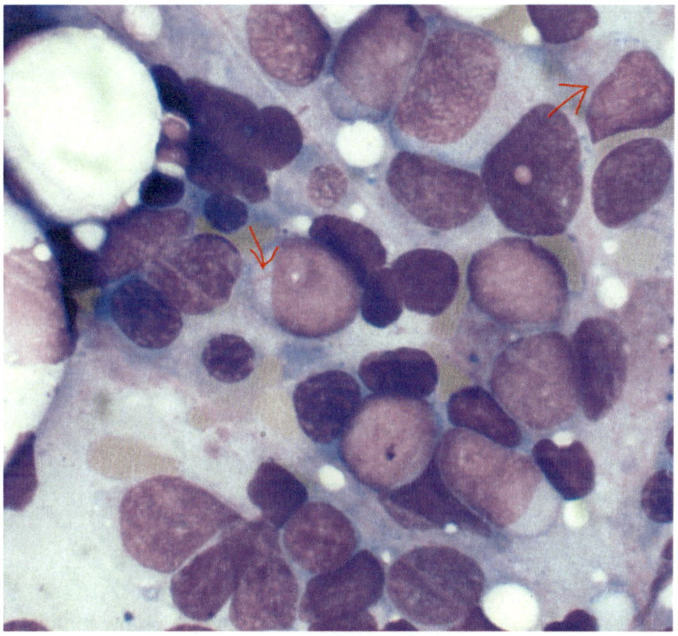

FIGURE 10.10.57 - Auer Rods in AML

IX. Acute Promyelocytic Leukemia
   A. t(15;17)
      1. Involves retinoic acid receptor (RAR)
   B. Treated with all-trans-retinoic acid (ATRA)
   C. Increased risk for DIC

X. Acute Monocytic Leukemia
   A. Proliferation of monoblasts
   B. Lacks MPO
   C. Blasts infiltrate gums

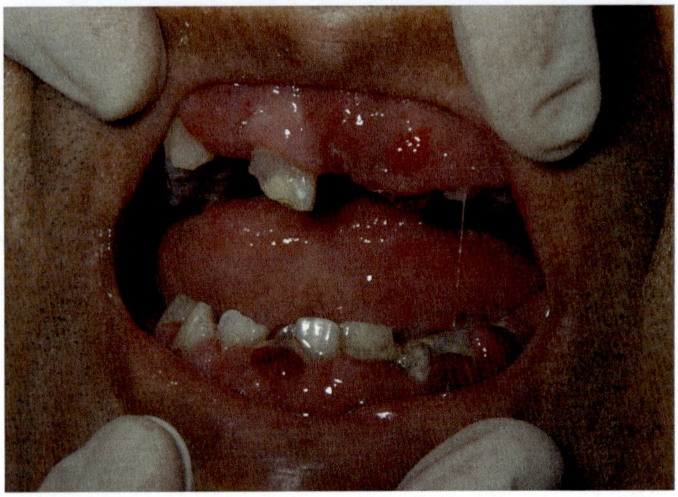

FIGURE 10.10.58 - Gum Infiltration in AML

XI. Acute Megakaryoblastic Leukemia
   A. Proliferation of megakaryoblasts
   B. Lacks MPO
   C. Associated with Down syndrome (before the age of 5)

REVIEW QUESTIONS

1. A 15-year-old boy with a 2-month history of fatigue and pneumonia presents with difficulty swallowing. Physical exam reveals decreased breath sounds on auscultation, decreased fremitus, and dullness on percussion. A complete blood count reveals 25% blasts. What markers are likely found on these blasts?

   - **The correct answer is TdT, CD2, CD3, CD4, CD5, CD6, CD7, and CD8, which are all markers for T-ALL.**
   - Notice that the patient is a teenage boy with fatigue (anemia) and pneumonia (infection), which are signs of leukemia. The patient also presents with dysphagia (difficulty swallowing), a pleural effusion (decreased breath sounds, decreased fremitus, and dullness on percussion), and a complete blood count that revealed 25% blasts.
   - This indicates that the patient may have developed T-ALL.

REVIEW QUESTIONS

2. A 40-year-old male presents to the emergency room with a complaint of large amounts of bright red blood in his stool. He reports gradual onset of fatigue over the past several weeks and the appearance of numerous small red dots on his skin the day before. Physical examination reveals tachycardia, tachypnea, orthostatic hypotension, pallor of the skin and mucous membranes, and numerous petechiae. Peripheral blood smear is positive for myeloperoxidase crystals. What condition is indicated by the clinical presentation and laboratory data?

   A. Chronic myelogenous leukemia
   B. Acute promyelocytic leukemia
   C. Acute lymphocytic leukemia
   D. Acute megakaryoblastic leukemia

   - **The correct answer is B.**
   - This 40-year-old patient has large amounts of bright red blood in stool (excessive bleeding), gradual fatigue (anemia), and numerous small red dots on his skin (thrombocytopenia). On physical exam, he has tachycardia, tachypnea, orthostatic hypotension, pallor of skin and mucous membranes (anemia), and numerous petechiae (thrombocytopenia).
   - Peripheral blood smear is positive for crystals staining for myeloperoxidase. Hopefully, from this information, it is clear that the patient has DIC as a result of acute promyelocytic leukemia. Remember that of the types of AML, only acute promyelocytic leukemia is positive for myeloperoxidase.
   - Acute promyelocytic leukemia is also associated with disseminated intravascular coagulation (DIC). Abnormal promyelocytes contain many primary granules that increase the risk for DIC. This results in bleeding, thrombocytopenia, and prolonged prothrombin and activated thromboplastin time.
   - Chronic myelogenous leukemia, acute lymphocytic leukemia, and acute megakaryoblastic leukemia are not associated with myeloperoxidase crystals or DIC, which makes A, C, and D incorrect.

Section XIII - Chronic Leukemia

I. Basic Principles
   A. Neoplastic proliferation of mature circulating lymphocytes
   B. High WBC count
   C. Gradual onset
   D. Seen in older adults

Type	Pathophysiology	Blood Smear	Clinical Findings
Chronic lymphocytic leukemia (CLL)	- Proliferation of naive B cells that express CD5 and CD20 - Transformation to diffuse large B cell lymphoma (rare)	- Increased lymphocytes - Smudge cells	- Generalized lymphadenopathy (due to transformation to small cell lymphoma) - Hypogammaglobulinemia (increased risk for infection) - Autoimmune hemolytic anemia (spherocytes on peripheral blood smear)
Hairy cell leukemia	- Proliferation of mature B cells - Bone marrow failure - Marrow fibrosis - Associated with *BRAF* mutations - Cells are positive for tartrate-resistant acid phosphatase (TRAP)	- Hairy cytoplasmic process	- Splenomegaly - Dry tap on bone marrow aspiration - Pancytopenia (anemia, bleeding, and increased risk for infection)
Adult T-cell leukemia/ lymphoma (ATLL)	- Proliferation of mature $CD4^+$ T cells - Cells infiltrate skin, lymph nodes, liver, spleen, and bone - Associated with HTLV-1 - Seen in Japan and the Caribbean		- Rash - Generalized lymphadenopathy - Hepatosplenomegaly - Lytic bone lesions with hypercalcemia
Mycosis fungoides	- Proliferation of mature $CD4^+$ T cells that infiltrate the skin	- Lymphocytes with cerebriform nuclei	- Localized skin rash, plaques, and nodules - Pautrier microabscesses - Progression to Sézary syndrome

TABLE 10.10.7 - Four Types of Chronic Leukemia

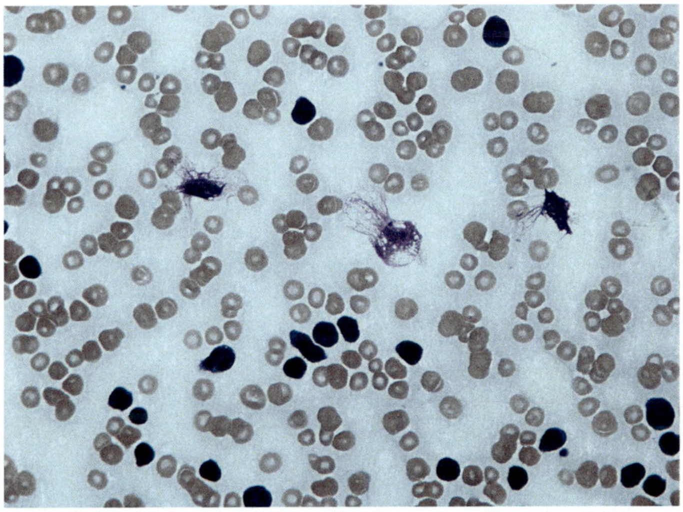

FIGURE 10.10.59 - Smudge Cells

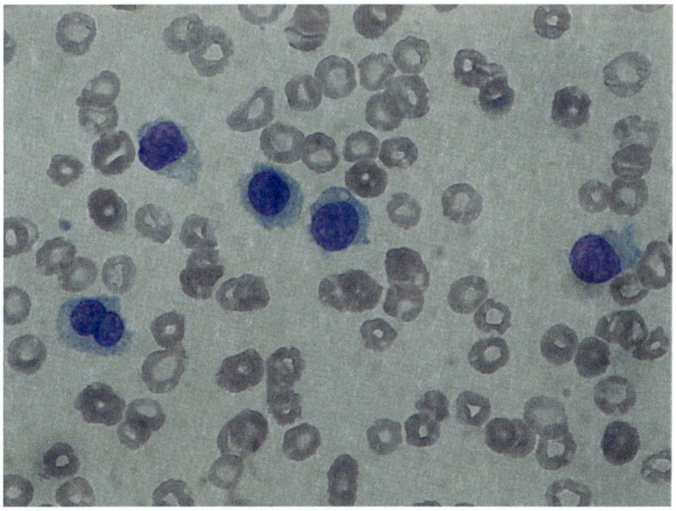

FIGURE 10.10.60 - Blood Smear of Hairy Cell Leukemia

II. Hairy Cell Leukemia: Treatment
   A. 2-CDA (cladribine)
      1. Adenosine deaminase inhibitor

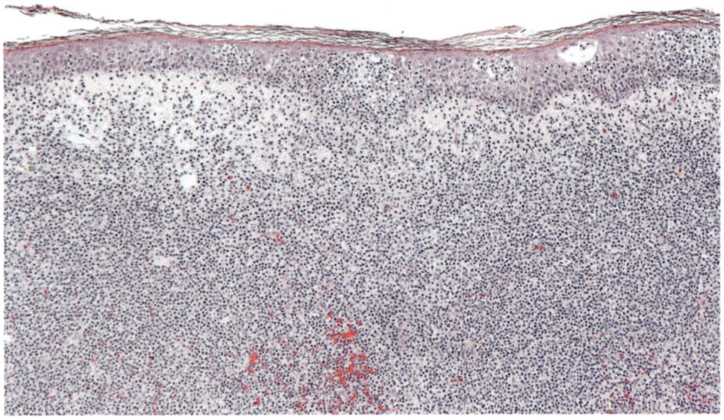

Photo Credit: Nephron / CC BY-SA (https://creativecommons.org/licenses/by-sa/3.0)

FIGURE 10.10.61 - Histological Slide of Pautrier Microabscesses

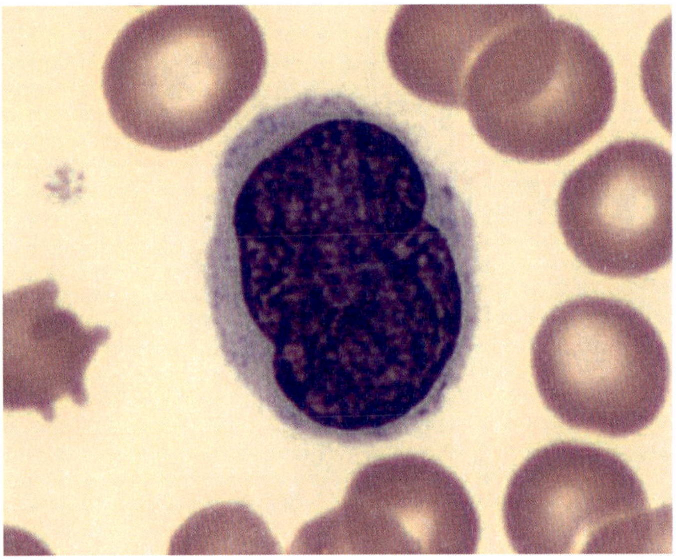

Photo Credit: El*Falaf / CC BY-SA (https://creativecommons.org/licenses/by-sa/3.0)

FIGURE 10.10.62 - Blood Smear Showing Cerebriform Nuclei

REVIEW QUESTIONS

1. A 65-year-old man with a 3-month history of fatigue presents to the emergency room following 2 consecutive cases of pneumonia. Physical exam reveals mucosal pallor. A peripheral blood smear reveals elevated lymphocytes and smudge cells. There is no generalized lymphadenopathy. What is the diagnosis? What would the diagnosis be if generalized lymphadenopathy were present?

REVIEW QUESTIONS

- **The correct answer is chronic lymphocytic leukemia in the presence of generalized lymphadenopathy and small cell lymphoma in the absence of generalized lymphadenopathy.**
- The patient presents with hypogammaglobulinemia (2 consecutive cases of pneumonia), anemia (mucosal pallor) and elevated lymphocytes and smudge cells on peripheral blood smear. Since there is no generalized lymphadenopathy, you can make the diagnosis of chronic lymphocytic leukemia. If there were generalized lymphadenopathy, then the diagnosis would be small cell lymphoma.

2. A 55-year-old woman presents with arthralgias, generalized weakness, and the inability to finish a meal. She reports gradual onset of fatigue over the past month. Physical examination is significant for conjunctival pallor and splenomegaly. A peripheral blood count reveals pancytopenia. Her blood tests positive for tartrate-resistant acid phosphatase. What diagnostic finding is most likely to be found on blood smear?

   A. Hairy cytoplasmic processes
   B. Spherocytes
   C. Smudge cells
   D. Cerebriform nuclei

- **The correct answer is A.**
- This 55-year-old patient presents with the inability to finish a meal, or early satiety, which indicates possible splenomegaly. She reports gradual onset of fatigue and generalized weakness, which should indicate anemia. Physical exam reveals conjunctival pallor, which also indicates anemia. Peripheral blood count reveals pancytopenia and tests positive for tartrate-resistant acid phosphatase. Hairy cell leukemia presents with splenomegaly, pancytopenia, and dry tap on bone marrow aspiration.
- B is incorrect because spherocytes are seen in cases of autoimmune hemolytic anemia, which is present in chronic lymphocytic leukemia. CLL does not present with splenomegaly, pancytopenia, or a positive tartrate-resistant acid phosphatase.
- C is incorrect because smudge cells are also seen in CLL.
- D is incorrect because cerebriform nuclei are found in mycosis fungoides. Mycosis fungoides would present with a rash and with anemia or pancytopenia.

Section XIV - Myeloproliferative Disorders

I. Definition
   A. Neoplastic proliferation of mature cells of myeloid lineage
   B. Most commonly presents around 50-60 years of age

II. Clinical Findings
   A. High WBC count with hypercellular bone marrow
   B. Cells of all myeloid lineages are increased

III. Complications
   A. Increased risk for hyperuricemia and gout
   B. Progression to marrow fibrosis
   C. Transformation to acute leukemia

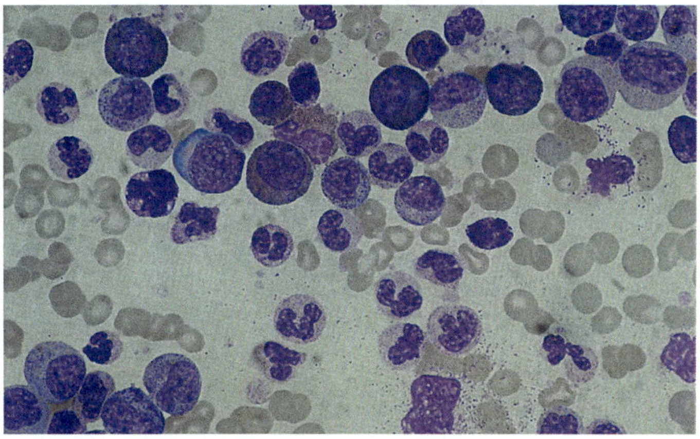

Photo Credit: Paulo Henrique Orlandi Mourao / (https://creativecommons.org/licenses/by-sa/3.0)

FIGURE 10.10.63 - Neutrophilia and Basophilia in CML

Type	Pathophysiology	Clinical Findings	Treatment
Chronic myeloid leukemia (CML)	- Neoplastic proliferation of mature myeloid cells, especially granulocytes and their precursors - t(9;22) → BCR/ABL fusion protein - Increased tyrosine kinase activity	- Splenomegaly - Increased basophils on blood smear - Negative leukocyte alkaline phosphatase (LAP) stain	- Tyrosine kinase inhibitor (imatinib)
Polycythemia vera	- Neoplastic proliferation of mature myeloid cells, especially RBCs - JAK2 kinase mutation - Increased tyrosine kinase activity - Hyperviscosity (can cause Budd-Chiari syndrome, peptic ulcer disease)	- Blurry vision and headache - Flushed face - Itching, especially after bathing - Decreased erythropoietin - Normal SaO_2	- Phlebotomy - Hydroxyurea
Essential thrombocythemia	- Neoplastic proliferation of mature myeloid cells, especially platelets - JAK2 kinase mutation	- Bleeding - Thrombosis	- Hydroxyurea - Systemic anticoagulation/aspirin
Myelofibrosis	- Neoplastic proliferation of mature myeloid cells, especially megakaryocytes - JAK2 kinase mutation	- Marrow fibrosis - Splenomegaly - Leukoerythroblastic smear	- JAK2 inhibitor (ruxolitinib)

TABLE 10.10.8 - Types of Myeloproliferative Disorders

Type	Causes	Erythropoietin (EPO) Levels	SaO_2
Polycythemia vera	- Neoplastic proliferation of mature myeloid cells, especially RBCs	↓	Normal
Appropriate absolute polycythemia	- Lung disease - Congenital heart disease - High altitude	↑	↓
Inappropriate absolute polycythemia	- Exogenous EPO - Malignancy (renal cell carcinoma, hepatocellular carcinoma)	↑	Normal

TABLE 10.10.9 - Types of Polycythemia

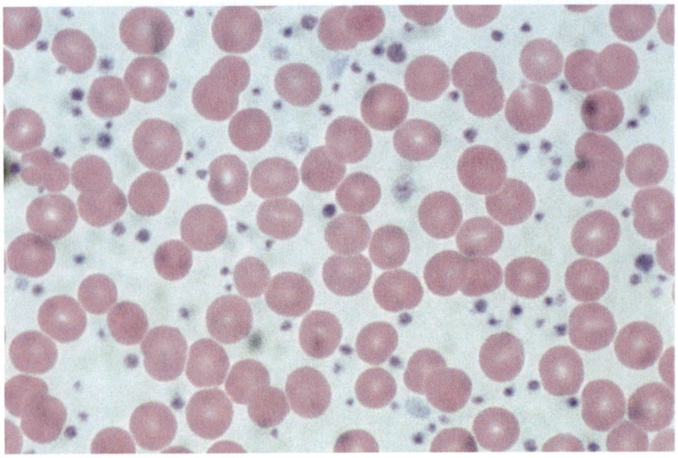

Photo Credit: Ed Uthman from Houston, TX, USA / CC BY (https://creativecommons.org/licenses/by/2.0)

FIGURE 10.10.64 - Blood Smear of Essential Thrombocytopenia

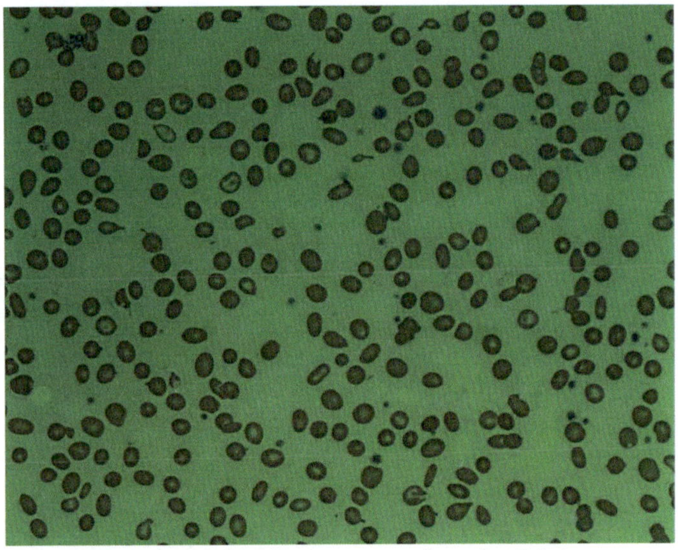

Photo Credit: Osaretin / CC BY-SA (https://creativecommons.org/licenses/by-sa/4.0)

FIGURE 10.10.65 - Leukoerythroblastic Smear in Myelofibrosis (Teardrop-Shaped RBCs)

REVIEW QUESTIONS

?

1. A 35-year-old man presents with blurred vision, confusion, and lightheadedness. He reports fainting earlier in the day after playing football with his friends. On physical exam, he appears pale and is disoriented. Pain is elicited upon palpation of the left upper quadrant of the abdomen. His blood pressure is 83/51 mmHg. A peripheral blood smear is negative for leukocyte alkaline phosphatase. What is the most likely cytogenetic finding?

- **t(9;22) is the most likely cytogenetic finding.**
- This man presents with blurred vision, confusion, fainting, and lightheadedness. He appears pale and disoriented and his blood pressure is 83/51. These are signs of shock. Now you have to figure out why he might be in shock.
- He was playing football earlier that day and is in pain upon palpation of the left upper quadrant of his abdomen. This indicates that he may have suffered a splenic rupture due to splenomegaly. Splenomegaly can result from a number of causes, but you are also told that his blood stains negative for leukocyte alkaline phosphatase.
- This makes the most likely diagnosis CML. CML is caused by a translocation between chromosomes 9 and 22.

2. A 23-year-old woman with a history of chronic headaches presents with painful swollen arms for the past week. She recently moved from Georgia to Colorado. Upon further questioning, she reveals itching after bathing. Blood smear reveals elevated RBCs. Erythropoietin levels are elevated and oxygen saturation is low. What most likely caused this patient's symptoms?

- **The most likely cause is high altitude.**
- This woman presents with chronic headaches, painful swollen arms, itching after a bath, and elevated RBCs. These signs point to polycythemia. But the erythropoietin levels are elevated, so it can't be polycythemia vera since EPO is low in this disorder.
- Oxygen saturation levels are also low, which rules out inappropriate absolute polycythemia. This leaves appropriate absolute polycythemia as the only option.
- Because she recently moved from Georgia to Colorado, the most likely cause is high altitude.

3. A 38-year-old man with a 6-month history of headaches, dizziness, and blurry vision presents with generalized itchiness after he takes a shower. Physical examination shows facial redness and splenomegaly. Laboratory studies show elevated hemoglobin and a decreased erythropoietin concentration. Which of the following is most likely responsible for this patient's condition?

   A. Exposure to a carcinogen
   B. Mutation of a tumor suppressor gene
   C. Presence of an oncogene
   D. t(9,22)

- **The correct answer is C.**
- This man presents with headaches, dizziness, blurry vision, itchiness after taking a shower, facial redness, and splenomegaly. Laboratory studies show elevated hemoglobin levels and a decreased erythropoietin concentration. The patient likely has polycythemia vera.
- Polycythemia vera is due to an activating mutation in JAK2 kinase, which is considered an oncogene. Remember that polycythemia vera is due to a JAK2 kinase mutation.
- A is incorrect because polycythemia vera is not due to exposure to a carcinogen.
- B is incorrect because polycythemia vera is not due to mutation of a tumor suppressor gene. Don't let the word mutation confuse you. *JAK2* is not a tumor suppressor gene.
- D is incorrect because the translocation between chromosomes 9 and 22 causes CML.

Section XV - Lymphadenopathy

I. Lymph Node Anatomy
  A. Outer cortex: B cells
    1. Primary and secondary follicles
  B. Inner cortex (paracortex): T cells
  C. Medulla:
    1. Cords: plasma cells and lymphocytes
    2. Sinuses: macrophages and reticular cells

III. Clinical Significance
  A. Outer cortex: B cells in follicles
    1. Called follicular hyperplasia
    2. Rheumatoid arthritis, Sjogren's, HIV, syphilis
  B. Inner cortex (paracortex): T-cells
    1. Viruses (EBV)
  C. Medulla:
    1. Sinuses: metastatic cancer

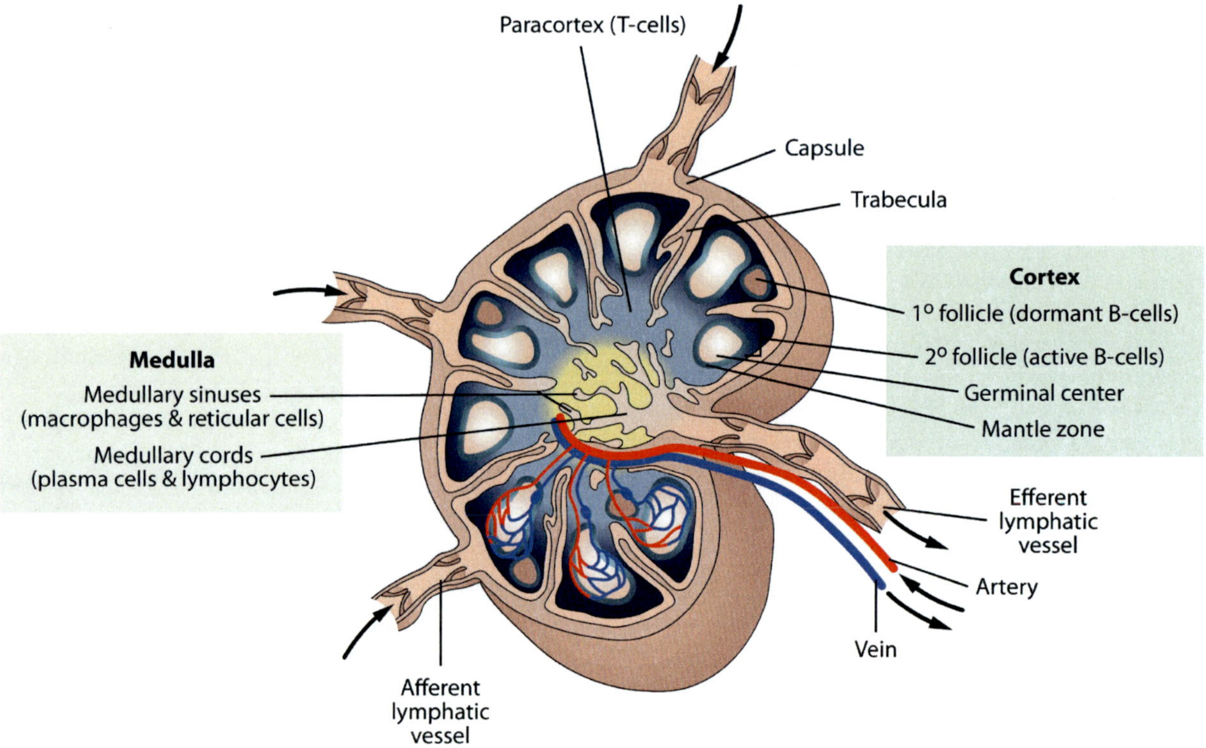

FIGURE 10.10.66 - Anatomy of a Lymph Node

II. Lymphadenopathy
  A. Definition: swollen lymph node
  B. Types
    1. Acute → infectious (painful)
    2. Chronic → inflammatory or cancerous (not painful)

REVIEW QUESTIONS

1. A 15-year-old male comes to the physician complaining of a sore throat and fatigue. His throat hurts all day but is worse when he swallows. No matter how much he sleeps, he always feels tired. He has a new girlfriend but he is not sexually active. On physical exam he has tender cervical lymphadenopathy. What part of the lymph node is enlarged secondary to this disease process?

   A. Outer cortex
   B. Follicles
   C. Medullary sinus
   D. Trabeculae
   E. Inner cortex (paracortex)

REVIEW QUESTIONS

- **The correct answer is E.**
- This is a 15-year-old male who has a sore throat and fatigue. He is not sexually active but does have a new girlfriend. Exam shows tender lymphadenopathy in the cervical region.
- This should make you concerned for EBV, a cause of infectious mononucleosis. This infection results in a large cellular response. In EBV, the inner cortex of the lymph node would be enlarged. This is where the T cells are found. Thus, choice E, inner cortex or paracortex, is correct.
- A and B are incorrect because this is where B cells are found and these areas are not enlarged in EBV. However, follicular hyperplasia can occur in the setting of autoimmune diseases, HIV, or syphilis.
- C is incorrect because the medullary sinuses would be enlarged in metastatic cancer.
- D is incorrect because the trabeculae are a site of drainage.

Section XVI - Non-Hodgkin Lymphoma

I. Lymphoma
  A. Neoplastic growth of lymphoid cells that form a mass
    1. May arise in a lymph node or in extranodal tissue
    2. Multiple lymph nodes involved
  B. Divided into
    1. Non-Hodgkin lymphoma
    2. Hodgkin lymphoma

II. Characteristics
  A. Non-contiguous spread
  B. Classified based on many factors
    1. Cell type
    2. Cell size
    3. Pattern of cell growth
    4. Expression of surface markers
    5. Cytogenetic translocations

III. Types
  A. Small B cell lymphoma
    1. Follicular lymphoma, mantle cell lymphoma, and marginal zone lymphoma
  B. Intermediate-sized B cell lymphoma
    1. Burkitt lymphoma
  C. Large B cell lymphoma
    1. Diffuse large B cell lymphoma

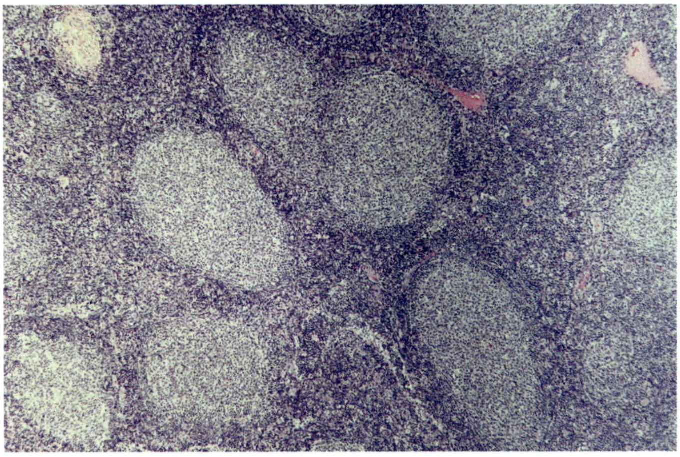

FIGURE 10.10.67 - Follicular Lymphoma

Type	Pathophysiology	Clinical Findings	Treatment
Small B cell lymphoma	Follicular lymphoma	- t(14,18) - *BCL2* expression in follicles - Neoplastic proliferation of small B cells (CD20+) that form follicle-like nodules	- Painless "waxing and waning" lymphadenopathy
	Mantle cell lymphoma	- t(11,14) - Overexpression of cyclin D1 - Neoplastic proliferation of small B cells (CD20+) that expands the mantle zone	- Painless lymphadenopathy
	Marginal zone lymphoma	- Neoplastic proliferation of small B cells (CD20+) that expands the marginal zone	- Associated with Hashimoto thyroiditis, Sjögren syndrome, and *H. pylori* gastritis
Intermediate B cell lymphoma	Burkitt lymphoma	- t(8,14) - Neoplastic proliferation of intermediate-sized B cells (CD20+) - Associated with EBV - Increased risk in patients with HIV	- Extranodal mass in child or young adult - African form involves jaw - Sporadic form involves abdomen
Large B cell lymphoma	Diffuse large B cell lymphoma	- Neoplastic proliferation of large B cells (CD20+) that grow diffusely in sheets - Arises sporadically or from transformation	- Enlarging lymph node or an extranodal mass

TABLE 10.10.10 - Groups of Non-Hodgkin Lymphoma

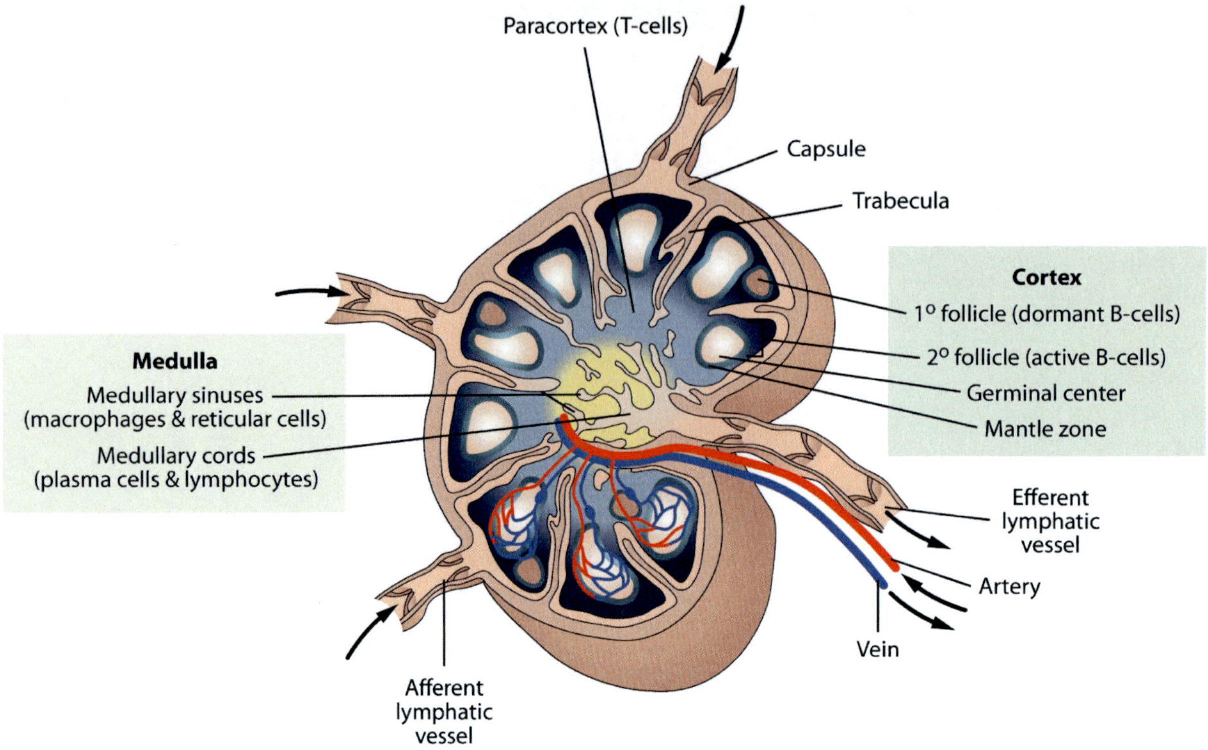

FIGURE 10.10.66 - Anatomy of a Lymph Node

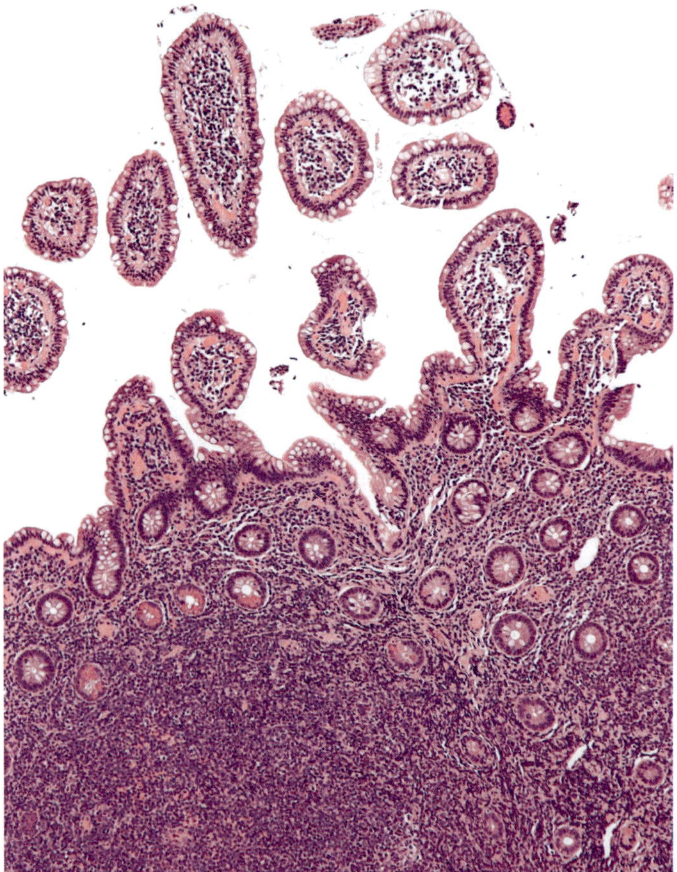

FIGURE 10.10.68 - Micrograph of Mantle Zone Lymphoma

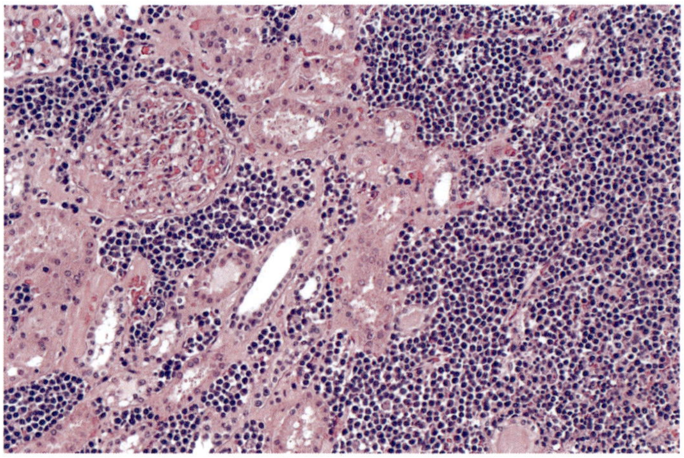

FIGURE 10.10.69 - Micrograph of Marginal Zone Lymphoma

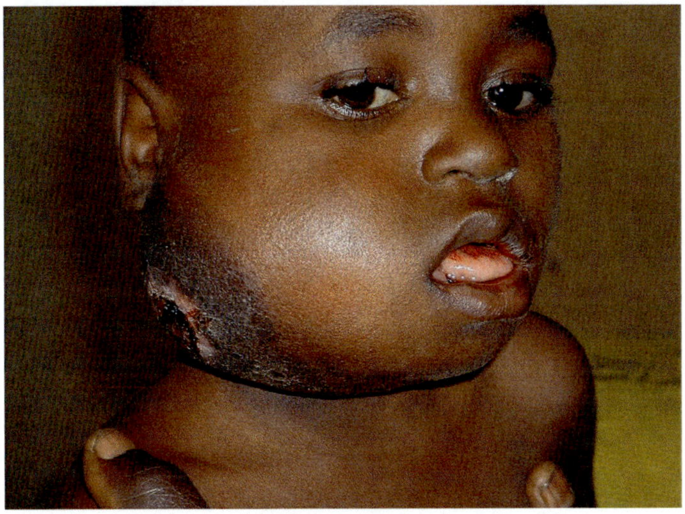

FIGURE 10.10.70 - Burkitt's Lymphoma

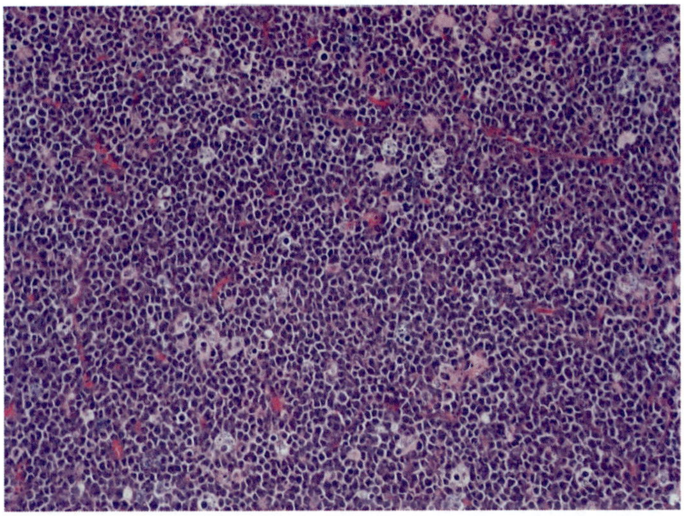

FIGURE 10.10.71 - Histopathological Image of Burkitt Lymphoma

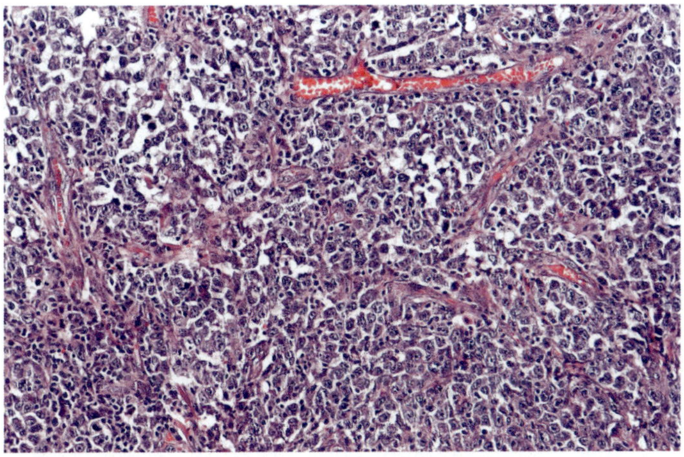

FIGURE 10.10.72 - Micrograph of Diffuse Large B Cell Lymphoma

REVIEW QUESTIONS

1. A 50-year-old woman presents with a fever and a sore throat. Physical exam shows tonsillar exudate and a nontender cervical lymph node that measures 5.5 cm in diameter. One week later, her symptoms have resolved. On several follow-up visits over the next year the patient remains asymptomatic and the size of the lymph node fluctuates, but it does not disappear completely. A biopsy of the lymph node is obtained. What cytogenetic change will most likely be seen?

   - **The correct answer is a t(14,18) translocation.**
   - This woman presents with a fever, sore throat with tonsillar exudate, a nontender cervical lymph node that fluctuates in size. This is likely follicular lymphoma and is due to a t(14,18).

2. A 20-year-old male presents with recurring night sweats, fatigue, and a loss of appetite. He experienced similar symptoms 6 months ago. Physical examination reveals nontender, enlarged cervical lymph nodes. A lymph node biopsy reveals sheets of lymphocytes with interspersed macrophages. What is the most likely cause of this patient's condition?

   A. Double-stranded DNA virus
   B. Single-stranded positive-sense RNA virus
   C. Single-stranded negative-sense RNA virus
   D. Single-stranded DNA virus

   - **The correct answer is A.**
   - This 20-year-old presents with night sweats, fatigue, a loss of appetite, and nontender, enlarged lymph nodes, which are classic signs of mononucleosis. He has also experienced similar symptoms in the past. The biopsy reveals a "starry sky appearance" or sheets of lymphocytes with interspersed macrophages, a classical description of Burkitt's lymphoma. With all of this information, we can determine that the patient's condition is due to EBV which can cause Burkitt's lymphoma. EBV is a double-stranded DNA virus.
   - B is incorrect because patients with HIV have an increased risk for Burkitt's lymphoma, but HIV does not cause Burkitt's lymphoma.
   - Both C and D are incorrect because they do not accurately describe EBV.

Section XVII - Hodgkin Lymphoma

I. Definition
   A. Neoplastic proliferation of Reed-Sternberg cells intermixed with reactive inflammatory cells
      1. Reed-Sternberg cells: large B cells with multilobed nuclei and prominent nucleoli; stain positive for CD15 and CD30
   B. Bimodal age distribution
      1. 20s and 60s

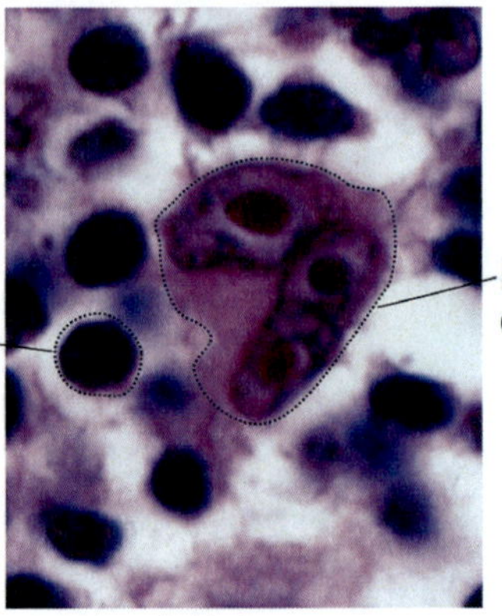

Photo Credit: National Cancer Institute / Public domain

FIGURE 10.10.73 - Hodgkin Lymphoma

II. Clinical Findings
   A. Fever, chills, weight loss, and night sweats (B symptoms)
   B. Enlarged lymph nodes
   C. Contiguous spread to adjacent node groups

III. Subtypes
   A. Nodular sclerosis
   B. Lymphocyte-rich
   C. Mixed cellularity
   D. Lymphocyte-depleted

IV. Nodular Sclerosis
   A. Most common
   B. Enlarging cervical or mediastinal lymph node in a young adult
   C. Females > males
   D. Lymph node subdivided by bands of sclerosis

V. Lymphocyte-Rich
   A. Best prognosis
   B. Composed primarily of reactive lymphocytes

VI. Mixed Cellularity
   A. Increased number of eosinophils
      1. Reed-Sternberg cells produce IL-5, which attracts eosinophils

VII. Lymphocyte-Depleted
   A. Most aggressive
   B. Seen in the elderly and HIV-positive patients

REVIEW QUESTIONS ?

1. A 20-year-old woman presents with a fever, chills, and a 10-lb weight loss over the past two months. She reports waking up in the middle of the night drenched in sweat. Physical exam reveals enlarged lymph nodes along her anterior neck. A peripheral blood smear reveals multi-nucleated cells with prominent nucleoli. Which of the following markers is most likely to be found on these cells?

   A. CD19
   B. CD45
   C. CD30
   D. CD5

- **The correct answer is C.**
- This 20-year-old patient presents with fever, chills, a 10-lb weight loss, and night sweats, which indicate cancer. Enlarged lymph nodes in her cervical region are suspicious of lymphoma. The peripheral blood smear reveals Reed-Sternberg cells, which indicates Hodgkin lymphoma. These cells classically express CD15 and CD30.
- A is incorrect, as CD19 is a B cell marker.
- B is incorrect, as CD45 is a general hematopoietic cell marker.
- D is incorrect, as CD5 is a T cell marker.

Section XVIII - Plasma Cell Dyscrasias

I. Multiple Myeloma
   A. Malignant proliferation of plasma cells
   B. Most common primary bone malignancy
   C. High serum IL-6
   D. Overproduction of IgG and free light chains

II. Multiple Myeloma: Clinical Features
   A. CRAB findings
      1. Hyper**C**alcemia
      2. Renal impairment (myeloma kidney)
      3. Anemia
      4. Bony lytic lesions/back pain
   B. Increased risk of infection
   C. Primary AL amyloidosis

III. Multiple Myeloma: Laboratory Findings
   A. Elevated serum protein
      1. M spike on serum protein electrophoresis (SPEP)
      2. Rouleaux formation of RBCs on blood smear
   B. Urinalysis: Bence Jones proteinuria
      1. Urine dipstick negative for proteinuria
   C. Bone marrow aspiration will show > 10% plasma cells
      1. "Clock-face" chromatin

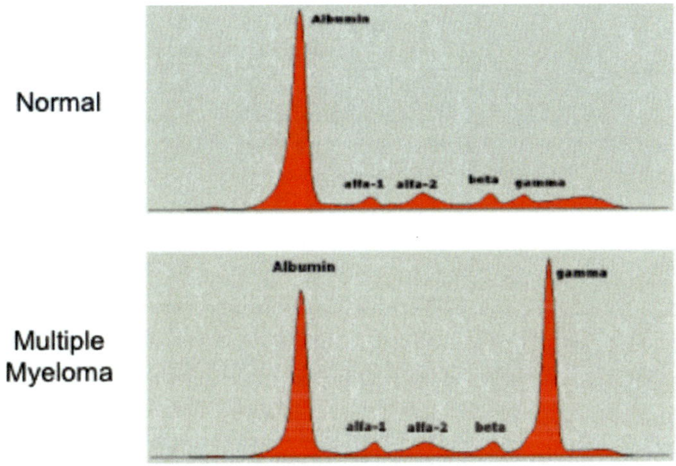

FIGURE 10.10.74 - Serum Protein Electrophoresis in Multiple Myeloma

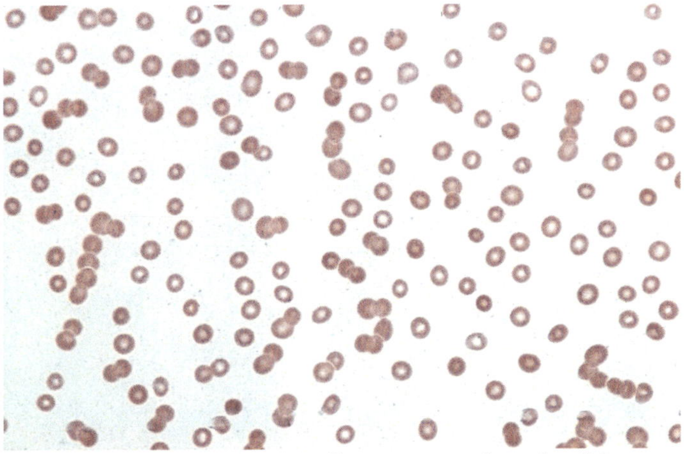

FIGURE 10.10.75 - Rouleaux Formation in Multiple Myeloma

IV. Waldenstrom Macroglobulinemia
   A. B cell lymphoma with overproduction of monoclonal IgM
   B. Autoantibodies against
      1. Myelin glycoprotein → neuropathy
      2. RBCs → Coombs-positive hemolytic anemia

V. Waldenstrom Macroglobulinemia: Clinical Features
   A. Hyperviscosity syndromes
      1. Visual impairment, stroke, and bleeding
   B. IgM deposition in kidneys, GI tract, and skin
      1. Proteinuria, diarrhea, and papules
   C. Lymphadenopathy
   D. Neuropathies
   E. No CRAB findings

VI. Waldenstrom Macroglobulinemia: Laboratory Findings and Treatment
   A. Increased serum protein
      1. M spike on SPEP (IgM)
   B. Bone marrow biopsy required for diagnosis
      1. > 10% small lymphocytes with intracytoplasmic IgM vacuoles (lymphoplasmacytic lymphoma)
   C. Plasmapheresis treats acute complications

VII. Monoclonal Gammopathy of Undetermined Significance (MGUS)
   A. Mild overproduction of any Ig subtype
   B. Asymptomatic
   C. Common in elderly
   D. Risk of progression to multiple myeloma

VIII. Monoclonal Gammopathy of Undetermined Significance (MGUS): Clinical Findings
   A. Increased serum protein
      1. M spike on SPEP
   B. Bone marrow biopsy: < 10% monoclonal plasma cells
   C. No CRAB findings

REVIEW QUESTIONS

1. A 68-year-old male with a past medical history of diabetes, hypertension, and obesity presents to the physician with back pain. The pain is localized to his lower back and is associated with a 10-pound weight loss in the past month. Vitals are within normal limits. A urine dipstick is negative. However, a 24-hour urinary protein is elevated. X-ray of the spine shows multiple radiolucent lesions within the lumbar and thoracic vertebrae. What would most likely be seen on blood smear and bone marrow biopsy?

    - **A peripheral blood smear will show RBCs in Rouleaux formation, and a bone marrow biopsy will show excessive plasma cells.**
    - The important thing to recognize here is that this patient is presenting with the classic symptoms of multiple myeloma: back pain, weight loss, lytic bone lesions, and elevated protein in the urine with a negative urine dipstick.

2. A 58-year-old male presents to the physician with a 1-month history of fatigue, weight loss, and headache and a recent loss of vision in his right eye. Physical exam reveals diminished sensation to light touch in his lower extremities. Serum protein electrophoresis shows an M spike of monoclonal IgM. What is the most likely cause of this patient's visual deficit?

    A. Large IgM pentamers
    B. Plasma cells inhibiting platelet aggregation
    C. Renal impairment from elevated serum free light chains
    D. Infectious thrombus from decreased IgG variability

    - **The correct answer is A.**
    - The important thing to recognize here is that this patient is presenting with neurological deficits and an M spike on SPEP with IgM. The M spike of monoclonal IgM is indicative of Waldenstrom macroglobulinemia.
    - Recall that one of the symptoms of Waldenstrom macroglobulinemia is visual impairment secondary to hyperviscosity syndrome. The underlying cause of hyperviscosity syndrome in Waldenstrom macroglobulinemia is due to the large size of the numerous IgM pentamers, which effectively "clog" the vasculature.
    - B is incorrect because the inhibition of platelet aggregation leads to an increased risk of bleeding, not visual impairment.
    - C is incorrect because CRAB findings are not seen in Waldenstrom macroglobulinemia. Renal impairment is a CRAB finding and would be seen in multiple myeloma.
    - D is incorrect because Waldenstrom macroglobulinemia has decreased IgM variability, not IgG. Decreased IgG variability is seen in multiple myeloma, and would not likely cause infectious thrombi.

Section XIX - Langerhans Cell Histiocytosis

I. Langerhans Cells
  A. Majority located in skin
  B. Myeloid lineage
  C. Specialized dendritic cells (APCs)
  D. Birbeck granules
    1. Tennis racquet-shaped
  E. Staining: CD1a and S100

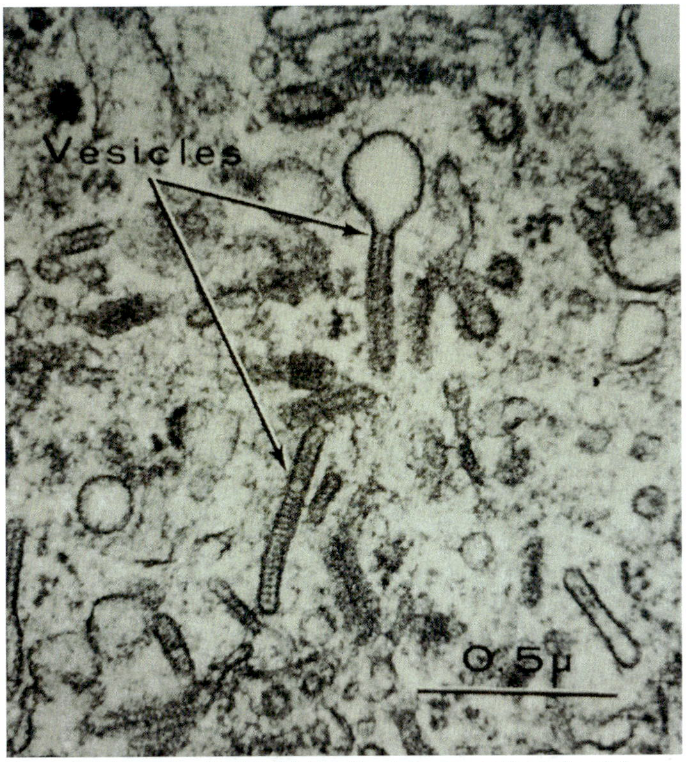

FIGURE 10.10.76 - Birbeck Granules Within Langerhans Cells

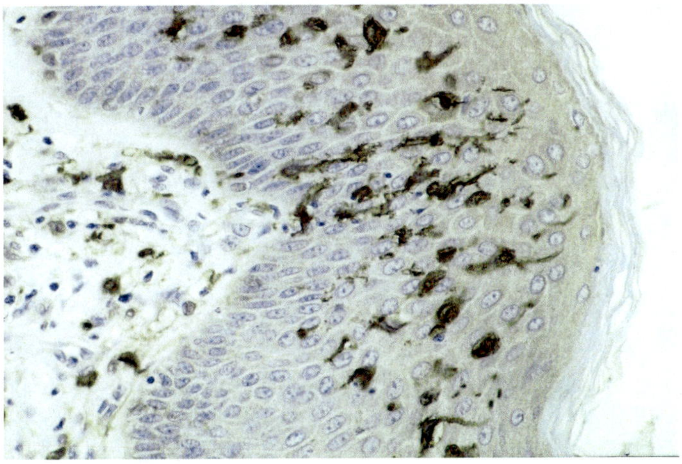

FIGURE 10.10.77 - Langerhans Cells with S100 Staining

II. Langerhans Cell Histiocytosis
  A. Excess growth of Langerhans cells
  B. Types
    1. Benign: eosinophilic granuloma
    2. Malignant: Letterer-Siwe disease, Hand-Schüller-Christian disease

III. Eosinophilic Granuloma
  A. Benign
  B. Children and adolescents
  C. Overgrowth of Langerhans cells in bones
  D. Osteolytic lesions → bone pain, swelling, pathologic fracture
  E. Biopsy: Langerhans cells and eosinophils
    1. Also other inflammatory cells

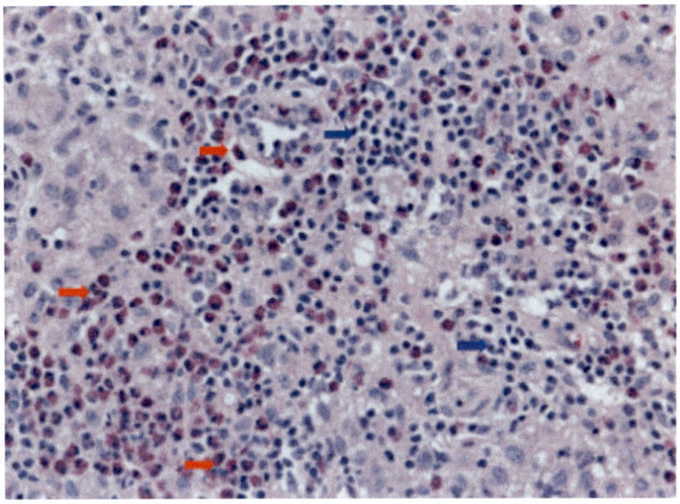

FIGURE 10.10.78 - Biopsy of an Eosinophilic Granuloma

IV. Letterer-Siwe Disease
  A. Malignant
  B. Worst variant → often fatal
  C. Infants under 2 years
  D. Osteolytic lesions (skull and other bones)
  E. Skin rash (purpura and ecchymoses)
  F. Hepatosplenomegaly

V. Hand-Schüller-Christian Disease
  A. Malignant
  B. Children and adolescents
  C. Triad
    1. Osteolytic lesions (skull)
    2. Exophthalmos (bulging eyes)
    3. Diabetes insipidus (polyuria and polydipsia)

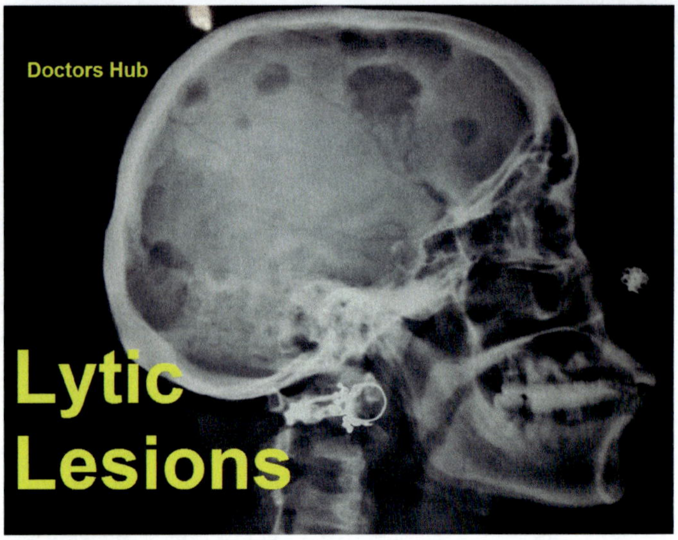

FIGURE 10.10.79 - X-Ray of Lytic Lesions of the Skull

REVIEW QUESTIONS

1. A 7-year-old boy comes to the physician for an exam. His mother says he has been getting in trouble at school because he has to go to the bathroom a lot. He reports drinking approximately 8 bottles of water during school hours and is "always really thirsty." Physical examination reveals eyes that appear to bulge out. TSH and HbA1c are normal. A skeletal survey is ordered. An X-ray of his skull reveals a lytic lesion. The lesion is biopsied. Which of the following is most likely to be found on microscopy?

   A. Eosinophilia
   B. Birbeck granules
   C. Positive S200 stain
   D. Negative S100 stain
   E. M. tuberculosis

- **The correct answer is B.**
- This is a 7-year-old boy who has symptoms of frequent urination and constantly being thirsty. This is described as polyuria and polydipsia. This can be a symptom of diabetes, but we are told his HbA1c is normal. He also has eyes that appear to bulge out, or exophthalmos. This can be a symptom of hyperthyroidism, but we are told his TSH is normal. However, he does have a lytic lesion on skull X-ray.
- We now have the classic triad of diabetes insipidus, exophthalmos, and osteolytic lesions seen in Hand-Schüller-Christian disease, a malignant variant of Langerhans cell histiocytosis.
- The question asks us what we would see on microscopy of the lesion. Since we know it is a Langerhans cell histiocytosis, we would expect to see Birbeck granules, which are characteristic of Langerhans cell histiocytosis.
- A is incorrect because eosinophilia would be found in a benign eosinophilic granuloma, which is a benign form of Langerhans cell histiocytosis.
- C is incorrect because the proper stain would be S100, not S200.
- D is incorrect because S100 stain would be positive.
- E is incorrect because Langerhans cell histiocytosis is not caused by *Mycobacterium tuberculosis.*

TABLES & FIGURES

Made in United States
Orlando, FL
06 November 2026

90243291R00245